Pharmaceutical Practice

FIFTH EDITION

Edited by

Judith A. Rees BPharm, MSc, PhD
Senior Lecturer, School of Pharmacy, Keele University, UK

Ian Smith BSc(Hons), MRPharmS, ClinDip, ILTM
Boots Teacher/Practitioner, University of Manchester, UK

Jennie Watson BSc, PG ClinDip, PGCert (LTHE), MRpharmS
Boots Teacher/Practitioner, School of Pharmacy and Biomedical Sciences,
University of Central Lancashire, Preston, UK

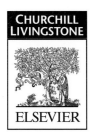

CHURCHILL
LIVINGSTONE

ELSEVIER

Edinburgh • London • New York • Oxford • Philadelphia • St Louis • Sydney • Toronto

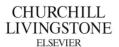

CHURCHILL
LIVINGSTONE
ELSEVIER

© 2014 by Churchill Livingstone, an imprint of Elsevier Ltd. All rights reserved.

First edition 1990
Second edition 1998
Third edition 2004
Fourth edition 2009
Fifth edition 2014

ISBN 978-0-7020-5143-2
International ISBN 978-0-7020-5144-9
Ebook 978-0-7020-5282-8

100714515X

British Library Cataloguing in Publication Data
A catalogue record for this book is available from the British Library

Library of Congress Cataloging in Publication Data
A catalog record for this book is available from the Library of Congress

Notices
Knowledge and best practice in this field are constantly changing. As new research and experience broaden our understanding, changes in research methods, professional practices, or medical treatment may become necessary.

Practitioners and researchers must always rely on their own experience and knowledge in evaluating and using any information, methods, compounds, or experiments described herein. In using such information or methods they should be mindful of their own safety and the safety of others, including parties for whom they have a professional responsibility.

With respect to any drug or pharmaceutical products identified, readers are advised to check the most current information provided (i) on procedures featured or (ii) by the manufacturer of each product to be administered, to verify the recommended dose or formula, the method and duration of administration, and contraindications. It is the responsibility of practitioners, relying on their own experience and knowledge of their patients, to make diagnoses, to determine dosages and the best treatment for each individual patient, and to take all appropriate safety precautions.

  your source for books, journals and multimedia in the health sciences
www.elsevierhealth.com

  Working together to grow libraries in developing countries

www.elsevier.com • www.bookaid.org

The Publisher's policy is to use **paper manufactured from sustainable forests**

Printed in China

Contents

In the five years since the publication of the last edition of *Pharmaceutical Practice*, the profession of pharmacy has once again changed and progressed. There are emerging new roles for pharmacists both within the traditional employment areas of hospital and community pharmacy, as well as other emerging roles to support the public health agenda, governance, risk management, prescribing and pharmacoeconomic areas. As well as changes in the content of this edition of *Pharmaceutical Practice*, Arthur Winfield, one of the original editors, made the decision to leave the editorial team after being involved in the editing of the previous four editions – what an accomplishment! He was an extremely efficient and experienced editor, whose retirement has left a big hole in the editing team. Fortunately, the other editors, Judith Rees and Ian Smith, have been joined by an enthusiastic and knowledgeable new editor, Jennie Watson. Together, this editorial team has been able to carry forward the original aims of the book, which are to provide the readers with an up-to-date knowledge base for all aspects of pharmacy practice presented whenever possible, in a way to encourage a professional attitude of always seeking to provide the highest standards of care for patients.

We have been fortunate with all our authors, who have produced up-to-the-minute information of their subject material to illustrate each of their chapters. We have recruited many new authors who have been chosen for their expertise and experience in their subject. Our authors include full-time practising pharmacists, academics experienced in teaching pharmacy and some pharmacists with joint appointments between hospital or community pharmacy and academic institutions.

Pharmacy continues to evolve as a profession and, while we are wary of saying that the next few years will be the most exciting ever for the profession, we certainly see great change and opportunity ahead. We have included many new chapters in this edition to reflect these newer aspects of practice, which will impact on areas of future pharmacy practice.

There are two companion volumes to *Pharmaceutical Practice*: *Aulton's Pharmaceutics: The Design and Manufacture of Medicines*, fourth edition (Churchill Livingstone 2013), edited by ME Aulton and K Taylor, which provides greater detail on the scientific principles that underpin the design and manufacture of dosage forms and medicines; and *Clinical Pharmacy and Therapeutics*, fifth edition (Churchill Livingstone 2012), edited by R. Walker and C. Whittlesea, which considers in greater detail, aspects of treatment with drugs and clinical practice by pharmacists. These three books complement each other and readers should realize that information cannot be compartmentalized. It is detrimental to patients to ignore any aspect of the total knowledge base – all must be integrated if optimum pharmaceutical care is to be provided.

We would encourage the readers to embrace the changes ahead, to move the profession ever further forward, to provide both the best care for your patients but also to provide you with the opportunity for job satisfaction and enjoyment.

JAR, IS, JW

Acknowledgements

The editors would like to take this opportunity to thank the many people who have helped to make this fifth edition of *Pharmaceutical Practice* possible. Since publication of the fourth edition, Dr Arthur J. Winfield has decided to 'retire' as an editor. Arthur was an extremely efficient, hardworking and experienced editor, who led the editorial team for several editions. We (JAR and IS) felt that he really was exceptional and irreplaceable. However, after much searching, we did find a willing and able replacement in Jennie Watson. She has been a pleasure to work with and has added new subject areas and direction to this edition.

New editors also bring new contacts, so we have been able to recruit many new authors for this edition. We are deeply grateful to all the authors for their willingness to contribute to this volume and for the time and effort they have spent researching their subjects and in preparing text. In particular, we would like to thank them for adhering to the very short time we gave them to complete their chapter(s).

Our special thanks are due to our families. Without their continued encouragement, support and assistance, an undertaking like this would not reach completion.

Those companies, organizations and individuals who have given permission to use or modify their materials or who have helpfully answered queries or provided information to our authors are thanked. Without this type of cooperation, any textbook cannot hope to present a worthwhile overview.

Thanks are also expressed to the publishers, in particular Fiona Conn and Julie Taylor, who have had to deal with our queries, misunderstandings, etc. but have provided guidance and timely support throughout the preparation of this fifth edition. Professional guidance is always necessary. We would also like to thank Fiona for encouraging us to use the publisher's electronic manuscript submission system. It has made life easier for us. Also thanks to the authors who keenly adopted the electronic system.

Finally, we wish to thank you, our students, past and present. We know that students do not appreciate how much their teachers learn from them, but we do! We hope that some of this is reflected in this book.

JAR, IS, JW

Contributors

Darren M. Ashcroft BPharm, MSc, PhD
Professor of Pharmacoepidemiology, Manchester
Pharmacy School, University of Manchester,
Manchester, UK

Christine M. Bond PhD, MEd, BPharm (Hons),
FRPS, FFPH, FRCPE
Professor of Primary Care, Centre of Academic Primary
Care, College of Life Sciences and Medicine, University
of Aberdeen, Aberdeen, UK

Derek G. Chapman BSc(Pharm), PhD
Retired Lecturer, Robert Gordon University, Aberdeen, UK

Victoria Crabtree BPharm (Hons)
Lecturer, Manchester Pharmacy School, University of
Manchester, Manchester, UK

Parastou Donyai PhD, BPharm, PGDPRM(Open),
PGCertLTHE, PGCertEBP
Lecturer in Pharmacy Practice, Department of Pharmacy,
University of Reading, Reading, UK

Isabel J. Featherstone MPharm, MBBS
Hospital Doctor, York District General Hospital, York, UK

Alison Gifford BSc (Hons), PGDip, MMedSci, PhD
Sessional tutor in Pharmacy Practice, School of
Pharmacy, University of Keele, Keele, UK

David Graham BSc, MSc, MRPharmS
Radiopharmacy Team Leader, Radiopharmacy
Department, Aberdeen Royal Infirmary, Aberdeen, UK

Felice S. Groundland BSc (Hons) Pharmacy
Boots Teacher/Practitioner, Strathclyde University,
Glasgow, UK

Jason Hall BSc, MSc, PhD
Reader, Manchester Pharmacy School,
University of Manchester, Manchester, UK

Lindsay Harper BSc(Hons), DipClin
Principal Clinical Pharmacist, Pharmacy Department,
Salford Royal NHS Foundation Trust, Salford, UK

Dyfrig A. Hughes BPharm, MSc, PhD, MRPharmS
Professor of Pharmacoeconomics and Co-Director of the
Centre for Health Economics and Medicines Evaluation,
Bangor University, Bangor, UK

Jenny Hughes MPharm
Lecturer, Manchester Pharmacy School,
University of Manchester, Manchester, UK

Alison Hunter MPharm
Boots Teacher/Practitioner, University of Huddersfield,
Huddersfield, UK

Sam Ingram BSc (Hons) Pharmacy, PGDipCommPharm,
PGCertHE, PGCert Vet Pharm
Boots Teacher/Practitioner, University of Brighton, UK

Janet Krska BSc, PhD, PGCert (Health Econ), FRPharmS
Professor of Clinical and Professional Pharmacy, Medway
School of Pharmacy, The Universities of Greenwich and
Kent, Chatham Maritime, Kent, UK

Liz Lamerton BSc(Hons) Pharmacy, DipClinPharm, PIP
Senior Clinical Pharmacist, Salford Royal NHS
Foundation Trust, Salford, UK

Alison Littlewood BSc, MSc
NW Lead Pre-registration Facilitator, Manchester
Pharmacy School, University of Manchester,
Manchester, UK

Brian Lockwood BPharm, PhD
Professor of Pharmaceutical Sciences, Manchester
Pharmacy School, University of Manchester,
Manchester, UK

Richard C. O'Neill LLB, LLM, BPharm, PhD
Head of Department of Pharmacy, University of
Hertfordshire, Hatfield, Hertfordshire, UK

Judith A. Rees BPharm, MSc, PhD
Senior Lecturer, School of Pharmacy, Keele University,
Keele, UK

Mary Rhodes MPharm
Lecturer, Manchester Pharmacy School, University of
Manchester, Manchester, UK

R. Michael E. Richards OBE, BPharm, PhD, DSc,
DPharmSci(Honorary), DPharmPractice(Honorary)
Professor Emeritus, Pharmacy, Robert Gordon University,
Aberdeen, UK; Professor of Pharmacy, Mahasarakham
University, Maha Sarakham, Thailand

Peter M. Richards BPharm (Hons)
Medicines Management Pharmacist, NHS West and
South Yorkshire and Bassetlaw, Commissioning Support
Unit, UK

Paul Rutter BPharm, PhD
Professor of Pharmacy Practice,
University of Wolverhampton, Wolverhampton, UK

Geoff Saunders BPharm, MPhil
Consultant Oncology Pharmacist, Christie Hospital,
Manchester, UK

Ellen Schafheutle MSc, MRes, FHEA, PhD, MRPharmS
Senior Lecturer in Law & Professionalism in Pharmacy,
Manchester Pharmacy School, University of Manchester,
Manchester, UK

Jenny Scott BSc (Hon), PhD, Cert Independent Prescribing
Senior Lecturer in Pharmacy Practice, Department
of Pharmacy & Pharmacology, University of Bath,
Bath, UK

Raminder Sihota BSc, PGDipCommParm, PGCertHE
Professional L&D Manager, Boots, UK

Ian Smith BSc(Hons), MRPharmS, ClinDip, ILTM
Boots Teacher/Practitioner, University of Manchester, UK

Megan R. Thomas BSc, MBChB, PhD
Consultant Community Paediatrician, Blenheim House
Child Development Centre, Blackpool Teaching Hospitals
NHS Foundation Trust, Blackpool, UK; Director, Research
and Development, Blackpool Teaching Hospitals NHS
Foundation Trust, Blackpool, UK

John Tucker BPharm
Weldricks Teacher/Practitioner, Bradford School of
Pharmacy, University of Bradford, Bradford, UK

Simon J. Tweddell BPharm, MRPharmS, FHEA
Senior Lecturer in Pharmacy Practice, Bradford School of
Pharmacy, University of Bradford, Bradford, UK

Jennie Watson BSc, PG Clin Dip, PGCert(LTHE), MRPharmS
Boots Teacher/Practitioner, School of Pharmacy and
Biomedical Sciences, University of Central Lancashire,
Preston, UK

Marjorie C. Weiss DPhil, MSc, MSc, BSc
Professor of Pharmacy Practice and Medicines Use,
Department of Pharmacy & Pharmacology, University of
Bath, Bath, UK

Simon White BPharm, MSc, PhD
Lecturer in Pharmacy Practice, School of Pharmacy,
Keele University, Keele, UK

Arthur J. Winfield BPharm, PhD
Retired Senior Lecturer and Head of Pharmacy Practice,
Robert Gordon University, Aberdeen, UK;
Retired Chairman of Department of Pharmacy Practice,
University of Kuwait, Kuwait

About this book

When we were asked by Elsevier to edit this new edition of *Pharmaceutical Practice*, our first task was to review the contents of the last edition. We soon realized that much had changed in pharmacy practice, in general, and that some individual chapters were rapidly becoming out of date and that newer developments in pharmacy practice were either nascent or not mentioned in the last edition. Certainly, it was evident that new developments in pharmacy practice were progressing rapidly as a result, in some cases, of changes in society, while other developments were the result of positive actions by the pharmacy profession or individual pharmacists.

Thus, it was necessary to decide which topics or chapters would be retained, and which new topics would be included in the new edition, always bearing in mind we had a limited word count and that no textbook can give total coverage of a huge subject such as pharmacy practice. What we aimed to produce was a book that would cover much of the widening topic of pharmacy practice. In order to achieve our aim, it was necessary to recruit new authors and persuade existing authors to revamp their chapters by rewriting the contents and/or bringing them up-to-date. We are very grateful to all the authors for writing the chapters in the very short timescale for completion and submission.

In view of the changes to the subject matter of some of the chapters, this has necessitated a reordering of the chapters into a logical sequence. We have also arranged the book into sections and in each section, we have grouped together chapters with related subject matter. These sections are not meant to isolate or compartmentalize the topics and indeed, we have cross-referenced, where appropriate, to similar subject material in another chapter or section. Not surprisingly, some topics underpin the development of other topics found in a separate chapter. Indeed, the ethos of the book was that no chapter stands totally alone. All chapters link in with one another, in the same way that pharmacists, whatever their role, need knowledge and skills that will be used by them in their role and by other pharmacists working in different roles.

The book consists of seven sections and four appendices:

- **SECTION 1: An introduction to pharmacy and its place in society**

In Section 1, the chapters address the wider aspects of pharmacy practice, the development of pharmacy and the emerging subject of pharmacy practice, as well as the influences of society on pharmacy practice and vice versa. The book opens with a detailed description of the development of pharmacy practice and the role it now plays within society and health care. The next two chapters cover the behavioural and sociological aspects of patients and their illnesses and treatment with drugs. An understanding of these two chapters will underpin later chapters, which consider patient choice, patient empowerment and self-care.

- **SECTION 2: Protecting the public**

The chapters in this section all consider the ways in which the pharmacy profession and the legal system have a duty to protect the public. The first chapter in this section describes the ways in which medicines are controlled by the legal system in order to protect the public and patients from freely accessing and using medicines which could be harmful to them. The second chapter in this section (Ch. 5) considers the ways healthcare professionals are regulated, again to protect the public from unscrupulous people. In order to maintain the standards of knowledge and skills of healthcare professionals, Chapter 6 focusses on continuing professional development (CPD) and revalidation. Chapters 7 and 8 together describe ethics and ethical dilemmas. Both these chapters underpin professional behaviour and are aimed at protecting the public. Clinical governance, which is considered in Chapter 9, describes the ways of providing quality in pharmacy services and health care, while Chapter 10 outlines the ways in which errors occur and the ways to manage risk and thus protect the public. Standard operating procedures described in Chapter 11 and audit in Chapter 12, are other ways of protecting the public by standardizing procedures used by professionals and then checking (auditing) that procedures actually do what they are meant to do. Public health considered in Chapter 13 aims to protect the public by promoting health by the efforts of healthcare professionals and informed choice by the public.

- **SECTION 3: Delivering professional pharmacy practice**

Chapter 14 starts off this section on delivering professional services, by describing the structure and organization of pharmacy, which supports this delivery. Chapter 15 considers the other members of the healthcare team and the importance of good management skills between pharmacists and their team. Chapters 16, 17, 18 and 19 describe the skills and understanding required by pharmacists to undertake the delivery of professional services. All pharmacy professions need to develop and maintain their skills to retrieve information (Ch. 16), to communicate with their team and patients as well as other healthcare professionals (Ch. 17) and to perform pharmaceutical calculations (Ch. 19). Chapter 18 describes concordance and emphasizes that pharmacists should gain an understanding of patients and their ability to choose if, and how they take their medicines.

- **SECTION 4: Access to medicines and their selection**

Section 4 considers access to medicines and their selection. In this section, the ways of obtaining medicines are described and the restraints on both their access and selection. Chapter 20 outlines the prescribing process and emphasizes the need for good prescribing to be based on sound evidence. Evidence-based medicine is a theme running through all the chapters in this section. Prescribing for minor ailments (Ch. 21) is based on a logical and rational approach to diagnose before considering whether a medicine needs to be prescribed or not. Chapters 22 and 23 consider how drugs are evaluated and whether they are value for money. This approach is then used to develop formularies to guide prescribers in their selection of effective and economical medicines. The impact of patient charges on the access to medicines is discussed in Chapter 23 and how to effectively provide advice and information in the selection of medicines is considered in Chapter 25. Nowadays, many people are moving away from conventional medicines and considering and using complementary

and alternative medicines. Chapter 24 provides the background and use of these medicines. Chapters 26 and 27 consider prescriptions, both the funding and requirements for medicines supply via a prescription. Lastly, the access and selection of veterinary medicines is considered in Chapter 28.

- **SECTION 5: Medicines and their preparation**

This section initially considers the many routes by which medicines are administered to patients and the dosage forms, which allow these methods of administration (Ch. 29). This is followed by a description of the dispensing techniques used to prepare extemporaneous preparations (Ch. 30). Chapters 33 to 39 each describe the methods of preparation and the use of necessary excipients to produce a different type of formulation. These methods, although only suitable for extemporaneous prepared products, are the basis of methods used in the pharmaceutical industry to produce the many medicines available commercially. Chapters 31 and 32 describe how to appropriately label and pack an extemporaneously produced medicine.

- **SECTION 6: Specialized pharmacy products and services**

Section 6 considers specialized pharmacy products and services provided by pharmacists. Chapters include an in-depth description of the production of sterile products (Ch. 40), followed by the types of parenteral products available and how they are prepared and packaged (Ch. 41). Chapter 42 considers in-depth ophthalmic products, the types used and their formulation including necessary excipients. Besides ophthalmic medicinal products, the chapter considers the types of products specially formulated for contact lenses and their users. Inhaled products are considered in Chapter 43, the different types of manufactured inhaled product, their specially designed packaging and how to explain to the patient how to use them. Parenteral nutrition and dialysis are two services provided in hospitals and often transferred into the community in which pharmacists are heavily involved in the preparation of the formulations and their use by patients (Ch. 44). Radiopharmacy is another specialized area in which pharmacists are involved in the production, packaging and use radio pharmaceuticals. These specialized methods and underpinning theory are described and explained in Chapter 45. Chapter 46 centres on the range, risks and benefits of medicines, which are aseptically compounded in hospital or specialized units by pharmacists. These pharmaceutical services include cytotoxic reconstitution and centralized intravenous additive services. Appliances dispensed by pharmacists including trusses and stoma products are described and explained in Chapter 47.

• SECTION 7: Pharmacy services

This section looks at some services which have increased in prominence in recent years. These include an acknowledgement that pharmacy provides public health interventions on a daily basis to an increasing number of the public. These pharmacy interventions are described in Chapter 48. Services to vulnerable people (Ch. 49) in the pharmacy setting have increased due, in some respects, to an increased number of government policies but mainly because pharmacists are well placed to access vulnerable people, when they require medicines. For many years, pharmacists have come into professional contact on a frequent basis with patients who misuse illegal drugs and substances. Chapter 50 describes the role of the pharmacist and the range of pharmaceutical interventions in operation for illegal drug and substance users. Monitoring the patient after they have received a medicine is the subject of Chapter 51. In this chapter, the methods of reporting adverse drug reactions are described as well as the role of pharmacists in medicine use reviews of patients.

• APPENDICES

Appendix 1 lists the abbreviations used throughout this book. This is followed, in **Appendix 2**, by a list of medical abbreviations that pharmacists may encounter during their careers. Latin terms and abbreviations frequently used in prescription writing are covered in **Appendix 3** and **Appendix 4** lists key references, including websites, and guidance to further reading for the chapters.

In producing this textbook, we have tried to cover as many aspects of pharmacy practice that is possible within the word count and realizing that subject matter should not be too brief an overview, but should have some substance. Clearly, each chapter is not a totally comprehensive description of the subject matter and readers requiring more information are directed to Appendix 4 for additional reading and then to Chapter 16 to practice their information retrieval skills.

Finally, we acknowledge that changes will take place in pharmacy practice between the writing and publishing of this text and this means that by the time the book appears in print, it will inevitably be out of date in places. This process of obsolescence will continue with time. Therefore, the readers are encouraged to keep up-to-date (your own CPD, see Ch. 6) by reading current pharmaceutical and medical journals and literature.

Section 1

An introduction to pharmacy and its place in society

The role of pharmacy in health care

Christine M. Bond

- The historical development of pharmacy
- The position of pharmacy within the National Health Service in the UK
- Recent developments in the services being provided by pharmacists
- The need for lifelong learning
- The public's attitudes to pharmacy

Introduction

Pharmacists are experts on the actions and uses of drugs, including their chemistry, their formulation into medicines and the ways in which they are used to manage diseases. The principal aim of the pharmacist is to use this expertise to improve patient care. Pharmacists are in close contact with patients and so have an important role both in assisting patients to make the best use of their prescribed medicines and in advising patients on the appropriate self-management of self-limiting and minor conditions. Increasingly this latter aspect includes OTC prescribing of effective and potent treatments. Pharmacists are also in close working relationships with other members of the healthcare team – doctors, nurses, dentists and others – where they are able to give advice on a wide range of issues surrounding the use of medicines.

Pharmacists are employed in many different areas of practice. These include the traditional ones of hospital and community practice as well as more recently introduced advisory roles at health authority/health board level and working directly with general practitioners as part of the core, practice-based primary healthcare team. Additionally, pharmacists are employed in the pharmaceutical industry and in academia.

Members of the general public are most likely to meet pharmacists in high street pharmacies or on a hospital ward. However, pharmacists also visit residential homes (see Ch. 49), make visits to patients' own homes and are now involved in running chronic disease clinics in primary and secondary care. In addition, pharmacists will also be contributing to the care of patients through their dealings with other members of the healthcare team in the hospital and community setting.

The changing role of pharmacy

Historically, pharmacists and general practitioners have a common ancestry as apothecaries. Apothecaries both dispensed medicines prescribed by physicians and recommended medicines for those members of the public unable to afford physicians' fees. As the two professions of pharmacy and general practice emerged this remit split so that pharmacists became primarily responsible for the technical, dispensing aspects of this role. With the advent of the NHS in the UK in 1948, and the philosophy of free medical care at the point of delivery, the advisory function of the pharmacist further decreased. As a result, pharmacists spent more of their time in the dispensing of medicines – and derived an increased proportion of their income from it. At the same time, radical changes in the nature of dispensing itself, as described in the following paragraphs, occurred.

In the early years, many prescriptions were for extemporaneously prepared medicines, either following standard 'recipes' from formularies such as the *British Pharmacopoeia* (BP) or *British Pharmaceutical Codex* (BPC), or following individual recipes written by the prescriber (see Ch. 30). The situation was similar in hospital pharmacy, where most prescriptions were prepared on an individual basis. There was some small-scale manufacture of a range of commonly used items. In both situations, pharmacists required manipulative and time-consuming skills to produce the medicines. Thus a wide range of preparations was made, including liquids for internal and external use, ointments, creams, poultices, plasters, eye drops and ointments, injections and solid dosage forms such as pills, capsules and moulded tablets (see Chs 32–39).

Scientific advances have greatly increased the effectiveness of drugs but have also rendered them more complex, potentially more toxic and requiring more sophisticated use than their predecessors. The pharmaceutical industry developed in tandem with these drug developments, contributing to further scientific advances and producing manufactured medical products. This had a number of advantages. For one thing, there was an increased reliability in the product, which could be subjected to suitable quality assessment and assurance. This led to improved formulations, modifications to drug availability and increased use of tablets which have a greater convenience for the patient. Some doctors did not agree with the loss of flexibility in prescribing which resulted from having to use predetermined doses and combinations of materials. From the pharmacist's point of view there was a reduction in the time spent in the routine extemporaneous production of medicines, which many saw as an advantage. Others saw it as a reduction in the mystique associated with the professional role of the pharmacist. There was also an erosion of the technical skill base of the pharmacist. A look through copies of the BPC in the 1950s, 1960s and 1970s will show the reduction in the number and diversity of formulations included in the Formulary section. That section has been omitted from the most recent editions. However, some extemporaneous dispensing is still required and pharmacists remain the only professionals trained in these skills

The changing patterns of work of the pharmacist, in community pharmacy in particular, led to an uncertainty about the future role of the pharmacist and a general consensus that pharmacists were no longer being utilized to their full potential. If the pharmacist was not required to compound medicines or to give general advice on diseases, what was the pharmacist to do?

The extended role

The need to review the future for pharmacy was first formally recognized in 1979 in a report on the NHS which had the remit to consider the best use and management of its financial and manpower resources. This was followed by a succession of key reports and papers, which repeatedly identified the need to exploit the pharmacist's expertise and knowledge to better effect. Key among these reports was the Nuffield Report of 1986. This report, which included nearly 100 recommendations, led the way to many new initiatives, both by the profession and by the government, and laid the foundation for the recent developments in the practice of pharmacy, which are reflected in this book.

Radical change, as recommended in the Nuffield Report, does not necessarily happen quickly, particularly when regulations and statute are involved. In the 28 years since Nuffield was published, there have been several different agendas which have come together and between them facilitated the paradigm shift for pharmacy envisaged in the Nuffield Report. These agendas will be briefly described below. They have finally resulted in extensive professional change, articulated in the definitive statements about the role of pharmacy in the NHS plans for pharmacy in England (2000), Scotland (2001) and Wales (2002) and the subsequent new contractual frameworks for community pharmacy. In addition, other regulatory changes have occurred as part of government policy to increase convenient public access to a wider range of medicines on the NHS (see Ch. 4). These changes reflect general societal trends to deregulate the professions while having in place a framework to ensure safe practice and a recognition that the public are increasingly well informed through widespread access to the internet.

For pharmacy, therefore, two routes for the supply of prescription only medicines (POM) have opened up. Until recently, POM medicines were only available on the prescription of a doctor or dentist, but as a result of the Crown Review in 1999, two significant changes emerged. First, patient group directions (PGDs) were introduced in 2000. A PGD is a written direction for the supply, or supply and administration, of a POM to persons generally by named groups of professionals. So, for example, under a PGD, community pharmacists could supply a specific POM antibiotic to people with a confirmed diagnostic infection, e.g. azithromycin for *Chlamydia*.

Second, prescribing rights for pharmacists, alongside nurses and some other healthcare professionals, have been introduced, initially as supplementary prescribers and more recently, as independent prescribers (see Ch. 4).

The profession

The council of the Royal Pharmaceutical Society of Great Britain (RPSGB) decided that it was necessary to allow all members to contribute to a radical appraisal of the profession, what it should be doing and how to achieve it. The 'Pharmacy in a New Age' consultation was launched in October 1995, with an invitation to all members to contribute their views to the council. These were combined into a subsequent document produced by the council in September 1996 called *Pharmacy in a New Age: The New Horizon*. This indicated that there was overwhelming agreement from pharmacists that the profession could not stand still. Four main areas in which pharmacy should make a major contribution to health outcomes were identified:

- Management of prescribed medicines. This covers drug development, provision of medicines, information and support, and ensuring patient needs are met safely, efficiently and conveniently so that they can get maximum benefit from their medicines.
- Management of chronic conditions. Here the need is to improve the quality of life and outcomes of treatment for the patient. Pharmacists may help by supplying medicines and advice, helping to develop local shared care protocols, ensuring that patients are taking or using their medicines properly and working as part of the healthcare team.
- Management of common ailments. Patients require reassurance and advice, with or without the use of non-prescription medicines and referral to other professionals if necessary (see Ch. 21).
- Promotion and support of healthy lifestyles. Pharmacists can help people protect their own

health through health screening, giving advice on healthy living and providing educational materials (see Ch. 48).

During the consultation process, pharmacists expressed their views on the way the profession should change. These, too, may be summarized under four main headings:

- *The strengths of pharmacy*. There was a high level of consensus that the knowledge base of pharmacy was very important. This is based on both the study of and experience with medicines and also in managing medicines and handling relevant information. A second strength which was seen as important was pharmacists' availability and accessibility in a wide range of different locations in the heart of the community, such as conventional high street premises, health centres, supermarkets, hospitals and in people's homes. This accessibility is strengthened by easy communication with both patients and other professionals, giving pharmacists a pivotal position. The growth of information technology could be a potential threat to this, although pharmacists are noted for their adaptability.
- *Demonstrating the value of pharmacy*. Pharmacy must claim its rights as a profession and accept the responsibilities which come with this. Thus high standards must be set and achieved. Additionally, evidence must be produced which demonstrates clearly the value of pharmacy in health care. This will require research and professional audit (see Ch. 12). Further support for this development will come from increased continuing education and recognition achieved by effective promotion of the profession.
- *Changes in practice*. Three main areas where there could be an increase in services were identified. These are: the enhancement of services to patients (advice, counselling, domiciliary visits, health promotion and non-prescription medicine sales); improved relationships with other healthcare professionals (closer support for prescribers, medicine management, liaison between hospital and community pharmacy and different community pharmacists, training for other professionals and carers); and practice research and audit, continuing education and better use of information technology (all required to support the other developments). There was also a

high level of support for a reduction in the mechanical aspects of dispensing, sale of non-health-related products and routine paperwork associated with the NHS and business activities.

- *A sustainable future.* These elements could make up a sustainable future for the profession. In particular, pharmacy would be concerned with advice and counselling, dispensing, health promotion, the sale of non-prescription medicines, medicines management and as a first port of call for health care. Some of these may require changes in the setting of pharmaceutical provision and others may require different types of employment for pharmacists. Other changes which would be required included changes to the system of payment under the NHS, a rationalization of pharmacy distribution and at least two pharmacists being employed per community pharmacy.

The main output of this professional review was a commitment to take forward a more proactive, patient-centred clinical role for pharmacy using pharmacists' skills and knowledge to best effect.

The NHS drugs budget

Health services are expensive to run and governments try to reduce expenditure as far as possible. In the UK, some medicines have been identified as being ineligible for prescribing on the NHS. The so-called Black List was introduced in 1984 to reduce the size of the NHS bill. Furthermore the introduction of computer technology into prescription pricing has enabled far more data to be produced than was previously possible. Doctors now receive a regular breakdown of the drugs they have prescribed and that have been dispensed and their prescribing costs, PACT (England) or PRISMS (Scotland)), and this information is also available on line (see Chs 22 and 23).

However, despite these moves, and in common with other developed countries, UK drug costs are inexorably rising due to the greater availability of new effective treatments, patient demand and changes in patient demography (more older people). This has made many governments look at other ways of controlling this item of expenditure, and there are two ways in which pharmacists can have a role.

First, it is recognized that not all prescribing follows the current best evidence for cost-effective practice. Pharmacists are seen as a profession with the necessary knowledge to support quality in prescribing at a strategic and practice level. At a strategic level they can appraise the evidence and make recommendations for the inclusion of a drug in a formulary. At a general practice level pharmacists can advise prescribers on the best drugs to prescribe for individual patients. Community pharmacists are well placed to monitor and review repeat prescriptions, which account for 80% of all prescriptions in primary care.

Second, in a move to promote self-care, pharmacists can encourage patients to be responsible for their own health care and, by implication, remove the cost of treating what is known as 'minor illness' from the NHS. Many drugs previously only available on prescription (POM) are now available over the counter from pharmacies (P) or from any retail outlet general sales list (GSL). These changes have resulted in many potent drugs now being available for sale from community pharmacies and the advisory role of the pharmacist has therefore been greatly enhanced (see Ch. 21).

The NHS workforce

As demand for health care grows, it is not only budgets that are stretched. Increasingly, there are insufficient trained professionals to deliver services, and innovative ways of working need to be introduced to maximize the skills of the different professionals in the healthcare team. This has resulted in recognition that many of the tasks previously undertaken by the medical profession, in both primary and secondary care, can be undertaken by other professions such as pharmacists and nurses. Thus, some of the professional roles originally identified by the profession, such as the management of chronic disease and a greater role in responding to symptoms are now supported by the wider healthcare community because they can contribute to more effective health care for the population. As a result, a team approach to managing health care has emerged.

The current and future roles of pharmacists

There are currently around 46 000 UK member pharmacists registered with the General Pharmaceutical Council, including those who are working in different sectors of the profession.

Approximately 70% work in community pharmacy, 20% in hospitals, 8% in primary care and 4% in the pharmaceutical industry.

Community pharmacy

As a result of the final recognition of the pharmacist's role beyond solely dispensing, new community pharmacy contractual frameworks were agreed for England and Wales, and for Scotland, in the early part of this century. In England and Wales, the contract is based on a list of essential services to be delivered from all NHS contracted pharmacies, and then an advanced service specification for specially accredited pharmacists operating from enhanced premises with private consultation areas. At the time of writing, there are four advanced services: the medicines use review (MUR) and prescription intervention service; the appliance use review (AUR); stoma appliance customization (SAC); and the new medicines service (NMS). Enhanced services, which are negotiated locally with individual NHS primary care organizations, are also delivered. These are summarized in Box 1.1. In Scotland, the new contract is similar, but there is an emphasis on all pharmacists delivering all of the four core service areas: these are the acute medicines service (AMS); the chronic medicines service (CMS); the minor ailment service (MAS); and the public health service (PHS). More detail on these is provided in Box 1.2. In Northern Ireland, a new contract is proposed but is not yet delivered. However, locally agreed contracts are supporting extended roles for community pharmacy, for example in providing smoking cessation services and Minor Ailment Services. In summary, whichever contractual framework pharmacists are operating under, the following generic services will be delivered to some extent.

Dispensing, repeat dispensing and medication review

Despite the recent contractual recognition of new clinical roles, which are described later, dispensing remains a core role of community pharmacy and would still account for the majority of a pharmacist's time. The preponderance of original pack dispensing means that, compared with even a decade ago, while the name may remain the same, the similarity ends there. The focus of dispensing now rests not only on accurate supply of medication, but also on checking that the medication is appropriate for the patient and counselling the patient on its appropriate use. All community pharmacists maintain computerized patient medication records which are a record of previous prescriptions dispensed. While not necessarily complete, since patients are not registered with an individual pharmacy, in practice, the vast majority of patients, particularly those on regular prescribed medication, do use one pharmacy for the majority of their supplies. Thus, pharmacists have a database of information, which will allow them to check on issues such as accuracy of the new prescription, compliance and potential drug interactions.

In the future, the dispensing role will be further enhanced as connection of community pharmacy into the NHS net becomes a reality. Electronic transmission of prescriptions is being implemented. Under this scheme, GPs send prescriptions to a central 'cyberstore' from which pharmacists can download the information using a unique identifier, and dispense the prescribed supplies or medications to the patient. Ultimately, this electronic link should allow access by the pharmacist to at least a selected portion of the patient's medical records, further enhancing the pharmacist's ability to assess the appropriateness of the prescription. It is hoped that there will also be a facility for pharmacists to write to the patient record, so that GPs will know whether or not prescriptions have been dispensed and what OTC drugs have been purchased.

A further enhanced dispensing role is in the management of repeat prescriptions, which until recently, have been issued from GP surgeries with little clinical review. Following research projects which demonstrated that when given this responsibility, community pharmacists could identify previously unrecognized side-effects, adverse drug reactions and drug interactions, as well as saving almost one-fifth of the costs of the drugs prescribed, this repeat dispensing service is now part of the new community pharmacy contract (see Boxes 1.1 and 1.2).

This opportunistic clinical input at the point of dispensing is also being developed in a more systematic way, in that patients with targeted chronic conditions, such as coronary heart disease, have formal regular reviews with the community pharmacist about their medication and other disease-related behaviours. Again schemes like this, with research evidence of benefit in small studies, are currently undergoing national implementation

Box 1.1

Community pharmacy contractual framework (England and Wales), introduced 2005

Essential services	Dispensing of prescribed medicine
	Repeat dispensing
	Disposal of unwanted medicines/waste management
Public health	Healthy lifestyle campaigns, prescription-linked healthy lifestyle interventions
Signposting	Provision of information to people visiting the pharmacy, who require further support, advice or treatment which cannot be provided by the pharmacy
Support for self-care	Provide advice on treatment of minor illness including OTC medicine sale, maintain records of clinically significant products purchased
Clinical governance	Provide in relation to public and patient involvement, monitoring by NHS, participation in clinical audit, undertaking risk management and supporting self and staff with education and professional development
	Appropriate use of information and compliance with statute such as the Data Protection Act 1998, the Human Rights Act 1998, the NHS Code of Practice on Confidentiality, the Disability Discrimination Act 1995 and Health and Safety legislation
	Maintenance of patient medication records
Advanced services	**Medicines use review**
	A service initiated by either the pharmacist, the GP or the patient in which accredited pharmacists undertake structured adherence centred reviews with patients on multiple prescribed medicines. The aim is to help patients understand and comply with their treatment, identify problems if any, and provide a report to the patient and the GP
	New medicines service
	A service to support for people with long-term conditions who have been newly prescribed a medicine, with the intention of helping them improve medicines adherence. The service is currently time limited until December 2013 at which point a decision will be taken whether to continue it, based on observed demonstrable value to the NHS
	Appliance use review
	The service aims to improve the patient's knowledge and use of any 'specified appliance' by establishing how they use it and advising on any changes required for optimum benefit.
	Stoma Appliance Customization
	This service aims to ensure the proper use and comfortable fitting of the stoma appliance and to improve the duration of usage, thereby reducing waste.
Enhanced services (locally negotiated)	A wide range of services such as alcohol screening, anticoagulation monitoring, asthma, care homes, care staff, controlled drugs, record cards, chronic obstructive pulmonary disease, databases, emergency hormonal contraception, gluten-free foods, *Helicobacter pylori* testing, minor ailments, needle and syringe exchange, needle collection, 'not dispensed scheme', out of hours, palliative care, Parkinson's disease, phlebotomy, point of care testing, prescription intervention, quality and outcomes framework, seasonal influenza, sexual health, smoking cessation, supervised administration (e.g. of methadone), vascular risk assessment, weight management and obesity

through the new contractual frameworks. Such services, called medicines management (see Ch. 20), MUR, NMS or CMS, are part of a more holistic approach often referred to as pharmaceutical care. Supplementary and independent prescribing will greatly enhance this role for pharmacy.

Responding to symptoms

Provision of advice to customers presenting in the pharmacy for advice on self-care is now an accepted part of the work of a pharmacist which, as described earlier, has been enhanced by the increased armamentarium of pharmacy medicines. Advertising

Box 1.2

New Scottish community pharmacy contract, introduced incrementally from 2006

There are four services delivered by all community pharmacies:

Minor ailment service (eMAS) (from mid-2006)	The provision of a range of pharmacy and general sale medicines (e.g. to treat skin problems, pain, coughs and colds) from the community pharmacy paid for by the NHS to patients registered with that pharmacy and meeting the eligibility criteria: • persons who are under 16 years of age or under 19 years of age and in full-time education • persons who are aged 60 years or over • persons who have a valid maternity exemption certificate, medical exemption certificate, or war pension exemption certificate • persons who get Income Support, Income-based Jobseeker's Allowance, Income-related Employment and Support Allowance or Pension Credit Guarantee Credit • persons who are named on, or are entitled to, an NHS tax credit exemption certificate or a valid HC2 certificate.
Public health service (from end 2006)	All interactions with patients should include provision of opportunistic healthy living advice, take part in four national campaigns a year, e.g. flu, vaccinations, meningitis by poster display and provision of health promotion messages, and offer smoking cessation service and emergency hormonal contraception supply.
Acute medication service (from July 2008)	Dispensing prescribed medicines, plus advice. Electronic transmission of prescriptions between GP and community pharmacy.
Chronic medication service	The management of long-term conditions by monitoring, medications review, adjustment of doses (by those with prescriber qualification), repeat dispensing. Patients 'opt in' to the service and are registered with the pharmacy.

There are also optional services:

National funded optional services	e.g. palliative care, prescribing clinics
Locally negotiated services	These will also continue, e.g. services for drug misusers (needle exchange and supervised consumption), flu immunization and drugs as per the English contract (see Box 1.1)

campaigns, particularly those by the National Pharmaceutical Association (NPA), have brought to public attention the advice which is available from the pharmacist, as have the commercial adverts from the pharmaceutical industry for their deregulated products. The increased emphasis on the provision of advice from community pharmacies has also extended to the counter staff, who require special training and must adhere to protocols (see Ch. 21).

The full contribution of this advisory role to health care has been limited, to some extent, to the more advantaged sections of the population, particularly since the deregulation of many potent medicines referred to earlier. Many of these newer P medicines are relatively expensive, and those on lower incomes, and particularly those who are exempt from prescription charges, may in the past have attended their doctor only for the purpose of obtaining a free prescription for the drug. This has now been circumvented. Under the contract in Scotland, all patients who meet certain criteria mostly related to age (e.g. <16 years of age or >60 years of age) or income (see Box 1.2) can access any medicine normally available from a pharmacy, without a prescription and on the NHS, from their local community pharmacist. Patients have to register with a community pharmacy to receive the service and all records are maintained centrally and electronically. Ultimately, they will be able to be linked to other patient information through a unique patient identifier, known as the CHI (Community Health Index). In England, similar schemes also exist under the new contract but they are an enhanced, locally negotiated service, rather than an essential service. At the time of writing, only about 12% of English community pharmacies provide this service.

Health promotion and health improvement

A large number of people pass through the nation's pharmacies in any one day; on the basis of prescription numbers, this is frequently said to be 6 million people per day in the UK. Another way of looking at this is that over 90% of the population visit a community pharmacy in any single year. Thus, the pharmacist is one of the best placed healthcare professionals to provide health promotion information and health education material to the general public (see Chs 13 and 48). This has now become part of the pharmacist's NHS contract and formalized as a core service to be delivered by all pharmacies in England and Wales, and Scotland. The service specification is generally limited to participation in healthy lifestyle campaigns and opportunistic intervention. More aspirational roles can also be delivered and there are extensive opportunities for proactive, targeted and specialist advice to be provided from community pharmacies. Pharmacists can give out patient information leaflets on healthy nutrition, which may reduce the development of disease which would otherwise occur and lead to the need for expensive treatment. Smoking is considered to be the single biggest cause of preventable ill health. Pharmacists have a successful record in supporting smoking cessation through tailored face-to-face advice and the supply of smoking cessation products such as nicotine replacement therapies (see Ch. 48), and the vast majority of pharmacies are engaged in local smoking cessation schemes. In Scotland, 70% of all quit attempts and 60% of all quits are delivered through community pharmacy. Studies to quantify the contribution community pharmacists can make to weight, exercise and alcohol consumption are ongoing.

Services to specific patient groups

Certain groups of patients have particular needs which can be met by community pharmacists more cost-effectively than by any other healthcare professional. One such example is drug misuse and its link to the spread of blood-borne diseases such as hepatitis and AIDS. Drug misuse is an increasing problem in society today (see Ch. 50). It is now generally accepted that drug misusers have a right to treatment both to help them overcome their addiction and to reduce the harm they may do, either to themselves or to society, until such time as they are ready to undergo detoxification. In particular, pharmacists have become involved in needle exchange schemes and in instalment dispensing and supervised consumption of methadone. Because of the urgent need for these important services, and to some extent because of the unwillingness of some community pharmacists to become involved, these services have unusually been recognized by specific locally negotiated remuneration packages.

Domiciliary visiting

Many pharmacists will visit a small number of patients in their own home to deliver medicines and provide advice on their use. This will now be extended to include other situations where patients could benefit, such as on discharge from hospital, including highly specialized services (often called the 'hospital at home') where patients may be on palliative care, cytotoxic agents, intravenous antibiotics or artificial nutrition (see Chs 44 and 46). As medicines' management services for people on chronic medication continue to evolve, and with more early hospital discharge, this could mean more domiciliary visits to housebound patients. There is also a separate but related need for services to be provided in care home settings, to include both advice on the storage and administration of medicines as well as clinical advice for individual patients (see Ch. 49).

Personal control

One of the requirements of the current regulations is that a pharmacist has to be in personal control/supervision of registered community pharmacy premises at all times. The principle is that the pharmacist should be aware of any transaction in which a medicine is provided to a member of the public and be able to intervene if deemed necessary. This requirement was intended to protect the public but it has been a barrier to innovative practice, and it has been interpreted as the pharmacist needing to be physically present in the pharmacy and aware of all transactions involving P and POM medicines. For single-handed pharmacists this has been difficult to combine with new roles undertaken outwith the pharmacy premises, such as domiciliary visits, or multi-professional meetings. In 2008, the Responsible Pharmacist Regulations were introduced which require that a retail pharmacy business must be in the charge of a named registered pharmacist who is the responsible pharmacist. Under these regulations, the responsible pharmacist can be absent for up to 2 hours per day; different activities can take place in the pharmacy when the pharmacist is present and absent, guided by whether not the physical presence of the pharmacist is required. For example the sale and supply of Pharmacy medicines requires the pharmacist to be present but the sale and supply of General Sales medicines does not. In general, there are moves to promote greater use of professional judgement, and this is reflected in the current Standards of Conduct, Ethics and Performance, which with successive editions, emphasizes principles and removes prescriptive details.

A further challenge to established practice will also come from the increasing use of the internet for personal shopping; and the acquisition of medicines, whether prescribed or purchased, will not be immune to such developments. Already mail order pharmacy and e-pharmacy are making small inroads into medicines distribution and supply, and challenge some of the Standards of conduct, ethics and performance and professional practice points which encourage personal counselling wherever possible. Again, the new Standards document has responded appropriately, with guidance to professionals on how they can still deliver the same standards of care as from face-to-face premises. Although online services are probably more developed in North America, such changes to practice are inevitable and need to be managed professionally, remembering that best care of the patient, rather than professional self-interest, must be the rationale of any decision-making.

Out of hours services

The NHS call centres: NHS 111 (England), NHS Direct (Wales) and NHS 24 (Scotland), handle health-related telephone enquiries from the general public and triage them on to appropriate services. Referral to community pharmacy is one of the formal dispositions included in the algorithms used by the call handlers. It is intended, therefore, that the community pharmacist will not be bypassed by the new telephone help lines. It should also serve to educate the public about the role of the community pharmacist and to increase general awareness that the community pharmacy is just as much a part of the NHS as is the general practice. Audits of calls have revealed that a high proportion are linked to medicines and could have been handled directly by pharmacists. As a result, pharmacists are now employed directly to provide online advice from NHS 111/NHS 24/NHS Direct phone lines, and there is also a recognized need to divert the public back to the community pharmacist as the port of call during normal working hours. Finally, there are moves to extend accessibility to face-to-face out of hours pharmaceutical advice through links between community pharmacies and out of hours centres.

Hospital pharmacy

Clinical pharmacy services have been established in the hospital setting for some time. In general, there is already a greater working together of the professions in the hospital setting compared with primary care, including pharmacists' involvement in medication history taking, active engagement in research and for the provision of 24-hour services. In 1988, the NHS circular 'Health Services Management: the Way Forward for Hospital Pharmaceutical Services' laid down the government policy aim as 'the achievement of better patient care and financial savings, through the more cost effective use of medicines, and improved use of pharmaceutical expertise obtained through the implementation of a clinical pharmacy service'. Two main components were identified. One is the overall management of medicines on the hospital ward. This is achieved through the provision of advice to medical and nursing staff, formulary management and ensuring the safe handling of medicines. The other component is the development of individual patient care plans. This is achieved through the provision of drug information and assisting patients with problems which may arise. In practice there are many stages and activities involved in these processes. A working group in Scotland published *Clinical Pharmacy in the Hospital Pharmaceutical Service: a Framework for Practice* in July 1996 (Clinical Resources Audit Group 1996). The framework advocates a systematic approach to enable the pharmacist to focus on the key areas and optimize the pharmaceutical input to patient care. One specific area where pharmacists have been called on to support better prescribing is in the appropriate use of antibiotics. Many hospitals have specialist antibiotic pharmacists whose role is to promote the correct use of antibiotics and hence reduce the spread of antibacterial resistance and associated problems, such as those caused by *Clostridium difficile* and MRSA.

There is growing awareness of the problems which arise at the interface between community (primary) and hospital (secondary) care. Patients move in both directions. Their medical and pharmaceutical problems also move with them. Over the next few years, it is hoped that a large proportion of these problems will have been resolved through the greater involvement of pharmacists at admission and discharge with effective (ultimately electronic) transfer of information, from hospital pharmacist to community pharmacist. As more patients are discharged early, and with more serious and specialized clinical conditions, there will need to be greater communication at this interface and possibly hospital pharmacists operating outwith their traditional secondary care base.

As in community pharmacy, the need for technical skills for local manufacturing of individual products is also now greatly reduced and the skills of hospital pharmacists are more utilized in decisions about the cost-effective and clinically effective selection of drugs, and contributing to drug and therapeutic committees, formulary groups and quality assurance procedures (see Chs 22 and 23). Issues of supply and efficient distribution of medicines are increasingly becoming automated.

Other NHS roles

Primary care pharmacy

During the 1990s, there was increasing evidence of close working between pharmacists and the rest of the general practice based primary healthcare team. Doctors realized that pharmacists had many possible additional clinical roles in primary care, beyond their traditional community pharmacy premises. Many pharmacists now provide doctors with advice on GP formulary development (see Ch. 23) and undertake patient medication reviews, either seeing patients face-to-face or through review of patient records, either globally or on an individual basis. They may also take responsibility for specific clinics following agreed protocols, such as anticoagulant and *Helicobacter pylori* assessment clinics. These pharmacists are known as primary care pharmacists. As community pharmacy develops and IT links become the norm, many of the tasks now done by primary care pharmacists will ultimately be carried out from the community pharmacy base.

Pharmaceutical advisers

Pharmaceutical advisers co-ordinate pharmaceutical care for primary care organizations, integrating community pharmacy into the delivery of core health care, and coordinating the primary care pharmacist workforce to achieve area wide goals in prescribing. As new NHS structures emerge involving GP-led commissioning bodies, the pharmaceutical advisor role may change.

Pharmaceutical public health

Strategic health authorities in England and NHS boards in Scotland administer large geographical areas. Many of these also have a senior pharmacist, operating at consultant level, as part of the public health team. They have a specific responsibility for local pharmacy strategy development, compliance with statutes and the managed entry of new drugs, as well as providing local professional leadership and advice on professional governance alongside other senior pharmacy colleagues. Increasingly, as professional boundaries begin to merge, they are also seen as public healthcare professionals and take their share of the generic public health workload.

The public's view

Increasingly, patient satisfaction with new services is monitored in formal health services research projects, as part of innovative pilot schemes and for ongoing routine quality control. Indeed, one of the requirements of the new contracts is that community pharmacists should 'have in place a system to enable patients to give feedback or evaluate services'. Large surveys of the public's opinion of community pharmacy services have also been conducted. In general, such surveys find that the public are satisfied with the service they receive, and that pharmacy is a trusted profession. Research also tells us the public regard community pharmacy services as an important resource for them to access when managing symptoms of minor illness, and that they prefer to seek such advice from a pharmacist rather than a GP or one of the NHS online services. However, it is also shown that they are more wary of hypothetical situations in which pharmacists become involved in the delivery of new roles which have previously been delivered by GPs or nurses working with GPs. In particular, older people are less open to new models of service, whereas younger people are much more positive. Once new services have been trialled, such as repeat dispensing, medicines management and prescribing, patient feedback is highly positive. Nonetheless, when asked whether or not they would prefer a doctor or pharmacist to provide the service, there is a status quo bias in favour of the GP. This is not really surprising, but the profession needs to be aware of this. New services have to earn their place in the public's esteem, building confidence in the quality of what they offer and the advantages of pharmacy delivered services. There is also a need for other healthcare professionals to value the pharmacist's new roles and to recognize their increasingly central place in the NHS team.

Clinical effectiveness

Clinical effectiveness is a term often used to describe the extent to which clinical practice meets the highest known standards of care. Clinical governance is a term used to describe the accountability of an organizational grouping for ensuring that clinical effectiveness is practised by all functions for which it is responsible (see Ch. 9). Central to this is the use of evidence-based guidelines and protocols, which have increased dramatically in the past decade. These guidelines are a way of increasing the quality of service because they are developed after systematic searches of the research evidence and make recommendations for 'best practice', which are easily understood and widely accepted.

The extent to which guidelines are actually applied in particular situations should be measured by clinical audit (see Ch. 12). Audit is also an important tool in the raising of standards of service delivery.

The roles of the Royal Pharmaceutical Society and the General Pharmaceutical Council

The RPSGB historically undertook an unusual dual role as a professional body and a regulatory body, being responsible for both developing and promoting the profession and the registration of pharmacists and premises, the maintenance of standards though a network of inspectors, and for disciplining those who do not meet the required standard. With increasing public concerns about standards of health care in general, the UK Council for the Regulation of Healthcare Professionals was established. As part of its review of the regulation of all healthcare professionals, a recommendation was made that the regulatory functions of the RPSGB would be delivered by an independent body, the General Pharmaceutical Council, and a new body for pharmacy was created to deliver the complementary professional role: the Royal Pharmaceutical Society. While membership of the GPhC is mandatory for all those wishing to practice as pharmacists, membership of the RPS is voluntary, although strongly to be encouraged.

Continuing education and continuing professional development

In such a rapidly changing profession, there is a need for continual updating of knowledge. The RPS through *The Pharmaceutical Journal*, has established a regular pattern of continuing education (CE) articles on a wide range of topics and introduced a formal web-based continuing professional development (CPD) initiative. The GPhC, through the standards of conduct, ethics and performance, requires that all pharmacists keep a record of their CPD and the GPhC can request this record be submitted to them for review at any time. There is a standard of a minimum of nine entries per year to reflect the context and scope of practice and describe how the CPD has contributed to the quality and development of the individual's practice. This approach is thus more about tailored personal and professional development (see Ch. 6).

Pharmacy education

Undergraduate education

Teaching of pharmacy was traditionally under four subject headings: pharmaceutical chemistry, pharmaceutics, pharmacology and pharmacognosy. This was seen as a restraint on the development of new ideas of teaching to make the course more relevant to the profession. The course has to have a firm science base, building on knowledge acquired in secondary school, but be relevant to practice. Pathology and therapeutics, law and ethics and the teaching of dispensing practice all have their place alongside clinical pharmacy, which is now accepted as a subject in its own right and one of the most important parts of the course. The course also includes social and behavioural science – a broad subject area which covers many sociological and psychological aspects of disease and patients – and communication skills. Although communication cannot be learned solely by studying a book, it is still useful to have an understanding of the underpinning theoretical framework when learning to put good professional communication into practice (see Chs 3, 4, 17, 25).

Most schools of pharmacy involve both primary and secondary care pharmacy practitioners in undergraduate teaching. The aim of utilizing these teacher–practitioners is to ensure that the university course is relevant to current professional practice. This reflects the situation in other healthcare professions such as medicine. Other ways of learning from current practice as part of course provision are also used, such as visiting lecturers, making GP practice and hospital visits, using part-time teaching staff, staff secondment to practice and joint academic/practice research studies.

Pre-registration training

The purpose of the pre-registration year is for the recent graduate to make the transition from student to a person who can practise effectively and independently as a member of the pharmacy profession. At the end of the year, the pre-registration trainee has to pass a formal registration assessment prior to entry to the register. Pre-registration training is carried out, in either hospital or community pharmacy practice, in a structured way with a competency-based assessment after 12 months. Some of the differences between community and hospital practice are becoming less distinct as pharmacists in the community take on roles which in the past have been common in hospital practice, such as prescribing advice to doctors. In the future, it may be that a combined pre-registration year may be introduced and interchange between the two areas of practice will become easier to achieve than it is at present (see Ch. 5).

Higher degrees and research

A wide range of taught MSc and Diploma courses are offered in the UK. Subject matter may be very specialized or more general. Study may be full-time or part-time. There are also distance learning courses for those who have limited opportunity to be away from their place of work. Additionally, taught PharmD courses are gaining in popularity and are provided in a small number of institutions across the UK. The programmes are intended to allow pharmacists to develop specialist skills in their chosen area, through formal learning, together with the conduct of either a substantive piece of research or work-based project.

Research has also developed, and research articles appear regularly in the *Pharmaceutical Journal* and the *International Journal of Pharmacy Practice*, as well as other academic journals from medicine and primary care. There are practice research sessions at the British Pharmaceutical Conference each year, and there is an annual dedicated Health Service and Pharmacy Practice Research Conference. Many students are now graduating with a doctorate for studies undertaken in aspects of pharmacy practice, and, reflecting the integrated multidisciplinary delivery of care, many pharmacists are carrying out research in multidisciplinary research teams. The development of the discipline of pharmacy practice research is something of which the profession should be justifiably proud. The generation of research evidence of the clinical and cost-effective contribution which pharmacists can make to health care has had a key part to play in the innovations in professional practice we have seen in the past decade, and which have been summarized in this introductory chapter.

Conclusion

During the twentieth century, pharmacy underwent major changes. This process has accelerated since the introduction of the NHS in 1948, the Nuffield

Report in 1986 and, most recently, the new plans for the NHS published at the turn of the century. As will be evident from reading this chapter, many changes are still ongoing, demonstrating the vibrant and dynamic nature of both the health service and of our profession. Pharmacists now deal with more potent and sophisticated medicines, requiring a different type of knowledge and a different skill set than was previously the case. At the same time, the public has become more aware of the services that are available from pharmacists. People are making increasing use of the pharmacist as a source of information and advice about minor conditions and non-prescription medicines. This is now extending to the general public regarding pharmacists as a source of information and advice about their prescribed medicines and seeking help from pharmacists with any medication problems they may encounter. This process is likely to develop further through the twenty-first century. We are also likely to see further changes reflecting the merging of professional boundaries and competency-based delivery of health care. Thus, generic healthcare professionals may emerge, and many may undertake tasks traditionally undertaken by one profession. In addition, in order to free up professional time, we can expect to see pharmacy technicians taking on greater responsibility for the technical aspects of the pharmacist's role, while qualified pharmacists concentrate on cognitive functions and interact directly with the patient.

Pharmacists need to have the knowledge and adaptability to take a lead in these processes, so that they can have a key role in ensuring that the health care of the public can be delivered as efficiently as possible. The undergraduate pharmacy courses must reflect these changes to ensure that their graduates meet the demands of the future NHS workforce.

KEY POINTS

- The UK NHS came into being in 1948
- Early developments in the NHS were in hospital services, but this has gradually changed to focus on community practice
- Publication of the Nuffield Report in 1986 marked a watershed for pharmacy in the UK
- New community pharmacy contracts in the UK are delivering the vision together with regulatory changes such as patient group directions and supplementary and independent prescribing
- Education at undergraduate and postgraduate levels reflects these changes and pharmacy graduates are well trained for their new roles
- The public values the pharmacist but still has some reservations about too much care being delegated from doctors

Socio-behavioural aspects of health and illness

2

Alison Gifford

STUDY POINTS

- The importance of social and behavioural sciences to pharmacy
- The meaning of health and illness
- Changing health-related behaviour and the related models
- How people behave when they are ill
- Behavioural aspects of health care
- Factors affecting the treatment process

Introduction

To develop a full understanding of the use of medicines by individuals and society and the role that pharmacy contributes to health care, an understanding of the sociology and psychology of health is required. These two factors are closely interwoven, and help the pharmacist to understand the influences on an individual's behaviour in relation to their health and any illness they encounter.

In pharmacy practice research, sociological and psychological influences on health have often been under researched, with research often focused on adherence in a mechanistic manner. However, if pharmacy as a profession wishes to understand and resolve medicine and medicine-related problems, we need to broaden our perspectives to incorporate relevant social and behavioural theory and research.

The purpose of this, and the following chapter is to provide the reader with a broad overview of the health-related issues from a health sociological and psychological perspective; emphasizing the need to understand the wider influences on individual

behaviour in order to enhance our pharmacy practice. The social sciences have a shared focus on understanding patterns and meaning of human behaviour, which distinguishes them from the physical and biological sciences.

Illness can be perceived as either a solely biophysical state, or a more comprehensive view may be taken, viewing illness as a human societal state where behaviour varies with culture and other social factors. It is argued that viewing illness as purely a malfunction of a physical process or structure underemphasizes the influence of the individual and psychosocial issues on their beliefs, thoughts and behaviour.

Pharmacists have to deal with many social and behavioural issues in their daily work, either directly or indirectly through health-related behaviour. The contribution of social sciences to pharmacy and pharmacy practice can be summarized in the following three areas:

- Analysing the practice of pharmacy – helping to identify important questions relating to the use of medicines, pharmacy practice and the pharmacy profession
- Providing conceptual and explanatory frameworks for understanding human behaviour in a social context
- Providing appropriate approaches to study the use of medicines and the practice of pharmacy.

It is impossible in two chapters to provide a comprehensive review of all the aspects of health sociology and psychology that may be relevant to pharmacy. Instead, the aim is to highlight the relevant key areas that may lead the reader to explore the sociological and psychological literature in more detail; a good starting point is the books and articles on the topic that are included in the further reading (Appendix 4).

This chapter will focus on defining health and illness and exploring the determinants of health and illness for an individual. It is important for a pharmacist to understand the influences and processes involved in illness behaviour and treatment to enable effective, patient-centred practice. In each area, the major concepts and theories that provide a deeper understanding of health and illness are briefly discussed.

An overall framework is presented in Figure 2.1.

Defining health and illness

Health and illness mean different things to different people, it is very subjective, and it is easy to take good health for granted. Commonly, health is seen as the absence of signs that the body is not functioning properly or absence of symptoms of disease or injury. Health is often perceived as a dichotomy; you are either healthy or you are not, but in reality, health is a continuum of different states, and both societal and individual perceptions influence our understanding of health.

However, disease, in contrast to illness, is something professionally defined. The organization of current health care around the world uses this concept of illness to frame its structures, yet research has shown that physicians and experts vary in their views on both physical and mental disease, such that it is difficult to argue that disease can be easily defined.

In reality, illness is more often a state defined by the individual patient based on their own subjective reaction to a perceived biological alteration of body or mind. It has both physical and social connotations. Our perception of illness is influenced by individual, cultural, social and other factors. Illness is also a socially defined condition, resulting in the individual being assigned a particular social status by other members of their society. Parson's concept of a societal 'sick role' and its effect on illness and health care will be explored in more detail.

It is important to understand that an individual may have a disease and not be ill, might be ill but not have a disease or might have both an illness and a disease.

The most widely used definition of health or wellness is that of the WHO, which states that: 'health is a state of complete physical, mental and

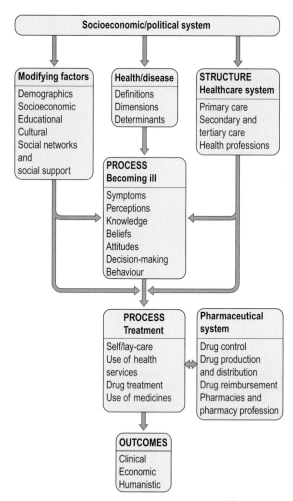

Figure 2.1 • A model of the social and behavioural factors involved in health and illness.

social well-being and not merely the absence of diseases and infirmity'. This definition incorporates all aspects of health and although holistic and widely quoted, it is used less by policy makers in the healthcare arena, as it does not provide guidance on which to base funding decisions.

The WHO definition offers a goal for health that is actively sought through positive actions and not merely through a passive process of avoiding disease-causing agents.

Dimensions of health

The WHO definition of health distinguishes between three aspects; physical, mental and social health, but very often healthcare systems use a narrower definition of health incorporating only physical and mental health to focus their resource allocation.

In utilizing the wider definition of health, there is a danger that we begin to 'medicalize' our society – issues such as loneliness, domestic violence and attention deficit disorder become the responsibility of medicine and public health, when they may not need medical treatment in the way that other diseases require. In opposing the argument, the broad definitions allow us to examine health issues in a holistic manner.

Physical health

Most of us see physical health as being free from pain, physical disability, acute and chronic diseases and bodily discomfort. However, our prior experiences of illness, our age, education and a variety of other personal and social factors will influence our perception of physical health. Health has to be understood to be subjective – what one individual may consider to be poor health may not be perceived as such by another. In dealing with patients and their health, the pharmacist needs to work to understand the individual's perceptions to facilitate effective interactions.

Mental health

Mental health comprises of an individual's ability to deal constructively with reality and to adapt effectively to change, to hold a positive self-image and to cope with stressors and develop intimate relationships. Furthermore, enjoying the pleasures of ordinary life and making plans for the future are important aspects of mental health.

Spiritual health

Spiritual health is considered by some as part of the mental health dimension, while others argue that it is a separate dimension. It should not be confused with religion or religiousness. A sense of spiritual well-being is possible without belonging to an organized religion. Spiritual health has been characterized as the ability to articulate and act on one's own basic purpose of life, giving and receiving love, trust, joy and peace, having a set of principles to live by, having a sense of selflessness,

honour, integrity and sacrifice and being willing to help others achieve their full potential. By contrast, negative spiritual health can be described by loss of meaning in one's life, self-centredness, lack of self-responsibility and a hopeless attitude.

Social health

The impact of social health on the well-being of the individual has been widely demonstrated. Social integration, social networks and social support have both direct and indirect influences on health. A low socioeconomic status defined by educational level, income and occupation is closely related to higher morbidity and mortality.

Determinants and models of health

Throughout history, the concepts of disease have changed. Early explanations involved evil spirits causing disease. Hippocrates (460–370 BC) suggested that the imbalance of the four body fluids caused disease, while during the Middle Ages, illness was seen as God's punishment.

Later in time, in the post-Renaissance period, René Descartes suggested that the body could be viewed as a machine and he theorized how action and sensation occur. In addition, he proposed that the body and mind were separate but could communicate, and that the soul leaves the human body at death.

Since Descartes' time, advances in science have led scientists to develop a more advanced understanding of the working of the body and the processes of illness and disease. The role of microbes and other agents in causing disease is understood, along with the effect of nutrition, hygiene and other lifestyle factors.

The biomedical model of disease proposes that all diseases and illness can be explained by disturbed physiological processes. The disturbances may be caused by injury, biochemical changes and bacterial, viral or fungal infection. This model separates the physical from the psychological and sociological influences on health. The biomedical model has dominated healthcare processes for a significant period of time, but in more recent years, there has been a recognition that it is not possible, or helpful, to separate out the components of an individual's life; the biopsychosocial model incorporates the interplay of biological, psychological and social aspects of a person's life on their health.

Individuals in both industrialized and less developed cultures continue to be influenced in their health behaviours by both cultural and religious beliefs. These may relate to 'bad' behaviour, weather, accidents, black magic, witchcraft, spirits and one or more Gods, to name but a few.

Genetic and biological determinants

In line with scientific developments, current medicine is interested in the genetic basis of disease and it does seem that it may be possible to determine an origin of many health problems in the human genes. Newspapers proclaim each discovery loudly, such as the possibility of genes that predispose to alcoholism and obesity, along with many others. This may lead to the belief that all health problems develop from a genetic 'fault' and these lie beyond the control of each individual, which may legitimize poor health behaviour. In reality, the picture is more complex, with health, and conversely disease, arising from an interaction of individual genetic, psychosocial and physical factors.

The scientific interest in this field lies in interactions between genetic predisposition and psychosocial factors encountered in early childhood. For example, research has shown that genetically predisposed, spontaneously hypertensive rat pups who were fostered to normotensive mothers did not develop hypertension as they matured, suggesting that genetic predisposition can be overcome by a favourable environment in the early years.

Behavioural determinants

The major leading causes of death in Western society today – heart disease, cancer, stroke and accidents – are all associated with behavioural risk factors. The origin of many chronic diseases such as diabetes and hypertension can be found in lifestyle factors. A sedentary lifestyle predisposes an individual to develop these diseases, regardless of genetic factors. Simple changes to behaviour, such as effective weight control, stopping smoking and regular exercise, will often prevent the onset of diseases such as heart disease and diabetes. It is possible, however, that for some individuals, the

inheritance of a protective genetic profile protects them from poor health caused by poor health-related habits.

Health psychology is a branch of psychology focusing on the behavioural and mental processes that contribute to health and illness. It focuses on cognition, emotion and motivation. Cognition involves perceiving, knowing, learning, remembering, thinking, interpreting, believing and problem solving. Emotion is a subjective feeling that affects and is affected by our thoughts, beliefs and behaviour. Emotions can be positive/pleasant or negative/unpleasant. Those individuals whose emotions are more positive have reduced incidence of disease and have much faster recovery times than those whose emotions are more negative. Motivation is the driver for individuals to behave the way that they do, influences individuals adopting new health-related behaviour, and the way they choose to take their medication or otherwise. Health psychology studies the effects of interpersonal relationships on individuals; our interactions with others, their thoughts, feelings and actions which in turn influences our own thinking and behaviour.

In studying a particular situation, there can be components of cognitive, affective (emotional), behavioural and interpersonal influences and separating these may be difficult. For example, an individual experiencing anxiety in a given situation may think that they lack control (cognitive), feel fear (affective), experience physical symptoms such as sweating palms and raised heart rate (behavioural) and seek out support and reassurance from others (interpersonal).

One of the major psychological issues that affects health is stress. Stress is an increasing factor in modern lives and arises when an individual experiences a situation in which they perceive that they are not able to cope with what is being asked of them, either physically emotionally or socially. Due to the interconnection of body and mind, the mental stress causes physical responses, including the release of catecholamines and corticosteroids, which may contribute to illness with continued exposure. The cardiovascular system can be affected and the emotional response to stress can result in anxiety and depression, which in turn have been shown to reduce the effectiveness of the immune system, putting the individual at risk of other diseases.

Stress can also affect an individual's health through altered health-related behaviour. People experiencing high levels of stress often consume more alcohol, drugs and smoke more than those with less stress, and they also experience more accidents.

Stress is therefore of concern when helping individuals to improve their health, and needs to be considered when advising patients in a pharmacy, as it will be affecting their behaviour and thinking.

Environmental determinants

Environmental factors (biological, chemical, physical, mechanical) that affect human health are widely understood and have been studied in detail. External contaminants can enter the body through the air we breathe, the items we ingest, either through direct contamination on food, or indirectly through the food produced from the soil.

The role of air-borne pollen in hayfever, other allergens such as pet dander and dust mites in asthma and the risks to health from contaminated water are well understood, but there are other contaminants from the environment that need to be considered, such as drug residues in the meat and meat products we eat, that can have an effect on health from the time of conception onwards.

Environmental risk factors can affect a far greater number of people at a given time than more individual factors such as genetic susceptibility or psychological responses. While individual risk factors can account for some of the differences seen in disease occurrence, they cannot account for all. Work to reduce individuals' risk factors for a given disease has only a limited impact on the disease occurrence, and Rose (1985) suggested that the causes of individual differences in disease may be different from the causes of differences between populations. Even where there is a strong link between a risk factor and the incidence of a disease, the disease may never develop in a particular individual.

Socioeconomic determinants

Socioeconomic determinants of health are socially situated factors that influence health, or may predispose an individual or population to poor health. Each society develops its own set of health-related values, both positive and negative, and these are reflected in the media used within the society. Western society sees being fit and healthy as 'good' and this exemplifies a positive value, while individuals in the public eye seen undertaking activities such smoking cigarettes or using illegal drugs exemplify a negative value. These societal values influence individuals and the way in which they behave, but the primary influence on an individual's behaviour is often their families.

An individual's family is the closest and most constant social relationship for the majority of people. Therefore, we learn and model many of our health-related habits, behaviours and attitudes on those of our close family. The degree of support or encouragement provided by family and friends when an individual undertakes a health-related activity can be an important factor in the potential for success.

The economic situation of an individual has been shown to have a great influence on their health. In developing countries, factors such as poverty, poor nutrition and poor resistance to pathogens are all interrelated in producing poor health status for the population, and in reducing the average life expectancy. Individuals living in the more industrialized, richer countries have improved health and greater life expectancy.

In addition to the international correlation between health and socioeconomics, the relationship between socioeconomic status and ill health can also be seen across the levels of the social hierarchy within a population. Those individuals who are wealthier within a society also have better health. Health is also linked to education, and those with better education levels tend to be healthier – their increased education level may also lead to a better financial situation, and this also correlates to improved health and longevity.

The relationship between socioeconomic status and health may therefore be related more to relative deprivation rather than absolute deprivation. Having less within your own society, even where this does not mean that the individual is deprived of the basic needs for life, or health care, still has a negative impact on your health. Better lifestyle habits may partially explain these social hierarchy differences, with those of a higher socioeconomic status potentially having healthier habits than those from lower socioeconomic groups, but does not provide a full explanation for the observed differences in health.

These differences in social situations that produce an effect on health are referred to as 'health inequalities'. Health inequalities within a society are often targeted with resources and interventions in order to try and produce population-wide improvements and equality in health (see Ch. 13).

Interaction of different factors

It is evident that no single influencing factor provides an explanation for the health of a nation, demographic group or individual. The factors discussed above interlink and provide a complex picture in which to determine the defining influences on the health. In considering an individual's health and illness, it is necessary to assess the impact of all aspects of a person's life as a total entity – this approach is called 'holism'.

There are models that try to describe the interactions between factors influencing health, and one such comprehensive model is the 'nested model of health'. This model consists of two levels of activity: the individual and the community level. The individual level is composed of five different categories:

- Psychosocial environment (e.g. personal relationships, housing)
- Microphysical environment (e.g. chemicals and noise)
- Work environment (e.g. work stress)
- Behavioural environment (e.g. smoking, alcohol use, exercise)
- Ethnicity, class and gender.

These categories are thought to affect each other and to affect and be affected by the individual. The individual level is nested/located in the centre of the community level.

This community level, which is the main focus of health policy decision-makers, is composed of four components:

- The political/economic climate (e.g. unemployment level)
- The macro-physical environment (e.g. air quality)
- Social justice/equity (e.g. social security system)
- Local control/cohesiveness (e.g. local planning efforts).

These four components are interrelated and changes in them are expected to lead to changes in the health of individuals.

This model shows the potential influences on the health of an individual and provides the healthcare professional with an idea of the complexity of the influences on an individual's health status.

Process of illness

Becoming ill

As pharmacists, we need to understand how and why people respond to illness in such differing ways. Health-related behaviour varies between individuals for all the reasons discussed above, and this may help to explain the subjective way in which patients respond to seemingly similar symptoms, such as pain or discomfort. Generally, individuals perceive themselves as 'well' if they have a feeling of well-being, experience no symptoms and are able to perform normal functions. This is the baseline situation against which any changes in health are measured. As an individual's health status changes, there will be a corresponding change in their health-related behaviour.

Kasl and Cobb in 1966 defined three types of behaviour that characterize three stages in the progress of disease:

- Health behaviour, which refers to 'any activity undertaken by people believing themselves to be healthy for the purpose of preventing disease or detecting it at an asymptomatic stage'
- Illness behaviour, which involves an activity undertaken by people experiencing illness, in order to determine their state of their health and receive appropriate treatment
- Sick-role behaviour, which refers to the activity that individuals, who consider themselves ill, undertake in order to get well.

Health behaviour is undertaken to benefit health, while illness behaviour and sick-role behaviour are aimed at minimizing the effects of illness.

Identifying and reacting to symptoms

Individuals can, and do react differently to symptoms of disease. Different symptoms may be perceived very differently, depending on the person, setting and situation. A behaviour which in some situations is regarded as normal and natural, can in other situations be regarded as a sign of illness. For example, being tired after a long day at work or after an exercise session is normal, while continuous tiredness without due cause may be a sign of illness.

We all use our current and past experiences of illness, our social exposure to illness, through family and friends and societal derived values to judge our illness, and these affect our health behaviour. The significance of symptoms is judged according to the degree of interference with normal activities, the familiarity and clarity of symptoms, the person's tolerance threshold, preconceptions about cause and prognoses, and the influence of friends and family. The presence of other stressors and life crises may also make the symptoms appear more severe to the individual. These subjective and psychosocial aspects may exert a greater influence over the individual's decisions and actions than the symptoms themselves.

The way in which an individual experiences illness involves affective and cognitive reactions, resulting in emotional changes in the person as they attempt to understand the illness. Bernstein and Bernstein have described these emotional reactions to illness and treatment in the following ways:

- Those directly related to illness or treatment, including fear, anxiety and a feeling of damage and frustration caused by loss of pleasure and enjoyment
- Reactions determined primarily by life experience before or during illness, such as anger, dependency and guilt
- Complications such as depression and loss of self-esteem.

These three emotional responses interact to produce the overall response in an individual and produce complex and varied reactions to illness.

In general, women are more likely to interpret discomfort as a medical symptom and they also recall and report more symptoms when consulting a healthcare professional. These differences may partly be explained by a higher interest in and concern with health issues among women.

An individual's family often plays an active role in the symptom identification process, as other family members may recognize some symptoms before the person does. The family also takes part in the interpretation process of symptoms.

The individual's cultural background is also an important factor influencing the process of symptom identification and evaluation. Some cultures more readily describe common symptoms as medical, while others tend to suppress signs of illness. There might also be differences between generations in this respect, in so much as symptoms previously considered as normal may today be seen as something requiring medical attention.

Sick-role behaviour

When people perceive themselves to be sick, they adopt the so-called 'sick-role behaviour'; a socially determined role. This includes the following components:

- The patient is not blamed for being sick
- The patient is exempt from work and other responsibilities
- The illness is seen as legitimate as long as the patient accepts that being ill is undesirable
- The patient is expected to seek competent help to get well again.

Not all people follow the patterns of the sick role but it does provide a general framework to help understanding illness behaviour. However, this framework is not able to explain variations within illness behaviour; it is not applicable to chronic disease, where getting better may not be realistic and often does not apply to mental illness. In addition, there may be certain diseases, such as alcoholism, where there might be unwillingness within society to grant exemptions from blame.

The role of personality in illness

Aspects of an individual's personality have been shown to be associated with illness and poor health. People who have high levels of anxiety, depression and anger/hostility traits seem to be more disease prone than others. Emotions, such as anxiety and depression may be a reaction to different types of stress. People handle stressful situations in different ways and an individual's approach to stress affects the impact of stress on their health. People who approach stressful situations more positively and hopefully, are less disease prone and also tend to recover in a shorter time if they get ill. Those who are ill will recover faster if they can overcome their negative thoughts and feelings.

Friedman and Rosenman in 1974 described differences in behavioural and emotional style, and their effects on health, when studying the behaviour of cardiac patients. They named the behaviour patterns they saw as 'Type A' and 'Type B'.

Type A behaviour pattern is characterized by:

- A competitive achievement orientation, with high levels of self-criticism and striving towards goals while not experiencing a sense of joy in achievements
- Time urgency, e.g. tight scheduling of commitments, impatience with time delays and unproductive time
- Anger/hostility which is easily aroused. Type A individuals respond faster and with more emotion to stress, often seeing stressors as threats to their personal control – this behaviour seems to be particularly detrimental to health.

The Type A pattern may also increase the person's probability of getting into stressful situations. The relationship between Type A behaviour and psychosocial factors is very complex. Type B individuals take life more easily with little competitiveness, time urgency and hostility.

Interestingly, the overall evidence for an association between Type A and Type B behaviour and general illnesses is weak and inconsistent. However, many studies, have shown a clear association between Type A behaviour and coronary heart disease.

Health knowledge, beliefs and attitudes

The concept of health knowledge may include a variety of components such as beliefs, expectations, norms and cognitive perceptions. Health knowledge is therefore more than merely having some factual knowledge about diseases and treatment.

Knowledge about a disease can improve a patient's health by improving their problem-solving capacity. Preventive behaviours, participation in the treatment process and taking medications all require a certain amount of knowledge. The current trend emphasizing guided self-care in chronic diseases such as asthma, diabetes and hypertension, requires a well-informed patient. The aim is to produce patients who actively participate in their own treatment. The starting point is providing the necessary information and improving the factual knowledge of the patient. It has been shown, however, that knowledge alone is insufficient to ensure behaviour change, which is often the goal.

In addition to improving patients' knowledge, there also needs to be a change in attitude in order for them to undertake new health-related behaviours.

Attitudes have been defined as states of readiness or predisposition, feelings for or against something, which predisposes to particular responses. They involve emotions (feelings) and knowledge (or beliefs) about the object and result in behaviour changes. Attitudes are not inherited but learned and, though relatively stable, are modifiable by education.

There are a number of models that have been suggested to explain the interaction between knowledge, beliefs, attitudes and behaviour in health:

The health belief model

The health belief model, developed by Rosenstock and colleagues in 1966, to predict the use of preventive health services, has been extensively used during the last two decades to try to explain various health behaviours. The model has been further developed to predict health behaviour in chronic diseases and compliance with healthcare regimens.

According to the model, the probability that a person will take a preventive health action – that is, perform some health, illness or sick-role behaviour – is a function of:

- Their perception of their own susceptibility to the health problem or disease (How likely am I to get it?)
- Their perception of the severity of medical and social consequences of the disease (How ill would it make me?)
- Their perception of the benefits and barriers (costs) related to the recommended behaviour (What will I gain and what will it cost me?).

All three of these aspects are based on subjective perceptions which can be modified, at least in theory.

According to the model, the more vulnerable the person feels and the more serious the disease the more likely it is the person will act. Various factors that result from the perceptions are expected to modify this motivating force. These factors include demographic, socioeconomic and therapy-related factors as well as the illness itself and the prescribed regimen. Prior contact with the disease or knowledge about the disease may modify the behaviour. Some incidents, so-called 'cues to action', are also expected to trigger the desired behaviour. These cues to action might include a mass media campaign, magazine article, advice from others or illness of a family member.

The concept of perception is important in the health-belief model. It is the patient's and not the pharmacist's perceptions that drive the decisions and behaviours of the patient. Once an individual has been diagnosed with an illness then their concept of personal susceptibility has been modified because they know they have an illness. Studies into health belief try to overcome these issues by examining the individual's estimate of or belief in the accuracy of the diagnosis. This concept has also been extended to measuring the individual's subjective feelings of vulnerability to various other diseases or to illness in general. Studies show that in hypertension, for example, the threat posed by hypertension and the perceived effectiveness of treatment in reducing this threat are important predictors of compliance. Likewise the perceived control over one's own health is important. There is some controversy about the chronology of these beliefs and whether they precede or develop simultaneously with health behaviour.

The health belief model and common sense might tell us that the patient's decision to seek health care, accept a diagnosis and engage in health-related behaviours would be related to the seriousness of the disease. Research indicates this may not always be the case. Patients' health behaviours are a function of many psychosocial variables. (Reasons why humans may behave illogically are dealt with below in 'The conflict theory' and 'Decision analysis and behavioural decision theory').

The theory of planned behaviour

The theory of planned behaviour offers an explanation of the factors that help to determine an individual's health-related behaviour. The actions of each individual are determined by their intention to perform, or not, any particular action; and their intention is determined by both personal and social influences. Two personal influences exert an effect on an individual's intentions. The first is 'attitudinal considerations', which are related to the individual's beliefs in the positive or negative effects of their behaviour, i.e. will it make me better or not? The second is the individual's perception of the ease or difficulty of performing the action, their 'perceived behavioural control'. The social influences, or 'subjective norm' relates to the pressure from the society in which they are present to undertake the behaviours or otherwise.

The pressure exerted by the normative beliefs acts independently of the individual's personal beliefs, and so may be in opposition to them. So in the case of individuals contemplating changing their behaviour, their own opinions on the new behaviour, and the illness it may avoid, will exert an influence over the chances of them undertaking the new behaviour, as will their perception of the difficulty or ease of doing this new activity or acting in a new way. They will also be affected by how their friends, family and society see the new behaviour; if positive and a good idea, then the individual is more likely to undertake it, while if they get negative comments these may justify not undertaking the new behaviour. In a situation where there is a conflict between the attitudinal considerations on one side, and the perceived behavioural control and subjective norms on the other, the action itself helps to determine which takes precedence in determining action or non-action.

The theory of planned behaviour proposes that the subjective norm and the attitude regarding the behaviour combine to produce an intention, which leads to the behaviour.

If behaviour is determined by beliefs, then what factors determine beliefs? Factors such as age, sex, education, social class, culture and personality traits all influence an individual's beliefs. These variables influence behaviour indirectly rather than directly. One of the problems with the theory is that people do not always do what they plan, i.e. intentions and behaviour are only moderately related. Another problem is that people do not always act rationally. Irrational decisions such as delaying medical treatment when symptoms exist cannot be explained by the model. Neither does the model include prior experiences with the behaviour, which might be an important factor to consider, since past behaviour is a strong predictor of future practice of that behaviour.

The conflict theory

The conflict theory has been used to explain rational and irrational decision-making. According to the model how a person arrives at a health-related decision involves five stages. It starts when something challenges the person's current course of action. It can be a threat (e.g. symptom) or a mass media alert about, for example, the danger of narcotics or an opportunity (e.g. free membership to a health club). The different stages of the conflict theory model are:

- Assessing the challenge, i.e. whether the risk is serious enough. The assessment may involve thoughts such as the risk is not real, it is irrelevant or inapplicable. If the risk is not considered serious enough, the behaviour continues as before and the decision-making process stops
- Assessing alternatives, i.e. the search for alternatives for dealing with the risk starts when the risk is acknowledged. This stage ends when the suitability of available alternatives has been surveyed
- Weighing alternatives, i.e. the pros and cons of each alternative are weighed to find the best option
- Making a final choice and committing to it
- Adhering despite negative feedback, i.e. after starting a new behaviour people may have second thoughts about it if the environment is not supportive or it gives negative feedback.

The decision process can be aborted at any point. Errors in decision-making are often caused by stress, which affects health, information overload, group pressure and other factors. According to the conflict theory, a person's coping with a conflict is dependent on the presence and absence of risks, hope and adequate time. Different combinations of these may result in different types of behavioural response. For example, when there are perceptions of high risk in changing the behaviour and no hope in finding a better alternative, a high level of stress is experienced. Denial and shifting responsibility to someone else are typical responses, with delays in seeking care. The perception of serious risk and belief in a better alternative, but also a perception of running out of time, also create high levels of stress. People search desperately for solutions and may choose an alternative hastily if promised immediate relief. The perception of serious risk, with a belief that a better alternative will become available, along with time to search for it, results in low levels of stress and more rational choices.

Locus of control

It has been claimed that individuals' perception of their ability to influence disease and their treatment is an important determinant of health behaviour. People have been categorized into two groups: those with an internal locus of control and those with an external locus of control. The former tend to perceive that they are in control of their own health by their actions and behaviour, while the latter consider that health is externally determined and their actions have little or no effect. Therefore those with a strongly internal locus of control should tend to practise behaviours that prevent illness and promote health. Research has shown that this is the case, but the relationship is not very strong. This locus of control is just one factor among many others that determine health behaviour. Belief in internal control is likely to have a greater impact among people who place a higher value on their health than among those who do not.

Self-efficacy and social learning

Sometimes performing a health action is hard to do because it is technically difficult or it may involve several steps. Therefore the belief in the success in doing something – called self-efficacy – may be an important determinant in choosing or not choosing to change behaviour. People develop a sense of efficacy through their successes and failures, observations of others' experiences and assessments of their abilities by others. People assess their efficacy based on the effort that is required, complexity of the task and situational factors, e.g. the possibility of receiving help if needed. People who think they are not able to quit smoking will not even try, while people who believe they can succeed will try and eventually some may succeed.

Those with a strong sense of self-efficacy show less psychological strain in response to stressors than those with a weak sense of efficacy. People differ in the degree to which they believe they have control over the things that happen in their lives. Those who experience prolonged, high levels of stress and lack a sense of personal control tend to feel helpless. Having a strong sense of control seems to benefit health and adjustment to sickness.

As environmental factors and expectations directed towards the individuals change, they must either intensify their activities or change their environment. Individuals have different capabilities of coping and different coping strategies. According to the Social Learning Theory, people change their environment with the help of symbols they choose in accordance with their values, norms and goals. On the other hand, the environment changes the individual's behaviour by rewarding beneficial activities and punishing or not rewarding activities that harm the environment. Through the socialization process the individual adopts the values and norms of the community, is socialized as its member and gains identity. Through this process the individual has learned to act efficiently in social systems.

Antonowsky has used the 'sense of coherence' concept, which is an extensive and constant feeling of an individual's internal and external environment being in harmony with each other. Every individual has characteristic psychosocial potentials that include material resources, intelligence, knowledge, coping strategies, social support, arts, religion, philosophy and health behaviour. Antonowsky calls a sense of coherence 'salutogenic' or health generating. Disease–health is a continuum, at one end of which is a high degree of coherence and health ('ease') and at the other end a low degree of coherence and illness ('dis-ease'). External factors that the individual considers threatening mobilize the defence mechanisms and cause stress conditions in the individual. Prolonged stress is disease generating and causes the condition 'dis-ease'.

Coping

Because of the emotional and physical strain that accompanies it, stress is uncomfortable and people are motivated to do things that reduce their stress. The concept of coping is used to describe how people adjust to stressful situations in their life. Coping is the process by which people try to manage the perceived discrepancy between the demands and resources they appraise in stressful situations. Coping means the ability to meet the demands of new situations and solve the problems with which one is confronted. Coping is determined by situational and personal determinants. At the individual level, external factors turn into stress factors if previous experiences together with personality traits, consciously or unconsciously, are considered as threatening or diminish self-esteem. Coping efforts can be quite varied and do not necessarily lead to a solution of the problem. It can help the person to alter his perception of a discrepancy, tolerate or accept the harm or threat and escape or avoid the situation.

Coping mechanisms

Coping can alter the problem or it can regulate the emotional response causing the stress reaction to the problem. Behavioural approaches include using alcohol or drugs, seeking social support from friends or simply watching TV. Cognitive approaches involve how people think about the stressful situation, e.g. changing the meaning of the situation. Emotion-focused approaches are used when people think they cannot do anything to change the stressful situation. Problem-focused coping is used to reduce the demands of the stressful situation or to expand the capacity and resources to deal with it. The two types of coping can also be used together. Commonly used methods of coping are:

- The direct method, i.e. doing something specifically and directly to cope with a stressor, e.g. negotiating, consulting, arguing, running away
- Seeking information and acquiring knowledge about the stressful situation
- Turning to others, i.e. seeking help, reassurance and comfort from family and friends
- Resigned acceptance, i.e. the person comes to terms with the situation and accepts it
- Emotional discharge, i.e. expressing feelings or reducing tension by taking, e.g. alcohol, drugs or smoking cigarettes
- Intrapsychic processes, i.e. cognitive redefinition, e.g. the 'things could be worse' attitude.

Decision analysis and behavioural decision theory

Decision analysis is a systematic way of studying the process of decision-making among patients and healthcare professionals. It is a widely used tool in pharmacoeconomics today (see Ch. 22) and usually involves assigning numbers to perceived values of therapeutic outcomes and the probability that the outcome will occur. This gives a utility of each outcome and the one with the highest utility would be chosen. One problem is that humans do not always make decisions logically or treat information as value free.

Why don't humans behave logically? One explanation that has been offered is that humans are biased when making decisions under uncertainty because we fail to appreciate randomness. We believe that there are known causes and effects for all phenomena and we have a need to be able to explain outcomes. It is easier to explain, even incorrectly, than to have to deal with uncertain situations. People also tend to be inconsistent in their judgement, often because of difficulties in remembering how a judgement was made. Another reason is that we seldom receive feedback from negative decisions, for example if we decide not to take the medicine, we do not know how effective it would have been.

Behaviour decision theory has been used to understand how patients make decisions about their medicine and health-related behaviour. These include acquisition of information, information processing, making decisions under uncertainty and interpreting outcomes of that decision. It has been found that patients are more likely to take a health risk to avoid an aversive situation than to gain a positive health outcome. Patients are more likely to choose a certain outcome than an outcome with a high probability of occurrence, even if the certain outcome is less valued than that one with a high probability of occurrence. When a person has already invested time and money on a product or activity, they are likely to continue it, even if it does not appear to be effective.

Hogarth has described different biases that influence decision-making, which may be helpful in understanding patient choices about health behaviour. Individuals tend to believe more in well-publicized events than in those that are less publicized – think about the consumer's choice of well-advertised OTC medicines rather than the cheaper generic alternatives. There is a tendency to selective perception, i.e. we believe what matches our existing beliefs and this has direct implications for health education in pharmacies. We tend to believe real incidents more than abstract statistics. Positive experiences from a family member quitting smoking is more likely to be effective than showing statistics about future (uncertain) consequences of smoking. Two incidents occurring close in time and place tend to be regarded as causal. Becoming ill after having taken a medicine, regardless of cause and effect, often triggers an aversive response with the same medicine in future. We are reluctant to change our beliefs, even when given new data. Very few instances of an occurrence are needed for us to form a new belief if it has a strong effect upon us and this has implications for an individual experiencing side-effects from drugs. We also believe something is more likely to happen if we want it to happen. A decision that was successful is more likely to be considered to be due to the knowledge and wisdom of the decision maker. On the other hand, a decision resulting in bad outcomes is likely to be blamed on others.

Theory into practice – the process of behaviour change

A lot of pharmacists' activities will focus on changing the behaviour of patients. Without going into the ethical aspects of behaviour change, we will concentrate on the process of change. It has been proved several times that merely using common sense is not enough to reach permanent behaviour change. Using a common-sense approach would assume that, given the facts, people will be able to change their behaviour in a direction anticipated by the healthcare professional. A simple example illustrates the limits of this approach – why do so many people still smoke cigarettes despite knowing all the negative consequences of smoking?

Even if many of the behavioural theories are far from complete or comprehensive, they may guide us in improving the outcome of behavioural interventions. Behaviour change includes a long list of steps that need to be taken before it is finalized:

- The process starts with *attention*. The person needs to be exposed to the message; via a counselling session by the pharmacist or a health campaign in the media. If the same message is repeated from different sources and these sources are regarded as credible, the likelihood of change grows. Therefore it is important that the information received from all healthcare professionals is congruent. If patients receive mixed messages they are more likely to ignore them
- Attention is followed by *motivation*. The person must feel motivated to change their behaviour. It is well known that immediate rewards are more motivating than anticipated rewards after several years
- Next the person has to *comprehend* the message to be able to act upon it, but they also need to learn some facts, i.e. improve their knowledge base. These facts need to be simple and match the local culture
- The following step is *persuasion*, i.e. the person needs to 'change their attitude'. Furthermore, they might need to learn some new techniques and skills in how to take or handle the medication. Demonstration and guided practice are the best ways of handling this step
- The person must also be able to *perform* the skills and *maintain* the learned skills, which

include self-efficacy training and feedback of success. Many experiments with a long enough follow-up show that positive results can be achieved with pharmacists' interventions, but when the experiment is over, the results soon deteriorate to pre-experiment levels

- *Continuous reinforcement* is necessary to maintain good results in any intervention, be it changing medicine-taking behaviour or modification of preventive health behaviour.

Pharmacists can help individuals change their health-related behaviour by providing information, advice and support as appropriate to each of the stages the individual will pass through. Pharmacist involvement in smoking cessation and weight loss has shown that the pharmacist can play an important role in helping individuals to live healthier lives.

The treatment process

Self- and lay-care

During the latter part of the twentieth century, a new trend emphasizing the role of the individual and patient in their own health care emerged as a part of a more general trend called 'consumerism'. People have become more committed to taking control of their own lives and assessing the impact of their behaviour on their health, resulting in various self-care and self-help movements. The same trend has been obvious internationally, although the starting time and speed of adoption has varied. At the same time, the dominant role of health-care professionals has diminished. Patients are asking more questions, seeking more information and taking a more active role in their health care. They have greater knowledge about their own disease and potential treatments.

These changes put increasing demands on pharmacists regarding their knowledge base, especially in therapeutics, and it also tests their communication skills. The priorities in treatment and the goals may differ between the patient and the prescribing professional and requires careful negotiation.

According to the self-care philosophy, people should be given more responsibility for their own health. One way this can be achieved is to emphasize the role of self-care in treating minor ailments using home remedies and an increasing number of self-medication products.

The most common 'action' in response to a perceived health problem has been to ignore the problem or wait for a few days. It is estimated that some 30–40% of health problems are dealt with in this way. Of those who take some action, 75–80% self-diagnose and use self-treatment, while only 20–25% seek professional care. Therefore a seemingly small change in this ratio (towards using more professional care) has a substantial impact and burden on the official healthcare system. Of those who use self-treatment, some 70–90% self-medicate, and of these, 80% use OTC drugs. Home remedies such as lemon, honey and garlic as well as different herbal products, vitamins and minerals, are widely used all over the world.

Before people decide to seek medical care for their symptoms, they seek advice from friends, relatives and co-workers. This lay referral network provides information and interpretation regarding the symptoms, home remedies, self-medication and gives advice on the need for professional help or consulting another 'lay expert' who may have had a similar problem.

The pharmacy is often the first place for people to seek help within the healthcare system due to its accessibility. The pharmacist can help distinguish between serious and non-serious symptoms and can refer on to other healthcare professions if needed. Certain situations may demand professional care without further delay caused by inappropriate self-medication practices. The lay referral network can in some cases be guilty of causing delay in seeking care. This treatment delay has been divided into three stages:

- Appraisal delay is the time it takes to interpret a symptom as a part of an illness. If friends and relatives do not see the symptoms as important, then the individual may delay seeking help
- Illness delay is the time between recognizing the illness and the decision to seek care
- Utilization delay is the time between the decision to seek care and actually using a health service.

There has also been concern about misuse of over-the-counter (OTC) drugs, including laxatives and codeine-containing pain relief. However, there is also a cost-saving in the reduced reliance on healthcare professionals. Pharmacists can help the public to become aware of the potential dangers of OTC medications, and can provide guidance on their safe and appropriate use.

Primary care

Simultaneously with emerging self-care, the concept of primary health care was introduced. In 1977, the World Health Assembly of the WHO adopted the concept of Health for All by the year 2000 and this concept was translated into the so-called 'Alma Ata Declaration'. The focus was on making health care more accessible and lowering healthcare costs leading to an improvement in quality of life for the whole population. According to the declaration, primary health care should include:

- Education about prevailing health problems
- Methods of identifying, preventing and controlling them
- Promotion of food supply and proper nutrition
- Adequate water supply and basic sanitation
- Maternal and child health care including family planning
- Immunization against the major infectious diseases
- Prevention and control of locally endemic diseases
- Appropriate treatment of common diseases and injuries
- Promotion of mental health
- Provision of essential drugs.

Primary health care focuses on principal health problems and must be part of national health policy and planning. The conference called for cooperation and commitment in striving for an acceptable level of health for all people by the year 2000. In 2003, the WHO undertook a review of the progress in achieving an improved health status for the world population. They found that there was an international commitment, across most governments, to primary health care and the Alma Ata goal. In countries where the development had not been successful, there was usually a lack of practical guidance on implementation, poor leadership to help achieve the change, insufficient political commitment, inadequate resources and unrealistic expectations of what could be achieved in a given timeframe.

The scope of public health is population based rather than individually based. Public health problems are considered in the context of the community. It is a public health problem to determine the prevalence of a disease in the community, compare that with figures from previous years and plan health services to reduce the prevalence. Public health includes enumeration, analysing and planning, as well as identifying the specific actions to be taken. Public health exists on two levels: the micro-level, for example performing some public health function such as immunization or preventing inappropriate use of illicit drugs, and the macro-level, with activities like planning or policy formulation (see Ch. 13).

Factors influencing the use of healthcare services

The structures of the healthcare systems in different countries have a lot of similarities but also a lot of differences. The system is the sum of historical development, culture and economic factors. In some countries, there are actually several different systems in place within the healthcare system. The country you happen to live in, the organization and financing of health care, the environment of medical care, social and cultural factors all influence the care that you will receive.

Demographic factors

Several important differences have been reported between different age groups and between genders. It is well known that women report more symptoms and are more likely to seek care. Men are more hesitant than women to admit to having symptoms and to seek medical care for these symptoms. This can be a result of perceived sex-role stereotypes – men should be tough and independent and ignore or endure pain. Women use physician services more than men in all age groups except for the first few years of life. Men have a higher mortality and shorter life expectancy at all ages.

In general, young children and the elderly use physician services more often than adolescents and young adults. Age differences in health behaviour cannot be explained by biological ageing alone. Elderly people have different views from other age groups and each other on health and illness, symptoms, healthcare use and drugs. Certain ideas are more prevalent among the elderly than the young. The differences can partly be explained by so-called cohort effects, meaning people of the same age have been exposed to the same kind of experiences and attitudes in society and therefore are also likely to share certain behavioural characteristics.

Cultural and socioeconomic factors

Ethnic and cultural background may explain some differences in symptom experience, how people seek medical care and how they take their medicines. A classic 1950's study about how people deal with pain found big differences between Italian, Jewish, Irish and Yankee (Old American) hospitalized patients. Italian and Jewish patients were more likely to respond emotionally and expressively to pain than Irish or Yankee patients, who tended to deny pain. Italian and Jewish patients showed their pain by crying, complaining and demanding, while the Irish and Yankee patients preferred to hide their pain and withdraw from others. More recent studies among immigrants in the USA found that the differences in willingness to tolerate pain diminish in succeeding generations. Other similar studies have shown cultural differences among European countries and the USA, e.g. in perception of fever and the need to medicate children with a fever.

There are also differences in seeking care according to social class, education and income – those who are better off access more healthcare services. Different models of why people seek or do not seek healthcare services have been proposed, but no one model appears to offer a full explanation of this aspect of people's behaviour.

Social support

Social environments and networks are important in the growth, development and health of individuals. Social support is an important factor in all phases of an illness and in the treatment process. Social support relates directly to the general and universal needs of people. Maslow's theory claims that, human needs are hierarchical, starting with basic physiological needs, followed by safety needs, belongingness and love needs, esteem needs, and finishing with the highest – self-actualization. Needs occupying the lower levels of the hierarchy need to be met before the individual will concern themselves with needs at a higher level. According to the Finnish sociologist, Erik Allardt, people's needs can be simplified to include standard of living ('having'), social relations ('loving') and forms of self-actualization ('being'). Social relations include social networks and belonging to them is the basis of one's identity and social existence. Social support is the term used for different forms of emotional and material support. The nature of social support is reciprocal. It can be support provided directly by one person to another or indirectly through the system or community.

Forms and levels of social support

- *Material or instrumental support* includes money, goods, auxiliary appliances and medicine
- *Operational support* includes service, transportation and rehabilitation
- *Informational support* includes advice, directions, feedback, education and training
- *Emotional support* involves the expression of caring, empathy, love and encouragement
- *Mental support* involves a common ideology, belief and philosophy.

Social support has two dimensions, a qualitative and a quantitative dimension and the quality of social support can be measured only by subjective assessments. When providing material support the quantitative aspect is more prominent (medicines are an exception to this); in the other support forms the qualitative aspect (including timing) is more important than the quantitative aspect. Thus a small functioning support network is better than a broad but passive one.

Social support has been divided into three levels based on the intimacy of the social relationships;

- Primary level includes family and close friends
- Secondary level includes friends, colleagues and neighbours
- Tertiary level includes acquaintances, authorities, public and private services.

Social support can be provided by a lay person (usually on the primary and secondary level) or a professional (usually on the tertiary level). Recently, different organizations have started training courses for lay providers of support aiming at strengthening the second level of support. Social support has both direct effects on health and well-being and indirect stress-buffering effects on coping in stressful situations.

Early research showed that lack of social support exposes people to recurrent accidents, suicide and risk of catching tuberculosis. Later the emphasis was on relationships between social support structures and health in communities. It was shown that the lack of social support increases the incidence of coronary heart disease, mortality due to myocardial infarction and total mortality in the population. It has also been shown that social support is important in perceived health and in reducing hypertension. Social support has a positive effect on physical, social and emotional recovery. It reduces the need for medication and speeds up symptom amelioration.

However, having too much support may make the patient passive, create dependence and reduce self-confidence and self-esteem. Social support needs to empower the individual and not remove all control to exert a positive effect on health.

KEY POINTS

- Social and behavioural issues can help explain non-biological aspects of health
- Illness is a person's reaction to a perceived alteration of body or mind, while disease is something which is professionally defined
- Health has been defined by the WHO
- Apart from biophysical factors, health is also affected by behavioural, environmental and socioeconomic determinants
- People react differently to symptoms as a consequence of many factors, including family, gender and age
- Certain behaviour types put the individual at increased risk of disease

- Knowledge influences an individual's response to illness
- According to the Health Belief Model, the patient's perception is of primary importance in determining patient behaviour
- The Theory of Planned Behaviour suggests that beliefs give rise to attitudes, which form intentions which lead to behaviour
- The Conflict Theory can be used to explain rational and irrational decision-making
- Humans may not reach decisions logically for many reasons
- Behaviour is seldom changed as a result of providing facts, but results from a series of stages of change
- The self-care philosophy encourages patients to be responsible for their own health and this opens up opportunities for pharmacists to influence health
- The 1978 Alma Ata Declaration defines the content of primary care which should be universally accessible
- Demographic, cultural and socioeconomic factors influence the use of health services
- Social support networks occur at different levels and all are important for the health of individuals

Socio-behavioural aspects of treatment with medicines

3

Alison Gifford

STUDY POINTS

- Functions of medicines
- Societal perspectives on rational use of medicines
- Factors affecting the treatment process with medicines
- Sociological and behavioural aspects of use and prescribing of medicines
- A sociological perspective of pharmacy and the pharmacy profession
- Measuring outcomes

Introduction

In attempting to understand the social and psychological aspects of treatment with medicines, we can to some extent apply the theoretical models for illness behaviour (see Ch. 2 and Fig. 3.1). The treatment process may be viewed from a macro- and a micro-perspective. The macro-perspective includes an analysis of the different systems and structural components in place to ensure a rational use of medicines, which is one of the primary goals of the system. The micro-perspective includes patient-related issues and the interaction between the patient and the healthcare professional.

When explaining patients' medicine-taking behaviour and the interaction with the environment we can, for example, use the social learning theory and the concept of self-efficacy. The health belief model has been used to explain patients' adherence in taking medicines. In addition, we need to understand the behaviour of the healthcare professional during the patient consultation and when prescribing medicines, and the interactions between healthcare professionals. Different models and theories provide different perspectives on the use of medicines, and the adequacy of the theory often depends on the question being addressed.

Functions of medicines

It has been proposed that medicines and the use of medicines serve important latent functions for the individual and society. In this context, it is important to have a wide definition of the word 'medicines'. The functions may be the same as the approved medical uses or may have hidden functions. Barber, and later Svarstad, identified a long list of medicine functions:

- Therapeutic function – the conventional use of medicines to prevent, treat and cure disease
- Placebo function – to show concern for, and to satisfy the patient

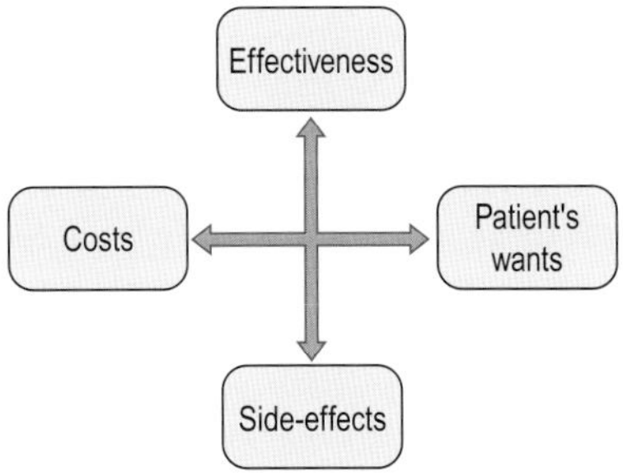

Figure 3.1 • The factors which must be balanced in treating patients.

- Coping function – to relieve feelings of failure, stress, grief, sadness, loneliness
- Self-regulatory function – to exercise control over disorder or life
- Social control function – to manage behaviour of demanding or disruptive patients, hyperactive children
- Recreational function – to relax, enjoy the company of others, experience pleasurable feelings
- Religious function – to seek religious meaning or experience
- Cosmetic function – to beautify skin, hair and body
- Appetitive function – to allay hunger or control the desire for food
- Instrumental function – to improve academic, athletic or work performance
- Sexual function – to increase sexual ability
- Fertility function – to control fertility
- Research function – to gain knowledge and understanding of human behaviour
- Diagnostic function – to help make a diagnosis
- Status-conferring function – to gain social status, prestige, income.

One medicine may fulfil one or more functions for an individual.

A societal perspective on the rational use of medicines

Defining rational use

The rational use of medicines has been defined as the safe, effective, appropriate and economic use of medicines. This definition seems to be clear and straightforward, but the definition of safe, effective and the other components needs consideration. Safety relates to aspects like relative and absolute safety. All medicines have side-effects, some less and some more, such that they may be viewed as more or less safe. Safety has to be assessed from many different angles, e.g. the severity of the disease, the available treatment options including medicines and other options, long or short-term treatment, whether the medicine is to cure or control symptoms, and over-dosage risks.

Effectiveness relates to the question of how well the medicine works in daily practice when used by unselected populations and patients having co-morbidities and other medications. Efficacy relates to the maximum effect of the medicine in a particular disease, particularly when it is optimally used in selected patients with as few confounding factors as possible, such as co-morbidities and other medicines used simultaneously.

Appropriateness refers to how a medicine is being prescribed and used in and by patients, including aspects such as appropriate indication, with no contraindications, appropriate dosage and administration. Duration of treatment should be optimal and the medicine should be correctly dispensed with appropriate and sufficient information and counselling (see Ch. 25). To achieve the intended effects, the medicine also needs to be correctly used by the patient.

The economic aspect refers to a cost-effectiveness approach which needs to be applied, where all factors are assessed (see Ch. 22). A somewhat more expensive medicine may be preferable to a less expensive medicine, for example, because it has better treatment outcomes or fewer side-effects. Additionally, hidden costs, such as a need for more extensive laboratory tests, may increase the total cost of a particular treatment.

National medicines policy (NMP)

The rational use of medicines requires that appropriate and effective structures and processes are in place. The starting point and frame of reference is the NMP, which, particularly in developing countries, defines the policies and key issues that need consideration and the policies relating to medicines and their usage. More developed countries often already have many key issues and policies regarding medicines and their rational use already in place and therefore, the NMP receives little attention. However, the global pressure on healthcare funding, especially the increasing medicines budget, has created the momentum to look more closely at medicine policies in industrialized countries too. When trying to understand the general principles that can be applied to all countries it is helpful to use the guidelines that have been proposed for developing countries, and from there, to understand how the system works and what might be the strong and weak points in each particular country.

The NMP can be seen as a guide for action, including the goals and priorities set by the government, and their main strategies and approaches. It also serves as a framework in the coordination of different activities. Depending on cultural, historical and socioeconomic factors there are differences in objectives, strategies and approaches between countries, but some common components can be identified. The goals for an NMP can be divided into:

- Health-related goals, which entail making essential medicines available, ensuring the safety, efficacy and quality of medicines, and promoting rational prescribing, dispensing and use of medicines
- Economic goals, which may include lowering the cost of medicines and providing jobs in the pharmaceutical sector
- National development goals, which may include increasing the skills of personnel in pharmacy, medicine, etc. and encouraging industrial activities in the manufacturing of medicines.

Ensuring the safety of medicines

Why is it important to regulate and control the medicine sector with special laws and regulations? The medicine sector is of concern to the whole population. Most citizens will use medicines and related services on a regular basis and therefore the functioning of the sector is of common interest. There are many parties involved – patients, healthcare providers, manufacturers and sales people – requiring detailed rules for interaction and functioning. The consequences from the lack of medicines or their misuse might be serious.

Legislation and regulation include different health-related laws, pharmacy law, trademark and patent laws, criminal law, international treaties (e.g. on narcotic and psychotropic drugs) and governmental decrees. Sometimes there may be a lack of political will or a weak infrastructure to enforce the laws. When looking at the legal situation in the medicine sector in different countries, the problems seem to be more often in the enforcement of legislation than in the lack of legislation.

Registration of medicines is a key tool in assuring the safety, quality and efficacy of a new medicine being introduced on to the market and in defining the legal status of the medicinal product. The infrastructure that will assure quality, safety and efficacy involves the licensing and inspection of manufacturers, distributors and their premises, and setting professional working standards. There is wide international cooperation in this field among the different component authorities. Nevertheless, every now and then the media have reports about counterfeit products and toxic products sold to the public, sometimes with disastrous consequences (see Chs 22 and 51).

Ensuring the availability of medicines

Medicines' availability is one of the key requirements in a well-functioning pharmaceutical system. This includes a functioning manufacturing and importation system of medicines, and good procurement and distribution practices. These functions are often taken for granted in industrialized countries, while in developing countries they are key issues for a functioning system. In developing countries the maintenance of a constant supply of medicines, keeping them in good condition and minimizing losses due to spoilage and expiry are issues that need to be solved to assure the availability of medicines to the population.

As medicines increase in sophistication, the prices increase, and many new products are too expensive for much of the population if no mechanisms like price control or reimbursement/insurance systems are in place in the country. Economic availability of medicines continues to be a major policy issue for all countries at the present time.

Use of medicines

Medicine (drug) use or utilization studies and pharmacoepidemiological studies have aimed to describe the users of medicines and quantify their usage. On a population, or macro-level, factors influencing medicine consumption include among others: size of population, age and gender distributions, occupational structure, income levels, availability of health services, number and type of health facilities and personnel, along with social insurance and reimbursement mechanisms.

Medicine use studies have been used to identify 'irrational medicine use', such as the overuse of psychotropics and antibiotics, where there has been inappropriate prescribing and unnecessary extended treatment periods. There has also been interest in the 'underuse' of medicines for major chronic diseases such as hypertension, diabetes and hypercholesterolaemia. Underuse of medicines, together with misuse, whether deliberate or unintentional, has been one of the main focuses of patient adherence studies. From these studies we know something about the use of medicines and the clinical, social and economic consequences.

The use of medicines should be seen within the context of a society, community, family and individual, recognizing cultural diversity in concepts of health and illness or how medicines work. To try and understand the medicine-related behaviour of patients, qualitative research methods such as in-depth interviews have been used. These studies have focused on people's thoughts about their medicines, their motivation to take or not take the medicine, their attitudes and beliefs about the medicines and their experiences of treatments. Some general consumer behaviour models have been used to explain non-prescription and prescription purchases. In one American study the medicine attributes that consumers rated as important included possible side-effects, physician recommendation, strength, prior use, price and the availability of generic versions. Medicines are not ordinary goods and consumers appear to understand this. According to one purchase theory, purchase motivations can also be characterized as being either transformational (positive) or informational (negative). Positive purchases are made to enhance or generate a positive situation or state of mind (e.g. clothes, music) and negative purchases to minimize or prevent negative situations (e.g. car service). Negative purchases are based on (rational) choices like perceived benefits and convenience (and therefore require more information), while positive purchases are more emotional and based on subjective appeal and positive shopping experience. Research has shown that OTC medicines and vitamins are neutral on the positive–negative dimension and oral contraceptives highly negative. This type of research is still not very well developed within the pharmaceutical field.

Like general illness behaviour, medicine use occurs in a social context. Choosing self-medication or consulting a healthcare professional to obtain prescription medicines is not based solely on symptoms or clinical aspects. The concept of 'social knowledge' has been used to describe collective understanding, arising in a group or population, which is based on available information and prior experiences. Family members, friends, work colleagues and their experiences, books and the media in addition to our own experiences, form the basis of social knowledge of medicines. Montagne in 1996 described some interesting social conceptions or fundamental principles about medicines in people's minds, which he calls 'pharmacomythologies'. It is a common belief among lay people that a specific medicine produces only one 'main' effect, which is positive. Other effects are considered as negative or 'side'-effects. Likewise, it is believed that a medicine produces the same main effect every time it is taken and in each person who takes it. This means that medicine effects are caused by the taken medicine and the effect of the medicine is a property residing inside the chemical compound and not a function of some change in a living human body. This perception leads to the belief that medicines cure diseases, rather than often only treating symptoms.

The general health behaviour models and theories previously presented – such as the health belief model, theory of reasoned action, social learning theory, conflict theory and behavioural decision theory – can all be used to explain certain types of behaviour related to taking medicines. Basic decision-making and problem-solving skills are important components of patients' seemingly rational and irrational behaviours. As presented earlier, the choices do not always follow the criteria of medical rationality, but can be justified as rational by the individual patient. It may be useful to consider rationality as a continuum rather than seeing something as either rational or not. The degree of rationality an individual exhibits is also influenced by social knowledge and the micro- and macro-environment, as described earlier, as well as the actual health problem.

Improving public understanding of medicines

During the last few years there have been attempts in both developed and developing countries to improve the knowledge and understanding about medicines among the general public. This can be seen as an attempt to influence and improve (from a medical point of view) social knowledge related to medicines and health in general. National campaigns such as 'Ask about your medicines' are good examples of this kind of activity. A more balanced partnership between consumer-patients and healthcare providers is one of the goals in such activities. This has been referred to as concordance (see Ch. 18). A better appreciation of the limits of medicines and a lessening of the belief that there is a 'pill for every ill' are examples of the goals of such efforts.

Advertising and other commercial information may fail to give objective information about medicines and patients need to be encouraged to be more critical of such information. Early education in schools about health and medicines would improve health knowledge, along with guidance on using appropriate information sources. To facilitate informed choices on the use of medicines, public education should be accompanied by supportive legislation and controls on the availability of medicines. Non-governmental organizations, community groups and consumer and professional organizations should be involved in the planning and implementation of such programmes to make them seem more relevant to their target audience. Healthcare professionals need to be prepared for their role in developing a partnership with their patient to optimize treatment options.

Prescribing

The process of prescribing has gained a lot of interest lately because of ever increasing medicine costs and the concern for rational prescribing from a clinical point of view (see Ch. 20). Previously, social scientists had studied aspects such as the decision-making process in prescribing and the adoption of new medicines, using the 'diffusion of innovations' theory.

The extension of prescribing rights, in some countries, to a wider range of healthcare professionals has also raised the issue of ensuring that prescribers understand their responsibilities in ensuring the safe and effective use of medicines.

Functions of prescriptions

Prescriptions are primarily issued to request the supply of a specific medicine to fulfil a treatment need. However, prescribers may sometimes use a medicine knowingly or unknowingly for other reasons too. According to Smith (2002), these can be either patient or physician centred. She presented a long list of latent functions of prescriptions in addition to their intended and recognized functions (method of therapy, legal document, record source and means of communication). Medicines may be used to stimulate the patient's expectations for recovery and to meet patients' expectations, e.g. the use of antibiotics for viral infections or boosting a patient's morale in intractable diseases. The prescriber may also want to gain some time to diagnose the condition more precisely. The medicine legitimizes the healthcare professional–patient relationship. The prescription is a sign of the prescriber's commitment to try to heal and care for the patient. Finally, the prescriber may use the prescription to communicate to the patient that the consultation is over.

For the patient, the prescription may legitimize their illness and confirms that they have fulfilled one of the obligations of the sick role, to try to become well again. There may be an expectation from the patient that they will receive a prescription and they may be reluctant to leave without one.

Prescribing can also raise ethical dilemmas, for example when purposely using placebos. Does the patient have the right to know what they are being given and in not informing the patient is the physician respecting the rights of the patient?

Choosing the right medicine

Therapeutic effect is of primary importance when the prescriber decides which medicine to prescribe. A second consideration is the incidence and severity of side-effects. Prescribers have been shown to concentrate on a few serious side-effects and ignore those that they perceive to be less important, even where this may not match the perception of the patient. Economic aspects have a lower priority than the first two dimensions, although if patients pay, the prescriber may give more attention to the cost of the medicine prescribed. Patient convenience and compliance may be decision criteria in situations when medically similar preparations are available, e.g. suppositories not being recommended when oral preparations are feasible. When prescribing for children, taste may be an important factor to consider (see Ch. 33).

Prescribers who work with others or are part of a professional network are often some of the first to use new medicines, while those who work alone adopt a new preparation more slowly than those working in group practices.

Barber summarized the areas that a prescriber considers and tries to balance, when deciding to prescribe a medicine (see Fig. 3.1):

- Maximizing the effectiveness of treatment
- Minimizing the side-effects
- Minimizing costs
- Taking into account patient's wants and wishes.

Models to study prescribing

Several studies have tried to determine if there are specific characteristics of prescribers and their work settings that would explain their prescribing behaviours. Three general models or approaches have been used to study prescribing:

- Models focusing on demographic and practice variables which give descriptive information about what and how prescribers tend to prescribe. These variables are often difficult or impossible to change, but these studies help to determine possible focal points for prescribing interventions
- Models focusing on psychosocial issues related to prescriber–patient interaction
- Models focusing on the cognitive theories that explain prescribing decisions. These studies focus on how prescribers evaluate product and clinical information and their decision-making processes.

These studies have shown some differences in prescribing behaviour, although the underpinning reasons are sometimes less clearly determined. Prescribing behaviour may be erratic, with a prescriber prescribing rationally in one area and less rationally in another. More recently graduated prescribers seem to prescribe more rationally and in line with clinical evidence than those who are older. It has been found that prescribers with a negative attitude towards the use of medicines for social problems tend to prescribe fewer psychotropic medicines. Where non-medicine, alternative treatments are available, such as with cognitive behavioural therapy for depression, there is a reduction in benzodiazepine prescribing. A study found that a more cosmopolitan attitude and a more critical attitude towards commercial information are associated with more careful prescribing of potentially risky medicines. Another study showed that 'less rational prescribers', defined as those with a high rate of benzodiazepine prescriptions, rely more on commercial information from the pharmaceutical industry than from other sources. Professional satisfaction and reading professional material seem to translate into better prescribing.

Personal experiences also influence prescribers, as they do patients. For example, previous experiences of adverse drug reactions may decrease the prescriber's willingness to prescribe a particular drug, and conversely, experiencing positive outcomes in other patients may encourage the prescriber to use the medication in future. Individuals may use positive personal experiences to legitimize their irrational prescribing decisions.

Certain patient factors also influence the probability of receiving a prescription for psychotropic medicines. The most widely studied factors have been age and gender. The elderly are usually prescribed more than younger people, which may be a reflection of a higher rate of symptoms and psychological distress and the nature of the longer-term conditions from which the elderly are more likely to suffer. Women are prescribed psychotropic medicines more often, possibly due to them being more likely to seek professional help.

The nature of the consultation process

In considering why some patients take medicines and why some do not, it is important to look at how the decision to prescribe is taken from the patient's perspective. In traditional, paternalistic models of prescribing, the prescriber decides on the treatment, prescribes a drug and the patient goes away and does as they are told. They must be compliant with the wishes of the doctor in order to get well, regardless of whether this fits into their life, respects their beliefs and values, or is what they want.

Including the patient in the decision over whether there should be a medicine prescribed, and if so, what this should be, is important in encouraging the patient to commit to the treatment protocol. This can be of particular importance where the illness does not manifest itself in symptoms on a daily basis, and therefore does not normally inconvenience the patient, such as hypertension.

Over the last 15 years, there has been a movement to encourage patients and prescribers to work together, as a partnership, to determine the appropriate treatment protocol for the individual and their lifestyle. This partnership has been termed 'concordance' and is seen as a move away from paternalistic compliance by the patient to the prescriber's instructions (see Ch. 18).

Ultimately, it is up to the patient whether or not they take their medication once they get home. There are a number of models that try to define aspects of the patient–practitioner relationship. Paternalism is at one end of the spectrum, where the power and decision making lies with the prescriber, and consumer choice at the opposite end, with all the power lying with the consumer or patient.

The model that relates most closely to the concept of concordance is the shared decision-making model. This model incorporates four fundamental factors that are required for shared decision making to occur:

- Both the prescriber and the patient must be involved in the decision-making process. Others may also be included, such as other healthcare professionals, carers, etc
- Information is shared by all the participants
- Both prescriber and patient participate and express their preferences with regards to treatment options
- The treatment decision needs to be agreed upon by both parties.

If the patient chooses to abdicate responsibility for treatment decisions to the healthcare professionals, this may be concordant. The important factor is that they have the option to participate fully.

Both the patient and the practitioner need to develop their relationship and skills to ensure that they can participate in the shared decision-making process. Pharmacists need to consider the communication skills that are needed to negotiate with the patient and gain their agreement to a mutually approved treatment plan.

It is entirely appropriate for the prescriber to provide the patient with evidence-based information for them to use in reaching their decision. This needs to be presented in a way that enables the patient to understand the information.

Individuals are influenced by a number of external factors when making decisions relating to their health and illness and this is also true in relation to their medicines. Concordance recognizes that individuals will value the various aspects they are considering subjectively and they will also vary in their willingness to take risks and deal with uncertainty

(see Ch. 18). Concordant discussions with patients were not the norm – equal sharing of views was not common.

It needs to be recognized that pressures on prescriber's time may not help with concordance. A 10 minute consultation period limits the scope for shared decision making. Pharmacists need to consider this when arranging appointments to discuss medication with patients. Time is needed for a concordant discussion and this may pay back in terms of more successful use of medication.

Influencing prescribing

Providing information and employing educational programmes to change prescribers' prescribing behaviour has become an integral part of the pharmacist's role. Pharmacists participate in this kind of activity as part of their daily work in community, hospital or primary care, and there have also been formal prescribing intervention programmes used in research studies. It has been shown that pharmacists who provide information and education for prescribers can produce positive effects on their knowledge and attitudes, but the effects on prescribing behaviour have usually been modest. However, interventions by healthcare professionals, such as pharmacists, are more effective than simply providing printed material alone, which does not influence prescribing habits.

Individual feedback coupled with one-to-one education is the method most likely to be successful. Prescribers are most receptive to education in their own practice base and the facilitators (often pharmacists) should be professional and well briefed, and the messages should be concise, clear and relevant to the prescriber. An ongoing programme with regular repeat visits is needed to maintain the contact and keep the messages up to date. Additionally processes and procedures, such as formularies which limit prescribing, hospital or regional drug and therapeutic committees providing advice on prescribing, drug utilization review, audit and treatment guidelines, also help to ensure rational prescribing.

The changing nature of prescribers

Another factor that may play an increasingly important role in prescribing behaviour is the extension of prescribing rights to other healthcare professions. In the UK for example, prescribers may now come from nursing, midwifery, pharmacy, physiotherapy and other healthcare professions if they have undertaken appropriate additional training (see Ch. 4). These individuals will have different backgrounds and experiences that may influence their prescribing habits. It may also be necessary to look at implementing wider education programmes for prescribers aimed at those from all backgrounds.

Pharmacies and the pharmacy profession

Historically, a pharmacy has been the place for preparing and dispensing medicines. The first known pharmacy was established in the year 766 in Baghdad. In Europe, the first pharmacies date back to the eleventh century. In ancient times, the same person acted as both doctor and pharmacist, i.e. diagnosed, prescribed and prepared the medicines for the patient. But in 1231, the German emperor and king of Sicily, Frederick II of Hohenstaufen in the edict of Palermo, legally separated the professions of medicine and pharmacy. Physicians were to diagnose and prescribe medicines, while pharmacists were to be responsible for preparing the medicines and providing these to the patients. Pharmacies were also designated to certain areas, where they had the monopoly of selling medicines. Frederick also laid down rules about the education of healthcare professionals. These and other provisions given by him were the basis of the legislation and practice of pharmacy in many European countries until the twentieth century.

Elsewhere, the distinction between the medical and pharmaceutical professions has not always been so clear. While medicine and pharmacy are clearly defined practice areas in the UK, there are still 'dispensing doctors' who both prescribe and dispense the medication for their patients from one premises. The system of dispensing doctors has been defended based on availability and grounds of patient convenience. The problems related to the system are an apparent conflict of interest, which is present when the income of the physician depends on the volume and price of medicines prescribed. Japan also has issues relating to dispensing doctors: they have one of the highest costs of medicines *per capita* in the world and prescription medicines in Japan are mainly distributed by physicians. The same conflict of interest is often mentioned in the context of the professional and business roles of the pharmacist, especially concerning sales of non-prescription medicines.

There has been much discussion in the literature about pharmacy and whether it is a true profession. Two major approaches have been used by academics in trying to answer the question. One approach is to look at the functions pharmacists perform for society, asking if they are vital for the society. The second approach is to look at certain characteristic traits of the occupation and determine whether they fulfil typical traits of a profession. During the last 50 years, different traits have been mentioned by different academics, but there are some common ones. The following are traits that characterize a profession:

- Registration or state certification embodying standards of training and practice in some statutory form
- A fiduciary practitioner–client relationship
- An ethical code
- A ban on the advertising of services
- Independence from external control.

Most authors agree that the basic traits of a learned profession are advanced and lengthy training in a highly specialized body of knowledge. This knowledge is to be used in the service of society and mankind. Research and abstract reasoning are the ways of expanding this unique body of knowledge. The services provided by a profession are related to the degree of impact or danger they may have on individuals or society. Besides the expert knowledge the professional possesses, he must also exert his professional judgement to the benefit of the client. Co-workers, in the same or related occupations, acknowledge the level of expertise of the profession, which is also important in legitimating the practice. There is a certain level of trust that the public must place in the work performance of the professional. Professionals themselves define which kind of activities are allowed and what privileges members may claim. They also define, through ethical codes and legislation which they have often themselves had an opportunity to draw up, the type of controls that guarantee the social privileges given to them (like autonomy of action, monopoly of practice, remuneration) are not abused. Pharmacy can be argued to fulfil all of the requirements above and therefore, in the practice of clinical pharmacy and providing clinical care for their patients, pharmacists are very much professionals.

International guidelines for good pharmacy practice by the FIP

The International Pharmacy Federation (FIP) has issued its guidelines for good pharmacy practice (GPP), stating that the mission of pharmacy practice is to provide medications and other healthcare products and services and to help people and society to make the best use of them. The concept of GPP is based mainly on the concept of pharmaceutical care. The patient and community are the primary beneficiaries of the pharmacist's actions and the pharmacist's first concern must be the welfare of the patient in all settings. The core of pharmacy activity is the supply of medication and other healthcare products of assured quality, along with giving appropriate information and advice to the patient and monitoring the effects of the medicine used. From an international perspective, a rather new aspect is the quest for the pharmacist's contribution to the promotion of rational and economic prescribing and appropriate medicine use. According to GPP, the objective of each element of pharmacy service should be relevant to the individual, clearly defined and effectively communicated to all those involved.

In satisfying GPP requirements, professional factors should be the main philosophy underlying practice. Economic factors are also important, but they should not be the driving force. Pharmacists should give their input to decisions on medicine use, and a therapeutic partnership with prescribers and good relationships with other healthcare professionals, including other pharmacists, are important. Pharmacists are also responsible for the evaluation and improvement of the quality of services given. There is a need to keep patient profiles and to record pharmacists' interventions. Pharmacists need independent, comprehensive, objective and current information about medicines. They should also accept personal responsibility for lifelong learning and educational programmes should address changes in practice. National standards of GPP need to be put in place and adhered to.

According to the guidelines there are four main elements of GPP: promotion of good health, supply and use of medicines, self-care and influencing prescribing and medicine use. It also encompasses cooperation with other healthcare professionals in health promotion activities, including the minimization of abuse and misuse of medicines. Professional assessment of promotional materials for medicines should also be carried out and evaluated, and appropriate materials should be disseminated to the public. Pharmacist involvement in all stages of clinical trials is also recommended. The guidelines include further areas within the four main elements that need to be addressed, such as national standards for facilities for confidential conversation, provision of general advice on health matters, involvement in health campaigns and the quality assurance of equipment used and advice given in diagnostic testing. In the supply and use of prescribed medicines, standards are needed for facilities, procedures and use of personnel. Assessment of the prescription by the pharmacist should include therapeutic aspects (pharmaceutical and pharmacological), appropriateness for the individual and social, legal and economic aspects.

Furthermore, national standards are needed for information sources, competence of pharmacists and medication records. Advice should be given to ensure that the patient receives and understands sufficient oral and written information. It is also important to have standards on how to follow up the effect of prescribed treatments and the recording of professional activities. When trying to influence prescribing and medicine use, general rational prescribing policies and national standards are needed. In research and practice documentation, pharmacists have a professional responsibility to document professional practice experience and activities and to conduct and/or participate in pharmacy practice research and therapy research. These guidelines form an international consensus on the current practice of pharmacy and point to the direction for national guidelines to improve it.

Outcomes of medical treatment

Evaluation and outcomes research

Evaluation and outcomes research are fairly new topics within pharmacy. They are integral elements of pharmaceutical care and much more effort needs to be put into these aspects of pharmacy practice and research in the future. Evaluation has been defined as making a comparative assessment of the value of the intervention, using systematically collected and analysed data, in order to make informed decisions about how to act or to understand causal mechanisms and general principles. One important aspect from society's point of view is the question 'What are we getting for our money?' According to the model originally proposed by Avedis Donabedian, evaluation of health care can focus on:

- Structure, e.g. facilities, equipment, money, number and qualification of personnel
- Process, e.g. activities by staff and patients such as prescribing and counselling
- Outcomes, e.g. intermediate outcomes such as patients' knowledge and behaviour, and final outcomes such as curing the disease.

Traditionally, evaluation has focused on structure and process and to a lesser extent on outcomes. More recently, a whole new research field has emerged within health care called 'outcomes research'.

One difficulty in health-related outcomes research is to demonstrate the links between the three elements of the model: structure–process–outcome. For example, will a new computer-based patient medication record system in the pharmacy (structure) improve the follow-up of a patient (process), so that the pharmacist is able to detect more efficiently a medicine-related problem in the use of the antihypertensive medicine with the outcome of lowered blood pressure and the patient feeling better and living a healthier, longer and happier life (outcome)? Even if there is little empirical evidence, it is the general view that good structure leads to a more appropriate process resulting in better outcomes.

Many of the interventions, treatments and procedures used in health care are still not backed by strong evidence for efficacy, effectiveness and safety. While new medicines are thoroughly tested and evaluated, there are older treatments for which the evidence of efficacy may be weak, and even when a medicine has a proven benefit, it still needs to be prescribed and taken correctly.

Within the pharmaceutical field a more comprehensive framework for the assessment of medicines and treatments has been proposed. This model, named ECHO, classifies outcomes in three categories: *economic*, *clinical* and *humanistic* outcomes. Clinical outcomes have been defined as medical events that occur as a result of the condition or its treatment. Economic outcomes are the direct, indirect and intangible costs compared with consequences of medical treatment alternatives. Humanistic outcomes include well-being, health-related quality of life and patient satisfaction. The ECHO model allows pharmaceutical interventions to be planned, implemented and assessed in a way that incorporates different perspectives, potentially providing a more complete assessment of the intervention.

Health-related quality of life

The primary objective of health care is to improve a patient's quality of life. To what extent this objective is achieved often remains unanswered. This may be due to a lack of proper measures, the knowledge and attitudes of healthcare providers or some other factors. The central feature and objective of pharmaceutical care is to achieve outcomes by identifying, solving and preventing medicine-related problems in order to improve a patient's quality of life. In experimental settings this has been shown to be the case but the extent to which this is achieved in ordinary everyday practice is still open to question, as not all studies of practice-based interventions have shown positive effects.

A classic list of outcomes in medical care has been crystallized in the 'five Ds' – death, disease, disability, discomfort and dissatisfaction. These include a wide range of different aspects, but are all negative terms. Utilizing the 'five Ds' to assess a patient's quality of life will give partial answers only but does not allow all the aspects that might be included in quality of life to be assessed. Quality of life is not just the absence of the negative but also incorporates a measure of the positive. The term 'health-related quality of life' has been used quite differently in the literature and daily practice. Explicit definitions are quite rare because of the multidimensionality of the concept. The domains of health-related quality of life usually include functional health (physical activity, mobility and self-care), emotional health (anxiety, stress, depression, spiritual well-being) social and role functioning (personal and community interactions, work and household activities), cognitive functioning (memory), perceptions of general well-being and life satisfaction, and perceived symptoms.

Health-related quality of life has been measured with disease-specific instruments and general or generic instruments, e.g. health profiles and measures based on utilities. Disease-specific instruments provide a greater detail concerning functioning and well-being in that particular disease. The disease-specific measures (e.g. those used in hypertension and asthma) can also be further categorized as population specific (e.g. elderly), function specific (e.g. sexual) and condition specific (e.g. pain). Examples of these instruments include the Asthma Quality of Life Questionnaire and the Diabetes Quality of Life Questionnaire.

The generic measures include health profiles, which constitute a number of questions covering the different aspects, giving separate scores for each domain of life. Examples include the Nottingham Health Profile, Sickness Impact Profile, McMaster Index and SF-36. The advantage of health profiles is that they provide a comprehensive array of scores that is multidimensional. If the measure used is sensitive enough, through the profile, we may be able to distinguish, for example, when a medicine influences the emotional domain while having no effect on the functional health domain.

The utility-based measures incorporate specific patient-health states while adjusting for the preferences (utilities) for the health state. The outcome scores range from 0 to 1, where 0 represent quality of life associated with death and 1 represents perfect health. The preferences have been empirically tested in different populations and have been through a validation process. These utility-based measures have been extensively used in pharmacoeconomics research and more specifically in cost–utility analysis (see Ch. 22).

The most accurate and comprehensive end result may be achieved by using both a generic and a disease-specific measure when possible. The focus in current medicine is more on patient-perceived impact on long-term morbidity than on limiting mortality. It is good to remember that medicines can both increase and decrease the quality of life. The goal of medical therapy is to improve health and make patients feel better. Physiological measures may change without people feeling any better, for example, treating mildly elevated blood pressure may show a change in measured blood pressure without the patient experiencing any change as they may have been asymptomatic to begin with. Nevertheless, treatment may improve subjective health without any measurable changes in clinical parameters. There may also be a trade-off between positive treatment outcomes and adverse events.

In trying to measure quality of life, many of the measurement tools change subjective experience into quantitative data. Given the subjective nature of quality of life this may simplify the reality for the patient.

Client and patient satisfaction

An important aspect when measuring the outcomes of pharmacy practice and pharmaceutical interventions is the satisfaction of clients and patients. Measurement of client satisfaction can be an important tool in quality assurance of pharmacy practice (see Ch. 12). There are difficulties in defining the quality of pharmacy services. One approach is to divide the quality into a technical dimension (i.e. what is offered) and a functional dimension (i.e. how it is offered). Different proposals have been made to cover different aspects of service provision in general. One comprehensive model is that by Parasuram: he distinguishes between 10 different dimensions: reliability, responsiveness, competence, access, courtesy, communication, credibility, security, understanding/knowing the customer and tangibles. Hedvall has presented a somewhat simplified model. She has proposed four dimensions: professionalism, commitment, confidentiality and milieu, which also contain the essence of that which Parasuram proposed. In assessing service provision, customers may have difficulty in distinguishing between all 10 dimensions and some of them tend to overlap. The proposed dimensions represent important aspects to both prescription and self-care clients visiting the pharmacy. These aspects also have a direct linkage to communication skills and pharmaceutical care.

Measurement of patient satisfaction has usually focused more specifically on aspects in providing care. Cleary and McNeil have listed the following dimensions that are typically covered in the measurements of patient satisfaction: accessibility and availability of care, convenience, technical quality, physical setting, efficacy, personal aspects of care, continuity and economic aspects. In these dimensions, we can distinguish a technical or cognitively based evaluation of the services offered and also an emotional or affective aspect – how well they are offered. The significance of client satisfaction can be correlated to patronage, patient adherence, and ultimately to the survival of the pharmacy profession.

KEY POINTS

- Medicines have a wider function than merely treating disease
- Rational use of medicines is defined in terms of safety, effectiveness, appropriateness and economics
- Society expects the medicines used to be safe and attempts to achieve this by employing legislation and regulation supported by pharmacoepidemiological studies
- Patients' medicine use behaviour is influenced by complex social and behavioural factors
- Prescribing is a complex process in which the prescriber has to balance cost, effectiveness, side-effects and the patient's needs and wants
- The professional status of pharmacy can be determined from its role in society and the service characteristics of pharmacists in society
- Evaluation of health care is achieved by measuring structure, process and outcomes
- Outcomes may be economic, clinical or humanistic
- Health-related quality of life can be assessed using disease-specific questionnaires or general health profiles

Section 2

Protecting the public

Control of medicines

Jason Hall and Judith A. Rees

4

STUDY POINTS

- Most countries place legal controls on their medicines
- All stages in the development, manufacture and distribution of medicines are controlled
- Medicines are classified to control their access to the general public
- Non-medical prescribing
- Patient group directions

Introduction

Modern medicines have transformed the world, but the drugs within them are powerful chemicals which have potentially harmful adverse effects. Medicines and drugs can be misused (see Ch. 50), abused and when taken as an overdose, which may be intentional, can sometimes be fatal. Self-treatment of the wrong drug for the wrong condition or disease can have severe consequences. For these reasons, most governments or states control all aspects of medicines from their first trials in animals, through manufacture and distribution to post marketing pharmacovigilance: together with who can supply and/or prescribe the medicine. This chapter explains this process in more detail and describes the controls placed on large organizations, such as the pharmaceutical industry, as well as the legal controls placed on the medicines and the professionals acting as suppliers/prescribers.

Control of medicines

Most countries have legislation in place to regulate and control medicines: in the UK, this is the Human Medicines Regulations 2012. The legislation will be administered through the legal system and government departments. Examples of these departments include the Department of Health (DH), which is headed by the Minister for Health in the UK, the Department of Health and Ageing in Australia and the Department of Health and Human Services in the USA. These Departments create agencies, which are responsible for the day-to-day regulation and control of medicines. The Medicines and Healthcare products Regulatory Authority (MHRA) in the UK is responsible for ensuring that medicines and medical devices work, and are acceptably safe. In Australia, the Therapeutic Goods Administration regulates medicines. In the USA, the Food and Drug Administration (FDA) aims to protect consumers and enhance public health by maximizing compliance of FDA-regulated products. These regulated products include medicines and medical devices. The FDA also deals with veterinary products, as well as human medicines. Veterinary medicines are regulated by the Veterinary Medicines Directorate in the UK (see Ch. 28).

In addition to the MHRA in the UK, advisory bodies have been set up including the Commission on Human Medicines, the Herbal Medicine Advisory Committee and the Advisory Board on

Registration of Homeopathic Products. These advisory bodies have expert panels which advise the Minister of Health on matters relating to their specialist products.

The MHRA is organized into divisions including: licensing, medical devices, vigilance risk management of medicines and inspection, enforcement and standards. These divisions ensure that medicines are regulated and their safety and efficacy are monitored, at both pre- and post-marketing stages.

Pre-marketing of medicines

Before medicines are marketed, the regulatory authorities in a country will place controls, usually in the form of licences or certificates, on the various development stages. In order to proceed to test a potential drug, the regulatory authority must grant licences before animal testing and human or veterinary clinical trials can be undertaken. If all these tests are successful and lead to a new medicine being developed, then the pharmaceutical company will need to obtain a Marketing Authorization (previously product licence in the UK) from the regulatory authorities. Only after obtaining this Marketing Authorization can a medicine be marketed in that country. Some medicines in the UK are licensed by the European Medicines Agency.

Any medicine imported into a country, will usually require a Marketing Authorization from the country of origin and an importation licence/certificate from the regulatory authority of the importing country.

Manufacturing and wholesaling of medicines

The manufacturing conditions employed by a pharmaceutical company in the production of medicines will be subject to controls by the regulatory authority. A system of inspection, enforcement and standards will be applied both before and after the granting of a Manufacturer's Licence. Inspection and standards will involve premises, equipment, record-keeping and suitability of staff employed. Legally, no manufacturer can produce medicines without a Manufacturer's Licence.

Manufacturers of medicines will normally be allowed to sell directly to the professional outlets for medicines, but usually sell though a pharmaceutical wholesaler. These wholesalers will be subject to controls by the regulatory authority, which will be similar to those applied to manufacturers. Again, inspection and application of standards will apply to premises, equipment and systems of transportation before the granting of a Wholesaler's Licence. Enforcement of standards will apply after the licence is obtained. No wholesaler of medicines can operate legally without a Wholesaler's Licence.

Post-marketing of medicines

The vigilance of medicines, after their marketing, with regard to their safety and efficacy will be monitored by the regulatory authority. Any medicine found to have adverse effects, which give rise to concerns over safety, can be withdrawn from the market immediately and, concomitantly, the Marketing Authorization removed (see Ch. 22).

Supply of medicines

The legal structure within a country will regulate the supply of medicines. Box 4.1 shows some of the controls on medicines.

Thus, the legislation controls healthcare professionals and their staff (see Ch. 5) and their professional premises, such as community pharmacies.

Legal classification of medicines

The legal classification used for medicines in a country will have a direct impact on how and where the general public can access their medicines.

Box 4.1

Ways in which legislation may control medicines

- Which professionals are involved in the supply of medicines
- Which medicines are available for purchase directly by the public
- Which medicines are only available on prescription
- Where medicines can be obtained by the general public
- Which medicines can be advertised directly to the public.

Most countries have additional laws to restrict access to narcotic analgesics and other groups of potent medicines and drugs of abuse.

Some countries have a two-tier classification of drugs:

- 'Prescription-only'
- 'Non-prescription' medicines, also called 'general sales' or 'over-the-counter' (OTC) medicines. These medicines are available from pharmacies and also from other retail outlets such as grocers, supermarkets, newsagents and garage forecourts.

Some countries further divide non-prescription medicines into 'pharmacy medicines' and OTC medicines. 'Pharmacy medicines' are available for sale to the general public, but only from a pharmacy and under the supervision of a pharmacist. Thus, pharmacists have a direct input into the sale of these medicines. Germany, Ireland and the UK are examples of countries which have this three-tier classification.

Australia has a three-tier classification, but has further divided pharmacy medicines into those that can be sold:

- Only under the direct supervision of a pharmacist in a pharmacy and cannot be self-selected
- In a community pharmacy on a self-selection basis.

The USA, Estonia and Saudi Arabia are examples of countries with a two-tier system in which pharmacists control access by the general public to prescription-only medicines.

Reclassification

In recent years, some medicines have been reclassified, usually from prescription-only to pharmacy or general sales classifications. This allows more medicines to become available, often with pharmacist input, to the general public for purchase. Such a process has given pharmacists a more professional image and increased the professional content of their work (see Ch. 21).

Prescribers

Any medicine classified as 'prescription-only' must have a prescriber to write the prescription before the patient can be supplied with that medicine. Traditionally, prescribers were doctors, dentists and veterinary practitioners (for animal medicines). In the last few decades, there has been a dramatic increase in the number of medicines available to treat disease and illness (see Chs 20 and 22) and this has resulted in an increase in the number of prescriptions provided by the traditional prescribers. In order to use the skills of other healthcare professionals, new methods of access to medicines have been introduced. These include non-medical prescribing, patient group directives (PGD) and minor ailment schemes (see Chs 21 and 49).

Non-medical prescribing

The review of prescribing, supply and administration of medicines chaired by June Crown in 1999 recommended that there should be two types of prescriber: the independent prescriber and the dependent prescriber, now termed the 'supplementary prescriber'.

Over the years, there have been many reports from the DH outlining the benefits of non-medical prescribing for patients, doctors and non-medical prescribers themselves (see Box 4.2). Many of these benefits stem from having the healthcare professional responsible for the care of a patient's condition also writing the prescription.

Independent prescribing

Independent prescribers (IP) are responsible for the diagnosis of the patient and can initiate prescriptions for patients without referring to other healthcare professionals. They have responsibility

Box 4.2

Anticipated benefits of non-medical prescribing

Patients

- Improved patient access to prescribers
- More accurate assessment of patient needs
- Better and quicker access to medicines

Doctors

- Saves time for doctors
- Clarifies professional boundaries

Healthcare professionals

- Improved use of healthcare professional's time
- Increased job satisfaction.

for monitoring and reviewing the patient's progress. In the UK, the first independent non-medical prescribers were the community practitioner nurse prescribers, introduced in 1994 in pilot sites and extended nationwide in 1999. These prescribers had a limited number of medicines which they could prescribe.

In 2002, a new class of nurse prescriber was created; they were originally called extended formulary nurse prescribers. This opened prescribing to any registered nurse. Nurses that chose this route to becoming a prescriber were required to complete a training course which consisted of 26 taught days and 12 days learning in practice, which included prescribing under the supervision of a medical prescriber. In 2006, many of the previous restrictions on extended formulary nurse prescribers were removed and their name was changed to 'independent nurse prescribers'. The independent nurse prescribers are able to prescribe any licensed medicine for any medical condition. Nurse independent prescribers must work within their own level of competence and expertise.

The changes in 2006 also paved the way for pharmacist independent prescribers, who can prescribe the same medicines and under the same conditions as nurse independent prescribers. Optometrists can also, with additional training, become optometrist independent prescribers. In this case they can prescribe any licensed medicine for ocular conditions affecting the eye and the tissues surrounding the eye, except controlled drugs or medicines for parenteral administration.

Supplementary prescribing

Supplementary prescribing is viewed by the UK DH as a voluntary partnership between the independent and the supplementary prescriber that has the agreement of the patient. Therefore, the patient must be informed regarding the underlying principles of the prescribing partnership by the independent prescriber and give their consent to the transfer of care to a supplementary prescriber. The patient does not have to give written consent, but once consent has been given, it should be noted in the patient's medical notes.

Providing the patient agrees, there is very little restriction as to what can be prescribed. Controlled drugs and unlicensed medicines were added to the list of drugs that can be prescribed by supplementary prescribers in May 2005.

An independent prescriber, who must be a doctor or a dentist, makes the diagnosis. If the independent prescriber thinks that the patient can be safely managed by a supplementary prescriber, then both the independent prescriber and supplementary prescriber agree a clinical management plan (CMP) for the patient. However, the independent prescriber does not discard all their responsibility and must still review the patient at suitable intervals, which should rarely exceed a year.

The CMP is central to supplementary prescribing in that it forms the agreement between the independent and supplementary prescribers that sets out what the supplementary prescriber is able to prescribe (Fig. 4.1). Each CMP must be drawn up for a specific named patient. The nature of the CMP can vary in terms of its detail and scope. At one end of the spectrum it could be very specific, allowing only relatively minor modifications to be made to the original prescription under specified criteria, such as increasing the dosage of an antihypertensive drug in order to reduce blood pressure to a specified level. At the other end of the spectrum it could be very open, allowing the supplementary prescriber to prescribe a wide range of drugs in accordance with a clinical guideline, such as the British Thoracic Society's guidelines for the management of asthma. The nature of the CMP will depend upon the confidence and competence of the supplementary prescriber in each therapeutic area and also the willingness of the independent prescriber to delegate the responsibility. The plan also sets out the circumstances that would require referral back to the independent prescriber.

The patients most likely to benefit from supplementary prescribing are those with chronic conditions requiring ongoing care, such as diabetes mellitus, asthma or hypertension. In addition, those with uncomplicated conditions, rather than those patients with multiple problems, are likely to be the most suitable candidates for supplementary prescribing. In practice, the supplementary prescriber is likely to continue prescribing the items initiated by the independent prescriber until there is a change in the patient's condition, provided such items have been included in the CMP. A change in the patient's condition could involve a deterioration of a chronic progressive condition. An example of managing the deterioration is stepping up therapy by prescribing an additional item such as a steroid inhaler to an asthmatic patient who is poorly controlled on a salbutamol inhaler alone (see Ch. 43).

Name of patient:			Patient medication sensitivities/allergies:		
Patient identification, e.g. ID number, date of birth:					
Current medication:			Medical history:		
Independent prescriber(s) (IP): Contact details: [tel/email/address]			Supplementary prescriber(s) (SP): Contact details: [tel/email/address]		
Condition(s) to be treated:			Aim of treatment:		
Medicines that may be prescribed by SP:					
Preparation	Indication		Dose schedule		Specific indications for referral back to the IP
Guidelines or protocols supporting clinical management plan:					
Frequency of review and monitoring by:					
Supplementary prescriber:			Supplementary prescriber and independent prescriber:		
Process for reporting ADRs:					
Shared record to be used by IP and SP.					
Agreed by independent prescriber(s)	Date	Agreed by supplementary prescriber(s)		Date	Date agreed with patient/carer

Figure 4.1 • Clinical management plan used in supplementary prescribing.

As supplementary prescribers do not diagnose conditions, one might assume that they would be unable to prescribe for patients presenting with acute conditions. However, they can prescribe items in response to changes in the patient's condition, provided such items have been included in the CMP. A change in the patient's condition could involve an acute exacerbation of a chronic condition. An example is prescribing an antibiotic for a chest infection for a patient with chronic obstructive pulmonary disease.

Patient group directions

An alternative way of getting medicines to patients without writing a prescription involves the use of a PGD. These allow pharmacists, or other healthcare professionals, to supply named products to patients who meet the inclusion criteria specified in the PGD. The legal definition of a PGD is: 'A written instruction for the sale, supply and/or administration of named medicines in an identified clinical situation. It applies to groups of patients who may not be individually identified before presenting for treatment'.

Under a PGD, pre-packed licensed medicines can be supplied to patients who meet the appropriate inclusion criteria and do not meet any of the specified exclusion criteria. The PGD must state the qualifications and training required of the staff administering the PGD, and it must name the medicine(s) that can be supplied. It must also list any advice that should be given to the patient, describe the referral procedure and state the action that should be taken in the case of a patient suffering an adverse drug reaction. The PGD must be reviewed and approved by a team containing a doctor and a pharmacist.

The DH has made it clear that the preferred route of getting medicines to patients is via the issuing of a prescription to a named patient by a trained and qualified prescriber and that PGDs should only ever be used where they offer clear advantages to patient care without compromising patient safety. Situations that could be suitable for PGDs are those that involve one-off or relatively short courses of standard treatment (i.e. the PGD operator does not have to select the drug, dose or formulation). An example of a PGD is the supply of emergency hormonal contraception through community pharmacies (see Ch. 48). PGDs have also been set up to supply medicines for weight loss, erectile dysfunction and smoking cessation.

Minor ailment scheme

Pharmacists have a long tradition of selling medicines over the counter to treat minor ailments. In some situations, pharmacists might have a choice regarding the method of supply of a medicine to treat a patient. This could be via an over the counter sale, prescribing a medicine as part of a minor ailment scheme (see Ch. 21) or supply through a PGD. In some of these situations the exact same product could be supplied and the only differences between the different methods might be who pays for the treatment and whether records have to be made. The pharmacist's duty of care to the patient does not vary between the different methods of supply and pharmacists should not treat an over-the-counter purchase of a medicine any differently than prescribing a medicine.

When recommending products to patients for OTC purchase, the pharmacist is acting as an independent prescriber, although they can only recommend general sales medicines or pharmacy medicines. As an independent prescriber, the pharmacist must go through all the steps of the prescribing process (see Ch. 20). The patient should be involved in the decision-making process to achieve concordance (see Ch. 18), and appropriate advice given to allow the patient or their carer to monitor the progress of their treatment and to know when to seek further help or advice (see Ch. 25).

Advertising of medicines

Many countries have strict controls on the advertising of prescription-only medicines. For example, advertising to anyone other than a healthcare professional is banned in the UK. These controls are to help protect the public from the potential misuse of medicines. However, in other countries, banning advertising is considered to be a constraint on trade and so advertising of prescription-only medicines is allowed, as for example in China. Nowadays, it is very difficult for any country to completely control the advertising of prescription-only medicines because the general public can access both advertising and information about prescription-only medicines via the internet. Some of the information on these sites may contain inaccurate information (see Ch. 16).

The advertising of pharmacy medicines and general sales medicines is usually permitted. However, most countries will have, as a minimum, some guidelines to ensure that advertisements are truthful and do not make excessive claims for their products. The advertising of pharmacy medicines may result in difficult patients who are not prepared for the pharmacist to advise against, or refuse to sanction, their purchase of a particular pharmacy medicine. Thus, the laws governing the advertising of medicines in that country will influence the everyday work of community pharmacists.

KEY POINTS

- Medicines are controlled by legislation
- Access to medicines is limited by their legal classification
- Non-medical prescribing has used the skills of healthcare professionals
- Patient group directions enable medicines to be accessed without a prescription
- Controls on the advertising of medicines are prejudiced by the internet

Control of health professionals and their staff

5

Jenny Hughes and Ian Smith

STUDY POINTS

- Why most nations control/regulate their healthcare professionals
- Healthcare regulation systems
- The role of the GPhC in UK Pharmacy regulation

Introduction

Most countries, usually by legislation, will control and regulate their healthcare professionals. Why do they do this? First, imagine the situation where anybody could call themselves a pharmacist, dentist, nurse, dietitian without the need for any relevant qualifications, skills and knowledge or integrity. Then, imagine if these self-named healthcare professionals could set-up in premises to offer services, advice and medicines. Would you want such an individual to drill your teeth, prescribe medicines or offer advice? Most certainly not is probably your reply. For this reason, all countries want their healthcare professionals to be suitably qualified, highly competent and with integrity. But how is this achieved? The normal process is to put in place an independent regulation system.

Healthcare regulation systems

Regulation aims to provide properly qualified and competent healthcare professionals. In the UK, although this is not dissimilar to other countries (see below), a system of regulatory bodies has been established. These bodies are independent of the profession they are regulating. The Professional Standards Authority for Health and Social Care, until recently the Council for Healthcare Regulatory Excellence (CHRE), scrutinizes and oversees the work of the individual regulatory bodies for healthcare and social work. In this role, it considers good examples of regulatory practice in one regulatory body and disseminates to all the other regulatory bodies. In addition, it will review and report on individual regulatory bodies on a regular basis.

Regulatory bodies may regulate just one profession, for example, the General Medical Council (GMC) regulates only medical doctors. Some regulatory bodies will regulate two professions, for example, the Nursing and Midwifery Council (NMC) regulates both nurses and midwives, which share a common pre-registration educational training. Other regulatory bodies regulate the whole of the professional team, for example, the General Dental Council (GDC), which regulates dentists, dental nurses, dental technicians, clinical dental technicians, dental hygienists, dental therapists and orthodontic therapists. Similarly, the General Pharmaceutical Council (GPhC) regulates the whole of the pharmacy profession, namely pharmacists and pharmacy technicians along with the premises in which they work. For healthcare professions with relatively small numbers of members, compared with some of the other professions, for example, medicine and pharmacy, it would not be efficient or cost-effective to have an individual regulatory body and so the Health and Care Professions Council (HCPC) has been established. This regulatory body covers about a dozen professions, including dietitians, paramedics, physiotherapists, radiographers and social workers.

In other countries, a similar system of regulation occurs. For example, in South Africa, pharmacists must register with the South African Pharmacy Council, which is the statutory, regulatory body. Its objectives include the control, promotion and maintenance of standards of pharmaceutical education and pharmacy practice. It also plays a role in the control and maintenance of the professional conduct of registered pharmacists. In Saudi Arabia, the Pharmacy Board of the Saudi Food and Drug Authority acts as the regulatory and registration body for pharmacy. In very small countries such as Bermuda, which does not offer its own pharmacy degrees, overseas trained pharmacists are employed, usually, with US, Canadian or UK degrees. They are required to undertake a 1-month pre-registration training to acquaint themselves with the Bermudan system before taking a pre-registration examination. Success in the examination will allow the individual to register as a pharmacist with the Pharmaceutical Council of Bermuda.

In many countries and in many professions, in addition to the regulator, there will be a professional body. For example, medical doctors have the British Medical Association (BMA) as their professional body. Similarly, pharmacists in England, Scotland and Wales are regulated by the GPhC and have the RPS as their professional body (see Ch. 14). Professional pharmacy organizations exist in South Africa, including the Pharmaceutical Society of South Africa, to professionally represent pharmacists. Similar professional bodies exist alongside the regulator in other countries and states, such as, New Zealand, Australia and Texas.

In Northern Ireland, the Pharmaceutical Society of Northern Ireland (PSNI) is both the regulator and the professional body. This dual system of regulator and professional body used to exist in the rest of UK and New Zealand up to a few years ago.

The work of regulatory bodies

The aim of any regulatory body is to protect the public by ensuring that their registrants are competent and remain competent to undertake their professional roles. Most regulatory bodies have a council which is made up of representative members from the profession and lay members, usually in an equal number. These members may be elected or, as is the case with the GPhC, can be appointed. The GMC, GPhC and GDC have a Chief Executive and Registrar who leads the organization. The Pharmacy Act of 2010 set-up the GPhC as the regulator for pharmacy.

A consideration of regulatory bodies shows that there are a number of common tasks.

Maintaining a register of members

All regulators maintain an up-to-date register of members, with members' names and addresses and date of first registration. These registers are available to employers and the public, so that a person, who claims registration, can be checked. In addition, these registers may include further relevant qualifications, for example, the NMC will identify specialist practitioners and nurse prescribers. The register of the GPhC will identify, by annotation, any further qualifications or responsibilities that the registrant has. Currently, these are qualifications as an independent and/or a supplementary prescriber. They will also indicate if the registrant is a superintendent pharmacist. A superintendent pharmacist has overall responsibility for all pharmaceutical issues within that organization. Any person who is registered with a regulatory body is allowed to use the legally 'protected title' of that body, for example, pharmacist, pharmacy technician, nurse, physiotherapist, etc. If the person is not registered with the regulator, it is an offence to use the 'protected title'. Normally, a registrant of a regulatory body has to renew their registration on an annual basis and pay a fee. The fee is used to pay the administration costs of the regulatory body.

Initial registration

Regulatory bodies require certain conditions to be met before initial registration can take place. These ensure that the person applying to be registered is competent to deliver the services they are required to deliver and do not have any reasons why they are unable to perform due to ill health. The regulator must also ensure that the person is of good standing and will uphold the professional standards by being a person of good reputation. In order to meet the required conditions, the person applying to the register must possess an accredited qualification, make some form of declaration about their health or have a medical review and make a declaration or have a police check to show that they have no convictions for any crimes.

In order to register as a pharmacist, an individual must have acquired a degree from an accredited degree course; have successfully completed 52 weeks of pre-registration training at an approved place with a recognized tutor; and have passed the registration exam. As part of the registration process, they must make declarations about their health and character. This whole qualification process must usually be completed within 8 years. On initial registration, some regulatory bodies allow full registration and others just provisional registration. The GPhC allows full registration, whereas the GMC only allows provisional registration with a licence to practice. After successful completion of Foundation programme year 1, the provisional registrant can apply for full registration.

Staying on the register

After initial registration, the registrant will have to re-register annually. Re-registration is not automatic and most regulators require certain conditions to be met before considering re-registration. These conditions will, usually, include a declaration of any conviction or warnings received from the Courts. Serious conviction could mean that re-registration may not be possible or be subject to certain restrictions (see later). Most regulators will require the applicant for re-registration to have undertaken some form and amount of CPD (see Ch. 6) during the previous year. CPD is rapidly becoming a mandatory requirement for continuing registration as a pharmacist in other countries, for example, Saudi Arabia requires 60 credits over 3 years. Other countries simply require the pharmacist to undertake CPD, while yet others, including the UK, require the keeping of written records which might then be reviewed by the regulator.

Some regulators will require evidence that the applicant has worked in practice for a certain, minimum, number of hours in the previous year or number of years. The NMC has strict requirements on hours of work in practice situations. All regulators will require a re-registration fee.

Revalidation

Revalidation is the process by which the regulator can be assured of a registrants fitness to practice. It is defined by the GPhC as: 'The process by which assurance of continuing fitness to practice of registrants is provided and in a way which is aimed primarily at supporting and enhancing professional practice'.

The GMC is the first UK regulator to require revalidation as part of the health re-registration process (see Ch. 6). The GMC claim it is a process to give patients 'extra confidence that their Doctor is up to date and fit to practice'. The revalidation takes place every 5 years and is based on an appraisal being conducted using a set of principles. Other regulators such as the GPhC and the HPCP, currently, have working parties considering the principles and methods of revalidation.

Leaving and returning to the register

Non-payment of fees or if a registrant is found not to be 'fit to practise' will mean removal of a person's name from the register. There may be reasons why a person might choose to have their name removed from the register. This might be a permanent removal, for example, when they retire, or it might be a temporary removal, for example, a career break or if they are leaving the country. Most regulators have a formal system of notification if a registrant wishes to remove their name from the register.

A person who has formally left the register can usually re-register under certain conditions. These conditions will depend on the time off the register and the regulator but, usually, involve a 'return to practice' course and/or some period of time under the supervision of registrant and/or some completion of CPD or even re-assessment.

Registration of non-UK healthcare professionals

All regulating bodies in the UK have systems in place for registering non-UK healthcare professionals. These overseas professionals are usually divided into those from the European Economic Area (EEA) and those applicants from elsewhere in the world. Each group is dealt with separately and will have to produce acceptable qualifications before being accepted onto a UK register. In some cases, the applicant may have to acquire an additional UK qualification or additional professional practice or sit English language tests or attend an induction course or a combination of these before being considered for registration. All applicants will require a police check from their home country.

EEA pharmacists

Pharmacists, and most other professions, who are registered or eligible to register in their own country are able to register in the UK. For pharmacists, they are required to complete an application form to be entered onto the register.

Overseas (non-EEA) pharmacists

In order to be registered in the UK, they must first have a pharmacy qualification and be registered or able to register as a pharmacist in the country from which they got their qualification. Then they must complete an Overseas Pharmacists Assessment Programme (OSPAP). This is a postgraduate qualification, which has been accredited by the GPhC. They must then follow the same route to qualification as a UK graduate by completing 52 weeks of pre-registration experience and the registration examination.

Recognition and accreditation of pre-registration qualifications

All regulatory bodies set standards for pre-registration qualifications, most of these being accredited degrees.

Accreditation of courses

The regulatory bodies will visit the educational institutions that offer professional qualifications, which entitle the student to register with that regulatory body. They do this in order to check that the course produces students that are suitable for registration. The accreditation process is rigorous and may impose conditions on the curriculum and the educational institution. In some cases, the educational qualification may include extensive placements in the professional setting and the development of a required level of competence.

Some accredited qualifications may allow the concomitant graduation and registration, for example, nurses, physiotherapists and dentists. Pharmacy in the UK is different from this, in that after obtaining an accredited degree in pharmacy, graduates have to undertake a year of pre-registration training under the supervision of a pharmacist and pass the registration examination before applying for registration with the GPhC. However, there are proposals for concomitant graduation and registration in pharmacy by integrating the pre-registration experience into the 4-year pharmacy degree, leading to a 5-year integrated degree.

In pharmacy, the accreditation process in conducted to a set of standards produced by the GPhC and involves appointed accreditors visiting the various Schools of Pharmacy on a 6-yearly basis, with an interim practice visit 3 years after the full accreditation visit.

A code of practice

All regulatory bodies have some form of code of practice or standards of conduct, performance and ethics. An overseas example is the South African Pharmacy Council, which produces 'Rules for Good Pharmacy Practice' and a list of products that should not be sold in a community pharmacy. These codes state the standards expected of registrants (see Chs 8 and 9). Breaches of the standards may constitute a Fitness to Practise (FtP) issue. Within England, Scotland and Wales, the GPhC produces the 'Standards of conduct ethics and performance', which includes seven principles for how a pharmacist or pharmacy technician should behave. Failure to meet these principles could lead to a pharmacy professional being removed from the register. In addition to this, the GPhC produces guidance to help pharmacy professions to understand the standards required around such topics as confidentiality and gaining consent.

A formal system of reporting registrants and dealing with FtP issues

In order to protect the public, all regulatory bodies have a reporting system, in which members of the public, employers, colleagues and other healthcare professionals can report a registrant if they consider they have acted in an unprofessional or criminal way or any other action that could bring the profession into disrepute. Each regulatory body will have a robust system to investigate such allegations that are reported to them. If an allegation is considered to be serious enough that it might affect the professional's FtP, then the allegation could be investigated by the regulator and if appropriate could result in the registrant appearing before a disciplinary committee, or if the allegation against a registrant is considered to be the result of a health issue, then a health committee. These committees will have various powers including the right to:

- Dismiss the case as the allegation is unfounded or warrants further action
- Issue a warning to the registrant which will then be used if a further allegation is raised
- Impose conditions on the practice of the registrant such that they are restricted in what they can do in practice
- Suspend or remove the name of the registrant from the register. Some regulators might suspend a registrant pending further

investigation of the allegation. Removal from the register is usually for a period of time and the registrant is informed what they have to do before they reapply to go back on the register or for how long they will be off the register before they can be considered for re-registration.

There is normally an appeal system which the registrant can go through if they believe they have been treated unfairly.

KEY POINTS

- The aim of all healthcare regulators is to protect the public
- All healthcare professionals must be registered with a regulator in order to practice
- The GPhC regulates UK pharmacy
- All regulators maintain a register
- All regulators have a code of practice for registrants
- All regulators have a system for disciplining registrants and removing them from the register

Continuing professional development and revalidation

6

Raminder Sihota

STUDY POINTS

- Continuing professional development (CPD) and why it concerns pharmacists
- The CPD cycle
- Recording evidence of CPD
- Revalidation

Introduction

This chapter is designed to develop an understanding of continuing professional development (CPD) and to consider the importance to pharmacists and pharmacy technicians of individual active engagement in an ongoing programme of CPD.

In the UK and many other countries, CPD is mandatory for pharmacists and pharmacy technicians. It is relevant to all pharmacists and pharmacy technicians, whether experienced or newly qualified and just starting a career, or working full-time or part-time. CPD is part of being a professional with an obligation on all to continue to enhance their own knowledge and skills throughout their career and working life.

CPD is related to, and indeed part of, clinical governance (see Ch. 9). Clinical governance is about both continuous quality improvement and being accountable for quality improvement. As such, CPD is an integral part of clinical governance and it involves all healthcare professionals. Those healthcare professionals working in the UK NHS will find there are specific requirements for clinical governance and CPD, which are mandatory. The Community Pharmacy Contract (England)

with the NHS states a clear need for community pharmacists to be undertaking and maintaining CPD records within the clinical governance requirements. In addition to this in the UK, the Standards of conduct, ethics and performance of the GPhC places further obligations on pharmacists. Before any service is offered, whether to prescribers, patients or others, a pharmacist must ensure that whoever is delivering the service has a relevant level of competence, skill or knowledge in that area. CPD allows the pharmacist to provide evidence and demonstrate competence.

What is continuing professional development?

The NHS defines it as 'a process of lifelong learning for all individuals and teams which meets the needs of patients and delivers the health outcomes and healthcare priorities of the NHS and which enables professionals to expand and fulfill their potential' (DH 1998). While this definition is accurate, it is somewhat lengthy. An easier option is to consider the three words individually:

- *Continuing*: this is about lifelong learning, an ongoing (or continuing) process regardless of the age of the pharmacist or the stage of their career
- *Professional*: this is focused on individual competence in a professional role, i.e. it is to do with the work of the pharmacist
- *Development*: this is about identifying and undertaking learning that improves the personal skills of the pharmacist to enhance patient care

and career development, i.e. it changes for the better the work of the pharmacist.

CPD can be defined as the process of reflection, planning, action and evaluation through which pharmacists and pharmacy technicians continuously develop their knowledge, skills, attitudes and behaviours throughout their professional careers.

The UK former pharmacy regulator (Royal Pharmaceutical Society of Great Britain) introduced a framework for CPD for pharmacists in 2002 in response to the requirements of the Health Act 1999.

Today, the concept of CPD is becoming a familiar process for the pharmacy profession. There is a formal (GPhC) requirement for CPD records to be completed and retained for the duration of a person's registration in order to demonstrate their competence to undertake the role they are working in at the time.

CPD gives a pharmacist and pharmacy technician the opportunity to demonstrate to their employer, the NHS, and to patients, that they are maintaining and building their own professional capability.

Background to CPD

The requirement for formal CPD in the UK arose from increasing pressure on the government to ensure healthcare professions operate in a 'professional' manner. Recommendations for ongoing professional development suggested that CPD should not focus solely on clinical skills but should encompass both attitudes and communication skills. CPD is now mandatory for all pharmacists and pharmacy technicians in the UK. This means that pharmacists and pharmacy technicians must keep a record which shows they are 'actively' keeping up-to-date with the knowledge they use day-to-day. The records need to reflect the scope of practice in which the individual works. By keeping up-to-date, they are able to demonstrate ongoing competence in their current role(s), and prepare themselves for roles that they wish to pursue in the future.

The GPhC format for recording CPD involves keeping a written record of an activity or event, demonstrating that the individual has learnt from a situation relevant to their professional role. This written record can be kept as a paper-based record or as an electronic record.

Pharmacists and pharmacy technicians gain from taking ownership of their CPD, since CPD is a personal activity: it is specific to each individual. No two individuals will have the same CPD records. CPD is designed to help an individual structure and plan ways to ensure that their skills are constantly being updated and renewed. CPD puts pharmacists and pharmacy technicians in control of their learning.

CPD cycle

CPD is defined as a systematic, ongoing, cyclical process of self-directed learning. It should enable pharmacists and pharmacy technicians to do their job more effectively and involves employers as well as individuals.

CPD is a four-stage process which helps individuals plan their learning and track, record and reflect on learning and development. The learning may be clinical or related to a skill, attitude or behaviour associated with their role. The four stages are often depicted as a cyclical process. The GPhC recording system is based on the four stages of the CPD cycle.

The four stages of the cycle are shown in Figure 6.1 and involve:

- Reflection on practice
- Planning
- Action
- Evaluation (reflection on learning).

Reflection on practice

Reflection involves the individual spending time reflecting on current performance and how work is undertaken. The reflection time helps in

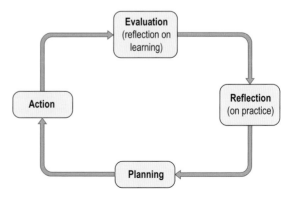

Figure 6.1 • The four stages of the CPD cycle.

identifying personal learning and development needs. Reflection involves thinking about how daily tasks are carried out, the areas in which the individual feels their knowledge or skills are weak or reflecting on events that have happened, which indicate a need to improve their knowledge or skills.

Sometimes a particular situation or event will draw the attention of the pharmacist to a weakness in knowledge, ability or systems of work which, if not addressed, could cause further problems. This is called a critical incident (see Ch. 10).

When reflecting, there are several questions which should be addressed:

- What knowledge gaps do I have when undertaking my current role?
- What areas do I need to develop to further progress my career?
- What have I done recently which I could improve next time?
- What do I want to be able to do?
- What extra skills can I offer my patients that would be of benefit to them?
- What skills could I develop that would help deliver my organization goals more effectively?

Other ways of identifying learning needs or knowledge, skill, attitude or behaviour gaps, include the pharmacist or pharmacy technician considering the following activities:

- Asking colleagues for feedback on one's own practice – how do they think you are doing? What do they think you could do differently?
- Participating in new activities
- Formulating a development plan to structure future development
- Questions from customers/patients
- Learning from a past event, sometimes referred to as critical incident analysis
- Appraisals
- Professional audit, measuring one's own standard against current competencies for a similar role.

An identified learning need is easier to address if broken down into bite-size pieces.

Planning

Having identified learning needs, the pharmacist or pharmacy technician needs to plan what can be done to meet these learning needs and how it can

be achieved. If several learning needs have been identified, then they should be prioritized.

If more than one learning need has been identified, then more than one CPD cycle needs to be started. When planning actions to meet learning objectives, the following should be considered:

- What level of competence needs to be reached?
- When does the learning objective need to be met by?
- What will be the impact of the learning on customers, colleagues, the organization and the pharmacist?
- What activities can be undertaken to best meet needs?
- What activities lead to the best learning? (This will differ for each individual.)

At this stage, there needs to be consideration of what the consequence of not undertaking the learning would be. If the learning need is no longer urgent or important, then it is appropriate not to take it any further.

When considering how to meet learning needs, there are a number of ways that learning can be undertaken. The list below is not exhaustive:

- Talking to a colleague
- Attending a course
- Reading a book, article or journal
- Research
- Work shadowing
- Coaching another individual
- Everyday experience (learning on the job)
- Talking to patients
- Computer assisted learning
- Deputizing for someone
- Audit.

Action

Action is simply carrying out the plan. The time taken to undertake the learning needs to be built into the plan and the timetable adhered to.

Questions to be asked while undertaking the actions are:

- What have I gained from this action?
- How might this action benefit my practice?

As these questions are answered, a record should be made of what has been learnt.

Evaluation (reflection on learning)

Evaluating what learning has been undertaken and how it has been undertaken is important. A series of questions should be considered during the evaluation process:

- Has the activity achieved what the original learning objective was?
- Has any learning occurred?
- Have any further learning needs been identified?
- Has an opportunity to apply the learning occurred? If so, was there any feedback?

In some cases, individuals may find that what has been learned is not what they set out to learn. In this case, there is a need to revisit the original learning need and consider if the requirement to undertake further actions is still necessary for their practice. If the learning need is still valid, then this will lead into a new CPD cycle or alternatively, the individual can go back a couple of steps in the cycle and add in different actions.

Assessing whether the learning undertaken has been effective

A further question that needs to be asked is: 'Can my practice now be shown to have improved as a result of the learning experience or is further learning required?' Realistically, true evaluation may not occur for some weeks or months, since an opportunity to apply the learning may not occur sooner.

Scheduled learning vs unscheduled learning

The CPD cycle is a circle – each stage flows into the next. There are three entry points into the cycle: 'Reflection on practice', 'Planning' and 'Action'. The exit (end point) is always 'Evaluation', when the impact of the learning undertaken is reviewed.

Scheduled learning is another term given to CPD which enters the process at 'Reflection on practice'. This is when someone or something leads the individual to identify a learning need or knowledge gap and plan ways that they can meet this need or gap. This can be as simple as someone asking a question that the individual does not know the answer to.

Unscheduled learning is learning that starts from 'Action'. This is learning that happens unexpectedly through someone or something. It is learning that was not planned and has not happened consciously.

All entry points into the CPD cycle are valid. Ordinarily, an individual would have a mixture of cycles, some starting at 'Reflection' or 'Planning', which indicates thinking about practice and planning appropriate actions, and some entries starting at 'Action', which indicates the individual is receptive to new ideas and concepts as they arise. The GPhC requires at least one-third of cycles to start at 'Reflection'.

Recording CPD

The CPD four-stage cyclical process should be documented to demonstrate learning is being undertaken, which meets the needs of the individuals and the organizations in which they work. The GPhC has issued guidance stating the requirement to record CPD in a specially designed format. It is advised that an individual focuses on the quality of the process and recording rather than the quantity, with a minimum of nine records requiring to be documented per year which reflect the context and scope of the practice.

Generally, the aim is to record at least one CPD entry each month. The time taken to undertake a CPD cycle may be hours, days, weeks, months or, for some learning needs, years. The length of time taken to record a CPD cycle is about 30 minutes. This time includes the recording and the thinking during the process. Pharmacists and pharmacy technicians have to submit their CPD records periodically for review to the GPhC. The method of review involves evaluating the records against a set of evaluation criteria.

In summary, CPD describes any activity that helps a pharmacist or pharmacy technician do their job better. What CPD does is to focus that learning on the needs of the individuals and the organizations which employ them.

Revalidation

While CPD has become embedded in the continued registration of pharmacists and pharmacy technicians in the UK and other countries, it does not necessarily show competence or the fitness of the individual to practice. Concerns have been expressed over the years that healthcare professionals in general are only assessed once in their career and that is at the point of registration. This situation was considered unsatisfactory and the UK government proposed that all statutorily regulated healthcare professions should have in place arrangements for the 'revalidation' of their professional registration. Revalidation would require demonstration by healthcare professionals of their continued competence to practice in order to maintain their registration.

The Non-Medical Revalidation group in 2008 published 12 principles on which revalidation should be based. These are: consistency, professional standards, remediation, patient and public involvement, CPD, quality-assured, equality, integration, UK wide, demonstrate benefit, information and incrementally introduced.

The RPS in 2009 proposed that in order to be successful, any future revalidation process should be effective and cost-effective; be standards-based; be proportional; be evidenced-based; be quality-assured; involve stakeholders; be equal and diverse; be remedial; be consistent and be implemented incrementally. These proposals incorporate and are based on the above 12 principles.

The GPhC has agreed a draft definition of revalidation which is: the process by which assurance of continuing FtP of registrants is provided and in a way which is aimed primarily at supporting and enhancing professional practice.

Any revalidation process introduced by any of the health professions will need to be supportive of the professionals involved and basis of revalidation will not be a one-off assessment which if 'failed' will mean immediate de-registration of the individual. The process will need to incorporate several sources of information about the individual, which may include annual appraisals, CPD activity, commentaries on complaints or errors, and multi-source feedback, including patient and colleague surveys. The details about these sources of information will need to take full account of the structure of the pharmacy workforce. For example, some industrial pharmacists may have little or no patient contact and so patient surveys would be inappropriate. Similarly who will conduct appraisals? Will it be a line manager who may not be a pharmacist or a fellow pharmacist or a more senior pharmacist working for another organization? What about a community pharmacist, who works alone or locum pharmacists? These are challenges which will need to be addressed if revalidation is seen to be an appropriate and fair process.

Conclusion

It is important for all pharmacists to be engaged in regular CPD regarding updating their knowledge of practice, regulation and legislative changes within their field of work.

KEY POINTS

- CPD is a feature of most professions
- CPD is part of clinical governance
- The CPD cycle involves reflection, planning, action, evaluation
- Entry into the cycle can be at any of the first three stages; exit is always at evaluation, but may lead into further cycles
- The UK pharmacy regulator requires pharmacists to record a minimum of nine CPD records each year which reflect the scope of practice of the pharmacist
- Revalidation has been defined by the regulator and in the future will be introduced for registrants

Ethics – the theory

7

Richard C. O'Neill

STUDY POINTS

- The major ethical theories and principles applied to decision-making in health care
- The key limitations of each ethical theory
- The distinction between morals, ethics and law
- Ethical decision-making frameworks
- Ethics relating to pharmacy

Introduction

The aim of this chapter is to introduce the concept of ethics, briefly explain ethical theories and principles and relate these to issues of relevance in pharmacy and healthcare practice.

Morals, values and ethics

The terms 'ethics' and 'morals', 'ethical' and 'moral', are often used interchangeably. They are almost synonymous in that an ethical action is one that is morally acceptable. However, they are not identical. Morals usually refer to practises; ethics is concerned with evaluating such practises. Morality is concerned with the standards of right or wrong behaviour, the values and duties adopted by individuals, groups and society. Personal morals arise from religious beliefs, political views, prejudices and cultural and family backgrounds.

Values are those ideals, beliefs, attitudes and characteristics considered to be valuable and worthwhile by an individual, a group or society in general. Personal values are acquired over a long period of time through interaction with family, friends, school, work, colleagues and role models, and develop and change throughout life. The way in which a person makes personal and professional judgements and choices is influenced by the way they organize, rank and prioritize values in a personal value system.

Ethics is the branch of philosophy that deals with the moral dimension of human life. Ethics deals with what is right and wrong, good and bad, what ought and ought not to be done. It is concerned with actions and judging whether an action is right or wrong and justifying this. The study of ethics is commonly grouped into three areas:

- Descriptive ethics simply describes the way things are – how people actually behave
- Meta-ethics is concerned with analysis of the language people use when they discuss a moral issue, e.g. the meaning of the words 'right' and 'wrong'
- Normative ethics is concerned with how things ought to be, how people should behave and how people justify decisions when faced with situations of moral choice. It attempts to generate the norms or standards of the right action.

Descriptive ethics is about facts while normative ethics is about values. One cannot argue from the one to the other. The way things are is not necessarily a guide to how they should be.

Ethical theories

Ethical theories provide a framework within which the acceptability of actions and the morality of judgements can be assessed. Absolutist theories rest on the assumption that there is an absolute right or wrong. Relativistic or reason-based theories rest on the assumption that right or wrong can depend purely on what any society, group or individual believes.

Normative theories of ethics

Normative theories are distinguished by the way in which they provide ethical guidance:

- Virtue ethics locate the highest moral value in the development of persons
- Consequentialist (or utilitarian) theories evaluate actions by reference to their outcomes
- Deontological theories hold that actions are intrinsically right or wrong.

These are summarized in Table 7.1.

Virtue ethics

The word ethics is derived from the Greek *ethos*, meaning a person's character, nature or disposition.

Virtue ethics has its roots in the work of Socrates, Plato and Aristotle, and places emphasis on the character of the person performing the action rather than on the action itself.

Virtue ethicists stress the importance of inner character traits such as honesty, courage, faithfulness, trustworthiness and integrity. Healthcare professionals are expected to demonstrate such characteristics or virtues.

Socrates (470–399 BC) taught the priority of personal integrity in terms of a person's duty to himself.

Plato (427–347 BC) emphasized four cardinal virtues: wisdom, courage, temperance and justice. Others virtues were fortitude, generosity, self-respect, good temper and sincerity. Hierarchies of virtues have changed over time.

Aristotle (384–322 BC) was concerned with what makes a good person rather than what makes a good action. He believed that being moral involved rationally applying good sense to find the middle way between one extreme and another, for

Table 7.1 Comparison of main ethical theories

Ethical theory	Virtue-based	Duty-based (deontology)	Consequentialism (utilitarianism)
Perspective	Actor-based	Action-based	Action-based
Features	Emphasis placed on character and motivation	Emphasis on the manner of the action; act out of a sense of duty; moral rules are those that pass the categorical imperative test; means count; never right to treat people as just means to an end	Emphasis on the outcome or outcome of the action; no action in itself is good or bad; ends count
Morally correct action	Right action is that which a virtuous person would do	Right action is that following duty	Right action is that with the greatest usefulness; greatest good for the greatest number
Strengths	More personal; supports actions done for virtuous reasons; not bound by rules	Sets clear rules/moral boundaries; follow duty not inclination; based on reason – no subjectivity; consistent	Practical; flexible; results orientated; no conflicting rules; moral form of democracy
Weaknesses	No universally agreed list of virtues; concerned with good character rather than the specific problem; difficulties in resolving moral conflicts or competing claims in practice; may do harm despite virtue	Questions about where rules originate; can be inflexible; not as simple as consequentialism; difficulties when rules conflict; follow duty regardless of results; ends cannot justify means even if outcome is good	Relies on single criterion when many factors need to be considered; difficulties in identifying who and what should be considered; difficulties quantifying utility; uncertainties in consequences of actions/speculative; can lack justice; does not consider individual rights; ends can justify means; bad or unjust acts permissible

Box 7.1

Examples of Aristotle's moral virtues and the golden mean

Excess	Mean	Deficiency
Rashness	Courage	Cowardice
Boastfulness	Truthfulness	Understatement
Irascibility	Patience	Lack of spirit
Vulgarity	Magnificence	Pettiness

example courage is the mean between cowardice and rashness (Box 7.1).

Modern Aristotelians believe that ethics should be concentrating more on how people should live their lives, advising which ethical characteristics people should try to develop and habituating people into having good dispositions so that moral behaviour becomes almost instinctive.

Consequentialism and utilitarianism

For consequentialists, whether an action is morally right or wrong, depends on the action's 'utility' or usefulness.

Utilitarians consider that an action should be judged according to the results it achieves. Jeremy Bentham (1748–1832) argued that actions are right if they maximize pleasure (good) and minimize pain (evil) for the majority of people. Since he believed everyone had an equal right to pleasure, everyone counted in the assessment of benefits of an action.

Later it was argued that not all forms of pleasure and happiness were equal and other values such as duty, love and respect should be considered. The goal of ethics is not only the pleasure (happiness) of the individual, but also the greatest pleasure (happiness) for the greatest number (John Stuart Mill 1806–1873).

Recent utilitarian theorists have advocated taking into account the preferences of persons concerned. This approach has become widely used in areas of applied and professional ethics and assumes that there should be equal consideration of interests. While accepting that not all have equal interests (animals compared with humans for example), all should be treated in a way that is appropriate.

The simplicity and practical usefulness of utilitarianism is one of its main benefits. If an act is likely to produce the greatest good for the greatest number, then it is right – if it does not, it is wrong.

Deontology

Deontology refers to a group of normative ethical theories that emphasize moral duties and rules. They are referred to as non-consequentialist, since some actions are inherently right or wrong, regardless of consequences. There are acts we have the duty to perform because these acts are good in themselves; and we have a duty to refrain from acts that are intrinsically bad or wrong.

Kantianism

Kantianism is the most comprehensive deontological ethical theory named after Immanuel Kant (1724–1804). He believed that people, not God, imposed morality because they were rational beings. Kant suggested that moral duty could be determined by the use of reason about the act in question. This categorical imperative exists as several versions, the two best known being:

- First version: 'Act only on that maxim through which you can at the same time will that it should become a universal law'

  This means that 'unless you are able to say that everyone must act like this, then you should not act like it'. Something is morally right, or wrong, only if it applies for everyone. It would be inconsistent and irrational to decide, for example, that you could steal from others, but they could not steal from you. Thus, reason demands that we do not steal unless everyone is allowed to steal.

- Second version: 'Act in such a way that you always treat humanity, whether in your own person or in the person of any other, never simply as a means, but always at the same time as an end'

  People must be treated as ends in themselves and not as a means to an end. This means that all people are equal and deserve equal respect. There are certain ways we must not treat people, no matter how much usefulness might be produced by treating them in those ways (e.g. not lying to a patient). A consequentialist, by contrast, does not believe it is wrong to use people as means – if the ends justify the means, lying is permissible.

  This second version has been very influential in medical ethics, as it can be translated as saying it is necessary to treat people as autonomous agents capable of making their own decisions. The concept of autonomy and respecting an autonomous decision demonstrates respect for the person as an 'end in itself'.

Ross's prima facie *duties*

WD Ross (1877–1971) recognized that a number of obligations present themselves in practical situations and that we must weigh up the various options available when deciding which course of action is morally correct (Hawley 2007). Ross distinguished duties as *prima facie* or 'actual' duties. A *prima facie* duty is one that is always to be performed unless it conflicts with an equal or stronger duty. The stronger duty becomes an actual duty that must be carried out for the action to be morally correct. The *prima facie* duty to keep a promise, for example, could be over-ridden if it was not in a person's best interests. Ross identified seven *prima facie* duties (see Box 7.2).

Conflict of duties can only be resolved by considered judgement in a particular situation: there is no general ranking of the duties. The morally correct action is the one that produces the greatest balance of *prima facie* rightness to *prima facie* wrongness. However, the principle of non-maleficence is considered to take precedence over the principle of beneficence when they come into conflict. Ross's theory has greatly influenced the 'four-principles' approach to medical ethics (see below), as it introduced the idea of sorting and weighing principles.

Box 7.2

Ross's *prima facie* duties

- Fidelity: duty to keep promises, honour contracts and agreements, tell the truth, be faithful
- Reparation: duty to rectify a wrong done to another
- Gratitude: duty to repay acts of kindness
- Beneficence: duty to make things better for other persons
- Non-maleficence: duty not to make other persons worse off
- Justice: duty to distribute pleasure or happiness, goods and benefits in accordance with the merit of persons concerned
- Self-improvement: duty to improve one's own condition.

Deontology and rights

The rights of persons are closely associated with duty. Using someone as a means to an end infringes that person's 'rights', such as rights to freedom and choice. This 'right' could be derived from the capacity to reason or to make choices, so that healthcare professionals, for example, are obliged to respect rational wishes of patients.

In every case, the deontological norm has boundaries. What lies outside those boundaries is not forbidden. Thus, lying is wrong while withholding a truth may be perfectly permissible. This is because withholding a truth is not lying. If more than one option is morally acceptable, the individual can choose which to carry out. By contrast, a consequentialist must always select the best option.

Principlism and the four ethical principles

'Principlism', introduced in the late 1970s, is now a widely applied bioethical framework for identifying key moral issues and as a starting point for looking at ethical dilemmas. It identifies four *prima facie* moral commitments relevant in health care and compatible with the major ethical theories. These enable a simple, accessible approach when the ethical theories themselves can be considered to be too general to guide particular decisions. Being conditional, the principles allow a stronger case to overrule a weaker one in a particular circumstance.

The four 'principles' are:

- Autonomy: self governance and respect for persons
- Non-maleficence: avoiding harm
- Beneficence: providing good
- Justice: fairness.

These are supplemented with four 'rules':

- Veracity
- Privacy
- Confidentiality
- Fidelity.

Autonomy

Autonomy encompasses the capacity to think, decide and act freely and independently. Respect for autonomy flows from the recognition that all rational beings have unconditional worth, and each has the capacity to determine his or her own destiny. People should be seen as ends in themselves and not treated simply as means to the ends of others.

Autonomy generally brings about the best outcome. Individuals should be allowed to develop their potential according to their own personal convictions provided these do not interfere with a like expression of freedom by others. A person's autonomy should be respected unless it causes harm to others. Liberty should not be limited on the sole grounds that a person's choice would harm them – competent adults should be free to risk their own health and well-being without interference. Respectfulness can be considered a characteristic of a virtuous person.

Three types of autonomy have been suggested:

- Autonomy of thought: thinking for oneself, making decisions, believing things, making moral assessments
- Autonomy of will (intention): freedom to do things on the basis of one's deliberations
- Autonomy of action: ability to act.

Autonomy is perhaps the dominant principle of medical ethics. Autonomy is the basis of informed consent and truthfulness, privacy and confidentiality. Other proposed 'principles' such as fidelity (faithfulness) and veracity (truthfulness) can be considered to come under the umbrella of autonomy. Autonomy means that patients can choose what type of treatment they would prefer given a choice, and even choose not to be treated. Autonomy also involves helping the patient to come to his or her own decision. Where a patient is able to make an informed decision, this should be respected, even when it appears to be detrimental, illogical or immoral. However, healthcare providers must also be able to recognize situations where a patient is unable to act autonomously. Of course, a person may even make an autonomous decision to leave decision-making to someone else.

Autonomy and patient preferences or wishes are not absolute and must be weighed against competing liberties and interests. The opposite of autonomy is paternalism. Paternalism over-rides the principle of respect for autonomy and involves making decisions on behalf of another, usually justified by appealing to the principle of beneficence (the duty to do good) or non-maleficence (the duty not to harm). In the past, paternalistic practise was common, but in modern society, it is less acceptable, although weak (soft) paternalism can be justified in some cases, such as when acting in the best interests of an incompetent patient. However, strong (hard) paternalism, ignoring or over-riding a competent person's wishes, is difficult to justify.

Non-maleficence

Non-maleficence means not doing harm, often expressed as 'First, do no harm' – a simplification from the Greek fourth century BC Hippocratic Oath.

Non-maleficence requires healthcare providers to do everything in their ability to avoid causing, and where possible actively avoid causing, either intentional or unintentional harm. This would include maintenance of competence through continuing education, always acting within the scope of practice and individual ability and doing everything to avoid making mistakes that can harm the patient. Healthcare providers have an ethical (if not legal) obligation to report behaviours by others that adversely (or could adversely) affect the health, safety or welfare of patients – an obligation to report others who are incompetent, impaired (such as from fatigue, alcohol, drugs or mental illness) or are unethical.

Beneficence

Beneficence is an obligation to do good. To benefit the patient is a fundamental goal of health care. Most people enter a healthcare profession because of the opportunity to help others and each profession will have its own definition of what 'good' means.

Beneficence and non-maleficence are often seen as two sides of the same coin. However, while there is a general positive obligation not to do harm, providing benefit (typically to a specific individual) is not always possible.

Desire to help others can come into conflict with the principle of autonomy, as when a patient chooses a course of action that does not appear to coincide with his or her best interest. Beneficence also frequently comes into conflict with non-maleficence. Most medical and therapeutic interventions are associated with some harm (e.g. the pain associated with immunization) and benefits have to be balanced against risks. In such instances, we rely on beneficence to ensure that any harm is performed for a greater good.

Beneficence involves doing what is best for the patient. This does raise the question of who should judge what is best. Conflicts between beneficence and autonomy can occur when a competent patient chooses a course of action that the healthcare professional does not consider is in his or her best interests.

Justice

Justice is often synonymous with fairness and equity: a moral obligation to act on the basis of fair adjudication between competing claims. All people of equal need are entitled to be treated equally in the distribution of benefits and burdens regardless of race, gender, religion and socioeconomic status, etc. Justice requires that only morally defensible differences among people be used to decide who gets what. Decisions should not be based on capricious or illogical reasons. The logical opposite of justice is discrimination.

Various factors can be used as criteria for the distribution of various resources (after Beauchamp and Childress 2001), e.g. to each:

- according to their need
- according to their merit
- according to their worth/contribution to society
- an equal share
- according to their effort.

Justice is about equal access to health care. Not all patients have an equal need and it is not always possible to provide the same level of care to all patients at all times. Consequently, a system has to be established to provide care as fairly as possible. For example, in emergency departments, a system of triage is applied in which the most critical patients are treated first on the basis of clinical need.

The four rules

Beauchamp and Childress (2001) analysed veracity, privacy, confidentiality and fidelity in the context of the professional–patient relationship.

Veracity

Veracity is the obligation to tell the truth and is an essential component of informed consent and hence, respect for autonomy. It is also closely linked to obligations of fidelity, trust and promise keeping. Veracity is not limited to cases of informed consent. Veracity provides for open and meaningful communication that is an absolute necessity in any moral relationship between two persons. The relationship between healthcare professional and patient needs to be based on mutual trust and honesty.

To Beauchamp and Childress, veracity is *prima facie* binding. It is not absolute, and non-disclosure, deceiving and lying could be justified when veracity conflicts with other principles such as non-maleficence. Non-disclosure or benevolent deception, but not involving lying, would be more easily justified, as it is less likely to threaten the relationship of trust.

With the complexity and uncertainties of modern medicine, complete honesty and 'whole truth' can be an oversimplification. Just what the truth is can be a matter of clinical judgement. Issues concerning how much information should be given, to whom and in what circumstances, create continuing difficulties for healthcare professionals. The obligation of veracity often conflicts with obligations of confidentiality and privacy.

Whistle-blowing, calling the attention of authorities to unethical, illegal or incompetent actions of others, is based on the ethical principles of non-maleficence and veracity.

Privacy

An obligation to respect privacy can be seen to come under the ethical principle of respect for a person's autonomy. Privacy relates to a right to restrict access to what a person regards as private and personal and not to be invaded. Beauchamp and Childress (2001) consider privacy to include decisions about sharing or withholding information about one's body or mind, one's thoughts, beliefs and feelings.

Confidentiality

Confidentiality relates to the duty to maintain confidence and thereby respect privacy. Beauchamp and Childress (2001) define privacy as allowing individuals to limit access to information about themselves and confidentiality as allowing individuals to control access to information they have shared.

Fidelity

Fidelity is the obligation of faithfulness and is concerned with acting in good faith, keeping promises, fulfilling agreements, integrity and honesty. Among the duties of fidelity is the duty of loyalty and an obligation to put the patient's interest first. Issues can arise when there are conflicts of interest or divided loyalties.

Principlist ethics and research

Principlist ethics have dominated the field of health research. The National Commission for the Protection of Human Subjects of Biomedical and Behavioural Research, in the Belmont Report of 1979, identified three basic ethical principles (the so-called Belmont principles):

- Respect for persons
- Beneficence
- Justice.

Respect for persons incorporated two ethical convictions: that individuals should be treated as autonomous agents; and that persons with diminished autonomy are entitled to protection.

Beneficence required that persons be treated in an ethical manner and their decisions respected and protected from harm. It incorporated the concept of non-maleficence by maximizing possible benefits and minimizing possible harms.

Justice required fairness in distribution of benefits and burdens associated with research and subject selection.

Morals and law

Both laws and morals can be considered to be guidelines for conduct. Laws establish minimum standards of behaviour that everyone must meet. The law is influenced by moral and ethical principles but they do not necessarily match. Laws may not necessarily be ethical and many things that are not illegal may still be wrong. Morality is a system of right and wrong enforced through societal pressure. Morals tend to be simple and general rather than precisely defined. They provide general rules that should be applied in particular instances according to circumstances and an individual's conscience. In general, morals correspond to what is done in a society and accord with customs and

traditions. Personal morals relate to the values and beliefs that provide the framework for an individual's decisions and actions. Ethics lies somewhat between law and morality. Ethical standards need to be precisely defined but are subject to individual interpretation. Ethics seeks ideal or maximal standards of behaviour.

All law has some moral basis, and in medicine, law, morality and ethics are inextricably linked. Many acts of parliament associated with health care are far from ethically neutral. There are many areas – research on embryos and embryonic stem cells for example – that are a source of deep moral divisions. Sometimes the law acts almost in a knee-jerk fashion, responding to society's moral disquiet, e.g. the Surrogacy Arrangements Act 1990, prohibiting commercialization of surrogacy; and the Human Reproductive Cloning Act 2001, prohibiting the planting of cloned embryos in a womb, were both rushed through parliament. Medical science and technology are continuously advancing and at a pace. Situations are having to be addressed before society has had time to thoroughly think them through.

Applied and professional ethics

Applied ethics is the branch of ethics that is concerned with the analysis of specific, controversial issues, arising in specific cases. It uses ethical theories and principles to form judgements. Applied ethics covers a number of areas including business ethics, environmental ethics and bioethics. Bioethics, a contraction of biomedical ethics, is concerned with the interface between the life sciences and ethics. It encompasses medical or healthcare ethics and focuses on issues that arise in healthcare or clinical settings. Professional ethics includes group standards and norms as well as individual ethics.

Ethical issues in health care

Advances and changes in health care and medical technology, the changing relationship between professional and patient and the changing interprofessional roles and their relationships all require an increased ethical awareness in healthcare professionals (see Ch. 15). Healthcare professionals need to be able to answer ethical questions, work out solutions to ethical problems and resolve ethical dilemmas. Some current issues such as medical research and resource allocation (rationing) appear to reflect a more utilitarian approach to ethics. Issues surrounding the beginning and end of life, cloning and reproductive technologies, and genetic testing clearly do not evoke utilitarian principles alone. In a pluralistic society, there are many different and strongly held moral viewpoints (moral pluralism) which apply to medicine, as is clearly demonstrated with issues such as abortion and euthanasia.

One area, for example, where significant challenges in ethics are likely to occur, is in relation to death and dying. The issue of euthanasia encompasses a number of concepts used in moral discussion, such as autonomy, the sanctity of life, quality of life, medical futility, best interests, acts and omissions, double effect and slippery slopes.

The doctrine of double effect embraces two effects, an intended good effect and an unintended secondary bad effect. This justifies giving pain-relief treatment to terminally ill patients, provided it is given with the primary intention of relieving pain, and excuses any unavoidable, but unwanted, life-shortening effect of doing so. The central core of the doctrine is the moral distinction between intention and foresight.

The moral distinction between passive and active euthanasia rests largely on the distinction between acts and omissions. To actively end life is both morally and legally wrong, whereas to withhold life-saving treatment could, in some circumstances, be seen as the right thing.

The slippery slope argument is one used against the practice of voluntary euthanasia. The sanctioning of some mildly objectionable practice inevitably leads to some highly objectionable practice. Thus, by permitting voluntary euthanasia this will lead down a slippery slope to involuntary active euthanasia.

Ethics and pharmacy

There are legal, ethical and professional implications to every decision and action taken by a pharmacist (see Ch. 8). While dramatic ethical dilemmas may not be the norm of everyday practice, each encounter with a patient raises ethical issues. Most do not present a dilemma. A dilemma arises from fundamental conflicts among beliefs, duties and principles. An expanded role and increased patient contact increases the opportunity for ethical issues to arise. Pharmacists need to become more comfortable with decision making in conditions of uncertainty. Ethics in practice involves such varied issues as pharmacist–patient relationships, empathy, responsibility and accountability, privacy and confidentiality issues, compliance and adherence, responding to errors, maintaining competence, supply of emergency contraception, abuse of over the counter medicines, supply of homoeopathic medicines, supply of unlicenced medicines, etc. (see Chs 5, 9, 15, 18, 21, 48, 50).

Ethical dilemmas are not restricted to clinical issues. Studies have reported a willingness of students to engage in some sort of academic dishonesty. This demonstrates the importance of nurturing and enhancing ethical behaviour in students and helping them to find their 'moral compasses'. Dilemmas may also arise in areas of practice, for example areas of possible conflict of interest, areas concerning NHS fees and remuneration (e.g. dispensing a prescription item at a loss), as well as personal behaviour, whistle-blowing and research, etc.

Professional ethics and law

Laws can be considered an empowering force in healthcare ethics. They define the legal aspects of practice, rights of patients and duties of healthcare professionals. Negligence involves a failure to meet obligations to others and, by attributing fault or blame, clearly has a moral dimension. Standards of care have a moral as well as legal and professional dimension. However, the law is seen as setting minimum standards, while the others aim for the maximum.

Professional ethics are concerned with the principles of professional conduct concerning the rights and duties of the profession and the professional person himself or herself.

Professional codes and oaths

Professional ethics are concerned with professional values and philosophies. Health professions articulate their profession's values and standards of conduct, and the rights and responsibilities of their members in an ethical code. Codes exist to encourage optimal behaviour and promote a sense of community between members. While codes tend

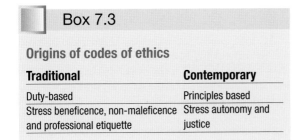

Box 7.3

Origins of codes of ethics

Traditional	Contemporary
Duty-based	Principles based
Stress beneficence, non-maleficence and professional etiquette	Stress autonomy and justice

Box 7.4

The Tavistock Principles

- Rights – people have a right to health and health care
- Balance – care of individual patients is central, but the health of populations is also our concern
- Comprehensiveness – in addition to treating illness, we have an obligation to ease suffering, minimize disability, prevent disease and promote health
- Cooperation – health care succeeds only if we cooperate with those we serve, each other and those in other sectors
- Improvement – improving health care is a serious and continuing responsibility
- Safety – do no harm
- Openness – being open, honest and trustworthy is vital in health care.

to emphasize duties and responsibilities (deontologically based), a feature of many is their aspirational nature – they strive for upper ideals. They make explicit, to both members and the public, the expectations and ideals central to the profession and so help ensure public trust and confidence in professional practice. Law and professional guidelines alone are unlikely to be an effective way of maintaining professional competence and behaviour. Standards of care are as much about ethics as they are about skills.

Various oaths and codes exist in health care (e.g. the Hippocratic Oath), their content having evolved (Box 7.3). Reference to autonomy and justice, as well as the obligation and virtue or veracity, has traditionally been ignored in medical codes and pharmacy codes.

Both law and ethics influence the formulation of the code of ethics and, more recently, so do the ethical principles: respect for people is related to autonomy, competence to non-maleficence and integrity to fidelity. The Standards of conduct, ethics and performance, published by GPhC, now adopts a principled approach, identifying ethical principles and including inherent value attitudes and behaviours that characterize a good pharmacist. The code is intended to promote professional judgement and support professional discretion.

Health care requires a multidisciplinary approach and healthcare professionals can be expected to share some common ethical rules. A shared code of ethics has been advocated and principles identified based on the Tavistock principles (Berwick et al. 2001) (see Box 7.4).

There has been a resurgence of interest in medical oaths in recent years (and such a personal professional pledge has been advocated in pharmacy). This could take the form of a personal affirmation encompassing the four ethical principles, some of the virtues such as integrity, honesty, compassion

and other key obligations concerned with working practice such as confidentiality and consent. Such pledges (or oaths) are used in some schools of pharmacy.

Ethical decision-making

In making ethical decisions, healthcare professionals can refer to law, professional codes and guidelines and to the principles and theories of ethics. Common sense, beliefs and values, intuition and experience also all play a role in influencing the decision. The first step in the process is to recognize that an ethical issue is involved and it is not purely a matter of law or professional etiquette. Ethical issues arise when there is confusion about competing alternatives for action, when interests compete and when none of the alternatives is entirely satisfactory. It typically prompts the question: 'What should I do?' or 'What ought I to do?' This requires a moral awareness or sensitivity. The next stage requires critical thinking and an ability to make ethical judgements. Typically this benefits from following a structured approach such as:

- Obtaining knowledge of all the pertinent facts
- Identifying the specific ethical issue(s)
- Framing these issues in the context of ethical theories and principles
- Considering – weighing up all available information in order to identify options

- Choosing an option
- Justifying the reasoning behind the decisions
- Reviewing and reflecting.

Wingfield and Badcott (2007) have set out in detail a methodology for ethical decision-making, based on a four-stage approach:

- Gather relevant facts
- Prioritize and ascribe values
- Generate options
- Choose an option.

Gathering relevant facts includes ascertaining what law (criminal, civil, NHS) applies and what guidance (codes and guidelines) is available. The second stage is identifying all the individual parties involved and attempting to balance their disparate interests. The third stage involves asking the question 'What COULD I do in this situation?' and the final stage, asking the question 'What SHOULD I do in this situation?' – recognizing that decisions may have to be justified. Finally, so as to develop decision-making skills, professional judgement and practice experience, once the decision has been made and any consequences realized, reflection is required.

When applying ethical principles, the principles involved should be identified, asking whether any of these are in competition, and whether one principle should take priority over another. The ethically correct option is typically one that fulfils the most principles. There may not always be right and wrong answers to situations, but there are better and worse ways of dealing with them. The better way would be to analyse an ethical problem by following a structured framework that enables the theories and principles to be critically reviewed and applied.

The importance of reflection cannot be emphasized enough. Most people make decisions at great speed and with little reflection. Experienced pharmacists often do not recognize the processes they use when making difficult choices. By slowing down the process, and breaking it up into stages and steps, it is possible to analyse how decisions were reached. An analysis of what was done, and why, can prove helpful the next time a situation presents with a difficult decision to make.

The virtuous pharmacist

Ethical principles do not in themselves solve ethical dilemmas but merely act as starting points to help identify the issues and concerns. Principles need to be supplemented with compassion, empathy and common sense.

At its simplest, the ethical principles become merely a checklist. Beauchamp and Childress (2001) were keen to assert that the principles-based approach was not designed to provide simple solutions to complex ethical dilemmas:

> Principles do not provide precise or specific guidelines for every conceivable set of circumstances. Principles require judgment, which in turn depends on the character, moral discernment, and a person's sense of responsibility and accountability ... Often what counts most in the moral life is not consistent adherence to principles and rules, but reliable character, moral good sense, and emotional responsiveness.
>
> (Beauchamp and Childress 2001: 462)

The four focal virtues

One or two virtuous traits do not amount to a virtuous person. A virtuous professional requires a virtuous character. To that end, they identified four focal virtues:

- Compassion: 'regard for the welfare of others. It combines an attitude of active regard for another's welfare with an imaginative awareness and emotional response of deep sympathy and discomfort at the other person's misfortune or suffering'
- Discernment: 'includes the ability to make judgements and reach decisions without being unduly influenced by extraneous considerations, fears, or personal attachments'
- Trustworthiness: 'Trust is a confident belief in and reliance upon the ability and moral character of another person'
- Integrity: 'means soundness, reliability, wholeness, and integration of moral character ... [it] means fidelity in adherence to moral norms'.

Mapping of values associated with pharmacy (Benson 2006; Benson et al. 2007; BMA 1995) have been undertaken in recent years and have identified some of the basic and ancient virtues.

Being a professional is concerned with personal development and striving for professional and moral excellence. In response to the question, 'What is a good doctor?', Tonks (2002) identified the following qualities:

- Compassion
- Understanding

- Empathy
- Honesty
- Competence
- Commitment
- Humanity.

The education of a healthcare professional is more than the acquisition of knowledge and skills. There is the need to learn professional behaviour and to acquire a new identity – a professional identity. From entering a professional programme, professionalism, the development of character traits and behaviours associated with professionalism, and the development of a commitment to ethical principles must be nurtured. This process continues throughout professional life.

Conclusion

Why is ethics important and why do healthcare professionals need to study ethics? Because it helps us to consider different perspectives, to respect others and the different needs of others. It helps us to take note of a patient's wishes. It helps personal and professional development. Autonomous professionals are required to make judgements and take decisions and it helps us to analyse these actions and their consequences.

Healthcare professionals have a responsibility to work ethically and personal standards, competence and high ethical standards are essential. Individual reflection on personal standards and ethics is vital. Excellence is not a state but a journey. It requires constant effort and never quite reaching the final destination. Aristotle recognized that it was not easy to be virtuous – otherwise we would not praise it.

KEY POINTS

- Ethics is associated with choices, judgements and decisions, encompassing concepts such as right and wrong, values, duty and obligation. Importantly, ethics is critically reflective and analytical
- Three main ethical theories inform biomedical ethics: utilitarianism, deontology and virtue theory
- Utilitarianism is the most prominent consequentialist theory and actions are judged by their usefulness
- Deontology emphasizes duty and motives
- Virtue theory stresses the importance of the actor's character
- The four key ethical principles in medical ethics are autonomy, non-maleficence, beneficence and justice
- Ethical principles serve as a stimulus to identify ethical conflicts and aid decision-making
- A coherent and consistent approach to ethical decision making is needed and requires critical analysis and reflective thinking

Ethics in practice and ethical dilemmas

8

Jennie Watson

STUDY POINTS

- What is an ethical dilemma?
- When legal problems become ethical dilemmas
- How to make ethical decisions
- Sources of help
- Who should take responsibility for decisions?

Introduction

As pharmacists, we are faced and deal with ethical dilemmas every day. Much of the time, we do not recognize them as dilemmas – just a situation that needs to be dealt with.

This chapter will build on the ethical principles described in Chapter 7 and help you ponder on what you need to consider as the best course of action in a given situation.

Towards the end of the chapter, there are some ethical dilemmas that have been faced by pharmacists in practice, together with some of the information you may need to gather to enable you to decide on the best outcome for both you and the patient.

Code of conduct, ethics and performance

The GPhC publishes 'Standards of conduct, ethics and performance' that pharmacy professionals must follow. The GPhC is clear in this document that pharmacy professionals are registered pharmacists and pharmacy technicians (see Ch. 5). The standards of conduct has seven principles.

As a pharmacy professional, you must:

1. Make patients your first concern
2. Use your professional judgement in the interest of patients and the public
3. Show respect for others
4. Encourage patients and the public to participate in decisions about their care
5. Develop your professional knowledge and competence
6. Be honest and trustworthy
7. Take responsibility for your working practice.

What is an ethical dilemma?

As professionals, every time we make a decision or take an action, we face a potential ethical dilemma. Often the situation is not dramatic and we do not always think in the moment that we have faced a dilemma. It is likely that many situations involving a person(s) has an ethical element and if there is more than one way to deal with the issue, then it is in effect an ethical dilemma.

It is also important to remember that we are pharmacists all day every day. We will sometimes be faced with a decision when we are not working, which because we are pharmacists, will have an ethical element to it, which may not need to be considered by others.

Example of an ethical dilemma

You are attending a party and several people at the party are drunk. You become aware that one of them is planning to drive home. As a non-pharmacist you will choose whether or not you want to get involved in the situation or ignore it.

If the driver is then involved in an accident, unless you were in the car with them, there is unlikely to be any personal consequence of your inaction.

As a pharmacist however, if you chose to ignore the drunken driver you may be in breach of the second principle of the standards of conduct, as you are not protecting the interests of the public and have not done your best to reduce risks to the public – this could mean that you are referred to the GPhC's FtP committee (see Ch. 5).

A legal issue or an ethical dilemma?

Scenario 1

You are working as a pharmacist and are presented with a prescription for a schedule 2 controlled drug; it is 4 pm on a Saturday afternoon. The prescription is not written correctly – there is no quantity on it. You have tried to get hold of the doctor as you have his mobile phone number but he is not answering. You are very clear that you cannot legally dispense this prescription. When you inform the woman who brought in the prescription, she tells you that it is for her mother who is terminally ill and does not have any of her painkillers left to take that night.

Scenario 2

It is Saturday morning, you are working in a small village pharmacy where the only other shops are the local grocers and the post-office. The village has been cut off by flooding and so your delivery has not arrived and won't be arriving before Monday. You have a number of drug-user clients who collect daily and you were relying on the delivery to ensure you had enough sugar-free methadone mixture to make up their daily doses. All you have left in the CD cupboard is methadone mixture DTF. You know that in law, the different methadone mixtures are different products legally and so substitution is illegal.

Considerations

Both of these situations have started as legal issues. However, if you leave either scenario at this point and choose not to supply anything for either patient, you are probably not complying with the first principle of the standards of conduct – make patients your first concern.

The law is very straightforward in pharmacy issues – you can either take certain actions under certain circumstances or you cannot. However, as a pharmacist you are also bound by the standards of conduct and so situations that are legally clear become ethical dilemmas when your compliance with the law is in conflict with the standards of conduct.

This is not to say that compliance with the standards of conduct is an excuse for breaking the law; it may, however, be an explanation of why you have made a certain choice in a particular set of circumstances.

Ethical decision-making processes

In many situations, you will make a decision without consciously working through a framework. However, in a more complicated or difficult situation, you may need to follow a structure to help you make the best possible decision. As an individual professional, it is inevitable that your process will be unique to you and will develop and change with time and with increased experience.

Your process should include the following:

Define the problem

- What do you believe the problem to be?
- Does anybody else involved in the situation have an opinion about the problem?
- If these two are different, what else do you need to know to truly identify the problem?
- Who else is potentially involved in the situation?
- Are there any other points that you need to consider?

Decide what information you need and obtain it

- Is there more clinical or legal knowledge you need?
- Where can you find this information?
- Should/could anyone else be involved in this process?

Reflect on values, conflicts of interest and if this is an ethical dilemma

- You need to identify the values involved in the situation so that you can check whether your own innate values may influence your thought process
- Does anyone involved in the process, including yourself, have a conflict of interest with anyone else in the process or with any elements of the process and what is the conflict?
- If values, ethics and beliefs are not involved in the situation it is unlikely to be an ethical dilemma.

Determine all available options

- Identify all potential options, including no action.

Decide if you need any other information

- Decide if any of your potential options are not entirely clear to you
- If so, identify what additional information you need and obtain it.

Identify the best option

- This is the best option for your patient, not for you.

Justify the chosen option

- Make sure you have reasons for choosing the option that you chose
- Make sure you have reasons for discarding the options that you did not choose.

Is making ethical decisions always a comfortable process?

Some ethical decisions are easier to make than others and some decisions will be easier for one pharmacist than another, because pharmacists are all individuals with different underlying beliefs and different life experiences.

Hopefully, you will choose a particular answer to a dilemma which you feel is the best option for your patient, even if this means the patient may be following a course of action that you would not be prepared to follow yourself.

An example of this is contraception and sexual activity outside of marriage. Your beliefs may mean that you believe that sexual activity should be confined to marriage and that you only believe in natural methods of contraception. As a pharmacist, you will be asked to advise about other methods of contraception and often, you will find out that the patient asking for advice is unmarried. Even if you have chosen not to supply contraceptives, the best option for the patient is that, in a non-judgemental way, you refer them to someone else who is able to help them, even if you feel that what they want is wrong.

Is there always a right answer?

In more complicated dilemmas, there is rarely a 'right' answer; your responsibility is to obtain enough information about the situation to enable you to decide, possibly with the patient, what is the best answer in that particular set of circumstances. If, after gathering the information, there is only one option available, then you are not facing a dilemma.

Can you justify what you have chosen to do?

If you have followed a robust decision-making process, then it should be very straightforward to explain your reasons for the outcome you have chosen. As a professional, you should always be prepared to justify and explain your decisions.

You may, on occasion, need to make these explanations some time after the decision was made. This may mean that you choose to make some notes about a particular situation at the time, so that you can remember your thought processes at a later date.

If you are making notes about an incident, you should only record factual information. You must also ensure that the notes are stored in a way that ensures patient confidentiality is maintained and access to them is restricted.

What is the difference between inaction and no action?

If you have followed your process, gathered your information and considered your options, you may on some occasions choose to take no action. You may decide this because it was one of your options and after considering all the other options, you decide that no action is your best choice and that you can justify this decision.

Inaction is different and rarely justifiable. Inaction is where you consciously choose not to engage in an ethical decision-making process. This may happen for one of the following reasons:

- The situation is uncomfortable for you personally
- You feel that any potential outcome would conflict with your values
- You do not have the courage to articulate your views.

Can you ask someone else's opinion?

Yes, is the simple answer. It is often useful as a professional to talk through complicated issues with a colleague. You have to be careful to make sure that you are not breaching other codes of practice, such as confidentiality, however, when discussing a situation. For example, another pharmacist does not need to know the patient's name as part of the discussion unless they were also involved in that patient's care.

As a professional, you should also consider what you would do if you discussed a scenario with several colleagues, all of whom pick the same outcome but this outcome is very different to the one

you had chosen. You should then reflect on why your choices are different to a group of your peers and whether you have considered all the information fully.

Can someone else make the decision for you?

Again there is a very simple answer to this – No. As a professional you are required under your code of conduct to take responsibility for your working practice. You cannot justify your actions by saying that you took them because someone else had done the same thing or someone else gave you a solution to a dilemma and you chose to follow it, without considering whether it was the right thing to do. This would also include following something you had read in a journal or book, without question. You have to be able to justify your *own* actions and thought processes for a specific situation.

Can someone else force you to make a decision?

If you have read the earlier parts of this chapter, you will know that the answer to this question is a resounding No. However, you need to be aware that on occasions, people try to put pressure on you to make certain decisions.

Patients

Occasionally, patients will try to influence you. Some people can be very manipulative and have an agenda that may not initially be clear to you. Some people will provide you with misleading or untrue information to help them achieve what they want. You will need to develop questioning techniques to ensure you get the most accurate information available (see Ch. 17).

Line managers

If you are an employee, you will have a line manager who will have their own set of values and beliefs. Sometimes your line manager will not be a pharmacist and have limited understanding of your ethical responsibilities. You may, therefore, feel at times that you are being pressurized to take a specific course of action that you do not agree with.

It will never be justifiable to follow a course of action unless you believe professionally it is the correct thing to do. You will, therefore, have to be prepared to explain your decision and stand firm about the correctness of it. Even if you feel that you are jeopardizing your job, this will not be an acceptable reason for not complying with the standards of conduct. You would need to be prepared to take further action to protect yourself and consider your position in terms of employment law and your employer's whistle-blowing policy.

Dilemmas to consider

For each of the dilemmas that follow, think about the following:

- Do you need any more information?
- What could you do next? This should be a series of options and you need to consider if there is a 'best' option.

After the scenarios below, are some thoughts about each, but remember in practice you will have to make your own decision, so there is no 'best' option chosen here for you.

Dilemma 1

A customer visits a community pharmacy and asks to buy a bottle of Phenergan elixir®. As part of the conversation, the following information is obtained:

The customer is the mother of a 10-month-old child

The customer wishes to buy the Phenergan® as the child keeps waking up in the night and disturbing her mother's sleep

During the discussion, the customer becomes quite agitated and verbally demands you sell her Phenergan® as she's entitled to decide the right course of action for her child.

Dilemma 2

You realize, over a period of weeks, that when one of your pharmacy technicians returns from her lunch each day, you can smell alcohol on her breath. It does not seem to be affecting her work. When, one day, you ask her if she could take a later lunch break she shouts at you and

says that you are not being fair and that she needs to go for her lunch at her normal time.

Dilemma 3

When the prescriptions arrive from the surgery, you realize there is one for your sister-in-law. From the medicines on the prescription, you think she is being treated for *Chlamydia*. She has been married to your brother for 12 years.

Dilemma 1 comments

Some of the information you may need:

- Is the drug suitable for the condition?
- Is the drug appropriate for this age of child?
- Is the product licensed for this condition in this age of child?
- Is the mother's reason for wanting the product in the best interests of the child?
- Why is the mother becoming agitated?
- Is the mother correct in her statement that she is entitled to decide what is right for her child?

Some options to consider (remember that none of these may be appropriate depending on the extra information you obtain)

- Sell the product – she is the child's mother
- Don't sell the product, it is not appropriate
- Tell her that the product is out of stock, it is easier than having an argument
- Think of different alternatives to help both mother and child
- Phone social services, the mother clearly wants to sedate her child inappropriately
- Explain why the product is not appropriate and try to come up with another solution
- If you decide not to supply her, contact the pharmacy across the road as you can see this is where the mother is now going, to let the pharmacist know about what has happened

What would you do?

Dilemma 2 comments

Some of the information you may need:

- Why is it so important to her to go for her lunch at her normal time?
- What does she do at lunchtime?
- Is she the type of person to shout at you?

- What would you do normally if a member of your team shouted at you?
- Is she drinking alcohol every lunchtime?
- Why do you feel her work is not affected – is this factually accurate?
- Does she have problems outside work that you are not aware of?

Some options to consider (remember that none of these may be appropriate depending on the extra information you obtain)

- Do nothing, she is obviously just having a bad day
- Talk to her to find out why she shouted and try to get her to open up about whether she is drinking alcohol in the middle of the working day and if she is drinking regularly or to excess
- Gossip with everyone else you both work with to see if they also think she is an alcoholic
- Report her to the GPhC
- Dismiss her, she must be dangerous and you do not want to miss a dispensing error she makes
- Talk to her and explain to her that you are concerned about her, but that she cannot work in the dispensary if you think she is under the influence of alcohol

What would you do?

Dilemma 3 comments

Some of the information you may need:

- Could the medicines be for anything else?
- Are you certain the prescription is for your sister-in-law and not your niece

who has the same name and still lives at home?

Some options to consider (remember that none of these may be appropriate depending on the extra information you obtain)

- Do nothing, you only have the information because you are a pharmacist
- Ask your brother if his wife is better, as you noticed she'd had a prescription for antibiotics
- Tell other members of your family that your sister-in-law is having an affair
- Talk to your sister-in-law and try to explain why you think your brother needs to know about the infection

What would you do?

KEY POINTS

- Dealing with ethical dilemmas is part of the everyday role of being a professional
- You must comply with the standards of conduct and use it to steer your decision-making processes and actions
- Different people will have different ways of dealing with situations
- It is important to be able to justify your decisions and actions
- There is unlikely to be one correct course of action to follow as a result of an ethical dilemma
- Your requirement is to identify the best available action

Clinical governance

Simon J. Tweddell and John Tucker

STUDY POINTS

- Clinical governance, what it is and why it is necessary
- The use of standards for delivering quality services
- The role of clinical governance in modern day pharmacy
- Regulation of pharmacists
- How to deal with errors made by the pharmacy team

Introduction

Clinical governance is defined by the DH as 'the system through which NHS organisations are accountable for continuously improving the quality of their services and safeguarding high standards of care, by creating an environment in which clinical excellence will flourish'.

Clinical governance

Why is clinical governance necessary?

Clinical governance was introduced in the UK following a series of well publicized lapses in patient quality in the 1990s as part of a broader government agenda to improve the quality of care delivered to patients by the NHS. It is a set of processes that healthcare professionals are expected to work within in order to learn from the successes and failures of both their own practice and those of others and to promote an open culture where experiences are shared to promote best practice for their patients.

When was clinical governance introduced?

The NHS document *A first class service: Quality in the new NHS* (DH 1998) introduced the term 'clinical governance', stating that, 'for the first time, the NHS will be required to adopt a structured and coherent approach to clinical quality, placing duties and expectations on local healthcare organisations as well as individuals. Effective clinical governance will make it clear that quality is everybody's business'.

What is clinical governance?

The NHS publication, *Clinical governance in the new NHS* (1999) outlines four main components of clinical governance. These are:

- Clear lines of responsibility and accountability for the overall quality of clinical care
- A comprehensive programme of quality improvement activities
- Clear policies aimed at managing risks
- Procedures for all professional groups to identify and remedy poor performance.

The publication also provides examples of quality improvement activities, including:

- Audit programmes (see Ch. 12)
- Ensuring evidence-based practice (see Ch. 20)
- Implementation of clinical standards
- Continuing professional development (CPD, see Ch. 6)
- Monitoring of clinical care and high-quality record-keeping (see Ch. 51)
- Research and development to promote 'an evaluation culture'.

Clinical governance should underpin the practice of all healthcare professionals as they strive for the best quality of care for their patients and continually seek improvement in their practice. Practicing good clinical governance ensures a consistent approach to decision-making, minimizes risk and ensures that patients are the priority and focus of the professional practice of pharmacists and all other healthcare professionals.

Quality: Three main elements for improving quality in the NHS

Creating standards for quality

Standards are set by clinical guidelines, such as National Service Frameworks (NSFs). These are documents that serve as a practical aid to the implementation of treatment and service guidelines in a specific therapeutic area. They are developed by groups of experts, which include healthcare professionals and patients, along with the support of NICE. With these, decisions to prescribe medicines can be based on the best available evidence (see Ch. 20).

Delivering quality

Quality health care should be delivered by well trained and motivated healthcare professionals who are well managed and are committed to lifelong learning through CPD (see Ch. 6). NHS staff should communicate openly with other healthcare professionals and should be encouraged to share best practice.

Monitoring quality

Quality of care should be monitored both nationally and locally through a process of clinical audit (see Ch. 12), with clear policies aimed at managing risks with involvement of patients in an open and transparent health service. NHS staff should be regularly appraised on their performance and underperformance should be identified and remedied. The NHS document, *An organisation with a memory* (DH 2000) requires that mechanisms are introduced for ensuring that, when errors or service failures occur and lessons are identified, the necessary changes are put into practice so that a wider appreciation of the value of analysing and learning from errors becomes the norm.

Clinical governance and pharmacy

The NHS document, *Clinical governance in community pharmacy* (DH 2001) first introduced clinical governance into community pharmacy, not as a terms of service requirement but by way of voluntary invitation to engage with clinical governance facilitators at a Primary Care Organization level. The NHS contract for community pharmacy launched in April 2005 included clinical governance requirements as one of the essential service components. Additional clinical governance requirements came into effect in July 2012 and include:

- Patient and public involvement programme: including a patient satisfaction survey, displaying the results and acting upon them
- Clinical audit: to check whether a service has reached required standards
- Risk management programme: including use of approved patient incident reporting system
- Clinical effectiveness programme: e.g. using protocols for appropriate self-care advice
- Staffing and staff management programme: to include training and CPD
- Premises standards: to ensure good design and cleanliness
- Use of information: via access to effective IT links and appropriate reference sources.

Professional governance

Professional governance in pharmacy can be defined as:

- The process by which the pharmacy profession works with its members to ensure that patients receive an optimal standard of pharmaceutical care and maintains confidence in the profession.

  Professional governance works in tandem with clinical governance, the aim of which is to:

- Ensure that pharmacists work to accepted standards of personal and professional conduct, put their patients' needs before their own and behave with integrity and probity.

Duty of care

Pharmacists have a duty of care to their patients and are required by law to ensure that the public is protected. The law would expect that pharmacists practise pharmacy to a level of competence expected by the profession, and indeed that practised by the 'average pharmacist'. Pharmacists are expected to exercise reasonable care when supplying the public and patients with medicines and professional advice.

In their practice, pharmacists are subject to criminal law (e.g. The Human Medicines Regulations 2012; Misuse of Drugs Act), administrative law (e.g. contractual agreements), civil law and the standards laid down by the GPhC in various documents.

The majority of care within the health service is of a high standard but it is inevitable that errors do occur. The vast majority of these are relatively minor and easily rectified without serious consequences. Unless a pharmacist causes deliberate harm to a patient, it is unlikely that he or she would be subject to criminal charges; although, in 2009 a pharmacist was given a 3-month jail sentence suspended for 18-months, following a dispensing error. The charge was brought under the labelling regulations of the Medicines Act 1968.

Negligence

If the mistake by a pharmacist causes harm, then a more likely charge of negligence may be pursued in a civil court. For a breach in a duty of care to be proven, then the prosecution must prove that a duty of care exists, that this duty of care has been breached and that the patient has suffered damages resulting from the breach. Often an expert witness from the pharmacy profession would be called to explain how a 'standard' member of the profession would have acted in this case.

The standards of conduct, ethics and performance

Pharmacists are also subject to the GPhC Standards of conduct, ethics and performance and should a pharmacist act in a manner that falls below the standards expected, then he or she may be subject to investigation by the GPhC.

Professional governance and regulation procedures in pharmacy

As mentioned above, one of the key components of clinical governance is that there must be 'procedures for all professional groups to identify and remedy poor performance'. This role in the governance of the professional is vital to ensure that patients are protected and confidence in the profession is maintained. Originally, the responsibility of the Royal Pharmaceutical Society (RPS), this role now falls within the remit of the GPhC, the independent regulator for pharmacists, pharmacy technicians and pharmacy premises, since September 2010.

The GPhC now has responsibility to:

- Set standards for pre-registration and post-registration education and training
- Set standards for the conduct and ethics expected of registrants
- Set standards for practice and performance
- Set standards for CPD
- Approve courses, institutions and qualifications
- Maintain registers of pharmacists, pharmacy technicians and premises
- Establish initial fitness to practise of potential registrants and continue to monitor after registration
- Investigate complaints and concerns and be prepared to adjudicate where there are issues of impaired fitness to practise.

Prior to the establishment of the GPhC, as a result of the publication of the Pharmacists and Pharmacy Technicians Order 2007, the RPS was tasked with setting up new committees to investigate 'fitness to practise' (FtP). This was a term used to describe a person's suitability to be on the register and to satisfy the principle of FtP; individuals must exhibit the skills, knowledge, character and health to be able to do their job effectively and safely.

Currently, all registrants must complete an FtP declaration each year when they renew their registration and any changes in this status must to reported as soon as the change occurs.

Fitness to practise can be influenced by circumstances of misconduct, including convictions of a criminal offence, ill-health or lack of competence.

Investigating committee

The Investigating Committee meets in private and considers whether allegations referred to it (see Box 9.1) should be dismissed or forwarded to the Fitness to Practise Committee. It also has the power to:

- Give a warning or advice to the person concerned or others in connection with any matter arising out of or related to the allegation
- Initiate criminal proceedings
- In relation to allegations of ill-health, order the person concerned to undergo a medical examination.

Fitness to practise committee

The Fitness to Practise Committee determines whether or not the FtP of the person of whom the allegation is made is impaired.

If the committee finds that fitness to practise is impaired it may:

- Issue a warning to the person concerned and advice to any other person or other body involved in its investigation of the allegation
- Give a direction that the person's registration shall be conditional upon compliance with

---

Box 9.1

Criteria for referral to the Investigating Committee

Cases will not be referred to the Investigating Committee unless threshold criteria have been exceeded. These are based around the seven principles of the GPhC Standards of Conduct, Ethics and Performance and examples are shown below:

From Principle 1: Make Patients your first concern
- There is evidence that the registrant was reckless with the safety and well-being of others.

From Principle 2: Use your professional judgement in the interest of the patient and the public
- There is evidence that the registrant put their own interest before those of their patient.

From Principle 3: Show respect for others
- There is evidence that the registrant failed to maintain appropriate and professional boundaries in their relationship with patients.

From Principle 4: Encourage patients and the public to participate in decisions about their care
- There is evidence that the registrant placed the best interest of the patient at significant risk by failing to communicate appropriately.

From Principle 5: Develop your professional knowledge and competence
- There is evidence that the registrant practised outside their current competence.

From Principle 6: Be honest and trustworthy
- There is evidence that the registrant behaved dishonestly.

From Principle 7: Take responsibility for your working practices
- There is evidence of health issues that impairs the registrant's ability to practise safely.

specified requirements that the committee thinks fit to impose for the protection of the public or in the person's own interests

- Give a direction that the person's registration shall be suspended
- Give a direction that the person concerned be removed from the register.

When things go wrong

Pharmacists are only human and, despite best intentions and safeguards, mistakes do happen. It is how mistakes are dealt with that will normally determine whether incidents are referred for further investigation.

When a dispensing error occurs, the pharmacist is ideally placed to determine the potential risk to the patient. When dealing with dispensing or prescribing mistakes, it is vital that pharmacists place the welfare of the patient first and seek immediate medical attention if necessary. An investigating committee would be unimpressed with a pharmacist who covered up a mistake, did not assess the risk of a mistake to the health of a patient or repeated mistakes where they have clearly not taken remedial action to prevent errors from recurring.

Dealing with errors

While this is not a comprehensive checklist, it may be helpful to consider the following when an error occurs:

- Is there any immediate risk to the welfare of the patient? If yes, refer to GP/Accident and Emergency, phoning ahead if necessary
- Who do I need to inform – e.g. patient's GP, superintendent pharmacist, family member of patient, GPhC inspector, primary care commissioner? It is better to proactively raise the error with these stakeholders rather than them to hear of it from the patient, patient's solicitor, etc.
- Document what happened in an incident report and describe all steps taken to remedy the error
- Make a report to the National Patient Safety Agency using their voluntary electronic reporting system
- If significant, conduct a root cause analysis (RCA) to help understand the underlying causes, behind those that are immediate and

obvious, and what could be done to prevent it re-occurring in the future.

Preventing mistakes

- Ensure standard operating procedures (SOPs) for the supply of medicines are in place, adhered to, evaluated and reviewed.

Consider the use of sensible safe practices, including the following:

- Ensure that one person is not responsible for all stages of processing prescriptions
- Ensure that medicines with similar sounding names or with similar company livery are not placed next to each other
- Separate different strengths of medicines from one another by placing another medicine between the two different strengths.

Recording and reporting medication errors

The document 'Building a safer NHS for patients' (DH 2004) suggested that to create a safer environment for patients, healthcare professionals needed to be more active in how they manage risk, including how pharmacy deals with errors.

Under the Pharmacy Contractual Framework, it is now a requirement to record medication errors, the level of which may depend upon the nature of the incident.

An error which has the potential for harm but does not actually reach the patient is termed a near-miss. The RPS created resources for recording these events and gives guidance on how teams working with pharmacies can review these logs for patterns and trends from which learning exercises can be made.

More significant events, especially where serious patient harm may have been caused, should be reported to the National Patient Safety Agency (NPSA) through its National Reporting and Learning System. Safety issues are collected and collated to allow analysis for the development of opportunities to reduce risk and improve patient care.

While all medication errors should be regarded as significant, the NPSA has provided definitions for grading patient safety incidents are shown in Box 9.2 (see also Examples 9.1 and 9.2).

Box 9.2

NPSA definitions for grading patient safety incidents

- No harm

  Incident prevented – any patient safety incident that had the potential to cause harm but was prevented, and no harm was caused to patients receiving NHS-funded care.

  Incident not prevented – any patient safety incident that occurred but no harm was caused to patients receiving NHS-funded care.
- Low harm

  Any patient safety incident that required extra observation or minor treatment and caused minimal harm to one or more patients receiving NHS-funded care. (Minor treatment includes first aid or additional therapy or medication)
- Moderate harm

  Any patient safety incident that resulted in a moderate increase in treatment and that caused significant but not permanent harm to one or more patients receiving NHS-funded care. (Moderate increase in treatment includes a return to the surgery or unplanned re-admission to hospital)
- Severe harm

  Any patient safety incident that appears to have resulted in permanent harm to one or more patients receiving NHS-funded care. (Permanent harm directly related to the incident and not related to the natural course of the patient's illness or underlying condition is defined as permanent lessening of bodily functions, sensory, motor, physiological or intellectual, including removal of the wrong limb or organ or brain damage)
- Death

  Any patient safety incident that directly resulted in the death of one or more patients receiving NHS-funded care. (The death must be related to the incident rather than to the natural course of the patient's illness or underlying condition)

 Example 9.1

You are a community pharmacist manager and you are asked to deal with a complaint from Mrs A.B. who claims she was supplied with the wrong medication for her mother yesterday. You establish that she was supplied with 28 amiodarone 100 mg tablets instead of 28 atenolol 100 mg tablets. What action should you take?

It is important to first of all establish whether or not the patient has taken any of the incorrect medication. If so, then you are best placed to use your knowledge of medicines to determine the risk to the patient. If there is any risk to the health of the patient then you must advise the patient to seek urgent medical attention. It may be necessary to telephone the A&E department in advance of the patient arriving to provide as many details as you can. It would also be good practice to telephone the patient's GP to inform them of the risk to the patient.

Mrs A.B. informs you that her mother did take one of the amiodarone tablets this morning.

You should advise her not to take any more and ask her to seek medical attention. You should then phone the patient's GP to discuss the incident. The Standards of conduct, ethics and performance require you to 'make the care of patients your first concern'. Once you have taken all reasonable steps to assure the patient's health and safety have been considered then it is important to apologise and offer to supply the correct medication. You should follow SOPs for recording and reporting errors.

How should you reflect on this incident and prevent it or similar errors from reoccurring?

Pharmacists and other healthcare professionals are only human and accordingly dispensing and prescribing errors do happen. What is important is to learn from them and take action to prevent this or other similar errors from occurring again. Good clinical governance involves auditing and reflecting on our own professional practice and when something goes wrong, taking action to improve systems and minimize risk.

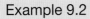

Example 9.2

You receive a letter from the PCO indicating that there is a member of the public purporting to be a medical practitioner who is contacting pharmacies in the area with a view to obtaining illegal supplies of prescription-only medicines (POMs) and controlled drugs (CDs). What action should you take now and what should you do if you find that you have supplied him with a medicine illegally?

Practising good clinical governance is not just about preventing mistakes from recurring, it is about auditing our policies and SOPs to ensure they protect the public and are robust enough to allow for all eventualities, including preventing medicines getting on to the black market.

In this case you should ensure that your SOP requires that all personal requests for prescription only medicines and controlled drugs by persons purporting to be medical practitioners, whether in person or by telephone, are dealt with personally by the responsible pharmacist and all early warning letters such as these are made available to all pharmacists practising from your pharmacy. It is essential that all unknown doctors are authenticated and if necessary confirmation verified by

a phone call to the medical practice and if necessary the General Medical Council.

While reviewing your procedures with the pharmacy assistants, a member of staff indicates that a doctor visited the pharmacy last Saturday requesting the purchase of a number of medicines. She informs you that the relief pharmacist dealt with the requests. You check the POM register but find no record of the sale of POM medicines to a GP last Saturday. What should you do now?

You must act on this information and assure yourself that POMs were not supplied illegally from the pharmacy. Although you were not the responsible pharmacist last Saturday you would be as culpable as the pharmacist who was if you later found out that the public was put at risk and you did nothing about it.

You should contact the pharmacist in charge on that day to ascertain the facts. If POMs or CDs were sold to a member of the public who was purporting to be a doctor then you must inform the police, the PCO, the superintendent pharmacist and the GPhC inspector. You should make a full record of the events that occurred and ask the relief pharmacist to do likewise.

KEY POINTS

- Clinical governance was introduced to improve the quality of care to patients
- The four main components are: lines of responsibility, programme of quality improvement, risk management policies and remedying poor performance
- Standards are set by NSFs
- Quality of care should be subject to clinical audit
- The 2005 contract for community pharmacists included clinical governance as an essential requirement

- During practice, pharmacists are subject to criminal, civil and administrative law
- Currently the GPhC has committees tasked with responsibility in these areas
- Mistakes will happen – how they are dealt with and learned from is important
- Errors or near misses should be recorded, reflected upon and shared with others. This process should be part of SOPs within the pharmacy
- When an error is made, the welfare of the patient is paramount

Risk management

10

Darren M. Ashcroft

STUDY POINTS

- The use of human error models to understand the causes of patient safety incidents
- Risk management techniques that can be used to understand the 'root causes' of an incident
- Some of the common risks in the pharmacy setting
- The National Patient Safety Agency's 'Seven Steps to Patient Safety'
- A structured approach to undertaking risk assessment in the pharmacy

Introduction

Risk – the probability that an adverse event will occur – is a normal part of daily life. We all continuously face risks and make decisions about them. Each day we decide when it is safe to cross the road and when it is more sensible to wait; we may choose to travel by car rather than walk. In these everyday choices, we assess the potential risks and benefits, and select a plan of action. Risk management is all about this process of anticipating potential hazards and reducing the likelihood of a problem occurring. However, before thinking about how to minimize or eliminate the possibility of errors, it is important to first consider how errors occur.

Human error models

Human error can be considered in two ways: the person approach and the systems approach. Traditionally, the person approach has been the dominant approach used in health care. This focuses on the errors of individuals, blaming them for forgetfulness, inattention, carelessness, negligence or recklessness. It has been widely acknowledged that blaming individuals does not encourage reporting and learning from errors, and the development of an effective risk management culture within healthcare settings depends critically on establishing an open reporting culture.

During the past decade, there has been increased interest to understand how management practices and other workplace factors impact on patient safety. The systems approach acknowledges that humans are imperfect and errors are to be expected, even in the best organizations. Rather than focusing on the individual, the systems approach concentrates on the conditions under which individuals work, trying to build defences to avoid errors or to mitigate their effects. James Reason (2000) classified medical errors into two types, *active* and *latent* failures, where active failures are unsafe acts (e.g. dispensing the wrong drug) committed by individuals who are at the 'sharp end' of health care, while latent failures are more distant from the actual incident and reflect failures in management or other organizational factors.

Active failures

Active failures take a variety of forms, such as slips, lapses, mistakes and procedural violations, as shown in Figure 10.1.

Slips occur when there has been a lack of attention, despite the fact that the individual has all the necessary skills to complete the task successfully. Lapses involve memory failures, such as forgetting

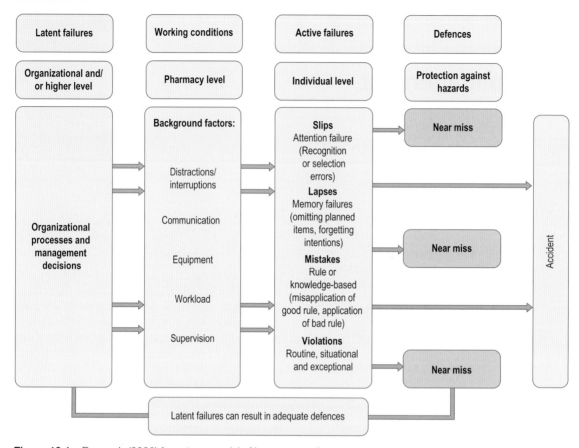

Figure 10.1 ● Reason's (2000) four-stage model of human error theory.

your intentions or omitting planned actions. In contrast, mistakes happen when we are in conscious control of the situation, but successfully execute the wrong plan of action. For instance, selecting the wrong plan can come about because of an incorrect assessment of the situation, such as arriving at the wrong diagnosis for an individual asking for an effective treatment for an 'upset stomach'.

Violations, on the other hand, involve deliberate deviations from the procedures or best way of performing a task, such as not following SOPs (see Ch. 11) within the pharmacy. Several types of violations have been described, which are outlined in Box 10.1.

Each of these error types (slips, lapses, mistakes, violations) requires different strategies to be implemented to avoid similar events occurring in the future. Better system defences, such as redesigning the workplace, can help to minimize slips and lapses. Improved training and rigorous checking procedures can prevent some mistakes. Developing relevant procedures and protocols,

ensuring effective implementation with the provision of the necessary resources and support are all important in promoting compliance and therefore avoiding procedural violations.

Box 10.1

Types of procedural violations

● *Optimizing violations* occur when skill and experience lead the individual to think that the rules do not apply to them
● *Routine violations* occur when it becomes accepted practice to break a rule within the organization
● *Situational violations* occur when the situation necessitates rule breaking, e.g. when there are not enough staff or there is not enough time to carry out all the required checks
● *Exceptional violations* arise when the rules that are in place are not able to deal with a novel situation

Latent failures

Latent failures are those whose adverse consequences may lie dormant, only becoming evident when they combine with other factors. These usually stem from poor decisions, made at a different time and place, by more senior members of the organization or people operating at a different level, such as the headquarters of a pharmacy chain. Latent failures have two kinds of adverse effect: they can lead to error and violation provoking conditions in the workplace (e.g. time pressures, understaffing, inadequate equipment, inexperience) or they can create weaknesses in the defences (e.g. unworkable procedures or design problems).

The investigation of many threats to patient safety has shown that there are usually multiple causes and they tend to occur when there is an unfortunate combination of active and latent failures. Reason (2000) proposed the 'Swiss cheese' model to illustrate how accidents can occur within systems. This analogy compares the defensive layers of the system to layers of Swiss cheese, each having holes that represent safety failures. The presence of holes in one slice may not result in an accident because the other slices act as safeguards. However, the holes in the layers may temporarily line-up, creating an opportunity for an accident. Figure 10.2 shows how multiple failures in the pharmacy setting can result in patient harm.

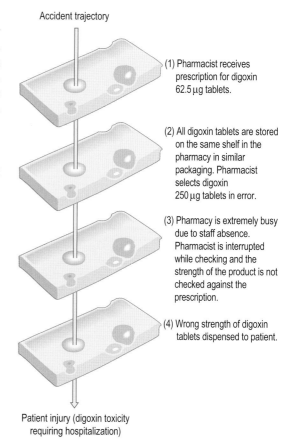

Accident trajectory

(1) Pharmacist receives prescription for digoxin 62.5 µg tablets.

(2) All digoxin tablets are stored on the same shelf in the pharmacy in similar packaging. Pharmacist selects digoxin 250 µg tablets in error.

(3) Pharmacy is extremely busy due to staff absence. Pharmacist is interrupted while checking and the strength of the product is not checked against the prescription.

(4) Wrong strength of digoxin tablets dispensed to patient.

Patient injury (digoxin toxicity requiring hospitalization)

Figure 10.2 • 'Swiss cheese' model showing how failures in the pharmacy can lead to patient harm.

Risk management tools

There are a number of useful techniques that can be used to help understand the underlying causes of adverse events and help identify actions that can be put in place to avoid similar events occurring in the future. For instance, root cause analysis (RCA) provides a framework to reflect on an actual or potential error, working back across the sequence of events. RCA aims to uncover the underlying, contributory and causal factors that resulted in an error, and also understand better the protective factors that may have prevented harm from occurring. It is important to include all those involved in the incident in order clearly to map out the chronology of events. The analysis is then used to identify areas for change and possible solutions, to help minimize the reoccurrence of the event in the future. Various methods can be used for RCA including the use of a 'fishbone diagram', in which each of the 'bones'

reflect different system failures, or the use of timelines where a chronological chain of events is mapped and tracked.

Failure modes and effects analysis (FMEA) is a systematic tool for evaluating a process and identifying where and how it might fail. It also assesses the relative impact of different types of failure and so prioritizes which areas need attention first. In addition, it can be used to assess the likelihood of the event reoccurring following changes to the system. The FMEA process involves:

- Mapping out the steps of the process through group discussion
- Identification of possible failure modes (what could go wrong?) by brainstorming
- For each error type or failure mode identified, a cause (why should failure happen?) and effect (what would be the consequences of each

failure?) are attributed, together with scores for likelihood of occurrence, likelihood of detection and severity.

Multiplication of these three scores generates a risk priority number (RPN), which can be used to prioritize changes within the pharmacy.

Risk to patients in the pharmacy setting

It is increasingly recognized that risks within healthcare organizations, including pharmacies, are diverse and complex, and not just confined to specific activities. An accurate estimate of the extent and causes of adverse events that originate from the pharmacy is difficult to obtain since different methods have been used to collect the data.

Research has, however, suggested that in the UK, for every 10 000 prescription items dispensed in community pharmacies, there are likely to be at least 26 dispensing incidents. Most threats do not result in actual patient harm, but have the potential to do so. The most common types of events include incorrect product selection (60%) and labelling errors (33%). Organizational factors are associated with the majority of these errors, including issues concerning distractions while assembling and checking prescriptions, poor communication, excessive workload and inadequate staffing.

Studies have also reported on practice variation in the way in which non-prescription medicines are sold and advice is communicated to patients in community pharmacies, suggesting that in some cases, pharmacy services may be deficient or suboptimal. Over the last decade, the Consumers' Association in the UK has repeatedly criticized deficiencies in the level of advice, questioning and referral of consumers to other healthcare professionals from community pharmacies.

It is also important to consider risks to pharmacy staff and customers through failures to comply with health and safety legislation. The Health and Safety at Work Act 1974 is the guiding piece of legislation placing responsibilities on employers and employees to carry out risk assessments. Pharmacies should have a health and safety policy in place, with responsibilities allocated to specific members of staff. Key areas of concern that are relevant to the pharmacy setting include having an effective procedures manual dealing with control of substances hazardous to health, fire precautions, workplace equipment, the pharmacy environment (such as unsafe furniture and fittings) and first aid.

Developments in health policy

In 2000, the Chief Medical Officer for England published *An organisation with a memory* (OWAM Report, DH 2000). This was a report of an expert group on learning from adverse events in the NHS, drawing on insights from human error and risk management as applied in other high-risk industries, such as aviation and nuclear power. The report presented international evidence on the scale and impact of adverse events and made reference to the lack of systems in the NHS that allowed there to be learning from adverse events. The expert group concluded that the NHS could benefit greatly by applying these risk management principles to health care.

The report also recommended as one of its four key targets, that there should be a 40% reduction in the number of serious errors involving prescribed drugs. In 2004, the Chief Pharmaceutical Officer for England published *Building a safer NHS for patients: improving medication safety* (DH 2004), which outlined strategies aimed at reducing the occurrence of prescribing, dispensing and administration errors drawing on experience and models of good practice within the NHS and worldwide.

More recent requirements, forming part of the essential services of the contractual framework for community pharmacy in England and Wales, has meant that SOPs covering the dispensing process need to be in place in pharmacies. In addition, all pharmacies should be able to demonstrate evidence of recording, reporting, monitoring, analysing and learning from patient safety incidents. Furthermore, pharmacists are now expected to be competent in risk management, including the application of root cause analysis (RCA).

National patient safety agency (NPSA)

Following the publication of the highly influential OWAM report, the NPSA was established in June 2001 to coordinate efforts to report and learn from patient safety incidents. The NPSA has published guidance for NHS organizations on the seven steps that they should take in order to improve patient safety (as described in Box 10.2). It is clear that risk management is firmly incorporated into this guidance.

Of particular interest, the NPSA has also published recommendations on the labelling and presentation of a dispensed medicine as well as suggestions on how to promote the safe use of medicines. In addition, it has also published recommendations on changes in the general dispensing environment that can improve patient safety.

The risk management process

The risk management process is about the planning, organization and development of a strategy that will identify, assess and ultimately minimize risk. The process can be represented by a sequence of steps but there is much overlap and often there is integration between all the steps.

Step 1: Establish the context

It is essential to identify all the legal and professional requirements for the pharmacy and to respond appropriately, since most of these will be needed for accreditation purposes or to satisfy

a risk insurer or commissioner of pharmaceutical services. For instance, pharmacies are routinely inspected by the regulatory body. Community pharmacies in England and Wales are also required to take part in monitoring visits from representatives of their commissioning body to check compliance with the community pharmacy controls assurance framework.

Step 2: Identification of risk

It is important to take into account things that have gone wrong in the past or near miss incidents that have previously occurred. Box 10.3 lists a variety of methods that can be used to identify risks in the pharmacy, and different approaches can be used in combination. Each method will identify different aspects about the frequency and nature of risks in the pharmacy.

Step 3: Analysis of risk

Once a risk has been identified, it should be analysed to determine what action needs to be taken. Ideally, the risk should be eliminated, but often this may not be possible and efforts need to be taken to minimize its potential impact. The use of rigorous risk management techniques such as RCA and FMEA can play an important role at this stage.

The following factors should be considered:

- The likelihood that an adverse event will occur
- Its potential impact (seriousness)
- The availability of methods to reduce the chance of the event happening
- The costs (financial and other) of solutions to minimize the occurrence of similar events in the future.

Box 10.2

Seven steps to patient safety

- *Build a safety culture* – create a culture that is open and fair
- *Lead and support staff* – establish a clear and strong focus on patient safety throughout the organization
- *Integrate risk management activity* – develop systems and processes to manage the risks and identify and assess things that could go wrong
- *Promote reporting* – ensure that staff can easily report incidents locally and nationally
- *Involve and communicate with patients and the public* – develop ways to communicate openly with and listen to patients
- *Learn and share safety lessons* – use root cause analysis to learn how and why incidents happen
- *Implement solutions to prevent harm* – embed lessons through practices, processes or systems

---

Box 10.3

Approaches that can be used to identify risks

- Direct observation of working practices within the pharmacy
- Incident reports of adverse events and near misses
- Interviews and questionnaires of patients and staff
- Complaints from patients, or other healthcare professionals
- Litigation and compensation claims

This will involve making decisions about risks that are rare but potentially very serious compared with risks that are very common but have a low probability of causing harm.

Step 4: Manage the risk

A range of choices is often available to manage the identified risks. The decision is largely determined by the financial cost of implementation balanced against the potential benefits (such as the cost of compensation if an adverse event occurred). The cost of preventing one major, but very rare, adverse event may be very great when compared with preventing hundreds of more minor adverse events.

Risk control

It may not be possible to eliminate all the identified risks, but preventative steps can be introduced that minimize the likelihood of an adverse event occurring.

Risk acceptance

This involves the recognition that the risk cannot be entirely removed, but at least it can be known and anticipated.

Risk avoidance

It may be possible to avoid the risk by understanding the causes of the risk and taking appropriate actions. An example is the recognition that company branding may result in different medications, such as digoxin tablets (see Fig. 10.2), being packaged in similar ways. This risk can be reduced by using different manufacturers so that different medications are clearly distinguishable.

Step 5: Auditing and reviewing performance

Finally, the effectiveness of the approaches used to identify, analyse and treat risks should be reviewed.

The role of audit is essential, in which risk management standards are set and monitored to see if the standards have been met. Following audit, the cycle of organizing, planning, measurement and review should reoccur to support continuous improvement within the pharmacy.

Conclusion

Risk management is an essential role for pharmacists to protect patients from harm. An understanding of human error models and risk management techniques can be used to analyse the possible risks in a working pharmacy environment and thus manage the risks.

KEY POINTS

- Risk is a normal part of daily life, but risk management attempts to minimize or eliminate risk
- Errors can be classified as active or latent
- Active failures are things like slips, lapses, mistakes and procedural violations by a pharmacist
- Latent failures often arise as a result of poor decisions by other, more senior people
- Techniques such as root cause analysis (RCA) are useful risk management tools
- A systematic tool such as failure modes and effects analysis (FMEA) has three main steps – mapping, identification and specifying cause and effect. Together they produce a risk priority number (RPN)
- Adoption of SOPs is a contractual requirement for community pharmacies
- Risk management processes have five essential stages: establish a context; identify the risks; analyse the risks; manage the risks; audit and review performance

Standard operating procedures

11

Alison Hunter

STUDY POINTS

- The reasons for standard operating procedures (SOPs)
- SOP requirements, adherence and review

Introduction

Standard operating procedures (SOPs) are written procedures or protocols to describe the way that tasks and activities within the pharmacy must be carried out. The NHS, and organizations contracted to them, must continually improve the quality of their services and ensure they are safeguarding the public by providing high standards of care. This is known as clinical governance (see Ch. 9). Every pharmacy must have an identifiable clinical governance lead, who is responsible for applying clinical governance principles to the delivery of all services. This will include the use of SOPs; recording, reporting and learning from incidents; participation in clinical audit and continuing professional development (CPD, see Ch. 6); and assessing patient satisfaction through surveys. Therefore, within clinical governance, SOPs are a legal requirement of the community pharmacy contract and of hospitals in England, Scotland, Wales and Northern Ireland, to ensure a high quality of service and patient safety.

Background to SOPs

In January 2005, it became a requirement for pharmacists to establish and operate within SOPs.

These SOPs were to be used in both hospital and community to cover the dispensing processes, including all the tasks that take place from the time that prescriptions are received in the pharmacy until the items are transferred to the patient.

In England, Wales and Northern Ireland, these requirements currently sit within essential services under clinical governance for core pharmacy activities. SOPs should, also, be produced to cover all advanced and enhanced services. In Scotland, SOPs are required within each element of the four core services and any local services. In hospitals, SOPs are the responsibility of the local trust.

It was recognized that there is a great deal of variance between each pharmacy, therefore no specific set of SOPs could be developed to cover all pharmacies. Each pharmacy can have individual SOPs, although larger companies may have a single SOP for each activity that covers all of their premises.

Regulations

The standards for owners and superintendent pharmacists of retail pharmacy businesses, published by the GPhC, specifies that SOPs should be in place for all aspects of the safe and effective provision of pharmacy services and that they must be maintained and regularly reviewed. Procedures must respect and protect confidential information about patients and employees in accordance with current legislation, relevant codes of practice and professional guidelines. The Pharmaceutical Society of Northern Ireland requires SOPs for dispensing services that the pharmacist provides or is responsible for.

Responsible pharmacists in the UK must ensure that pharmacy procedures are established (where not already established) and SOPs are in place, to ensure the safe and effective running of the pharmacy. These procedures need to be maintained and regularly reviewed.

Reducing risk to patient safety

Set up as part of the process of assuring clinical governance, SOPs should be designed to reduce risk and the chance of harm to patients. They should allow for continuing improvement to the standards of service offered to the public. Pharmacists should be able to ensure that their teams are working consistently to the safest method possible. SOPs should enable pharmacists to delegate and therefore, fully use the expertise of all pharmacy team members. The qualifications and capabilities of individual members of staff will determine the extent to which individual tasks can be delegated. This may in turn create efficiencies to free up time for other tasks and for talking to patients about their care. SOPs will also help to advise locums and new members of the pharmacy team where guidance is needed, which will reduce the chance of mistakes happening.

Content of the SOP

SOPs should be pharmacy specific and will always be dependent on the level of competence of the team members working in the pharmacy. A set of SOPs will be required even where no dispensary support staff are employed and the pharmacist is working single-handedly. The SOPs should cover all aspects of the dispensing process from receiving the prescription to transfer of products to the patient, including delivery. Patient confidentiality must be maintained at all times. SOPs can be drafted in many different formats, e.g. detailed information, algorithm-based or bulleted points.

SOPs should include:

- The date of preparation
- A full and clear description of each part of the process and how it should be carried out
- Activities that must be carried out by the pharmacist
- Activities that can be delegated to identified and competent support staff

- Any contingency plans, where appropriate, to specify any changes to the SOP in the event of any situation that leads to reduced staffing levels
- Other useful information including, e.g. the auditing of the SOP or references to any documents or computer-based information
- How and when the SOP will be reviewed.

It is good practice to keep a record of those members of the team that have read the SOPs and been signed off as competent by the pharmacist. As new members join the team they should read the SOPs for the activities they will be undertaking as a priority. The pharmacist should always check with each team member after they have read the SOPs to ensure they have fully understood the procedure. By asking questions or observing the team member, they can confirm that they are satisfied that the procedure will be adhered to in day-to-day practice. Where the team member shows a lack of competence, further training must be given to ensure compliance. Similar arrangements should be made for any amended SOPs and it may provide a good opportunity to define roles within the team and is good for staff development.

Regular reviews must take place to ensure that SOPs are current and relevant to the practice in the pharmacy. These reviews should take place regularly to allow for changes to practice or circumstances. These changes may be due to a change in the premises or team members, or to external factors, e.g. changes to legislation or new services. In the absence of any obvious changes, these reviews should take place at least once every 2 years.

Non-conformance

Once SOPs are in place, there may be circumstances where it is necessary to work outside of an established SOP, either by changing the process or by asking a member of the team with different qualifications to complete the activity. A responsible pharmacist must always use professional judgement in these situations to minimize risk to the patient.

A responsible pharmacist should always be aware that any amendments to a SOP may introduce risk and all team members must be made aware of the necessary changes.

An example of this could be where a pharmacist decides to allow an untrained counter assistant to put the dispensary delivery to shelf on a day they are low on staff. Although the counter assistant is

Process steps	Responsible	Additional Points
1. Greet the patient and ask them for the name of the patient whose prescription is being collected. 2. Locate the prescription and collect any additional items such as fridge lines or controlled drugs (CDs). 3. Ask the patient for the address and check the prescription and the bag of medication to confirm the name and address on the prescription. Do not give the address for them to confirm as this may lead to the patient receiving the wrong medication or a breach of patient confidentiality. 4. For CD items follow the CD SOP and record all the information in the CD register. 5. For insulin items confirm that the item dispensed is the insulin that the patient is expecting. 6. Inform the patient/representative of any owed or part-supplied items. Hand over any notes and follow the relevant SOP. Take a telephone number in case there are any issues with the owed medication. 7. Check that the back of the prescription has been correctly completed and take any payments. 8. Relay any counselling points from the pharmacist to the patient/representative and ask if they have any questions about the medication. 9. Refer to the pharmacist if you are unable to provide the required further information. 10. Hand over the bagged prescription items 11. File the prescription	Pharmacist/ Dispenser/ Technician/ Healthcare assistant	Where a representative collects a CD it is good practice to request some identification.

Accountable signature	Date:	Date review due:
M. A. Matn	2 Feb. 2013	2 Feb 2015

Figure 11.1 • Handing out of dispensed medicines to the patient or patient's representative.

not named on the SOP, due to the lack of time the pharmacist allows the counter assistant to put the stock away without any training or reading the SOP. The counter assistant does not realize the difference between different drugs and strengths, and the medicines with similar packaging become mixed on the shelves. As the staff are busy in the pharmacy, the dispenser selects the wrong medication and the error is missed in the final check. The patient takes the medication and it causes harm. This is just one example of how non-compliance with SOPs can introduce significant risk to the patient.

Where possible, contingency plans should be written in to the SOP to ensure the safest alternative is always used. On those occasions where it is necessary and appropriate to amend a procedure, it is good practice to record the incident. These amendments can then be used during the audit to review the SOP.

Examples of SOPs

How to dispense a prescription in both a community and hospital setting can be split into a number of stages:

1. Receiving the prescription
2. Clinical and legal checking
3. Interventions and problem-solving
4. Labelling and assembly of the product(s)
5. Accuracy checking
6. Transferring the prescription item(s) to the patient or their representative
7. Dealing with 'owings', where the full amount of medication prescribed is not in stock and cannot be supplied, and any procedures to be followed during the second dispensing.

Each stage will need a separate SOP and individual issues within the stages may need a separate SOP, e.g. the supply of 'specials', dealing with queries from another healthcare professional or additional safety guidance for high-risk medicines.

Figure 11.1 contains an example of an SOP for handing out dispensed medications to the patient or their representative, variations of which could be used in both hospital and community settings.

SOPs, in just a few years since their introduction, have become an integral part of pharmacy practice.

KEY POINTS

- SOPs are written procedures or protocols to describe the way that all tasks and activities within the pharmacy must be carried out
- SOPs are a requirement in both hospital and community pharmacy to ensure the safe and effective provision of pharmacy services
- SOPs should be pharmacy specific and will always be dependent on the level of competence of the team members working in the pharmacy
- Regular reviews must take place to ensure that SOPs are current and relevant to the practice in the pharmacy

Audit

Janet Krska

- Audit as part of clinical governance
- The relationship between practice research, service evaluation and audit
- Types of audit
- Structures, processes and outcomes which may be audited
- The stages in the audit cycle: standard setting, data collection, comparison with standards, identifying problems, implementing change, re-audit
- Learning from audit

Introduction: what is audit?

Audit concerns the quality of professional activities and services. Audit is carried out to determine whether best practice is being delivered and, equally importantly, to improve practice. Audit is part of clinical governance (see Ch. 9) – probably the key part – therefore it forms part of the quality improvement work which takes place within all NHS organizations. It can be described as 'improving the care of patients by looking at what you do, learning from it and if necessary, changing practice'. In England, quality improvement is now part of the QIPP agenda: Quality, Innovation, Productivity and Prevention, which is a major programme of work, aiming to transform the NHS; improving quality of care and making efficiency savings.

Audit is based around standards of practice. The hallmark of a professional is that they maintain standards of professional practice, which exist to protect the public from poor-quality services.

Audit provides a method of accountability, both to the public and to the regulator, which demonstrates that standards are being met or, if not, that action is being taken to remedy the situation. It also provides managers with information about the quality of the services their staff deliver. Although this may seem somewhat threatening, ultimately the aim of audit is to improve the efficiency and effectiveness of services, to promote higher standards and to improve the outcome for patients. It also allows changes in practice to be evaluated. Therefore it is an essential component of any professional's work and an integral part of day-to-day practice.

Most healthcare professionals' activities have an impact on patients, either directly or indirectly, so can be described as a clinical service. Audit of these services is therefore clinical audit. Clinical audit is defined by NICE as 'a quality improvement process that seeks to improve patient care and outcomes through systematic review of care against explicit criteria and the implementation of change'. All NHS trusts in the UK must support audit, so should have a central audit office which provides training and help in designing audits and collates the results of clinical audits. All NHS staff are expected to participate in clinical audit and the GPhC requires pharmacists to organize regular audits to protect patient and public safety and to improve professional services pharmacies. Community pharmacists in England must participate in two clinical audits each year, one based on their own practice and one multidisciplinary audit organized by their local primary care organization. Hospital pharmacists are required to be involved in clinical audits of Trust performance in areas of national priority.

There are few instances where pharmacists provide a clinical service to patients in isolation from other healthcare professionals. Providing advice and selling non-prescription medicines are examples of services which could be audited to comply with the requirement. Many services will impact on or be affected by services provided by other professionals, so can be regarded as multidisciplinary. Audit of these clinical services should ideally also be multidisciplinary. Users of services should also be involved in audit whenever possible, perhaps by asking patient representatives to join the audit team. They can provide important insight into what aspects of a service would benefit from audit and can help to set the criteria against which performance will be audited.

Relationship between practice research, service evaluation and audit

It is important to understand the relationship between practice research, service evaluation and audit. Practice research is designed to determine best practice. An example of this would be a randomized controlled trial of pharmacists undertaking a new service compared with normal care. In a controlled trial, patients are often carefully selected, using inclusion and exclusion criteria, special documentation and outcome measures are used, which may differ from those used in routine practice and all aspects of the service being studied must be standardized.

To implement a new service into routine practice, further development will be required. Many aspects of a new service are likely to differ from those used in a research situation and may differ between practice settings. All new services will then need to be evaluated, which may involve determining the views of service providers and users, collecting data on the outcomes for patients who use the service and finding out if publicity is adequate. Changes may be necessary if problems are identified during service evaluation.

Once a service is running smoothly it should then be subject to audit. This will involve setting standards for the service and measuring actual practice against these standards.

Although there are many similarities in the methods used to obtain data for research and for audit, there are important differences. In research, it is important to have controlled studies, to be able to extrapolate the results and to have large enough samples to demonstrate statistical significance of any differences between groups. None of these applies to audit. Audit compares actual practice to a predetermined level of best practice, not to a control. The results of audit apply to a particular situation and should not be extrapolated. Audit can be even applied to a single case; large numbers are not required and so the number included in an audit should be practical, to ensure resources are not wasted in carrying it out.

Types of audit

Audit may be of three types, depending on who undertakes it. These are:

- Self-audit
- Peer or group audit
- External audit.

Self-audit is undertaken by individuals and is part of a professional work attitude in which critical appraisal of actions taken and outcomes is continuous. While anyone can do self-audit, it is most likely to be used by pharmacists who work in isolation, such as in single-handed community pharmacies. There are many areas where self-audit can be conducted, e.g. smoking cessation services, owing and out of stock items and waste medicines.

Peer audit is undertaken by people within the same peer group, which usually means the same profession. Peer audit involves joint setting of standards by an audit team. For example, pharmacists from several hospitals which provide similar services could get together and audit each other's service. Another way of doing this is benchmarking – a process of defining a level of care set as a goal to be attained. Here, standards may be set against those identified by a leading centre, such as a teaching hospital. Benchmarking in prescribing may involve the use of prescribing indicators (see Ch. 22) or comparators. A wide range of these has been developed to benchmark or audit good prescribing practice, available from the QIPP section of the DH website.

External audit is carried out by people other than those actually providing the service and so is perceived as threatening by those whose services are being audited. It may be more objective in its

Table 12.1 Audit example: Dementia care in hospitals, conducted as part of the National Clinical Audit and Patient Outcomes Programme

Aspect of service	Structure/ process/ outcome	Data collection method
Service structures, policies, care processes and key staff providing services for people with dementia	Structures, processes	Checklist
Medical records of patients with dementia, audited against a checklist of standards covering admission, assessment, care planning/delivery and discharge	Processes	Retrospective case note review, using data collection form
Staffing, support and governance	Structures, processes	Checklist
Physical environment known to impact on people with dementia	Structures	Checklist
Staff awareness of dementia and support offered to patients with dementia	Structures, processes	Questionnaire to staff
Carers'/patients' experience of the support received and perceptions of the quality of care	Outcomes	Questionnaire to carers/patients
Quality of care provided to people with dementia	Processes	Data collection through direct observation

Audit standards were derived from: national reports, guidelines, recommendations of professional bodies and service user/carer organizations. Adapted from report available at: http://www.hqip.org.uk/national-audit-of-dementia.

criticisms than self or peer audit, but there may be less enthusiasm for corrective action to improve services. If standards are imposed, there is a perceived threat if an individual's performance is not of the standard required. Involving the providers of services to be audited in deciding what best practice should be and in making improvements makes external audit more acceptable. Multidisciplinary audit is the most common type of group audit and is usually preferred for clinical audit, but it is essential to ensure that one subgroup is not auditing the activities of another subgroup. This would lead to tensions and be counterproductive. For example, in an audit of doctors' prescribing errors detected by pharmacists, pharmacists cannot set the standard for an acceptable level of errors without involving the doctors. If they are not part of the audit team, there is little chance of improvement. Pharmacists are often involved in carrying out audits of clinical practice, for example audit of prescribing against NICE clinical guidelines. NICE produces tools for clinical audit, baseline assessment and self-assessment to help organizations implement NICE guidance and audit their own practice. Pharmacists should work with prescribers in setting local standards for these audits.

In England, a National Clinical Audit and Patient Outcomes Programme, managed by the Healthcare Quality Improvement Partnership, enables national clinical audits to take place. Data are collected locally and pooled, but also fed back to individual Trusts, so that they can identify necessary improvements for patients. Pharmacists may be involved in collecting data for such audits. An example is shown in Table 12.1. This is an example of a clinical audit, for which data were collected from many centres and which has the potential to change practice.

What is measured in audit?

There are three aspects of any services and activities which can be audited. These are:

- The structures or resources involved
- The processes used
- The outcomes of the activity.

Structures are the resources available to help deliver services or carry out activities. Examples are staff, their expertise and knowledge, books, learning materials or training courses, drug stocks, equipment, layout of premises.

Processes are the systems and procedures which take place when carrying out an activity and may include quality assurance procedures and policies and protocols of all types. Examples are: procedures for dealing with patients' own medicines in hospital, prescribing policies and disease management protocols.

Outcomes are the results of the activity and are arguably the most important aspect. In pharmaceutical audits of activities such as drug procurement, distribution or dispensing, outcomes should be easily identified and measurable. In many clinical audits, some outcomes are relatively easily measured, e.g. changes in parameters such as blood pressure, INR (international normalized ratio) control and serum biochemistry. Surrogate outcomes can also be used, such as the drugs or doses prescribed or patient perceptions of service quality. Outcomes such as health status, attitude or behaviour can also be included, but changes may be very difficult to achieve and to measure.

Any individual audit can examine structures, processes and outcomes individually or together. (See Table 12.1 for an example which involved all three aspects.)

The audit cycle

Audit is a continuous process, which follows a cycle of measurement, evaluation and improvement. The basic cycle is shown in Figure 12.1, but audit can also be seen as a spiral in which standards are continuously raised as practice improves.

Before starting an audit, first identify its purpose. This will derive from the desire to improve the quality of the service. For example, the purpose may be 'to improve the dispensing turnaround time' or 'to increase the proportion of patients counselled about their new medicines'. It may be appropriate to conduct a 'baseline assessment' to find out if indeed there is a need to improve service quality through audit. This means conducting a small study before setting standards. Once you decide audit is needed the audit cycle incorporates:

- Setting standards for practice
- Measuring actual practice
- Comparing the two
- Finding out why best practice is not being achieved
- Changing aspects of practice to improve performance.

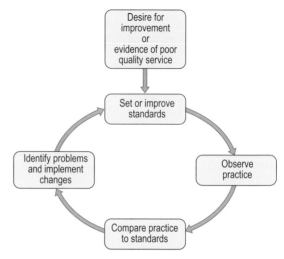

Figure 12.1 • The audit cycle.

Although the process is continuous, it is not practicable to audit all activities or services all the time. A baseline assessment helps to decide whether improvements are possible and routine monitoring may be instituted instead of repeat audits to ensure that best practice, once attained, is maintained.

Setting standards

All audits should be based on standards which are widely accepted (i.e. best practice). Examples of useful documents for helping to set standards are the Medicines, Ethics and Practice guide, national service frameworks and clinical guidelines. Several standards are usually set for any individual audit, relating to resources, processes or outcomes.

Because audit is about comparing actual practice to standards of best practice, numerical values are needed. A guideline may suggest a criterion, for example that patients receiving warfarin should be counselled about avoiding aspirin. For this to form a useful standard for audit, it needs to be clarified whether this applies to all patients, i.e. 100%. This numerical value is the target, which, together with the criterion, forms the standard or 'level of performance'. It is then easy to measure whether this occurs in practice. Many clinical guidelines suggest audit standards and criteria.

A target level of 100% is termed an ideal standard but may not be achievable. The level set may need to be a compromise between what is desirable and what is possible, since resources may be limited. This would be an optimal standard. Using the previous example, it may be considered at the outset that there are insufficient staff to ensure that 100% of patients receiving warfarin could be counselled about avoiding aspirin. A compromise could be that 100% of patients prescribed warfarin for the first time receive this advice. Another type of standard is the minimal standard, which, as its name implies, is the minimum acceptable level of service and is often used in external audits.

If there are no published guidelines or standards, they will need to be devised. This may involve searching the literature, for example recent journals, textbooks or educational material. Whether devising standards from scratch or making guidelines into standards, it is important that the whole audit team is involved in devising them. This may include doctors, nurses, health visitors, technical staff, receptionists or porters, and patients or their carers. Inclusion avoids the potential feeling of threat which may be created by audit. Once standards have been set, the next stage of audit involves collecting data on actual practice.

Observing practice

Many audits require a simple form onto which data from other sources are transferred. Checklists are often most useful for auditing structures and processes but other types of data may also be needed, while auditing outcomes may require methods such as questionnaires (see Table 12.1). As with any data collection, the information obtained must be able to answer the questions asked, which may be relatively simple, such as 'What percentage of patients receiving warfarin are counselled?'

It is often useful to incorporate some measure of potential factors which may influence practice within the data collection. So, in addition to finding out whether local guidelines are being used by examining medical records, it is worth issuing a questionnaire to those expected to use the guidelines to find out their views on whether the guidelines are readily available, are in an acceptable format and meet their needs. In an audit of warfarin counselling, it is useful to collect data on how busy the pharmacy is when each patient presents their prescription and how many staff trained to provide advice were available. This may mean that the data collection procedures may need to

anticipate some potential causes of failing to provide best practice.

Before setting out to devise a data collection form, it is always worth finding out whether a similar audit has been done before, so you can adapt or modify the data collection procedures used. (See NICE or RPS websites for examples of audit documents.) If you do need to design a new procedure, the data collection must fulfil some basic requirements (Box 12.1). First the data collected must be able to address the purpose of the audit. The method of data collection must be valid and reliable. If sampling procedures are used, they too must be appropriate, avoiding bias and must be feasible.

Validity is the extent to which what is measured is what is supposed to be measured. To use the warfarin counselling example, the standard was about advice concerning aspirin. If the only data collected involved the number of patients who were counselled and not what advice they were given about aspirin, these data would be invalid, since they did not measure what they set out to measure.

Reliability is a measure of the reproducibility of the data collection procedure. It can be difficult to achieve reliability in measuring outcomes, so it is important to use recognized measures wherever possible. Reliability may also vary among individuals collecting data, despite their using the same data collection tool. It is important to check this, provide training if necessary and ensure everyone understands what is required.

Sampling is important in collecting data for audit, because the data should be unbiased and representative of actual practice. It may be that the numbers and time involved are small enough that

Box 12.1

Requirements for data collection procedures

- Provide information required
- Validity
- Reliability
- Controlled for bias
- Adequate sampling technique
- Feasible
- Quantitative or qualitative
- Retrospective or prospective
- Routinely or specially collected
- Pilot study.

all examples of the activity are included in data collection procedures. If numbers are large, it may be necessary to include a proportion in the audit. If so, a sampling plan is needed to ensure cases selected are representative. Many different sampling methods could be used, including random (using number tables or computer) or systematic (such as every tenth patient presenting a prescription for warfarin). Another way is to decide in advance that a certain proportion of the total population (a quota) will be sampled, usually ensuring that they will be typical of the population in important characteristics. These techniques require that the total population size within the audit period is known. A large population may need to be stratified into subgroups first before sampling, for example patients with new prescriptions and patients with repeats.

Since audit is about a particular service or activity, carried out by one or more particular individual professionals, the audit needs to strike a balance between having enough in the sample and not taking too much time. It must be possible, i.e. feasible, to collect the data required to answer the question. It is often necessary to incorporate data collection for audit into routine work, so the time needs to be minimized. Some data for use in audit may already be collected on a routine basis, e.g. data on PMRs or from MUR records. Some pharmacies routinely log the time when prescriptions are handed in and given out, so an audit of turnaround time could easily be carried out using these data. Routinely-collected hospital data on length of stay and number of admissions, discharges and deaths, may be useful.

Data for audit can be either quantitative or qualitative. Qualitative data can be useful in obtaining opinions about services or for assessing patient outcomes and large numbers are not required. It may be useful to undertake qualitative work to help design a good data collection tool to be used quantitatively, such as a questionnaire targeting larger numbers. Quantitative audit may generate large amounts of data, which require subsequent analysis. Usually only simple descriptive or simple comparative statistics are needed.

Whether the data collected are retrospective or prospective depends to a large extent on the topic of the audit and the data available. Retrospective audit can only be undertaken if good records of activities have been kept. Prospective audits should ensure that the data required are recorded, even if only for the audit period. There is a possibility of practice changing during the audit period simply because the audit is being undertaken. This may not always be a problem if practice is better than usual and if audit is continuous, since the ultimate aim is to improve services. It is more important to be aware of this effect if practice is measured periodically.

In large audits, piloting the data collection tool using a sample similar to those to be included in the audit is a valuable way of finding out if it is suitable. This should avoid discovering too late that there were difficulties in interpretation or that vital information has not been recorded.

Comparing practice to standards

This is the evaluation stage of audit, in which actual practice is compared to best practice. First the data obtained must be analysed and presented. Most audit data require only descriptive analysis, such as percentages, means or medians, along with ranges and standard deviations to show the spread of the data. Comparative statistical tests are useful for looking at one or more subgroups of quantitative data. This could be for different data collection periods (audit cycles) or for subgroups within one audit. Examples where comparison may be useful are three different pharmacies' prescription turnaround times or the counselling frequencies for patients presenting prescriptions for warfarin for the first time compared to those who have taken it before. The statistical test must be appropriate for the type of data. Chi-square is used for non-parametric data, such as frequencies. For parametric data which are normally distributed, t-tests can be used. When using statistics, it is important to consider the practical significance of the data. An improvement which is statistically significant may not always be of practical significance and vice-versa.

Results should be presented to the team or to those involved in collecting audit data, using simple graphics, such as pie charts or bar charts. Data collected for audit purposes relate to the activities of individual professionals and to their effects on patients. It is therefore essential to maintain confidentiality. Permission is required before any information about one individual's practice is given to other members of the audit team. Managers who may need this sort of information should be part of the audit team. In presenting audit results therefore, it is important to ensure that no individual practitioner or patient can be identified. This is essential if the audit is to improve services, as it will help others to learn and allow comparisons to be made.

When comparing the results of audits between centres, there will most probably be differences – perhaps in staffing levels, population served, case mix and so on – which could account for differences in apparent performance. Any unusual situations which occurred during the audit and which may have affected performance should be highlighted. Also any errors in data collection must be identified, which may mean data have to be excluded from analysis as they could be unrepresentative of what should have happened. It is most important to remember that the results of any audit should not be extrapolated beyond the sample audited. Audit applies to a particular activity, carried out by particular individuals and involving particular patients.

Providing the standards for the audit have been set appropriately, it should be relatively easy to determine whether they have been achieved. Often the most difficult part of audit is finding out why best practice is not being delivered and ensuring that improvement occurs.

Identifying problems

It is little use simply finding out that a service fails to meet an agreed standard. The underlying causes of failure need to be established and the data collection procedures should have attempted to identify some of these. Suboptimal practice can arise for a variety of reasons, such as inadequate skills or knowledge, poor systems of work or the behaviour of individuals within a team. Each should be examined as a possible contributory factor to disappointing results of an audit. Simple lack of awareness, e.g. about local clinical guidelines can contribute to their lack of use. Lack of skill may be related to infrequency of carrying out a particular activity or need for training. Both are relatively easily remedied. Both behaviour and the way in which work is organized are more difficult to change. The strategies adopted for effecting change will need to differ depending on which of these underlying causes is present.

Implementing changes

Achieving improvement in practice requires a change in behaviour. Change can be threatening simply because of its novelty. It may also involve increased work and is often resisted. This is why everyone whose work pattern may need to change should be active members of the audit team from the start. Change must be seen as leading to improvement in performance and ultimately patient benefit. The changes proposed to improve practice must be closely tailored to the underlying cause of the suboptimal audit results. They should be specific to the situation which has been audited, rather than general. They should be non-threatening and may need to be introduced gradually. Change may require resources, including time. It may also have other knock-on effects which need to be anticipated. The effect of changes must be monitored, to see whether they have been successful. This can be done by re-audit or by continuous monitoring if routinely collected data can be used.

Re-audit

Sometimes it may be appropriate to reconsider the standards before undertaking a further period of data collection.

Standards which were set too high may always be unattainable, although this may not have been apparent before practice was measured. It is equally possible to have used low standards and to have found they were exceeded. In this case it may be appropriate to raise them, which is a good way of improving practice. Whether or not the standards remain the same, a second period of measuring practice is needed if changes have been implemented, so that the effectiveness of these changes can be determined.

It is always difficult to change behaviour and improvements in practice may be short-lived. It may therefore be necessary to repeat audits at regular intervals to reinforce the desired practice and maintain the improvement in service.

Learning through audit

If the prevailing view of an audit which shows performance to be less than the standard set is that there are lots of reasons which could excuse this result, then little has been learned from undertaking the audit. Evaluating your service may be difficult, but it may also teach you a lot about yourself and the staff with whom you work. For example, it is of little use to suggest that the reason there were so many dispensing errors during the audit was that there was a new locum employed for part of the time. It is much more valuable to consider what information you have available for locums about your dispensing procedures and indeed whether your dispensing procedures are adequate.

If the results of an audit were suboptimal, but much as expected, is this because staff have been willing to accept poor practice in the past? Have staff been aware of the need for improvements in systems but felt unable to suggest changes? Have staff been wanting more training but known that there is no money available to pay for it? All these are hypothetical situations, but help to illustrate how conducting audit may have more learning than just what needs to be done to improve services. In this way, carrying out audit can contribute to continuing professional development and so has benefits both for you and, ultimately, for the patient.

KEY POINTS

- Pharmacists need to audit their practice to show that they meet appropriate standards
- The main aim of audit must be to improve standards of service and outcomes for patients
- There are similarities and differences between audit, service evaluation and practice research
- The three main types of audit are self-, peer and external audit
- An audit may examine structures, processes or outcomes
- Criteria should be formulated into standards for audit which may be ideal, optimal or minimal
- Standard setting should involve at least all those involved in delivering the service being audited
- Data collection must address the purpose of the audit and have the potential to identify reasons for failure to meet the standard
- Sampling must ensure that the data collected in an audit are representative of the total activity
- Piloting the data collection tool ensures that it is suitable and comprehensive
- Comparison with standards will normally involve very simple descriptive or statistical analysis
- Confidentiality must be respected, but outcomes should be shared with all the audit team
- Implementing change is a key part of audit
- Re-audit tests whether changes have led to improved achievement of standards

Public health

13

Simon White

STUDY POINTS

- The principles of public health
- The concept of public health pharmacy
- The determinants of health and lifestyle influences on health
- How pharmacists can be involved in public health pharmacy

Introduction

While pharmacists have increasingly received wide recognition for their considerable knowledge, skills and expertise in working with patients to resolve medicines-related issues, they appear to have struggled with the concept of contributing to the wider public health agenda. This is ironic, given that for many years pharmacists have addressed a range of public health issues by giving lifestyle advice, among other services, to the populations they serve on topics such as smoking cessation, diet, substance misuse, sexual health, alcohol and exercise.

However, in recent years, pharmacy has started to recognize its public health contribution, following the publication of key government strategies to develop public health pharmacy. Working with other agencies as part of a multidisciplinary team to address population-wide public health issues is a relatively new challenge that requires additional knowledge and skills, but this has provided new opportunities for pharmacists to become involved in developing and delivering new initiatives to promote healthy living. This chapter will help the reader to understand better the principles of public

health and the partnerships required to deliver the public health agenda and identify what the pharmacist can contribute.

What is public health pharmacy?

There are many definitions of public health in common use but perhaps the one most widely used in the UK is:

> The science and art of preventing disease, prolonging life and promoting health through the organized efforts and informed choices of society
>
> (Acheson 1998).

Central to this definition is the concept that promoting public health is not solely an application of evidence-based science, such as epidemiology. For those working in public health, there is also a need to understand different sociological groupings within society and work with others to support and encourage the population or particular sectors of society to make changes that are likely to bring health benefits. To achieve this, those employed in public health typically work across organizations such as local health service bodies, local authorities and local communities in settings that range from acute hospital trusts and local health organizations to local authorities, social services and the voluntary sector. Much of the work is long term and it may take several years before any outcomes materialize that can have a lasting impact on health. Indeed, this could be viewed as being a 'health service', in contrast to the current healthcare system that may more closely resemble an 'ill health service'. This is because resources are used to encourage people to adopt a healthy lifestyle and protect them from communicable diseases, rather than being primarily targeted at people who are ill.

As a corollary to the definition of public health presented above, public health pharmacy can be defined as:

> The informed application of pharmaceutical knowledge, skills and resources to promote public health
>
> (Walker 2000).

This definition reflects a pragmatic approach to public health pharmacy and has proved useful to help understand what pharmacy can contribute, but it has mis-led some to believe that public health pharmacy is a discipline in its own right. Rather, public health requires a multidisciplinary team approach and pharmacy is only one of the contributors, often with a strong focus on medicines-related issues.

Pharmacy should always be in a position to make an impact on public health, even if it restricts its contribution to medicines-related issues. However, to make an optimal contribution to public health, pharmacy needs to also influence the wider determinants of health. This is more challenging and requires an appreciation that more than 70% of the factors that determine a person's health lie outside of the domain of health services and instead in their demographic, social, economic and environmental conditions. For example, there is limited opportunity to help a patient with asthma improve their health by advising them on the correct use of their inhaler when wider public health issues also influence treatment outcome. The patient may live in poorly heated, damp, infested accommodation, have a low paid job that involves working in a dusty or dirty environment, be poorly educated, have few or no friends or family to support them and have poor mental health. In addition, they may continue to smoke cigarettes, take little exercise and eat too many foods with a high fat content. It is clear that these factors will impact on good disease management, but the influential factors are often much less obvious than described above. Being aware of the wider determinants of health is important, as each carries a significant health burden, many of which are linked to deprivation. A number of these are summarized in Table 13.1.

Table 13.1 Examples of indicators that have been shown to have a significant association with deprivation

Domain	Indicator	Increased deprivation significantly associated with indicator
Lifestyle health determinant	Smoking	Yes
	Excess alcohol consumption	No
	Diet	Yes
	Physical inactivity	Yes
Health status	Obesity	Yes
	Physical functioning	Yes
	Bodily pain	Yes
	General health	Yes
	Vitality	Yes
	Social functioning	Yes
	Role – emotional	Yes
	Mental health	Yes
	Low birth weight	Yes
Illness and injury	Depression and/or anxiety	Yes
	Hearing	Yes
	Eyesight	Yes
	Limiting long-term illness	Yes
	Arthritis	Yes
	Back pain	Yes
	Respiratory disease	Yes
	Asthma	Yes
	Diabetes	Yes
	High blood pressure	Yes
	Heart disease	Yes
	Angina	Yes
	Heart failure	No
	Cancer registrations	Yes
	Pedestrian injury 4–16 years reported to police	Yes
	Pedestrian injury 65+ years reported to police	Yes
	Pedestrian injury 5–14 years hospital inpatient	Yes

Table 13.1 (Continued)

Domain	Indicator	Increased deprivation significantly associated with indicator
Use of health service	Dentist	Yes
	Family doctor	Yes
	Hospital inpatient (persons)	Yes
	Coronary heart disease admission	Yes
	Angiography	Yes
	Revascularization	Yes
	Hip replacement	Yes
	Knee replacement	No
	Lens replacement	No
	Infant mortality	Yes
Deaths	All-cause persons	Yes
	All-cause females	Yes
	All-cause males	Yes
	All cancer	Yes
	Colorectal cancer	Yes
	Lung cancer	Yes
	Breast cancer	Yes
	Coronary heart disease	No
	Stroke	Yes
	Respiratory disease	Yes
	Unintentional injury	Yes
	Road traffic injury	Yes
	Unintentional fall	Yes
	Suicide	Yes

Wider determinants of health

Most measures of population health have shown marked improvement over the past 150 years. For example, life expectancy in England and Wales has improved in every decade since the 1840s. In 1841, life expectancy for males was 41 and this had increased to 78.7 years by 2011. The equivalent improvement for females was from 43 to 82.6 years of age. Much of the improvement seen has been the result of environmental and social changes rather than developments in medicine and health care. Despite these overall improvements, social inequalities have widened, with improvements in the health of the most disadvantaged groups being relatively small. To illustrate these inequalities, we can look at the life expectancy of those who live in the most and least deprived areas of our big cities. In Scotland, for example, people living in the most deprived districts of Glasgow have a life expectancy 12 years shorter than those in the most affluent areas. In London, boroughs a few miles apart have markedly different life expectancies. Each of the eight tube stations on the Jubilee line from Westminster to Canning Town represents a decline of one further additional year in life expectancy for the resident population.

The landmark work of Dahlgren and Whitehead in 1991 highlighted the main factors that determine the health of a given population (Fig. 13.1). The age, gender and genetic make-up of an individual clearly influence the health potential of that individual, although each is fixed and non-modifiable. Other factors that influence health and which can be modified to have a favourable impact include addressing individual lifestyle factors such as smoking, diet and physical activity. Improving interactions with friends and relatives, and developing mutual support within a community can help sustain health. Other wider influences on health include living and working conditions, food provision, access to essential goods and services, and the overall socioeconomic, cultural and environmental conditions. There are too many factors to discuss in detail here, but a number of the relevant, key determinants are outlined below. However, the simple message is that, whether attempting to evaluate mortality, morbidity or self-reported health, and regardless of whether it is income, class, house ownership, deprivation, social exclusion or a similar indicator or combination of indicators that is used as the socioeconomic indicator, those who are worse off in society have poorer health.

Employment and unemployment

Both employment and unemployment can be associated with adverse effects on health. Job security has

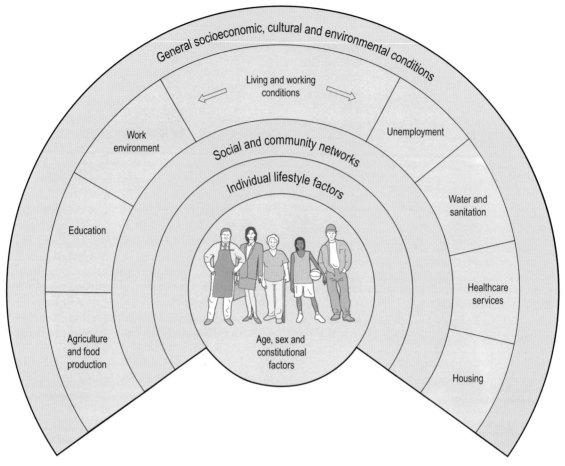

Figure 13.1 • Schematic model of the determinants of health (Dahlgren and Whitehead 1991).

also been recognized as important for well-being. The trend towards less secure, short-term employment affects everyone but is a particular problem for less skilled manual workers. Unemployment imposes a number of health burdens on the unemployed and some of these are summarized in Box 13.1.

In addition to job security, there is considerable evidence that greater control over work is associated with positive health such as lower coronary heart disease, fewer musculoskeletal disorders, reduced mental illness and less sickness absence. The relationship between status in the workforce and health has been demonstrated across the gradient from the top jobs to those at the bottom. The landmark studies with civil servants in Whitehall, London demonstrated that even those in the next grade down from the top had worse health than those in the top posts. Despite being in well paid

---

Box 13.1

Examples of the health burden on individuals who may be unemployed

- Increased smoking
- Increased alcohol consumption
- Reduced physical activity and exercise
- Increased use of illicit drugs
- Increased sexual risk-taking and sexually transmitted diseases
- Increased weight gain
- Reduced psychological well-being, e.g. self-harm, depression, anxiety
- Increased morbidity
- Increased premature mortality from diseases such as coronary heart disease
- Social exclusion and isolation

and relatively secure posts, a health gradient was observed across a range of disorders when compared to those in the top posts.

A confounding issue when trying to interpret the effect of unemployment on health is that people with poorer health are more likely to be unemployed. This is particularly true for people with long-term conditions, although this does not fully explain why the unemployed have poorer health.

Environment air quality

Some of the most enduring images of poor air quality are the photographs taken in the 1950s of London in dense smog. Pollution arising from the burning of domestic coal accounted for a significant number of premature deaths among Londoners. In the London smog of 1952 there was almost a three-fold increase in death in the over 65s, while deaths from bronchitis and emphysema rose 9.5-fold, pneumonia and influenza increased 4.1-fold and myocardial degeneration increased almost three-fold, along with associated increases in hospital admissions. Although the sulfur dioxide and black smoke from domestic coal is now a thing of the past, other pollutants have taken their place, notably from burning petrol and diesel in cars and other forms of transport. Ambient levels of air pollution continue to be associated with raised morbidity and mortality and are particularly hazardous to the elderly, children and those with pre-existing disease.

Crime

Crime affects not only the health of the victim but also that of the community involved. Fear of crime is a real phenomenon that impacts on both health and well-being. As a consequence of crime or the perception of crime, people make adjustments to their lifestyle and behaviour such as not going out after dark, not going out alone, avoiding certain areas, not using public transport and avoiding young people. Because crime is often concentrated in particular neighbourhoods and the avoidance measures outlined above are adopted, this can weaken social ties and undermine social cohesion in these neighbourhoods.

Energy and housing

It is recognized that energy obtained from fossil fuels must be reduced to meet international

Box 13.2

Examples of the health burden of poor housing

- Increased respiratory infections
- Increased cardiovascular morbidity (cold housing)
- Increased risk of infection due to overcrowding
- Increased risk of accidents due to faulty wiring, dangerous appliances, lack of smoke alarms, cluttered conditions
- Increased risk of infestation with rats and cockroaches and the associated health risks
- Increased risk of indoor pollutants, e.g. carbon monoxide, radon, lead

commitments on global warming and reduce their associated adverse impact on health. In many UK cities, the trend is for falling use by industry but increased use by transport.

Heating of houses must also become more energy efficient. Typically housing for low income families is the most inefficient with the use of electric fires at standard tariff prices costing three times more than gas central heating. There is a fuel poverty strategy in the UK which seeks to provide heating and insulation improvement for those who spend 10% or more of their income on heating their home. Cold homes exacerbate many existing illnesses such as asthma and make the individual prone to respiratory infections (Box 13.2). In addition, fuel poverty brings opportunity loss. Low income families spend a disproportionate amount of their income in keeping warm and this has an adverse effect on their social well-being, ability to adopt a healthy lifestyle and overall quality of life.

Lifestyle determinants of health

The individual lifestyle determinants of health represent the areas in which pharmacy has traditionally made its most significant contribution to public health (see Ch. 48). These continue to be key ways that pharmacies can promote healthy living. It is therefore important to appreciate that behaviours that can have an adverse impact on health may be associated with one or more of the wider determinants of health, especially social and economic disadvantage. For example, socially and economically disadvantaged people are less likely to eat a good diet and more likely to have a sedentary lifestyle, be obese and abuse alcohol. Cigarette smoking has one of the strongest associations with social disadvantage, with higher levels recorded in more deprived sectors of the population, and this in turn has the greatest cost in terms of premature death.

Smoking

Tobacco smoking remains one of the main avoidable causes of premature death in the UK, estimated as being responsible for more than 81 000 deaths among adults aged 35 and over in 2010 alone. Smoking causes a wide range of serious illnesses including cancer of the lung, respiratory tract, oesophagus, bladder, kidney, stomach and pancreas; respiratory disease, including chronic obstructive lung disease and pneumonia; circulatory disease, such as heart disease, strokes and aneurysms; and digestive disorders, such as ulcers of the stomach and duodenum. Second-hand smoke also puts others at risk and has been linked to lung cancer, strokes, respiratory disorders and infections, particularly in children.

In 2007, before the introduction of the ban on smoking in public in England, Wales and Northern Ireland (smoking in public was banned in 2006 in Scotland), approximately 28% of men and 23% of women were smokers, accounting for up to 10 million people in England alone. In 2011, this was reported to have fallen to 22% of men and 20% of women. Smoking therefore remains a significant problem, despite the decline in prevalence seen over the past 30 years from the 53% of men and 42% of women who smoked in the mid-1970s. Factors that continue to predict the likelihood of smoking include challenging material circumstances, cultural deprivation and stressful marital, personal and household circumstances.

To reduce the health burden of smoking, a number of public health strategies have been put in place and these include reducing the public's exposure to second-hand smoke, providing more support for smokers to stop, raising public awareness of the health effects of smoking and the benefits of stopping smoking and reducing tobacco advertising and the impact of tobacco promotion, and regulating the sales and design of cigarette packets.

With respect to the no smoking agenda the major contribution of pharmacy is in raising awareness of the harm caused by smoking, supporting strategies to reduce the adverse impact of smoking on health, identifying smokers who want to stop and providing these individuals with behavioural support or referring them to alternative sources of smoking cessation support.

Weight management

The UK is experiencing one of the world's fastest growing rates of obesity. In 2010, obesity was considered to be at epidemic proportions with over 26% of men and women over 16 years of age and 16% of children classified as being obese. Such classification is often based on determining the body mass index (BMI: defined as weight in kilograms divided by the square of height in metres) of an individual. A BMI in the range of 25kg/m^2 to 30kg/m^2 indicates the individual is overweight while a BMI of $>30 \text{kg/m}^2$ indicates obesity.

Being overweight can seriously affect an individual's health and may lead to high blood pressure, type II diabetes, cardiovascular disease, many cancers including colorectal and prostate cancers in men and breast or endometrial cancer in women, osteoarthritis, poor self-image and decreased life expectancy.

Increasingly, the measurement of waist circumference is being undertaken as it presents a simple way of assessing someone's risk rather than measuring BMI. Men are at an increased health risk if their waist measurement is $\geq 94 \text{cm}$ and at substantially increased health risk if the measurement is $\geq 102 \text{cm}$. Equivalent waist measurements for women are $\geq 80 \text{cm}$ and $\geq 88 \text{cm}$.

Raising issues of weight management can be difficult but opportunities for the pharmacist to intervene may arise when a person complains of being unhappy with their weight, short of breath or having mobility problems associated with back or hip pain.

Alcohol

Excessive alcohol intake is associated with a range of health problems including serious liver disease, disorders of the stomach and pancreas, anxiety and depression, sexual problems, high blood pressure and cardiac disease, involvement in accidents, particularly car crashes, a range of cancers, including those of the mouth, throat, liver, colon and breast and becoming overweight or obese.

Alcohol misuse currently accounts for approximately 22 000 deaths each year, with consumption above the recommended limits of 3–4 units/day for men and 2–3 units/day for women being exceeded by 22% of adult females and 39% of adult males. Of equal concern is the fact that 20% of the population in England drink to get drunk (binge drinking). This is defined as consuming more than 8 units for men and more than 6 units for women and is strongly associated with involvement in accidents and with cardiovascular disease.

Most people are sensitive about revealing the details of their drinking habits; however, opportunities for pharmacy staff to raise awareness of sensible drinking may arise when individuals present with a hangover, headache, indigestion or complain of insomnia, excessive tiredness, depression, stress, being overweight or report having been involved in a minor accident. Requests for alternative medicines/complementary therapies that may be used to treat alcohol-related problems or supplying a prescribed or over-the-counter medicine known to interact with alcohol, are further opportunities that may allow discussion with the individual.

Exercise

Regular exercise for adults that is equivalent to at least 30 min/day of moderate physical activity on 5 or more days of the week, can help prevent or manage a range of disorders including cardiovascular disease, type II diabetes, musculoskeletal disorders, mental illness and a range of cancers. Children are required to undertake at least 60 minutes of moderate activity each day to promote healthy growth, development and psychological well-being. Recent surveys have shown less than 37% of adult men and 24% of women undertake sufficient exercise to gain any health benefit. Older people need to maintain their mobility and undertake regular daily activity, and attempts to improve strength, coordination and balance may be particularly beneficial.

Clearly the amount of physical activity an individual needs to undertake will be influenced by their daily routine and nature of their job. Opportunities for pharmacy staff to raise issues relating to physical activity may arise when people are unhappy with their weight, complain of being short of breath or tired, have mobility problems, suffer from depression or stress or have difficulty sleeping. Similarly, the purchase of support equipment, e.g. for knees, requesting alternative or complementary medicines to provide energy or obtaining prescribed or purchased medicines for blood pressure may be additional opportunities.

Changing habits and lifestyle

To assist people in making changes to their habits and lifestyle, there is a need to recognize the part played by sociocultural influences and the environment. There are many models that are used to help understand the change process. One that has found use within public health is the 'three Es model for lifestyle change'. In this model three stages are identified:

- Encouragement
- Empowerment
- Environment.

Encouragement involves raising awareness and may include the use of adverts, leaflets, one-to-one advice and targeted campaigns, among other approaches. This stage of the change process is used to act as a trigger for people to make healthy choices or at least consider the healthy options. However, by itself, encouragement is unlikely to bring about sustained change in the population without empowerment and changes to environmental factors.

Empowerment involves the education and development of the individual and the community. Central to empowerment is the development of knowledge, life skills and confidence that will enable individuals, groups or populations to make the healthy choice. This process can be enhanced by pharmacy staff who can instill confidence in patients rather than undermining them, and by making changes to environmental factors.

Environment changes are targeted at the social, cultural, economic and physical surroundings in which people live and work. These changes aim to make the healthy choice the easy

> ## Box 13.3
>
> **Examples of public health roles that could be undertaken by most pharmacies**
>
> - Develop closer working relationships with local authorities and other non-pharmacy bodies to influence the wider determinants of health
> - Develop healthy living champions from within pharmacy
> - Develop pharmacy services in deprived areas to provide additional pharmaceutical support and tackle health inequalities
> - Provide information and advice to the public on health improvement and health protection
> - Improve medicines and health literacy of patients, public and carers
> - Provide access to, or signpost, health information resources and services
> - Provide lifestyle advice for individuals with disease risk factors
> - Provide services to promote self-care
> - Promote health literacy and participate in national campaigns
> - Provide stop smoking services
> - Provide sexual health services, e.g. emergency hormonal contraception (EHC), *Chlamydia* screening, free condoms
> - Provide healthy weight programmes
> - Provide safe use of alcohol services
> - Provide health screening services
> - Encourage immunization uptake and provide immunization services
> - Monitor and track safe use of medicines including reporting of adverse reactions
> - Promote safe, efficient and effective use of prescribed and purchased medicines
> - Develop medicines management programmes for those with chronic conditions
> - Make pharmacies more accessible for difficult to reach groups, e.g. men, teenagers

option. Initiatives aiming to make environmental changes tend to be most effective if instituted on a national basis (e.g. bans on smoking in public places).

A good example that can be used to illustrate the three Es approach to the process of lifestyle change is the need for the wider population to reduce their intake of salt to <6 g/day. 'Encouragement' could involve a campaign to raise awareness of the daily intake of salt and the harmful effect of excessive intake; 'empowerment' might target the labels on food and ensure they are easy for everyone to understand and to know what they are consuming; changes to the 'environment' could involve a reduction in the salt content of prepared foods by manufacturers and the availability of low salt options in supermarkets and restaurants, thereby making it easier for consumers to reduce dietary salt intake. It is important for pharmacists to recognize that there are numerous ways that public health pharmacy can contribute to this process at both local and national levels.

Conclusion

This chapter has highlighted the key determinants of health and focused on areas of lifestyle advice where pharmacy has traditionally contributed to the public health agenda. Hopefully it is apparent to the reader that to make a substantive contribution to public health, pharmacy will need to build on its traditional roles. Some public health pharmacy roles, such as assessing the health and social needs of communities through involvement in surveillance, surveys and information gathering exercises, acting as an advocate for local communities on health issues, and building sustainable communities or working in partnership with relevant statutory and voluntary services to promote and protect the health of the public, may be seen as roles best undertaken by individuals who choose to specialize in public health. Nevertheless, a large number of public health activities can be undertaken from any pharmacy, whether it is located in the community or hospital sector. Some of these are identified in Box 13.3.

KEY POINTS

- Pharmacists have many opportunities to promote health
- Public health pharmacy can be defined in many ways
- More than 70% of the factors affecting an individual's health are outside the domain of the health services
- Public health has improved markedly during the past 150 years
- During this time, social inequalities have widened, with disadvantaged groups showing little improvement

- A wide range of factors affect the health of an individual, some of which are fixed, while others can be modified
- Both employment and unemployment are associated with adverse health effects
- Air pollution is associated with raised morbidity and mortality
- It is with individual lifestyle determinants that pharmacists have had a traditional role
- Community pharmacists may offer support with smoking cessation, weight management, exercise and problems with alcohol
- To help people change lifestyle or habit, think – encouragement, empowerment, environment

Section 3

Delivering professional pharmacy practice

Structure and organization of pharmacy

14

Mary Rhodes and Jennie Watson

STUDY POINTS

- How pharmacy is structured on a global and national basis
- How pharmacy within the NHS is currently structured
- The difference between primary, secondary and tertiary care
- The different roles and jobs undertaken by pharmacists
- The UK organizations which support pharmacy

Introduction

All countries of the world have medicines to treat ailments and maintain the health of their populations. The aims of each country will be to vaccinate even the youngest child against childhood diseases and provide medicines to treat them and the adult population. Generally, the pharmacist is the trusted healthcare professional that is given the responsibility for safe guarding and supplying medicines to the individual patient within the legal system of that country. Clearly, some countries will have more developed systems than others to control and supply their medicines and this will depend, to some extent, on the wealth of the country and its political stability. Concomitantly, the countries with more developed systems will have more pharmacists and more supply outlets for medicines. But with pharmacy and pharmacists worldwide, what structures and organizations are available to administer and support both countries and pharmacists in their endeavours to supply medicines to their populations? This chapter will consider global, state and local structures that organize and support aspects of pharmacy and pharmacists.

Global organizations

There are two major organizations that have an involvement in pharmacy worldwide. These are the World Health Organization (WHO) and International Pharmaceutical Federation (FIP).

The WHO is a directing and coordinating authority for health within the United Nations (UN). It provides leadership on global health matters, setting norms and standards, shaping health research agendas, articulating evidence-based policy options, providing technical support to countries and monitoring and assessing health trends. It employs pharmacists in advisory and operational capacities. In the pharmaceutical sector of the WHO, the essential medicines concept was developed for low income countries and a Model List of Essential Medicines was produced. The essential medicines concept encourages countries to focus on access to those medicines that represent the best balance of safety, quality, efficacy and cost to meet the priority health needs in a country. The Model List of Essential Medicines was developed in the 1970s and has been revised regularly. The list consists of a 'core' of medicines that are the minimum required for a basic healthcare system, for example this would include analgesics and antibiotics, and a 'complementary' list, including essential medicines for priority diseases which may be cost effective but not, necessarily, affordable. Currently, the Essential Medicines List contains about 350 individual medicines and it is designed to guide the development of national and other essential medicines lists.

The WHO has a 6-point agenda to address health objectives, strategic needs and operational approaches. Currently, it is involved in patient safety campaigns and research, international health regulations, global vaccine safety initiatives and the role of pharmacists in tuberculosis care, among others.

FIP is a global federation of national pharmacy associations representing approximately 3 million pharmacists and pharmaceutical scientists worldwide. It has annual conferences and aims to set global pharmacy standards, through professional and scientific guidelines, policy statements and declarations, as well as collaborating with WHO and the UN. It publishes statements of policy on a wide range of subjects such as:

- Quality assurance of pharmaceutical education
- Pharmacists role in promoting a future free of tobacco
- Role of pharmacists in the presentation and treatment of chronic disease
- Quality of medicines used in children
- Counterfeit medicines.

It also has projects on such topics as education initiatives on tuberculosis and patient safety, as well as producing a series of pictograms for labels to be used by patients without a working knowledge of a language.

Organization of pharmacy at a national level

Most countries will have a government, which will need specialist advice on all manner of subjects, including transport issues, financial issues and usually including health issues. And thus, the government will have specialist departments, for example, a department of health which will employ health professionals to advise the government ministers as and when the need arises. This section of the chapter will concentrate on the organizations in England, but similar arrangements exist in many other countries.

The Department of Health (DH), headed by the Minister of Health, is a department of the UK government which is responsible for health and social care matters and for the NHS in England. It develops policies and guidelines to improve the quality of care and to meet patient expectations. Among its employees, there is a Chief Pharmaceutical Officer to advise on pharmaceutical matters. It also employs other pharmacists in specialist capacities. A number of publications, such as the BNF and BNF for Children are published under the authority of the DH and the Joint Formularies Committee, which consists of representatives of doctors and pharmacists. The British Pharmacopeia Commission, which is responsible for the British Pharmacopeia (a collection of legally enforceable standards of quality for UK medicinal substances) recommends publication to the Minister of Health.

The Medicines and Healthcare Regulatory Authority (MHRA) is a UK government agency set up under the auspices of the DH (see Ch. 4). It regulates medicines and medical devices to check whether they work and are acceptably safe.

The National Patient Safety Authority (NPSA) monitored patient safety incidents including medical and prescribing errors. The key functions and expertise for patient safety developed by the NPSA has now transferred to the NHS Commissioning Board Special Health Authority. An off shoot of NPSA is the National Clinical Assessment Service (NCAS), which was set up to investigate concerns over the performance of individual doctors and dentists, but now pharmacists are included in their remit. The NCAS is currently hosted by the National Institute for Health and Care Excellence (NICE) and, in future, will be part of the NHS Litigation Authority.

NICE is currently a Special Health Authority and in the future will become a non-departmental public body. NICE currently publishes guidelines on:

- Health technologies, such as the use of new and existing medicines and treatments
- Clinical practice, such as the treatment and care of people with specialist diseases and conditions
- Guidance for public sector workers on health promotion and ill health avoidance.

In the future, NICE will, also, produce quality standards for people and services involved in providing social care.

The NHS Confederation is a membership body for the full range of organizations that commission and provide NHS services. The membership includes hospital trusts, commissioning bodies and independent and voluntary organizations that deliver services to the NHS.

Health Education England is part of the NHS and is a national leadership body responsible for ensuring that education, training and workforce development drives the highest quality public health and patient outcomes. Pharmacy and pharmacists come under the remit of Health Education England. At a more local level, there will be Local Education and Training Boards (LETB) which are tasked with developing the NHS workforce at a local level.

The Pharmaceutical Services Negotiating Committee (PSNC) is recognized by the DH as the representative negotiating body representing community pharmacy contractors on NHS matters. This committee negotiates the remuneration that community pharmacy contractors receive for NHS dispensing services and other pharmaceutical services, such as MURs (see Ch. 51).

The Veterinary Medicines Directorate, is an agency of the Department of Environment, Food and Rural Affairs and aims to protect the public health, animal health, the environment and promote animal welfare by assuring the safety, quality and efficacy of veterinary medicines in the UK (see Ch. 28).

Structure of the NHS in the UK

In the UK, health care is primarily accessed via the NHS, which was launched in 1948 with the underlying ideal that 'good health care should be available to all, regardless of wealth'.

The NHS is funded through public taxation and is managed by the DH. The Secretary of State for Health heads the department and is answerable to Parliament on all issues relating to health.

Some Members of Parliament have a special interest in pharmacy and belong to The All Party Pharmacy Group, whose stated purpose is 'to raise awareness of the profession of pharmacy and to promote pharmacists' current and potential contribution to the health of the nation'.

Within the DH guidance on professional pharmacy issues is provided by the Chief Pharmaceutical Officer.

The NHS is divided in to three main sectors, primary care, secondary care and tertiary care.

Primary care

Primary care is the largest sector of the NHS providing the main stay of patient care. It is, currently, structured into a number of local commissioning bodies throughout the UK which are responsible for organizing and commissioning services provided in both primary and secondary care. Most primary care is delivered via a local practice where a patient will be registered for treatment by a number of healthcare professionals including general practitioners (GPs) and community nurses. Patients can also access other healthcare services via other healthcare professionals such as dentists, optometrists and chiropodists at their respective practices. Community pharmacists are the main stay of medicine supply and advice on the use of medicines in this sector.

Secondary care

Secondary care is organized into different levels and types of services for patients known as 'Trusts' (mainly hospitals), which together deliver a comprehensive service for patients. There are a greater variety of healthcare professionals working in secondary care including doctors, nurses, pharmacists, radiographers, physiotherapists and dietitians, etc. Most patients will be seen in secondary care through a referral from primary care for diagnosis and treatment or they may also present to secondary care as an emergency through the accident and emergency department.

Tertiary care

Tertiary care includes more specialized medical centres and includes specialist centres in paediatric cardiac surgery or cancer care.

Pharmacists and pharmacy technicians work within all three of these areas providing advice, guidance and the supply of medicines and appliances.

The other way of obtaining medicines in the UK is through dispensing doctors. In rural areas where patients live over a mile from a pharmacy, patients can choose to have their medication dispensed by their GP as part of their NHS service. GPs will often employ a dispenser or pharmacy technician to support them in this role.

Private health care is structured in a similar way, as patients can access private care in the community through GPs and other healthcare professionals. These practitioners may provide, solely, private services or joint NHS and private services. Private secondary care is provided in private hospitals and treatment centres in a similar way to the NHS.

Pharmacy in the UK

Regulation and training

Pharmacy in the UK is regulated by a regulatory body called the General Pharmaceutical Council (GPhC) whose main functions are to maintain the safely of patients and the public by regulating pharmacy and pharmacists (see Ch. 5).

There are a number of general organizations that support and represent pharmacy and pharmacists, such as the Royal Pharmaceutical Society (RPS) a professional body whose aim is to promote pharmacy and support its members (Table 14.1).

Table 14.1 Some general pharmacy organizations

Organization	Role
Royal Pharmaceutical Society	Professional leadership body in the UK. Hosts many specialist groups
Local Practice Forums	Bring together providers of pharmacy learning, employers and pharmacists
Centre for Pharmacy Postgraduate Education (CPPE), Wales Centre for Pharmacy Professional Education (WCPPE), NHS Education Scotland (NES)	Providers of post-graduate pharmacy education
Pharmacist Support	Independent charity providing support to pharmacists and their families
Pharmacists' Defence Association (PDA)	Defends their members when faced with conflict and lobbying organization. Provides indemnity insurance to pharmacists
International Pharmaceutical Federation (FIP)	Federation of national associations
UK Clinical Pharmacy Association (UKCPA)	Promotes excellence in clinical practice and medicines management, hosts specialist clinical groups

The four main fields of pharmacy are: community pharmacy, hospital pharmacy, industrial pharmacy and primary care pharmacy; however, there are many other roles for pharmacist in other sectors.

Community pharmacy

The community pharmacist is one of the main providers of medicines and medicines advice in primary care. They are based in pharmacies either on the high street, in supermarkets or attached to GP practices. This sector has the largest proportion of registered pharmacists working within it. The business may be anything from an independently run single pharmacy, small chains of pharmacies, or a large multiple chain of pharmacies. The community pharmacy is a privately run business which is contracted to deliver NHS services including the dispensing of NHS prescriptions and other NHS services.

The NHS community pharmacy contract for England and Wales outlines all the NHS services to be provided by a community pharmacy. There are three levels of service to be delivered by pharmacies; essential service, advanced services and enhanced services (see Chs 9, 48, 49 and 50). The Drug Tariff (DT) outlines the remuneration structure that community pharmacies receive for providing these services.

Community pharmacies also deliver some healthcare services privately. This may take the form of dispensing prescriptions written by a private practitioner, the sale of over the counter medicines or the provision of private services for which the customer and not the NHS pays, e.g. Flu vaccination.

Various organizations provide support for pharmacists working in community pharmacy and some of these are covered in Table 14.2.

Hospital pharmacy

The hospital pharmacy is usually based within the hospital in question; this may be an NHS or private hospital and is the second largest employer of pharmacists. The pharmacist's role within the hospital is more specialized than that of the community pharmacist and, usually, there is more than one pharmacist working in the same hospital. They work closely with other healthcare professionals in the hospital to ensure the safe use and delivery of medicines to the patient regardless of the type of hospital.

Hospital pharmacists are responsible for the purchase, manufacture, dispensing and supply of all the

Table 14.2 Some community pharmacy organizations

Organization	Role
National Pharmacy Association (NPA)	Trade body for community pharmacists
Company Chemists' Association (CCA)	Represents the views of the nine largest multiple pharmacy chains
Association of Independent Multiples (AIMp)	Represents the views of smaller more regional pharmacy chains
Pharmacy Voice	An umbrella organization of the NPA, CCA and AIMp working to share best practice and represent most community pharmacies
Local Pharmaceutical Committee (LPC)	A statutory body representing community pharmacy in a locality to negotiate with local commissioners
Pharmaceutical Services Negotiating Committee (PSNC)	Negotiates nationally with government in England on contract and payment issues (comparable bodies in Wales and Scotland)

Table 14.3 Some hospital pharmacy organizations

Organization	Role
Guild of Healthcare Pharmacists	Provides a voice for employed pharmacists working in hospitals and primary care
Supported by either RPS or UKCPA for various specialisms	Specialisms include oncology, mental health, nutrition, technicians, HIV, palliative care, radiopharmacy, critical care, neonatal and paediatrics

medicines used in the hospital. One of their main roles is to advise other staff on the most safe and effective use of medicines for individual patients including the selection of the drug, dose, formulation, administration and monitoring of that drug.

During ward rounds hospital pharmacists will speak to patients to improve patient understanding and concordance with their medicines during their stay and before they leave the hospital and some pharmacists will develop specific clinical specialisms to support this work. Other pharmacists will work in other areas of hospital pharmacy (see Chs 16, 40, 41, 45 and 46).

Depending on the area the pharmacist works in they may belong to various organizations that relate to their specialism (Table 14.3).

Pharmacy industry

Privately run industrial companies are the main source of research and development for medicines worldwide. The pharmaceutical industry is largely responsible for the identification and development of new medicines and ensuring the safety of the medicine. Pharmacists have a number of roles within industry including identifying a compound which could become a medicine, testing its safety, formulating it into a usable medicine and marketing the final product for sale and distribution.

Primary care pharmacy

One of the newer roles in pharmacy is the primary care pharmacist. They are employed by the local commissioning body. This role entails medicines management, prescribing advice, working with GPs and being clinical governance leads. The aim of medicines management is to maximize the benefit and reduce the risks of medicines but also take in to consideration cost-effectiveness. Pharmacists use evidence-based medicine to develop formularies and prescribing guidance for use in primary care (see Ch. 20). They may also be involved in budgeting and the development of new services in the community.

Other pharmacy roles

Pharmacists as the experts in medicines are useful to a number of different organizations and have developed many different roles outside the main four already discussed.

Veterinary pharmacists are experts in the supply of medicines for the use in household animals or livestock (see Ch. 28).

Pharmacists may also work in a prison pharmacy supplying medicines and pharmaceutical care to inmates. This role combines aspects of both hospital and community pharmacy and pharmacists will often have trained to prescribe and run clinics within the prison. Within the prison setting, a higher percentage of the population will have mental health and addiction problems than in the wider community which often steers the specialism of the pharmacist. Both legal and illegal drugs can have 'value' within the prison, so the pharmacist will have to be able to advise on the production of the formulary within the prison to reduce the risk of increasing drug misuse (see Ch. 23).

Some pharmacists will work in teaching and training capacities. They could be based in a University, teaching pharmacy students or on other related courses, e.g. non-medical prescribing. Others will design and deliver training within sectors of the profession.

Regulatory pharmacy provides career opportunities for a small number of pharmacists. They may work for a pharmacy regulator, such as the GPhC, in industry, for either a drug company or the MRHA and in a more general healthcare regulator, e.g. the Care Quality Commission in the UK.

Another area that pharmacists work in is with the armed services. Armed services provide medical services for personnel and their families on bases both within the UK and abroad. Personnel also need medical services when they are on tours of duty. Pharmacy will need to be part of these teams. Services pharmacists will be commissioned as officers within the service they have joined and in the UK, the Army sponsors some pharmacy students who are then required to serve for 6 years within the Army on qualification.

Within in all sectors, pharmacists have the opportunity to move into management roles. Groups that support these areas of work are listed in Table 14.4.

Conclusion

There is wide variability in the delivery of health services around the world; how it is delivered within any particular country will depend on many factors. The supply of medicines in any country invariably involves a pharmacist or pharmacy technician to ensure the

Table 14.4 Areas/groups covered by other pharmacy organizations

Area covered
Locum pharmacists
Overseas pharmacists
Rural pharmacy
Secure environment pharmacists
Pharmacy students
History of pharmacy
Pharmacist prescribing
Veterinary pharmacy
Science and research
Qualified persons
Management
Pharmacy law and ethics

safety of the public and compliance with local regulations. Health care in the UK is mostly delivered through the NHS using a wide range of healthcare professionals, though private care is also available. Pharmacists work in the NHS and private care in a number of different capacities with the main role of ensuring the safe supply of medicines to patients.

KEY POINTS

- Pharmacy works in different ways in different countries
- Different countries have different legislation and training requirements relating to pharmacy and pharmacists
- The majority of pharmacists work as community or hospital pharmacists
- A wide variety of groups provide links, networking opportunities and support to pharmacists working in different areas of the profession

Relationship with other members of the healthcare team

15

Felice S. Groundland

STUDY POINTS

- The other members of the healthcare team that work directly with the pharmacist
- The roles played by the other members of the healthcare team and how the pharmacist interacts with them
- The role of technicians, dispensers and medicine counter assistants and their qualifications
- The importance of leadership, delegation, negotiation and teamworking and how to achieve these

Introduction

Nowadays most pharmacists work as part of a team with other healthcare workers. If this team is to function efficiently to provide good pharmaceutical services to the public, then a good working relationship needs to be developed between all the members of the healthcare team. In many situations, the pharmacist will be the manager/supervisor or responsible person for the team. In other situations, the pharmacist may be part of a team but not responsible for the team, for example as a member of an ethics committee or team developing educational materials for use by ward staff in a hospital.

The relative position of the pharmacist in a team will determine the skills required to undertake an efficient role. If the pharmacist is responsible for the team, then the required skills will be leadership, managing/supervising and delegation. In order to delegate, the pharmacist must be confident the team has the required skills. If not, then an assessment of training needs and subsequent training

will need to be organized. Negotiating skills will be needed and crucial if the pharmacist is part of, but not responsible for, a team. In such a situation, the pharmacist must be a good teamworker.

What is teamwork?

Teamwork can be defined as the process whereby people work together cooperatively to deliver goals. The goals will vary depending on the type of team but it is essential that these goals are well defined. In any team it is important that each member knows the role they play and how they contribute to the goals. The introduction of SOPs (see Ch. 11) has gone a long way in helping define each member's role and responsibility as well as fulfilling UK clinical governance criteria (see Ch. 9).

The following skills and attributes are desirable for successful teamwork:

- *Listening skills* – within any team all members should be encouraged to speak out and offer suggestions for improvement which in turn may trigger other ideas from the other team members.
- *Questioning skills* – to always question why things are done the way they are and not to blindly accept something because that is the way it is always done.
- *Respect* – treat others as you would want to be treated yourself. This comes back to being an effective leader. Effective leaders command respect. However, all members of the team should be treated with respect by the team leader and other team members for the role that

they play in the team. All members and their role in the team are necessary for a productive, efficient team.

- *Helping* – this is the true essence of teamwork and ensures that everyone is involved in reaching the goals.
- *Sharing* – this means sharing ideas and information. If one person keeps important information to himself or herself, then the team will not function properly. Sharing also means that no one person should take the glory for the team's efforts as everyone has had a part to play.
- *Collaborating* – all members are encouraged to participate in the team and when there is a high level of collaboration an effective team emerges. This requires elements of trust, shared goals and clarity of roles.
- *Communication* – a skill required in all areas including by e-mail, at meetings where face-to-face communication is important or the written word. It is crucial not to be misunderstood at any level.

The healthcare team

The healthcare 'team' can be defined in a number of ways and will depend on the work environment of the pharmacist.

In community pharmacy, the immediate team that the pharmacist works with on a day-to-day basis is made up of:

- Pharmacy technicians
- Accuracy checking technicians
- Dispensing/pharmacy assistants
- Medicines counter assistants or healthcare assistants/advisors.

The terminology will vary depending on the individual company or business.

The community pharmacist will also be involved with external people, depending on their job role – the extended 'team':

- A pharmacist providing services to residential or nursing homes will be in constant communication with the care home staff and a variety of clients, e.g. the elderly, children and psychiatric patients
- Communication will take place with the GP practices and their staff on a regular basis depending on requirements, e.g. receptionists, practice managers, practice nurses, practice physiotherapists, asthma and stoma nurses, etc.
- The pharmacist will be in contact with healthcare professionals in the local area, for example, community/district nurses, health visitors, psychiatric nurses, Macmillan nurses, physiotherapists
- The community pharmacist may liaise with the local drug misuse teams depending on the services provided in that pharmacy
- Other groups of professionals the pharmacist may have contact with include dentists, chiropodists and optometrists and social workers
- Community pharmacists will have to work with local commissioners and their pharmacist representatives on clinical governance matters and contract negotiations.

This list is not exhaustive but gives an idea of the variety of people/professions the community pharmacist has to interact with on a daily basis when dealing with specific problems related to individual patients' care, selection of drugs by the healthcare professional, dealing with drug interactions, etc.

In a hospital pharmacy, the pharmacist will interact with the pharmacy team as well as the healthcare professionals directly involved in the patients' care on a daily basis and with far more ease of contact than the community pharmacist has with the GP. When dealing with the junior doctors and nursing staff in hospital, the pharmacist will have a teaching/supportive role while assuming an advisory role on the use and side-effects of drugs when dealing with more experienced staff. Hospital pharmacists will have contact with other professionals with regard to discharging patients into the community, such as social workers, physiotherapists, occupational therapists, dentists and the local drug misuse team. Within the hospital environment the pharmacist may have to become involved with the various hospital committees, e.g. drug safety, ethics, general administration, formulary, etc. and interact with a range of professional as well as administrative staff. In addition, hospital pharmacists will be in contact with community pharmacists to ensure a seamless supply of medicines to those patients discharged from hospital on specialized drug regimens.

The changing role of the pharmacist (see Ch. 1) has made it even more important that the pharmacist depends on their healthcare team to free up the time to allow them to deliver the various services required by the new pharmacy contracts. The pharmacist is moving further away from the traditional role of dispensing to advising patients and customers on their medicines and offering additional services.

The community healthcare team

Medicines counter assistants/ healthcare assistants

From 1 July 1996 it has been a professional requirement in the UK that each member of staff whose work in a pharmacy will regularly include the sale of medicines, must have completed a course or be undertaking an accredited course relevant to their line of work. The regulatory body for England, Wales and Scotland, set the requirements for these courses and undertake a quality assurance process which leads to the course being accredited.

There is a requirement that the member of staff should be enrolled on an appropriate course within 3 months of starting their role and have completed it in 3 years.

The following training programmes for medicines counter assistants/healthcare assistants have been accredited by the GPhC:

- Boots UK: 'Healthcare Advisors' Programme'
- Buttercups Training: 'Medicines Counter Assistant Course'
- Chemist and Druggist (UMB Medica): 'Counterpart'
- CIG Healthcare Partnership: 'Counterintelligence'
- National Pharmacy Association (NPA): 'Interact'
- Scientia Skills: 'Medicines Counter Assistant Programme'.

Medicines counter assistants/healthcare assistants will primarily be found in community pharmacy. Their training usually takes the form of 'workbook-led on-the-job learning', meeting the above requirements for accreditation with the pharmacist acting as the tutor. This allows the relationship to develop and the pharmacist to realize the potential and limitations of these members of staff.

Dispensing/pharmacy assistants

The training required is much more in-depth than for the medicines counter/healthcare assistant to reflect the variation in role and responsibilities. The job title will vary depending on the sector of pharmacy the person works in and indeed the company/ business they work for – dispenser, dispensing assistant, pharmacy assistant, assistant technical officer, etc. Regardless of which sector of pharmacy they are working in, what they all have in common is that they are working under the supervision of the pharmacist.

Since January 2005, there has been the professional requirement that dispensing/pharmacy assistants are competent in the areas in which they are working to a minimum standard which is equivalent to the Pharmacy Services Skills S/NVQ level 2 (QCF) qualification or are undertaking such training.

This applies to staff working in the following areas:

- Sale of OTC medicines and the provision of information to customers on symptoms and products
- Prescription receipt and collection
- The assembly of prescribed items including the generation of labels
- Ordering, receiving and storing pharmaceutical stock
- Preparation for the manufacture of pharmaceutical products, including aseptic products
- Manufacture and assembly of medicinal products, including aseptic products.

To fulfil this requirement, a training programme relevant to the job needs to be completed within a 3-year time period and the member of staff should be enrolled on such a course within 3 months of starting their role. Exemptions to the minimum training requirements exist and include:

- Pre-registration trainee pharmacists
- Students currently studying for a pharmacy degree
- Students currently studying on an Overseas Pharmacists' Assessment Programme (OSPAP).

The dispensing/pharmacy assistant is a key member of the healthcare team, as they free up the pharmacist from the assembly processes involved in the dispensing of prescriptions.

Pharmacy technician

A pharmacy technician is someone who has undertaken a course that involves completing both knowledge and a competency-based qualification. The GPhC will either accredit programme providers such as the NPA and Buttercups or will recognize the qualifications provided by various awarding bodies, i.e. Edexcel, City and Guilds and SQA, which can be undertaken at various colleges and centres throughout the UK.

Once qualified, the pharmacy technician has to register with the GPhC if they want to practise as a Pharmacy Technician (a title protected by Law) in England, Wales and Scotland. Pharmacy Technicians are bound by the Standards of conduct, ethics and performance and must participate in continuing professional development (see Ch. 5).

The pharmacy technician may work in hospitals, community pharmacy, health centres, primary care trusts, prisons and the armed forces and in the pharmaceutical industry. We will focus on community and hospital pharmacy.

Community pharmacy

Pharmacy technicians are required to make up the prescriptions issued by doctors. These are checked by the pharmacist for accuracy and to make sure that the dosage and treatment are safe for that patient, i.e. a clinical check.

The role of the technician involves:

- Reading prescriptions and translating doctor's instructions
- Counting solid dosage forms and measuring specific quantities of liquids
- Preparing accurate labels for medicines
- Selling medicines and other complementary preparations
- Referring to the pharmacist when appropriate
- Small-scale or individual preparation of extemporaneous products as requested by the doctor which are not supplied as ready to use by manufacturers
- Maintaining and managing stock within the pharmacy
- Record-keeping and audit
- Being aware of the legal requirements relating to prescribing and supply of medicines.

There is considerable overlap with the dispensing/pharmacy assistant role, but with additional responsibilities. In community pharmacy, this may include training and development and management of other staff.

The pharmacy technician may choose to become an accuracy checking technician (ACT). This will require them to undertake a further period of study and the development of a portfolio of evidence to demonstrate their competence in this area. The requirement for most ACT courses is that the trainee must have successfully checked 1000 items error free in a defined period of time (usually 4 weeks), while keeping a diary of all items checked and any errors made while checking or dispensing and completing any assignments required by the employer. There is usually a final assessment, which requires them to check the accuracy of a set number of prescriptions.

An ACT plays a valuable role in the dispensing process. They will accuracy check prescriptions after the pharmacist has clinically checked them. This has not only been shown to be more accurate than pharmacist checking but also, more importantly, frees up the pharmacist to carry out other additional services.

Hospital pharmacy

The work in the hospital pharmacy setting for a pharmacy technician has many similarities to that in the community sector. However, the work has greater variation due to the different areas for care within hospital. These include:

- Visits to the wards to take orders for medicines
- Preparation of radioactive materials or working on clinical trials
- Production of medicines in special sterile units
- Working in manufacturing or production units.

The hospital pharmacy also employs ACT pharmacy technicians.

Other members of the pharmacy team

There are other people who can play an important role in the pharmacy team but they are not present in every pharmacy team at all times. These are pre-registration pharmacy trainees and also pharmacy undergraduates, either taking part in a period of vocational placement or working on a part-time basis in the pharmacy setting.

Pre-registration pharmacy trainees will have obtained an accredited degree in pharmacy (see Ch. 5). During the pre-registration year, the pharmacy trainee becomes a valuable member of the team as they learn to apply their university knowledge. The pre-registration pharmacy trainee is given guidance from their tutor throughout this period.

Pharmacy undergraduates may join the pharmacy team at any time; some working on a part-time basis at weekends, others for a period of time during the university breaks to gain experience of career pathways.

Role of the pharmacist in teamwork

The role of the pharmacist, both in the primary and secondary care setting, is changing. No longer can the pharmacist work in isolation; they must learn to become integrated members of both their immediate and extended teams, and so it is essential for the pharmacist to recognize that team leading, delegation, negotiation and teamworking are essential skills that they must possess.

Leadership

There have been many studies carried out to determine what it is exactly that makes good leaders. The majority of these studies lead to the conclusion that leadership is about the behaviour of the leader first and the skills that they possess second. It is about recognizing that people need to trust and respect you before they will listen and act on what you ask them to do.

In any one environment, there can be a number of different teams working together and sometimes one particular team will outperform the others. Why is this?

In all cases, it is attributable to the person leading the team and the fact that they possess such qualities as integrity, honesty, humility, courage, commitment, sincerity, passion, confidence, positivity, wisdom, determination, compassion and sensitivity. This makes their staff willing to go that 'extra mile' for them. Some people are naturally born with these behaviours already well developed but others, recognizing that these behaviours are important, can work to develop this side of their behaviours to achieve great leadership qualities.

A good leader will be able to use a number of different leadership styles depending on the situation they are faced with. Again some people have a dominant style of leadership, but to be truly great they need to look at all the other styles of leadership and develop these also.

As a pharmacist, it is crucial to know your own strengths and weaknesses and build on the weaknesses. This is where continuing professional development (CPD) is important (see Ch. 6). The correct behaviour, especially towards your team, is the key to being an effective leader and the following are some tips towards being respected as a leader:

- Honesty and integrity: without this no-one in your team will respect you (see Ch. 7)
- Never shout at people no matter how angry you get as this only serves to break down the relationships built with the team
- Always lead by example: if you are not seen to be 'doing' then the message that sends to others is that it is not important to be hard working
- Recognize when you need to work with your team to get tasks done: nothing should be beneath you and you should never be afraid to 'get your hands dirty'
- You need to treat all members of the team fairly and based on merit, not singling people out because they like the same football team, for example
- You need to be seen to be dealing with any bad or unethical behaviour of team members. Ignoring this type of behaviour is giving out the message that you condone it
- Listen to your team and try to understand their point of view: it is sometimes important to place yourself in someone else's shoes to see their point of view. This does not mean you have to agree with everything but it will give you a better understanding of where they are coming from
- Accept the responsibility for when things do not go as planned: do not blame the team or individuals within the team
- Always give credit where credit is due, even for your own successes, because you would never have got there without your team behind you ('Behind an able man there are always able men' – Chinese proverb)

- Provide support for the team so they know that they can trust you to act in their best interests
- Always ask for opinions and ideas from the team so that they feel that they are involved in the decisions you may make, especially if things need to change. It is easier to handle change if the team members have been involved from the beginning
- If you agree to do something then make sure you follow through: do not make empty promises as you will quickly lose the trust of your team
- Encourage the development of your team, giving them responsibility for certain tasks that stretch their abilities without putting undue pressure on them
- Be positive, even about things that have gone wrong: we can always learn from this and make things better the next time
- Have fun in the workplace: your staff should feel happy in the work they do and in the environment they work in as they spend so much time there; there is no point being miserable
- Smile!
- Remember why you are all there: what is the job in hand?
- Seek feedback from others to find ways you can develop and improve your skills and behaviours and recognize that we never stop learning.

No pharmacist can do all the tasks themselves, so it is essential that they recognize that many tasks need to be delegated to the other team members.

Delegation

Good delegation will save you time, will develop your team and generally motivates all involved. It is not just a technique to free up time. Poor delegation will lead to frustration, demotivation among your team and failure of the task(s) involved, so it is essential that delegation is effective.

When delegating tasks one should follow the SMARTER mnemonic. To ensure success on completion then all delegated tasks must be:

- *Specific* – if it is unclear what the task is, then how can it be completed effectively? Can this task, in fact, be delegated?
- *Measurable* – you have to be able to measure when the task has been completed to know that success has been achieved. What is the end goal

or measure to demonstrate this? This needs to be clearly defined.

- *Agreed* – all parties must be in agreement to the task otherwise this is where frustrations and resentments start to form. Is the individual or team capable of doing the delegated task? Do they understand the bigger picture and where they fit in?
- *Realistic* – if the task is not achievable, either because of timescales or lack of the necessary skills or resources, then this will only serve to demotivate the person involved.
- *Timebound* – the task should not be so great that it cannot be completed in the timescales agreed; is it realistic? If it is an ongoing task then specific review dates need to be in place and adhered to and agreed outcomes clearly defined, e.g. generation of reports, targets reached, etc.
- *Ethical* – you should not be asking your team to carry out a task that goes against their professional or moral ethics.
- *Recorded* – this is important to celebrate the successes of your team if you keep a record of the tasks that have been completed and it also helps to learn from tasks that have not been completed and enables you to provide constructive feedback to your team when things do not go as planned.

It is extremely important for the pharmacist to be able to delegate various tasks within the pharmacy to suitably trained persons because it is no longer cost-effective for the pharmacist to be carrying out tasks that others are more than qualified to complete. Thus, this frees the pharmacist to get on with their job and leads to job satisfaction for all staff involved.

In order to get the members of the immediate and extended teams on board the pharmacist has to be aware of, and if necessary develop, their negotiation skills.

Negotiation

Negotiation is something that we do all the time in and out of the working environment and maybe do not realize it, e.g. deciding what to see at the cinema, where to go out to eat, what shift someone should work and for how long, etc.

Negotiation is usually considered as a compromise between people to get what we want. To be really effective in the team environment the compromise should allow both parties to be satisfied with the eventual outcome. The only time you may want to consider the win–lose negotiation is if you do not need to have an ongoing working relationship with the other party. This is something that is going to be very unlikely in the pharmacy setting. If the pharmacist always negotiates to 'win' then the working relationship within the team will eventually break down and the working environment will suffer. Ultimately, patient care deteriorates as no one works together.

Communication is the key link that will be used to negotiate and as such can be in a variety of ways (see Ch. 17). Body language is another area that the pharmacist may wish to develop as body language significantly influences a conversation.

For successful negotiation to occur the following should be considered:

- Goals: what do you need to get from the negotiation and do you know what the other party wants? You need to be really clear why you are negotiating and think about what you will accept before entering into the negotiation.
- Separate people from the problem: do not get caught up in personalities and relationships and focus on what the actual issues are. It will be a lot easier to justify a decision reached if the results are based on objective criteria.
- Generate a variety of possible solutions – no matter how ridiculous they might first sound – before going on to decide the best option to meet everyone's needs. Sometimes asking the other party 'What do you think?' might allow them to actually come up with a solution that you had not thought about but which fulfils everyone's needs.

Pharmacists in both the primary and secondary care sector are now required to work very closely with their teams to deliver the government targets for access to health care. Pharmacists are dependent on the skills of their immediate teams to be able to fulfil these new roles and demonstrate that they meet the clinical governance requirements. This requires a great deal of teamwork both within the immediate teams and the extended teams.

Conclusion

Pharmacists may work well in their immediate teams but if they are to embrace the changing role of pharmacy and health care, then they need to extend their teamworking across a wide variety of healthcare professionals.

It is essential that pharmacists start to maintain a formal record of all their contributions and interactions within the wide variety of teams to demonstrate their invaluable contribution to patient care.

KEY POINTS

- Pharmacists need to work with a wide variety of other healthcare staff
- Good communication skills are required to be an effective member of a team, together with the ability to respect, help, share and collaborate with others
- A healthcare team will be either an immediate or an external team
- The immediate team will be trained to carry out specific responsibilities
- External team members could include many other healthcare professionals, other professionals and administrators
- There are detailed requirements for qualifications required of different levels of pharmacy support staff
- Some pharmacists will occupy leadership roles, which require a wide range of skills
- Delegation has to be effective and achievable.
- Negotiation is part of making progress in a healthcare team

Information retrieval in pharmacy practice

16

Parastou Donyai

STUDY POINTS

- How to categorize health- and medicine-related information
- Relevant search and retrieval processes
- Organizations that can help with information retrieval
- How, practically, to apply the suggestions in this chapter

Introduction

The current era is characterized by man's inordinate ability to store, retrieve and transmit large volumes of information using computer technology. Albert Einstein proposed that the secret of success is 'to know where to find the information and how to use it'. Most pharmacists would probably agree. This chapter aims to provide the reader with a theoretical understanding of how to source health- and medicines-related information in the present information age. While the quality of retrieved information is considered, guidance on the detailed evaluation of what is known broadly as 'clinical evidence' is found elsewhere (see Ch. 20).

In the GPhC's Standards of conduct, ethics and performance, the knowledge and provision of health- and medicines-related information, specifically, is considered in the following manner. In relation to their own knowledge and competence, pharmacists must develop their skills in-line with their area of expertise, keeping up-to-date with relevant progress through CPD (see Ch. 6). In relation to the provision of medicines-related information to

those who want or need it, pharmacists are expected to be able to provide accurate, reliable, impartial, relevant and up-to-date information.

Yet with thousands of medicinal products, dressings and appliances on the UK market, pharmacists are highly unlikely to hold in-depth knowledge of all health- and medicines-related issues at all times. Therefore, the ability to retrieve relevant health- and medicines-related information in a timely and efficient manner becomes central to the practice of all pharmacy professionals (Box 16.1).

Where does information exist and how can it be retrieved?

Information retrieval is the tracing and recovery of stored information. Information can range from patient information to drug monographs, to more

Box 16.1

Pharmacy activities that might involve information retrieval

- Solving clinical problems
- Critical evaluation/appraisal of literature
- Effective provision of information to the public
- Guideline development
- Drug policy management
- Preparation of bulletins and newsletters
- Adverse drug reaction/event management
- CPD

sophisticated health technology assessments. It can exist in many forms from the archives of a drug company to the worldwide web. Effective information retrieval requires an understanding of the range of relevant information available, where it exists and how it might be sourced.

Pharmacists sourcing information are likely to use the internet at some point during their search. The expanse of information on the Web and its apparent accessibility has integrated the internet into most work routines. While, on the whole, the seemingly endless material may not suit most pharmacists' information needs, there are specific online resources that pharmacists can browse. These include websites operated by governments, professional, practice, regulatory or academic bodies, as well as websites belonging to patient groups and the pharmaceutical industry. However, the fluid nature of the internet, the vast array of information available, plus the variable nature of each query will probably involve pharmacists in some degree of internet searching. This necessitates an understanding of search engines and search strategies. There are databases on the net and on CD-ROM which act as directories for scientific papers and other publications and, as such, can be used to search for available material.

Before widespread use of the internet, the principal source of health-related information was the printed book. Books still contain a vast array of indispensable information and reputable ones play a vital role in information management. Although individual pharmacies may not keep the full range of essential books, specialist centres will have access to these and to other resources.

The internet

The internet in its current form came into being in 1983 and the web came into widespread use from the mid-1990s onwards. From the beginning, it acted as a place where large numbers of files and documents could be stored for download, circulation, discussion and communication. These days, many thousands of documents and other items are added to the web every hour and so it is not possible to create a comprehensive directory of the web. Most people create their own directory of useful websites or search the internet for the information they need.

The web address

The term 'website' is used to denote a set of themed, linked web pages, usually accessed via a 'homepage'. Web pages are written in hypertext markup language (htm/html). A web page is a collection of text, graphics, sounds and/or video that corresponds to a single window of scrollable material. Web pages are stored on a web server, which hosts the website and 'dispenses' the pages in response to a web browser. The web browser displays web pages after communicating with the server. There are a large number of browsers.

Each page on the web has a distinct web address known as the uniform resource locator (URL). The URL can be a good clue as to the quality of the information found on a website. The 'locator' in URL can also give an indication of where one is within a website and indicate the source of the information being viewed.

A web address or website name appears on the address bar. All website names are part of the domain name system (DNS) and look similar to this: http://www.dh.gov.uk/.

Box 16.2 breaks down this address and examines the individual parts.

Directory of useful websites

Table 16.1 provides a list of some of the established health-related websites, although web addresses or pathnames can change or more useful sites can be created. To help order the directory, similar websites are grouped together. The list is not exhaustive and it should be used as a starting point.

Bookmarking

Once a number of relevant websites have been identified and authenticated for inclusion, these can be stored as a saved text file, using hyperlinks to connect each typed URL address in the document to the address bar on the browser and therefore the desired web destination. Hyperlinks are, usually, in a different colour to the rest of the document or are underlined and can be activated by a mouse click.

Hyperlinks provide a way of finding and bookmarking useful websites. Websites normally have a directory of related websites as 'links'.

Box 16.2

Individual components of a typical domain name system

A web address: http://www.gov.uk/government/publications

PROTOCOL.   http:// shows us that we are looking at a website with http meaning 'hypertext transfer protocol', the set of rules used by the computer to access and deliver web pages. The variation https:// indicates a secure connection to the site in question

SERVER AND ORGANIZATION'S NAME.   www.dh informs us that we are viewing a website held on a computer or a web server known as www belonging to an organization called 'dh', in this instance the Department of Health

DOMAIN AND COUNTRY.   gov.uk tells us that we are looking at the website of the UK government. This part of the web address is the 'domain', other examples of which are .edu (educational); .com (commercial); .co (a company); .ac (academic); .org (non-governmental, non-profit making organizations). Sometimes domains are followed by a country code that indicates the location of the computer holding the website

PATHNAME AND DOCUMENT NAME.   Beyond the homepage of an organization's website, other pages are ordered in a hierarchy of folders. In this example, /government/publications indicates we are looking at a folder in which we will find another folder containing publications

FILE EXTENSION.   The file extension usually identifies the type of data found in the file. For example, the extension .htm (or .html) indicates a file that contains code expressed in the hypertext markup language used to develop pages that are to be placed on the web. There are countless other examples; the extension .txt indicates a file containing textual data; the extension .pdf indicates a file in portable document format.

Table 16.1 Directory of 'established' websites that can be accessed via the internet for health-related information

Name of website and web address	Brief description of content
Government and regulatory bodies	
Department of Health http://www.dh.gov.uk/	Contains material produced by and for the Department of Health, of relevance to health professionals
European Medicines Agency http://www.ema.europa.eu/	Website of the European Union body responsible for issuing European marketing authorization and for regulating the safety, quality and efficacy of medicinal products
Medicines and Healthcare products Regulatory Agency http://www.mhra.gov.uk/	Information about the regulatory processes for medicines and medical devices in the UK, including news about initiatives in Europe and beyond. Allows online reporting of safety problems. Look at drug safety updates, news on Safety of Herbal Medicines, and Drug Analysis Prints (DAPs) – a complete listing of the suspected ADRs
NHS bodies, evidence-based medicine and guidelines	
AHFS Drug Information	Drug information provided by the American Society of Health-System Pharmacists; electronic access available via Medscape: http://www.medscape.com/
Bandolier http://www.medicine.ox.ac.uk/bandolier/	Academic department providing collection of abstracted evidence (systematic reviews of treatments, of evidence about diagnosis, epidemiology or health economics) under various subheadings
British National Formulary http://www.bnf.org/bnf/	The BNF provides UK healthcare professionals with authoritative and practical information on the selection and clinical use of medicines in a clear, concise and accessible manner

(Continued)

Table 16.1 Continued

Name of website and web address	Brief description of content
DIAL www.dial.org.uk/	Website of an information service, based at Royal Liverpool Children's NHS Trust (Alder Hey), offering advice on the use of medicines in children, to healthcare professionals working in the UK and Eire
Drug and Therapeutics Bulletin http://www.dtb.org.uk/	Subscription-based publication of the British Medical Journal group providing independent evaluations of, and practical advice on, individual treatments and the overall management of disease
DrugScope http://www.drugscope.org.uk/	Independent centre of information and expertise on drugs of abuse in UK
Evidence in Health and Social care www.evidence.nhs.uk	This is operated by the NICE and contains a general search engine for evidence based reviews relevant to the NHS
Health Protection Agency http://www.hpa.org.uk/infections/	Provides support and advice to various bodies and NHS professionals to protect UK public health. Remit includes communicable disease surveillance, microbiology and major emergency response
Health Technology Assessment programme http://www.ncchta.org/	Independent research into the effectiveness, costs and broader impact of healthcare treatments and tests for those who plan, provide or receive care in the NHS
Immunization Against Infectious Diseases (the Green Book) http://immunization.dh.gov.uk/category/the-green-book/	Provides the latest information on vaccines and vaccination procedures for all the vaccine-preventable infectious diseases that may occur in the UK
IPPF Directory of Hormonal Contraceptives http://contraceptive.ippf.org/	Website of International Planned Parenthood Federation, recommended and used by the RPS Information Service to identify foreign contraceptive pills
Malaria Reference Laboratory http://www.malaria-reference.co.uk/	Based at the London School of Hygiene and Tropical Medicine, the Malaria Reference Library provides malaria prevention guidelines
Medicines and Prescribing Centre http://www.nice.org.uk/mpc/index.jsp	New website which came about as a result of integration of the former National Prescribing Centre into the National Institute for Health and Care Excellence (NICE)
National Horizon Scanning Centre http://www.hsc.nihr.ac.uk/about-us/	The centre provides advanced notice to the DH and national policy makers in England of selected key new and emerging health technologies
The National Institute for Health and Care Excellence http://www.nice.org.uk/	Responsible for providing national guidance on the promotion of good health and the prevention and treatment of ill health, produces guidance on areas of public health, health technologies and clinical practice
National Library for Health http://www.library.nhs.uk/	NHS electronic library. Aims to be the best, most trusted health-related knowledge service in the world
National Travel Health Network and Centre (NaTHNaC) http://www.nathnac.org/	Funded by the DH, the centre has been created to promote clinical standards in travel medicine
National Treatment Agency's Orange Guide www.nta.nhs.uk/uploads/clinical_guidelines_2007.pdf	UK guidelines on clinical management of drug misuse and dependence
Palliative drugs.com http://www.palliativedrugs.com/	Created by palliative care practitioners, the website aims to promote and disseminate information about the use of drugs in palliative care
Prescription Pricing Authority (Division) http://www.nhsbsa.nhs.uk/prescriptions	Provides pricing information for NHS prescriptions dispensed in England and related services with associated usage statistics. Monthly NHS electronic drug tariff available on this site at www.ppa.org.uk/ppa/edt_intro.htm

(Continued)

Table 16.1 Continued

Name of website and web address	Brief description of content
Prodigy http://www.prodigy.clarity.co.uk/home	Formerly this was known as Clinical Knowledge Summaries for 'minor-ailment' type guidance and was commissioned by the NHS. Prodigy is marketed as a reliable source of evidence-based information and practical 'know how' about the common conditions managed in primary care
Royal College of Obstetricians and Gynaecologists http://www.rcog.org.uk	Makes available a range of guidelines on women's health
Scottish Intercollegiate Guidelines Network http://www.sign.ac.uk/	SIGN develops and disseminates national clinical guidelines containing recommendations for effective practice, based on current evidence
UK Medicines Information (UKMi) http://www.ukmi.nhs.uk/	The website hosts UKMi strategy, policies, clinical governance standards and training materials
Pharmacy organizations and associations	
General Pharmaceutical Council http://www.pharmacyregulation.org/	The independent regulator for pharmacists, pharmacy technicians and pharmacy premises in Great Britain
National Pharmacy Association http://www.npa.co.uk/	Trade association for UK community pharmacy owners. Provides professional and commercial support and represents community pharmacy at national negotiations
Royal Pharmaceutical Society http://www.rpharms.com/	The professional body for pharmacists and pharmacy in England, Scotland and Wales
Continuing professional development	
Postgraduate Pharmacy Education https://www.cppe.ac.uk/; http://www.nes.scot.nhs.uk/; http://www.wcppe.org.uk/	Funded by the DH to provide continuing education for pharmacists and pharmacy technicians providing NHS services in England, Scotland and Wales
Pharmaceutical industry	
The Association of the British Pharmaceutical Industry http://www.abpi.org.uk/	Trade association for UK companies producing prescription medicines. Also represents companies engaged in the research and development of medicines for human use
Electronic Medicines Compendium http://emc.medicines.org.uk/	Associate website of the ABPI. Provides electronic copies of Summaries of Product Characteristics (SPCs) as well as patient information leaflets (PILs) for members' products licensed in the UK
The Proprietary Association of Great Britain http://www.pagb.org.uk/	Trade association for UK producers of over-the-counter medicines and food supplements
Patient information	
Best Health http://besthealth.bmj.com/x/index.html	Website produced by the BMJ Publishing Group based on clinical evidence in a patient-friendly format
Family Planning Association http://www.fpa.org.uk/	Website of Family Planning Association, a leading sexual health charity
Medicines Guides http://medguides.medicines.org.uk/	Produced by an independent not-for-profit group, the Medicine Guides are being developed in partnership with NHS Direct to provide people with information about medicines, conditions and different treatment options
NHS Direct http://www.nhsdirect.nhs.uk/	Official NHS website for 24-hour delivery of information and advice about health, illness and health services to the public
Patient UK http://www.patient.co.uk/	Authored by GPs, the website aims to provide non-medical people in the UK with good quality information about health and disease

An accepted method of bookmarking relevant pages is to use an internet browser with functions such as 'Favourites'. A marker points at a website which then enables the user to quickly return to that site without having to remember and type in its URL. Browsers usually offer the facility for organizing the bookmarks into folders and subfolders.

There are also innovations such as the social bookmarking website http://delicious.com/, which provides a means of storing personal bookmarks online instead of within the browser, thus enabling bookmark information to be accessed and shared online.

Searching the internet

Accessing a list of useful websites and following the links therein is one approach to finding information on the internet, but is unlikely to be productive unless the query falls specifically within the remit of a known website. With the web containing over 40 billion pages, at some point it is likely that the website containing the required information is simply unknown to the user and it has not been possible to reach it via 'browsing' the internet. For that reason, it is essential to have a good appreciation of internet search options.

Commercial search engines

The internet is not controlled or owned by any individual or organization, and plays host to a multitude of material with limitless authors. The manner in which information is stored on the internet is quite unique. There is no central catalogue of the internet.

A variety of websites concentrate on providing internet search facilities. Some are set up as web portals with the aim of providing a complete resource for everything on the web that they consider to be worthwhile. Portals display their own editorial material, news headlines and other up-to-date information, as well as links to commercial partners and paid advertisements. They are good for general or commercial information but most will fail to identify websites for non-profit organizations, such as the NHS. Web portals also provide a search facility. Search engines attempt to search all the text on all the pages of the web. Software seeks out and indexes web pages, storing the results in sizeable databases. When a user types a

query, the search engine searches its database for pages that contain words matching the query and displays the results as a list of links (Box 16.3). Each search engine ranks results according to its own criteria and so different search engines can give different results for the same query.

Effective use of search engines

Before beginning a new search, the user should take time to consider what they already know, knowledge gaps and information required. It is advisable to have a plan that focuses the search. The user should select a set of keywords that best reflect the information need and narrow the search to a particular subject or topic. Results should be compared to the original information need. If appropriate

Box 16.3

Search engines are essentially made up of three interconnected parts: the crawler, the indexer and the query processor

The crawler (spider)	This is a specialized programme, a form of robot that constantly travels the web similar to a browser, following links with absolute diligence, returning a copy of each page it finds for the indexer
The indexer	This program maintains an extremely large database of computerized records. For any given website, the index will list all the pages on that site alongside other relevant information. The database is then inverted so that a typed phrase will lead to relevant URLs. Indexes are analysed in a manner that ranks the search results, giving preference to what are thought to be web pages more relevant to the user's inquiry. Tagged and analysed pages are ultimately handed over to the query processor
The query processor	This program moves between the user interface and the indexer. The query processor is designed to make it user-friendly, and to enable it to make an intelligent guess about the user's intentions in making their query

material is found on the first page of the search then the activity need go no further. It is important to know when to stop searching, especially when there is limited time.

When, however, the results do not match the information need, it is advisable to pause and reflect. The user should consider what they are searching for; can the search be refined by changing keywords, perhaps adding, taking away or replacing them? The keywords must match the information needed. One additional approach is to subtract any redundant words from the search query. These include words such as 'a', 'an', 'the', 'and', etc. It might also be helpful to rearrange the search so that the more important search terms are placed first, to give more influence when the results are ranked.

Boolean terms for academic databases are described in more detail later. In Google™, the Boolean terms AND and NOT are not used in the traditional sense. Google™ will automatically link a series of words using the AND operator, instead of NOT, to eliminate a word from the results. A space should be left after the word that is needed and a minus sign (−) should be typed immediately before the word that is to be excluded. The term OR can, however, be used in Google™ by typing OR between the words. Google™ can also be forced to link words by using a plus sign (+), especially where one of the words is a common word that might normally be ignored. The search engine can also be asked to search for a string of words in a particular order, e.g. 'Community-acquired pneumonia'. The user should examine search engine tools to make the most of any advanced features. Sometimes, the search engine itself may need to be changed or the basis of the search re-examined.

It is important to recognize that search engines do not necessarily index the whole of each document they retrieve. A search engine may upload each page in full, but it may only use the first few thousand characters for indexing and so vital information further down the web page will escape being indexed. Where a search engine does return a link to a site, sometimes it is not possible to access the content if the user is behind their organization's 'firewall'. Search engines do not locate everything on the web first-hand. It might be that a general search engine finds another site that is a more appropriate starting point, for example a health services directory. In that way, the search is narrowed automatically.

Some public web pages are protected from search engines through use of a file (robots.txt) that blocks access to the robot. This normally relates to personal, sensitive, interactive, timely or premium (subscription, or paid for) content. Another place that search engines cannot always reach is commercial data collections, or collections of valuable, copyrighted content, such as subscription-based academic journal databases and other specialized databases, information in professional directories, patents and news articles.

Assessing the quality of information on the web

There is no restriction on what is placed on the web or by whom. There is certainly no process of editorial or peer review for material placed on the web. Apart from the Advertising Standards Authority, which recently gained the authority to regulate marketing material on UK websites, no UK organization is currently responsible for regulating health- and medicines-related information on the internet. Under these conditions, there is always the danger that an internet site contains incomplete, inaccurate, irrelevant, obsolete or even hoax information. As a result, the utmost care should be taken in making use of health-related information from the internet. An informed approach must include a system for evaluating the quality of the information found against the intended use of that information. Factors listed below can all affect the quality of an information source; they are not mutually exclusive and must be considered in combination (see Table 16.2).

Context of the website

The user must identify the scope of the website (what it aims to cover), as well as the intended audience (at whom the information is aimed). Knowledge of URL nomenclature helps to contextualize the information found. For example, information on a product licensed in the USA may not be applicable in the UK market.

The user should also assess the authority and reputation of the author(s) and website providing the information. Authority is based primarily on the perceived knowledge, qualifications and expertise of the author(s) as well as the reputation of the parent organization.

Table 16.2 Evaluating the quality of an internet-based website for health- and medicines-related information

Activity	Purpose
Follow internal links	To find out as much as possible about the resource, e.g. the scope of the material; the intended audience and coverage; the origin of the information; who is responsible for the content; involvement of others in the production of material; any access restrictions
Analyse the URL	To find out where the information comes from and to judge if they are qualified to provide the information, e.g. the individual or group that has taken responsibility for the website
Examine the information contained	To find out the subjects and types of materials covered; comprehensiveness of coverage; notable omissions; notable indicators of accuracy; editorial procedures; research basis to the information; creation date; the frequency and/or regularity of any updating
Consider the presentation	To find out if the resource is frequently unavailable or noticeably slow to access; any access restrictions (e.g. by geographical region, hardware/software requirements); whether there is a registration procedure and whether this is straightforward; whether the available content is free or subscription based; the copyright statement and copyright restrictions; whether the site is particularly difficult or easy to use; presence or absence of user support facilities and/or help information
Obtain additional information	To find out if an individual or group has taken responsibility for the website; whether they are qualified to provide this information; whether the resource is well known (e.g. recommended via links), reviewed and/or heavily used
Compare with other similar websites	To find out if a resource is unique in terms of content or format and any differences between mirror and original sites for the same materials

Reputation is created when others endorse the value of a website by using it. The user should consider and draw inferences from the popularity of a website. Establishing the provenance of a source can also help assess its potential quality, for example, knowing when the website was first established. A final consideration is how the website compares with rival material and whether it offers anything unique.

Content of the website

The reputation and popularity of a site, or even the expertise of an author, do not guarantee the quality of content. Here, the key questions relate to the accuracy, currency and coverage of the health-related information found. The likely accuracy of a website is inextricably linked to its perceived authority. Users will rely on a number of markers to judge accuracy, including: whether the information has been edited or peer reviewed; the basis of the information; possible bias and the overall impression provided by a website.

It is important to find out when the information found was produced (and updated) and whether the frequency of updates can provide up-to-the-minute information. A final consideration is the coverage provided by material found on the website. The relevance of this factor depends very much on the user's information needs. The quality of coverage includes the comprehensiveness of a resource and links to further information.

Format of the website

As well as a marker of immediate usefulness, the format of a website is important when considering its potential use. Three distinct factors can be considered here; accessibility, presentation and usability. In relation to accessibility, some resources are not available to the public; may require special software or hardware for accessing content; require subscription; some websites contain material with copyright restrictions; and some are not written in English. Also, overwhelming demand, server unreliability and heavy use of graphics can all impede access to an otherwise good website.

Most probably, users will intuitively form an impression of a website based on its design and interface. This might be based on such factors as sensible use of hypertext links and other navigation aids, indexes, menus and search facilities. Usability is, of course, related to accessibility and presentation. A good website should allow the user to navigate the site and find the required information. Another important consideration, nowadays, is the presentation of a website on mobile devices.

User-generated content

Recent times have seen an upsurge in what is known as user-generated content on the internet. Users have no difficulty publishing their output if they can find a way to put it on the internet, where it is instantly available to a global audience and where it can be found by search engines. Many kinds of user-generated content exist. A particular example is a wiki, a type of website that allows the visitors to easily add, remove, edit and change some available content, sometimes without the need for registration. An important example is Wikipedia. This is a vast online reference work that is written and edited by its users. It can be changed at will by anyone, so cannot be an authoritative reference source. Yet, because it is easily accessible and provides wide coverage, students will (erroneously) use websites such as Wikipedia in preference to good, authoritative textbooks.

The sequence of information

Information is often repackaged, re-versioned and developed for different audiences and different uses. Health-related information has by tradition been categorized on the basis of an accepted chronology of inception and development. As such, information is labelled, as belonging to a primary, secondary or tertiary reference source. Primary reference sources are those in which new information is published, usually in the form of research, such as papers in biomedical journals. Secondary reference sources, such as academic databases, act to index and/or abstract literature from primary sources. Tertiary sources provide an overview of a topic in a condensed readable form and include textbooks, drug compendia and formularies; with authors drawing on the primary literature for material. An awareness of this can help pharmacists identify where to look for the most appropriate type of information for their particular information needs (see Table 16.3).

Primary reference sources

The primary literature is the basis of the information hierarchy. The term primary literature is used in essence to refer to original publications and normally entails research papers published in journals, although it can include other material. Preliminary research findings are sometimes presented at conferences and a record of these is normally published in the conference abstract book or the conference website.

The publication of research papers

Primary research enters the public domain once the researchers write and submit their work to a primary reference source, such as a journal publication. Authors aim to create accurate, clear and easily accessible reports of their studies that can be considered for publication. Each journal is headed by an editor who is the person responsible for its entire editorial content, although some journals also have an independent editorial advisory board to help establish and maintain editorial policy.

Most health-related research papers based on empirical methods, such as observational and experimental studies, follow a conventional style, such as that advocated by the International Committee of Medical Journal Editors (ICMJE). The text of these papers is usually divided into sections with the headings: Introduction, Methods, Results and Discussion, and sometimes Conclusion. This so-called 'IMRAD' structure is not an arbitrary publication format, but rather a direct reflection of the process of scientific discovery. Specific research designs have additional reporting requirements (see Table 16.4).

Abstracts and keywords merit a special note, since abstracts are the only substantive portion of articles indexed in many electronic databases and the only portion many readers read. Keywords assist indexers in cross-referencing the article. Abstracts should reflect the content of the article accurately and provide the context or background for the study, stating the study's purposes, basic procedures, main findings and principal conclusions. The abstract should emphasize new and important aspects of the study or observations. Terms from the medical subject headings (MeSH) list of Index Medicus should be used if available or current terminology may be used.

Once a manuscript is received, a process known as 'peer review' is used by editors to help decide

Table 16.3 Advantages and disadvantages of primary, secondary and tertiary reference sources

Source	Advantages	Disadvantages
Primary	Contains current, original and 'cutting-edge' information	Potential for bias and not guaranteed to be without errors
		Interpretation and critical appraisal required by readers
		Time lag from publication to widespread acceptance
Secondary	Rapid access to the primary literature	Time period between article publication and inclusion in secondary sources
	Large spectrum of information on specific topics	User needs to have access to primary sources
	Journals covered generally of a high standard	The number of journals indexed by each system
	Ability to link concepts to perform complex searches	Command language varies between databases
	Most resources have a facility for provision of routine updates on selected topics	The user needs to be familiar with a particular database's structure and terminology and to have proficient search skills in order to search effectively
		Need for user to be proficient in sifting through the sources listed on a particular subject to find the most relevant information
		Not suitable for browsing
		Can be expensive to access relative to tertiary sources
Tertiary	Present users with a manageable digest of a vast amount of published information	Out of date almost as soon as published – exceptions include electronic books with frequent updates
	Easy to handle, readable, contain concise information and indexed	Information in textbooks sometimes not comprehensive. Poorly referenced. Opinion of author

Table 16.4 Reporting guidelines for specific study designs

Initiative	Type of study	Source
CONSORT	Randomized controlled trials	http://www.consort-statement.org/
STARD	Studies of diagnostic accuracy	http://www.stard-statement.org/
PRISMA	Systematic reviews and meta-analyses	http://www.prisma-statement.org/
STROBE	Observational studies in epidemiology	http://www.strobe-statement.org/
MOOSE	Meta-analyses of observational studies in epidemiology	http://www.consort-statement.org/resources/downloads/other-instruments/

which manuscripts are suitable for their journals. Peer review also helps authors and editors in their efforts to improve the quality of reporting. A peer reviewed journal is one that has submitted most of its published research articles for outside review. However, even the 'best' journals contain some material that has not been refereed.

The quality of health-related journals is variable. Some journals do not adopt a peer-review process and can publish studies that are not scientifically robust. High-impact factor journals such as the *British Medical Journal* and the *New England Journal of Medicine* are considered prestigious publications. Primary reference sources of particular relevance to pharmacy practice include the *Pharmaceutical Journal* and the *International Journal of Pharmacy Practice*.

Because a primary reference source presents the paper in its original form, the reader has the opportunity to critically appraise and analyse the study or article in order to develop a conclusion on its merits.

Open access academic information

Traditionally, authors write-up their research into a paper and submit it to a journal, the paper is peer-reviewed to ensure quality, and the publisher then publishes the paper in the journal. An alternative to this model now exists in the form of open access publishing. In this publishing model, the authors make the research available on the web, via a repository or in a freely accessible journal, with authors paying for this privilege. This process bypasses the publisher completely. There are differing views on whether open access publishing is a good thing or not.

Additionally, universities in the UK are now expected to maintain an open archive of the peer-reviewed literature they have produced.

Secondary reference sources

Secondary reference sources are searchable resources that index and/or abstract from the primary literature. Some are equipped with alerting systems, which scan selected journals as soon as they are published and send summarized abstracts directly to users to help them maintain knowledge of new developments from a large pool of journals. Nowadays, the data format used for providing users with frequently updated content is known as a web feed. A recent addition to web feeds is the RSS (really simple syndication) feed, which contains either a summary content from an associated website or the full text.

Secondary reference sources are, generally, searchable electronically but may also be available in hard-copy format. Secondary reference sources include commercial academic databases, resource gateways (collections of sites that have been reviewed), as well as the more recent academic search offerings of internet search engines such as Google™, Scholar and Microsoft® Live Academic.

Academic databases

An academic database is a well-designed catalogue created and maintained by trained personnel. A database, in essence, is a set of searchable records. Nowadays, records are commonly maintained as a set of virtual cards in a computer database. Two main categories of academic database exist: the 'bibliographic' database contains information in summary form (the abstract); the 'full-text' database provides access to electronic versions of the full text of documents.

The purpose of an academic database is to enable users to systematically search the records so that specific search terms can ultimately 'unearth' relevant items. In the case of a scientific paper, for example, its record might contain details of title, authors, journal name, date of publication, keywords, abstract and so on. Each of these categories in a database is called a 'field'. The record then is a collection of several fields of information about the item, be it a book or a journal article. The process of creating and adding records to an academic database is known as indexing and each record is called a citation.

Some journals ask for submitting authors to provide a set of 'keywords', usually corresponding to MeSH headings, for the purpose of indexing and classification. MeSH is the National Library of Medicine's controlled vocabulary thesaurus. It consists of sets of terms naming descriptors in a hierarchical structure that permits searching at various levels of specificity. MeSH descriptors are arranged in both an alphabetical and a hierarchical structure. At the most general level of the hierarchical structure, are very broad headings such as 'Anatomy' or 'Mental Disorders'. More specific headings are found at more narrow levels of the 11-level hierarchy, such as 'Ankle' and 'Conduct Disorder'.

Many academic databases now exist, and although their search interfaces might at first look very different, similar tools are usually found on each. To the novice user, academic search interfaces can appear somewhat intimidating; the form looks quite complex and appears as an advanced search screen. But the format of the academic database search screen enables the user to simultaneously search for something specific (e.g. the keywords) in any of the database's fields. Sometimes, each text entry box in the interface corresponds to a field. For example, restricting the keywords to particular fields such as the title or abstract can help focus the search by returning only those articles where the

Box 16.4

Checklist for exploring the search interface and other features of an academic database

The user should take the time to find out:

- How to combine keywords
- How to search in different fields
- How to limit searches
- How to keep track of useful citations
- How to export citations
- What format the information can be viewed in
- How the items might be retrieved
- Whether full text is available
- Whether there is a browse feature for scanning specific journals
- Whether an article's references are also available as links or in full text
- Whether there is a 'cited by' option
- How easy it is to move between articles

Box 16.5

Boolean operators that can be used when searching academic databases

AND	Combines search terms so that each search result contains all of the terms
OR	Combines search terms so that each search result contains at least one of the terms
NOT	Excludes terms so that each search result does not contain any of the terms that follow it

keywords are a prominent feature. A new database resource can be explored by examining helpful features that enhance efficiency (see Box 16.4).

Boolean logic defines logical relationships between terms in a search. The conventional Boolean search operators are AND, OR and NOT. They can be used to create a very broad or very narrow search (see Box 16.5). To make better use of Boolean operators, one can use *parentheses* to nest query terms within other query terms, as they specify the order in which they are interpreted. The information within parentheses is read first, followed by the information outside the parentheses. For example, when one enters (aspirin OR ibuprofen) AND analgesic, the search engine retrieves results containing the word aspirin or the word ibuprofen together with the word analgesic in the fields searched by default.

Once a search is conducted and results returned, most databases offer a facility for marking and exporting useful records. Users can then decide which references are worth retrieving as full papers. Most databases, traditionally classified as 'bibliographic', will automatically help retrieve the full paper through icons such as 'Check for Full Text' and 'View Full Text'.

Citation indexes and impact factors

As referred to above, citation indexes and impact factors can be used to help assess the quality of a publication. A citation in a paper is the formal acknowledgement of intellectual debt to previously published research. It generally contains sufficient bibliographical information to uniquely identify the cited document. An obvious example of a citation is a reference listed at the end of a scientific research paper.

Citation and article counts are taken to be important indicators of how frequently current researchers are using individual journals. The impact factor in brief is the average number of times that articles from the journal published in a specific period have been cited by others. The notion, well accepted in the scientific community, is that the higher the impact factor, the 'better' the journal.

Box 16.6 lists some relevant databases.

Tertiary reference sources

Information from primary reference sources, perhaps retrieved using a secondary reference source, can in due course come to be included in textbooks and similar tertiary publications. As mentioned above, tertiary reference sources provide an overview of a topic in a condensed readable form with authors drawing on the primary literature for material. Examples are textbooks, drug compendia and formularies. Key publications include *Martindale: The Complete Drug Reference*, and the *British National Formulary* (BNF). There are also textbooks covering specific subject areas. Table 16.5 lists some of the key tertiary drug information resources for practising pharmacists in the UK.

Textbooks are important for locating established knowledge or information that is not rapidly changing. The information in a tertiary source is updated

Box 16.6

Secondary reference sources for health- and medicines-related publications Each database may be searchable via a number of interfaces

BioMed Central provides full access to its portfolio of journals

The Cochrane Library is part of the Cochrane Collaboration, an international independent organization, dedicated to making up-to-date, accurate information about the effects of health care readily available worldwide. There is a collection of databases to search. One the Cochrane Database of Systematic Reviews (CDSR) represents a high level of evidence on which to base clinical treatment decisions

Embase is a major biomedical and pharmacological database, produced by Elsevier Science. It indexes over 7600 biomedical journals from around the world. Coverage dates back to 1947 and it includes over 24 million records

International Pharmaceutical Abstracts (IPA) is a comprehensive collection of pharmacy literature including information on drug use and development, pharmacy practice and education

Iowa Drug Information Service (IDIS) indexing/full-text system, is a bibliographical database 200 premier English language medical and pharmaceutical journals but only those articles relating to drug therapy in humans are indexed

Medline is widely regarded as the premier database for bibliographical and abstract coverage of biomedical literature. It is created by the US National Library of Medicine (NLM®), and uses MeSH (medical subject headings) indexing

Natural Medicines Comprehensive Database provides evidence-based, clinical information on natural medicines

Pharm-line® is a database for medicines management, pharmacy practice and prescribing produced by medicines information pharmacists at Guy's and St Thomas' Hospital, London. About 11000 new records are added each year. All MI centres in the UK have access to Pharm-line

Reaxys© is a chemical information solution, covering over 200 years of primary literature. The database contains data on structures, reactions, facts and citations for more than 11 million compounds

Science Direct contains over 25% of the world's science, technology and medicine full-text and bibliographical information. It offers a journal collection of over 2500 titles.

TICTAC is a visual drug identification database provided by Virtual Health Network. It covers medicines, illicit drugs, veterinary products, vitamin and food supplements, herbal remedies and products that might be mistaken for drugs such as confectionery. It contains detailed information on over 24000 tablets and capsules or related products, with over 65000 high-quality images of those products

against new information or knowledge documented in the primary literature only once every 3–4 years, when the book is updated and published as a new edition. Thus it can take 5 years or more for new research findings to filter into medical textbooks. In addition, most books are out of date almost as soon as they are published. Because the knowledge base in many areas of therapeutics is rapidly changing, the information contained in textbooks may be too old to be useful. This problem does not apply usually to those textbooks available in electronic full texts. Another important exception is the BNF, which is updated and published as a new edition every 6 months.

Tertiary references should be the starting point when trying to find background information on a subject. With the advent of the electronic age, it is easy to forget that information can be found quickly and easily in a book. Books are easy to handle, readable, contain concise information and are indexed.

Having said that, the reader must also be aware that the information presented in a textbook is subject to the opinion, evaluation and bias of the author. It is often assumed that what is written in a textbook must be accurate; in fact, the author(s) may not have comprehensively searched, analysed or interpreted all information. The information contained in textbooks may also not be as comprehensive as the reader would like. But, especially in comparison to user-generated websites such as Wikipedia, good textbooks are an important and reliable resource and they should not be overlooked.

Organizing and citing references

For academic work, it is often necessary to store a relatively large number of retrieved citations. It is always advisable to implement some system for keeping track of the information amassed. Bibliography management systems exist for this

Table 16.5 Key tertiary drug information sources for pharmacy inquiries (further details available on publishers' websites)

Type of resource	Authors/editors	Publisher
Core resource		
Martindale: The Complete Drug Reference	Sweetman SC	Pharmaceutical Press
British National Formulary	N/A	Jointly by British Medical Association and the Royal Pharmaceutical Society of Great Britain
Monthly Index of Medical Specialities (MIMS)	N/A	Haymarket Business Subscriptions
The OTC Directory	N/A	Proprietary Association of Great Britain
Chemist and Druggist Directory	N/A	CMP Medica
Therapeutics		
Clinical Pharmacy and Therapeutics	Walker R, Whittlesea C	Churchill Livingstone
Clinical Medicine	Kumar PJ, Clark ML	Elsevier
Merck Manual of Diagnosis and Treatment	Porter RS	Merck and Co
Adverse drug reactions		
Meyler's Side-Effects of Drugs: The International Encyclopaedia of Adverse Drug Reactions and Interactions	Aronson JK, Dukes MNG	Elsevier
Children's doses		
British National Formulary for Children	N/A	British Medical Association, Royal Pharmaceutical Society of Great Britain, Royal College of Paediatrics and Child Health
Complementary therapies		
Stockley's Herbal Medicines Interactions: A Guide to the Interactions of Herbal Medicines	Williamson EM, Driver S, Baxter K	Pharmaceutical Press
Dietary Supplements	Mason P	Pharmaceutical Press
Contraception		
Contraception: Your Questions Answered	Guillebaud J	Churchill Livingstone
Cytotoxics		
The Cytotoxics Handbook	Allwood M, Stanley A, Wright P	Radcliffe Medical press
Dictionaries		
Concise Medical Dictionary	Martin EA	Oxford University Press
Drug administration		
Handbook of Drug Administration via Enteral Feeding Tubes	White R, Bradnam V	Pharmaceutical Press;

(Continued)

Table 16.5 Continued

Type of resource	Authors/editors	Publisher
NEWT Guidelines for Administration of Medicines to Patients with Enteral Feeding Tubes or Swallowing Difficulties	Wrexham Maelor Hospital	North East Wales NHS Trust
Injectable Drugs Guide	Gray A, Wright J, Goodey V, Bruce L	Pharmaceutical Press
Drug interactions		
Stockley's Drug Interactions	Baxter K	Pharmaceutical Press
Evidence-based medicines		
Evidence-based Medicine: How to Practice and Teach it	Straus SE, Glasziou P, Richardson WS, Haynes RB	Churchill Livingstone/Elsevier
Legal and ethical		
Dale and Applebe's Pharmacy Law and Ethics	Applebe GE, Wingfield J	Pharmaceutical Press
Palliative care		
A Guide to Symptom Relief in Palliative Care	Regnard CFB, Dean M	Radcliffe Medical Press
Pharmacokinetics		
Basic Clinical Pharmacokinetics	Winter ME	Lippincott Williams and Wilkins
Pregnancy and lactation		
Drugs During Pregnancy and Lactation	Schaefer C, Peters PWJ, Miller RK	Elsevier
Prescribing in Pregnancy	Rubin P, Ramsay M	Blackwell Publishing
Psychiatry		
Maudsley Prescribing Guidelines in Psychiatry	Taylor D, Paton C, Kapur R	Blackwell Publishing
Renal or hepatic impairment		
Drugs and the Liver: A guide to drug handling in liver dysfunction	North-Lewis P.	Pharmaceutical Press
The Renal Drug Handbook	Ashley C, Currie A	Radcliffe Medical Press
Wound management		
Formulary of Wound Management Products	Morgan D	Euromed Communications

purpose including, but not exclusively, RefWorks, EndNote®, Reference Manager® and ProCite®. These products help users create personal databases for written academic work such as projects, reports and papers.

A number of referencing styles exist for citing retrieved information. Most academic institutions and publications have standardized requirements. Whatever style is used, accuracy, clarity and consistency are the key factors when citing information sources.

Avoiding plagiarism

As discussed, a citation is the formal acknowledgement of intellectual debt to previously published research. Therefore, referencing is a way of ensuring that due credit is given to other people's work. While common knowledge does not need a citation or reference, taking someone's work and not indicating where it came from is termed plagiarism and is regarded as an infringement of copyright. Higher education institutions invest in plagiarism detection software to scan assessment material.

Information services

Pharmacists are expected to be able to provide accurate, reliable, impartial, relevant and up-to-date information on a wide range of issues. A number of organizations exist to help. Unlike libraries, pharmacy information services can provide tailor-made answers to specific enquiries using analysis and interpretation. In the UK, the best known facility is the Medicines Information (MI) service based in NHS hospital pharmacies.

Most information services will work to standardized procedures to ensure quality in enquiry answering. Pharmacists working in any sector of the profession should follow similar methods. The same basic information should be collected from the enquirer (see Box 16.7). Ideally, the full manner in which enquiries are handled should be documented to provide an audit trail for quality assurance purposes. Clear and comprehensive documentation is necessary for legal and ethical reasons, in order to ascertain exactly what information was provided, by whom and what resources were used. Appropriate documentation also ensures that an enquiry can be located at a later date, to save time in dealing with future enquiries.

Medicines information services

The NHS MI service is provided by a network of 220 local MI centres based in the hospital trust pharmacy departments, as well as 14 regional centres and two national centres (Northern Ireland and Wales). The aim of MI is to support the safe, effective and efficient use of medicines through the provision of evidence-based information and advice on therapeutic use of medicines. The centres are staffed by pharmacists and technicians with clinical

Box 16.7

Headings for documenting medicines information enquiries

- Full name and contact details of enquirer
- The date and time the enquiry was received
- Full identity of the person receiving the enquiry
- Mutually realistic agreed timescale for provision of answer
- Enquirer's preference for method of reply
- Clear account of the enquiry in sufficient detail to allow a third party to tackle the enquiry without further contact with the enquirer
- All relevant background information for patient-specific enquiries to include: patient age; sex; weight; medication (including dose and duration of therapy); diagnosis; relevant medical history; liver and renal function; history of adverse drug reactions; whether pregnant or breast-feeding
- Annotation of enquiry at various stages with the date and signature
- The search itself in the order the resources have been searched with clear identification of resources
- Evaluation of the information, consideration of practicality of advice and detail of answer
- Summary of answer given
- Completion date and/or time
- All other relevant information

expertise. Centres provide an enquiry answering service, to patients and healthcare professionals, on all aspects of drug therapy. Over half a million enquiries are handled by the service each year.

In addition, the UK Medicines Information (UKMi) network produces a range of resources available through its own internet site (www.ukmi.nhs.uk/) or that of the National electronic Library of Medicines (NeLM) (http://www.nelm.nhs.uk/en/).

RPS information centre

This is based at the Royal Pharmaceutical Society (RPS) in London and comprises the Library and Technical Information Service, providing a service for members. The information pharmacists can help answer scientific and technical questions relating to pharmacy practice or continuing education from members. The subject scope includes advice on the usage and availability of proprietary and other medicinal products, adverse drug reactions and interactions, and the identification of medicines from overseas.

NPA information services

The National Pharmacy Association (NPA) has an information service for members only. The department is a complete reference centre, skilled at assisting members with a wide range of pharmacy practice-related questions. In addition, the NPA information department includes a specialist library of British and foreign reference books and a range of technical CD-ROMs.

The pharmaceutical industry medical information departments

All pharmaceutical companies are able to provide certain types of information on their products. This source of information can be particularly important for new products, when there is often a lack of published information.

Conclusion

The ability to retrieve relevant health-related information in a timely and efficient manner is central to the practice of all pharmacy professionals. The advent of the electronic age and the expanse of available information can make information retrieval appear a daunting task. However, categorizing information, developing an understanding of search and retrieval processes, knowing who to approach for help, as well as groundwork and deliberation can all help facilitate the process.

KEY POINTS

- As part of their work, pharmacists handle a large amount of information. In order to do so efficiently they must know how to find and evaluate information sources
- While the internet gives access to a vast resource, but of variable reliability, printed books still play an important role
- Commercial search engines give access to web pages, but to use them effectively it is necessary to understand their operators
- No search engine will give access to all relevant websites
- There is no control over material placed on the web, so its reliability must be evaluated by the user
- User-generated websites, such as Wikipedia, are less reliable
- Information sources are classified as primary, secondary or tertiary
- Primary reference sources are original research publications which normally follow a conventional layout style
- Secondary sources are searchable indices or abstracts which lead to primary sources
- Keywords are often used for searching, especially in academic databases
- Tertiary sources present an overview of a topic
- Textbooks are quick and easy to use, but are inevitably out of date and may be subject to bias or be incomplete
- NHS information services are based, mainly, in hospital pharmacies in the UK
- The UK Medicines Information (UKMi) network produces resources which are available through its website

Communication skills for pharmacists and their team

Judith A. Rees and Isabel J. Featherstone

Introduction

Josie is a community pharmacist. At the end of the working day she thinks back to what has happened that day. She has discussed with customers their purchases of medicines; advised patients how to use their prescription medicines; conducted a medicines use review; phoned the local GP about a potential drug interaction; supervised a methadone addict; spoken briefly to the district nurse; negotiated with her boss about a day off; interviewed a potential sales assistant; exchanged pleasantries with the delivery person; and had been introduced to the new chairman of the local pharmaceutical committee at lunchtime.

Ravi, a hospital pharmacist, similarly looked back at his working day. He had spent time on the wards discussing drug-related matters with junior doctors; undertaken medication histories; and talked to a patient about their discharge medication. The latter task involved phoning the patient's GP and local pharmacist to arrange a continuity of medicine supply. He had given a seminar for fellow pharmacists. Later he had attended a committee meeting, with other healthcare professionals and administrators on developing policies for the safe use of medicines. He had finished off his day supervising the dispensary, and dealing with a complaint from a prescriber.

From the above descriptions of two pharmacists' very different working days, it can be seen that while each is performing pharmaceutical tasks, all of these tasks required the use of communication skills. In fact, almost everything we do in life depends on communication. Pharmacists spend a large proportion of each working day communicating with other people – patients, doctors, other healthcare professionals, staff and others. Poor communication has the potential to cause a range of problems, from misunderstandings with healthcare professionals to inappropriate or incomplete advice on the use of medication to a patient/customer.

Thus, there is a need for effective communication skills for pharmacists. But how effective is our communication? Good communication demands effort, thought, time and a willingness to learn how to make the process effective. Some people find that good communication is difficult to achieve and an awareness of this fact is an important first step to improvement.

This chapter considers some of the elements of successful communication, looking at our assumptions and expectations of people and at the processes involved in communication, listening and questioning skills. A total model for an effective pharmacist–patient consultation is outlined, followed by the barriers to effective communication in pharmacy. The importance of confidentiality is emphasized.

Assumptions and expectations

When we meet somebody for the first time, we make assumptions about that person. We often put people into categories and the assumptions lead to expectations of their behaviour, job and character.

This initial judgement of a person is often based purely on what we see and hear and includes appearance, demeanor, speech, dress, age, gender, race and physical disabilities. It is important that we are aware of these assumptions in order to avoid stereotyping people. For example, the impression we have of a person wearing a hooded jacket, baseball cap and jeans may be very different from that of the same person wearing a designer shirt and smart trousers.

What is communication?

Communication is more than just talking. It is generally agreed that in any communication, the actual words (the talking) convey only about 10% of the message. This is called verbal communication. The other 90% is transmitted by non-verbal communication which consists of how it is said (about 40%) and body language (about 50%).

The communication process

Argyle (1983) describes the message process as a sender encoding a message, which is then decoded by the receiver:

> Mistakes can be made by both sender and receiver. The sender may not send the message they wished to send or they may sometimes intentionally seek to deceive. At the receiving end the message may not be decoded correctly. Poor communication skills contribute to these mistakes in encoding and decoding. Messages are not normally one way and if we send a

message then we generally expect a reply, and so in replying the receiver becomes the sender and the sender becomes the receiver. While the messages may be going backwards and forwards between two people, effective communication becomes a helical model. In other words, what one person says influences how the other person responds in a spiral fashion with reiteration and repetition, coming back around the spiral.

Pharmacists tend to see contact with patients/customers as either getting information or imparting advice. However, this ignores the vital purpose of communication, which is to initiate and enhance the relationship with their patients/customers. If this can be achieved, then pharmacists will be perceived as more 'patient friendly' and more supportive of patients. Indeed, good communication skills will make it easier for a pharmacist to seek information and to advise patients.

Listening skills

Communication is not just about saying the right words; it involves listening correctly. If we do not listen properly, then it means we are not decoding the message that is being sent to us. However good the patient is at telling the pharmacist their symptoms, if the pharmacist does not listen correctly, then the patient may be given the wrong diagnosis, medicine or advice. Listening and hearing are different. Hearing is a physical ability, while listening is a skill. Listening skills enable a person to make sense of and understand what another person is saying. The listening process is an active one that consists of three basic steps, namely:

- *Hearing*: listening enough to catch what the person is saying
- *Understanding*: understanding the message in his or her own way (this may not be what was intended by the speaker)
- *Judging* takes the understanding stage and questions whether it makes sense. Do I believe what I have heard? Is it credible? Have I really understood what I have been told or have I misinterpreted the meaning?

How to be a good listener

Listening, like other skills, takes practice. Tips for developing good listening skills are shown in Box 17.1.

Box 17.1

Tips for being a good listener

- Always look attentive at the person who is speaking. Maintain eye contact and stand/sit facing them. Try not to fidget or move around too much. Do not stare at the floor or look at some other object in the room
- Focus your mind on what is being said. Do not let your mind wander, even if you think you know what is going to be said or you think you have heard it all before
- Always let the speaker finish what they are saying. Do not interrupt – speakers prefer to finish what they were trying to say. In addition, interruption tends to imply that you were not listening
- Let yourself finish listening before you start to talk. Listening is an active process and you cannot really listen if you are busy thinking of how to reply
- Listen for the main ideas of the message. The main ideas may be repeated several times by the speaker
- Ask appropriate questions or repeat what has been said in your own words if you are not sure that your understanding is correct
- Give feedback to the speaker by nodding to show you understand (but only if you do). It may be helpful to smile, laugh, grimace or just be silent to let the speaker know that you are listening. Leaning towards the speaker may show you are interested in what the speaker has to say and give them encouragement
- Do not forget the non-verbal side of communication. The speaker may be demonstrating many non-verbal clues and gestures, which may indicate their true feelings. So in the listening process, use your eyes as well as your ears.

In a pharmacy, avoid listening across a barrier such as a counter or desk or getting too close and invading a patient's 'intimate zone'

Questioning skills

Pharmacists need effective questioning skills to obtain information from patients/customers. Examples of situations in which questioning skills are used include:

- Drug-history taking
- Requests for treatments for minor ailments
- Probing a patient's knowledge of how they take/use their medicines
- Determining the need for an emergency supply.

Box 17.2

PQRST symptom analysis

- **P** = Precipitating/palliative factors
  Ask: What were you doing when the problem started? Does anything make it better/worse, such as medicine or change in position?
- **Q** = Quality/quantity
  Ask: Can you describe the symptom? How often are you experiencing it? What does it feel/look like or sound like?
- **R** = Region/radiation/related symptoms
  Ask: Can you point to where the problem is? Does it occur or spread anywhere else? Do you have any other symptoms? (These symptoms may be related to the presenting symptoms)
- **S** = Severity
  Ask: Is the symptom mild, moderate or severe? Asking the patient to grade on a scale 0–10 may help
- **T** = Timing
  Ask: When did the symptom start? How often does it occur? How long does it last?

Effective questioning skills involve the use of different types of questions, namely open and closed questions.

Effective questioning should be used in assessing a patient's presenting symptoms. The mnemonic 'PQRST' provides key questions which will help pharmacists to obtain an overview of symptoms, although additional questions can be added, for example, 'Is the patient taking any concurrent medication?' The PQRST approach to symptom analysis is shown in Box 17.2.

Questioning skills do not apply only to pharmacist–patient/customer situations. Good questioning skills are required in staff training, implementing procedures and other management tasks, as well as dealing with other healthcare professionals and administrative staff.

On many occasions, questioning may not be a face-to-face situation. Often, a pharmacist has to communicate by telephone with, e.g. another healthcare professional. The major drawback of this type of communication is that reliance is put solely on good verbal communication skills and not on the non-verbal aspect of communication. In these circumstances, it is vital to obtain the information as efficiently as possible. For example, when a GP phones to order a prescription medicine for a patient, the pharmacist is required to ask specific questions to ensure that all information is accurate. As another example, a patient phones about a prescription item – using good questioning skills, the pharmacist should check the prescription information, identify the patient's concerns and be able to take appropriate action.

A model for guiding the pharmacist–patient interview

The Calgary–Cambridge model was developed in 1996 to aid the teaching of communication skills. Since that time, it has been adopted widely (see Ch. 18). The Calgary–Cambridge model is designed to specifically integrate communication skills with the content skills of traditional medical history and thus the approach can be used by pharmacists for their core tasks, such as drug history taking and the interviewing of patients to determine the best treatment for presenting minor ailments.

The Calgary–Cambridge model has five main stages:

- Initiating the session
- Gathering information
- Physical examination
- Explanation and planning
- Closing the session.

Concomitantly, and alongside these stages, the model provides for two further ongoing stages:

- Providing structure to the interview
- Building the relationship.

Providing the structure to the interview involves:

○ *Summarizing* at the end of a line of enquiry to make sure there is mutual understanding between the pharmacist/prescriber and the patient/customer, before continuing

○ *Signposting* – in other words indicating to the patient when moving from one section to the next, e.g. gathering information and explaining

○ *Sequencing* – this means developing a logical sequence which is apparent to the patient, in other words do not interrupt information gathering to explain and then go back to information gathering

○ *Timing* – this means keeping to agreed time, being able to close the session and not having to close abruptly because the time has run out.

Building the relationship during the interview involves:

○ *Developing rapport* – being aware of non-verbal behaviour clues and involving the patient in the interview process. Developing rapport has four areas:

  ▪ Acceptance of the patient, their views and feelings and being non-judgemental

  ▪ Empathy with the patient by showing an understanding and appreciation of the patient's feelings or predicament

  ▪ Support which expresses itself as concern for the patient, a willingness to help, an acknowledgement of their coping efforts and self-care, e.g. use of OTC medicines, and offering a partnership approach

  ▪ Sensitivity, which includes dealing sensitively with embarrassing and disturbing topics.

Some sensitive areas can be seen in Table 17.1.

An awareness of non-verbal behaviour is the next step in building the relationship. The awareness relates to the interviewers themselves – Are they demonstrating good eye contact and other features of positive non-verbal behaviour? Are they picking up on any cues displayed by the patient's non-verbal behaviour? Any note taking or reading (or use of computers) should not interrupt or affect the dialogue.

In building the relationship, it is important to involve the patient and to share thoughts with them (e.g. 'I think we are looking for a medicine that doesn't cause drowsiness'), to provide a rationale for questions (e.g. explain why you need to know about concurrent prescribed medicines when recommending an OTC cough medicine), and to explain and ask permission if a physical examination is necessary.

We will now consider in more detail the stages of the interview process relevant to current pharmacy practice, according to the Calgary–Cambridge model.

Initiating the session

Preparation involves the interviewer (the pharmacist) preparing him- or herself and focusing on the session. The pharmacist will need to focus on meeting the patient. It is important to establish initial rapport by greeting the patient, introducing yourself, the role and nature of the interview (e.g. a pharmacist conducting a drug medication history) and obtain consent, if necessary. The next step is to identify the

Table 17.1 Types of patients' problems and the communication difficulties which they present

Problem type	Examples	Communication difficulties
Embarrassing problems	Contraception; disorders of the reproductive system; hyperhydrosis; skin conditions	Obtaining privacy in the pharmacy. Establishing a common language of understanding. Demonstrating empathy and understanding. Establishing trust and confidentiality. Not exhibiting negative non-verbal behaviour
Emotional/ psychological	Anxiety; depression; marital problems; drug abuse and dependence; stress	Demonstrating empathy and understanding. Insufficient time for counselling. Evaluating patient's immediate needs. Establishing the nature and amount of advice to be given. Establishing two-way listening
Problems of handicap Sensory Physical Communicative Mental Psychological Social	 Blindness, deafness Paralysis, congenital deformity Speech impairment Educationally subnormal Personality disorders Introversion	Making inaccurate judgements regarding personality, intellect, etc. Providing effective explanations. Listening and taking sufficient time with patient. Overcoming social barriers
Terminal illness		Knowing what to say and how to say it. Establishing patient's feelings
Financial problems		Interpreting cues given off by patient. Not embarrassing the patient regarding cost of medicines

reasons for the consultation by an opening question such as, for a patient requesting to see the pharmacist, 'I understand that you would like to speak to me – how can I help?' The patient's answer must be listened to attentively and then the pharmacist needs to check and confirm the list of problems/queries/ issues with the patient. During this stage, the pharmacist should pick up on any verbal and non-verbal behaviour cues and help facilitate the patient's responses. To complete this stage, an agenda for the interview is negotiated (e.g. 'So you would like me to recommend a medicine to help relieve your cough that doesn't make you drowsy? Is that right?').

Gathering information

An initial exploration of the patient's problems, either disease or illness, is necessary and the patient should be encouraged to 'tell their tale' in their own words. The pharmacist needs to listen attentively and question appropriately (open and closed questions) and suitable use of language (e.g. avoiding jargon and very technical language). The pharmacist needs to be aware of verbal and non-verbal cues and the possible need to facilitate responses. It may be necessary to clarify what the person is saying (e.g. 'What do you exactly mean by a stomach cold?'). Certainly it will be necessary to periodically summarize to check your own understanding of what the patient has said. This summarizing also allows the patient to correct any misinterpretation. A further exploration of the disease framework may be necessary and this may include symptoms analysis (see, e.g. the PQRST symptoms analysis in Box 17.2), and more focused closed questions. The patient's perspective is taken into account by the Calgary–Cambridge model at this stage in the interview, when a further exploration of the illness from the patient's perspective is undertaken. This further exploration investigates the following:

- The patient's ideas and concerns, i.e. the patient's beliefs on the causes of the illness and their concerns about each problem, e.g. the idea that taking medicines might make them addicted to the medicine
- The effects on the patient's life of each problem, e.g. concern that a medicine may make them too drowsy to drive

- The expectations of the patient, e.g. that a medicine will instantly make them better
- The patient's feelings and thoughts about the problems, e.g. feeling that no medicine is strong enough to take away the symptoms.

The above are important and may indicate if a patient is unwilling to take, or is untrusting of, modern medicines. They may also indicate that the drug regimen and formulation would be totally unsuitable for the patient and should be changed. These are important issues for compliance and concordance (see Ch. 18).

Explanation and planning

This is the next stage of the interview, which has three areas, all of which are very appropriate to pharmacists (see Ch. 25):

1. To provide the correct amount and type of information
   - To give comprehensive and appropriate information
   - To assess each individual patient's information needs and to neither restrict nor overload
   - To make information easier for the patient to remember and understand.
2. To achieve a shared understanding: incorporating the patient's illness framework (see Ch. 3)
   - To provide explanations/plans that relate to the patient's perspective of the problem
   - To discover the patient's thoughts and feelings about the information given
   - To encourage an interaction rather than one-way transmission.
3. To plan: shared decision-making
   - To allow the patient to understand the decision-making process
   - To involve the patient in decision making to the level they wish
   - To increase patients' commitment to the plans made.

All of the above stages, although designed for medical interviews, are very relevant to pharmacists. Patients need to be involved in decisions about any treatment with medicines, and they need to be given sufficient information on what the medicine is used for and how to take it, in a way that is achievable in their lifestyle. Also, patients should be offered some information on side-effects, so that they can make an informed choice (see Ch. 18).

Closing the session

At the end of the session, it is important to summarize what has taken place and the joint decisions made. The patient should also be informed about the next stage; for example this could be seeing how the medicine works and coming back to the pharmacy if the patient feels the medicine is not working. Ensure the patient knows what to do if the problem/symptoms do not resolve (e.g. go to see the doctor), and finally, check whether the patient agrees and feels comfortable with the chosen plan or needs to discuss any other issues.

Patterns of behaviour in communication

A number of terms are used in connection with behaviour during communication:

- *Assertive behaviour* may be defined as standing up for personal rights and expressing thoughts, feelings and beliefs in direct, honest and appropriate ways which do not violate another person's rights. Being assertive involves listening to others and understanding their feelings. People who behave assertively deal with other people as equals. An assertive communicator will find a mutually acceptable solution. An important part of being assertive, therefore, is to formulate your aims and objectives clearly.
- *Aggressive behaviour* violates others' rights as the aggressive person seeks to achieve goals at the expense of others. Aggressive behaviour is often frightening, threatening and unpredictable. It will bring out negative feelings in the receiver and communication will be difficult.
- *Passive–aggressive behaviour* usually involves a person giving a mixed message; that is, he may agree with what you are saying but then raise his eyebrows and pull a face at you behind your back.
- *Submissive behaviour* is displayed by people who behave submissively, have very little confidence in themselves and show poor self-esteem. They often allow others to violate their personal rights and take advantage of them.

Assertiveness is a positive way of relating to other people – a means of communicating as effectively as possible, particularly in potentially awkward situations. Assertive behaviour is useful when dealing with conflict, in negotiation, leadership and motivation, when giving and receiving feedback, in cooperative working and in meetings. Assertive communication can give the user confidence, and a feeling of more control over situations.

People who behave assertively usually achieve what they set out to do. This is in comparison to those who act aggressively, who think that they have achieved their goal – but usually at the cost of respect and loyalty from those around them. Submissive people rarely achieve what they want.

Barriers to communication

In a pharmacy setting, there are a number of factors which can be of benefit to, or can detract from, the quality of any communication. Common barriers which exist can be identified under four main headings:

- Environment
- Patient factors
- The pharmacist and their team
- Time.

Environment

Community and hospital pharmacies and hospital wards are some of the areas where pharmacists use their communication skills in a professional capacity. None of these areas is ideal for good communication, but an awareness of the limitations of the environment goes part of the way to resolving the problems. Some examples of potential problem areas are illustrated below.

A busy pharmacy

This may create the impression that there appears to be little time to discuss personal matters with patients. The pharmacist may appear to be too busy to devote his full attention to an individual matter. It is important that pharmacists organize their work patterns in such a way as to minimize this impression.

Lack of privacy

For good communication to occur and rapport to be developed, it should take place in a quiet environment, free of interruptions All pharmacies, whether hospital or community, should have counselling rooms or areas. Lack of these facilities, such as in a busy hospital ward, requires additional communication skills.

Noise

Noise within the working environment is an obvious barrier to good communication. People strain to hear what is said, comprehension is made more difficult and particular problems exist for the hearing impaired. Conversely, a patient may feel embarrassed having to explain a problem in a totally quiet environment where other people can 'listen in'.

Physical barriers

Pharmacy counters and dispensing hatches are physical barriers which may dictate the distance between pharmacist and patient. This can create problems in developing effective communication. Similarly, a patient in bed (or in a wheelchair) and a pharmacist standing offers a different sort of barrier for effective communication. Ideally, faces should be at about the same level.

Patient factors

One of the main barriers to good communication in a pharmacy can be patients' expectations. They may not expect the pharmacist to spend time with them checking their understanding of medication or other health-related matters. However, once the purpose of the communication is explained, most patients realize its importance and are quite happy to enter into a dialogue.

Patients with hearing and sight impairment

Such patients must be considered carefully when adopting questioning skills. Sight-impaired people will have difficulty or may not be able to read any written material, unless it is in Braille. Special Braille labels are available. Many customers who come into pharmacies will suffer from a degree of hearing impairment. Recognizing the profoundly deaf is usually simpler than recognizing those who have hearing impairment.

A person with hearing difficulty is likely to do one or more of the actions listed in Box 17.3. Having recognized a customer with hearing impairment, the guidelines in Box 17.4 are helpful. Listening, and being able to demonstrate that you are listening by using non-verbal responses, e.g. nods of the head, is very important for customers with hearing loss.

Comprehension difficulties

Not all people come from the same educational background or have the same native language and care must be taken to assess a patient's level of understanding and choose appropriate language. Information leaflets in appropriate languages can be provided for patients with language difficulties and pharmacists may be able to access translator services from local primary care organizations.

Illiteracy

A significant proportion of the population, both in the UK and in other countries, is illiterate. For these patients, written material is meaningless. It is not always easy to identify illiterate patients, but additional verbal advice can be given and pictorial labels can be used. For example the United States Pharmacopoeia has designed a range of pictograms for this purpose.

The pharmacist and their team

Not everybody is a natural, good communicator. Identifying strengths and weaknesses will assist in improving communication skills. Some of the weaknesses which can be barriers to good communication are:

- Lack of confidence
- Lack of interest
- Laziness
- Delegation of responsibilities to untrained staff
- A feeling of being under pressure, especially time pressure
- Being preoccupied with other matters.

If any of these characteristics is present, the reason for it should be identified and resolved, if possible.

Confidentiality

Matters related to health and illness are highly private affairs. Therefore it is important that privacy and confidentiality are assured in the practice of pharmacy.

The public expects pharmacists to respect and protect confidentiality and have premises that provide an environment where you can communicate privately without fear that personal matters will be disclosed. This concerns the whole staff of the pharmacy, not just the pharmacists.

Time

In many instances, time, or the lack of it, can be a major constraint on good communication. It is

Box 17.3

Actions usually associated with people with hearing difficulties

- Speak in an unusually loud or soft voice
- Turn their head to one side or cup a hand to their ear while listening
- Concentrate on lips while being spoken to
- Give inappropriate responses to questions
- Have a blank or confused expression during conversation
- Frequently ask speakers to slow down or repeat information
- Are unable to hear a conversation when they cannot see the speaker's mouth
- Are unable to carry on a conversation in a noisy environment

Box 17.4

Guidelines when speaking to the hearing impaired

- Ask them how they wish to communicate
- Make sure that background noise is at a minimum
- Look directly at the person and do not turn away
- Make sure sufficient light is on your face
- Do not hide your face or mouth behind hands, pens, etc.
- Do not shout
- Keep the normal rhythm of speech but slow down slightly
- Articulate each word carefully and exactly, particularly emphasizing consonants
- If a sentence is not heard, rephrase it or write it down
- Do not change the subject in mid-sentence

always worthwhile checking what time people have available before trying to embark on any communication. That way, you will make the best use of what time is available.

Not all barriers to good communication can be removed, but an awareness that they exist and taking account of them will go a long way towards diminishing their negative impact.

Conclusion

Good communication is not easy and needs to be practised. We all have different personalities and skills, which mean that we have strengths in some areas and weaknesses in others. If we can become aware of, and maximize, our strengths and work to minimize our weaknesses, we will become better communicators. Being articulate and able to explain things clearly is of great importance to a pharmacist. However, listening with understanding and empathy is of equal, and in certain situations of greater, importance. We may all hear the words being said, but are we really listening to the complete message?

KEY POINTS

- Communication consists of both verbal and non-verbal communication
- Assertive behaviour treats other people as equals, and is not to be confused with aggressive behaviour, which violates other people's rights
- Questioning and listening skills are equally important
- In the working environment there are many potential barriers to effective communication, including the environment, patient and pharmacist and the time implications
- Confidentiality must be assured in the practice of pharmacy
- Pharmacists need to maximize their strengths and minimize their weaknesses of communication

Concordance

18

Marjorie C. Weiss

STUDY POINTS

- What is meant and understood by the term 'concordance'
- How concordance differs from compliance and adherence
- The concordance model and the relationship with patients
- The need for good communication skills in developing a concordant relationship
- Concerns about using a concordance approach with patients

Introduction

'Mrs Jones is being a non-concordant patient [sigh] again'. Or is she? Concordance offers a way forward when we, as pharmacists, notice that patients are not taking their medicines as prescribed. Yet concordance can fundamentally challenge our assumptions about the role of patients in a professional–patient interaction. It states that patients have a legitimate and valuable perspective on taking their medicines and that healthcare professionals should encourage patients, should they wish it, to become involved in decisions about their treatment. For these reasons, concordance is about a consultation process and not individual patient behaviour. Mrs Jones cannot be non-concordant on her own: it takes at least two, professional and patient, to have a non-concordant (or successfully concordant) encounter. The consultation could have been non-concordant but Mrs Jones, on her own, cannot have been. Mrs Jones can be non-compliant or non-adherent with her medicine but these have a distinctly different meaning from concordance.

What is concordance?

Concordance occurs when 'the patient and the healthcare professional participate as partners to reach an agreement on when, how and why to use medicines, drawing on the expertise of the healthcare professional, as well as the experiences, beliefs and wishes of the patient' (Marinker et al. 1997). It arose from the recognition that throughout the decades of research investigating interventions to help patients follow prescriptions for medications, there was still a high level of non-adherence. In a review by Haynes et al. (2001), interventions that used a combination of approaches in helping patients take their medicines, such as providing more convenient care, giving patients more information, providing reminders or offering medicine counselling, did not lead to large improvements in adherence rates. From this synthesis of research findings, there was a call to investigate more innovative approaches to assist patients with taking their medicines. Concordance is one such innovative approach.

This is not to say that terms like adherence and compliance can no longer be used. When referring to the extent to which patients take medicines as prescribed by their doctor or other healthcare professional, the words 'adherence' and 'compliance' are appropriate terms to be used. As a concept distinct from compliance or adherence, concordance may affect adherence although it is mainly concerned with improving the quality of health care through a shared understanding between professional and patient on treatment choices. Yet there are difficulties with words like adherence and compliance, which have overtones of the patient being disobedient or 'naughty' in not following the doctor's instructions. Conceptually, terms like 'compliance' and 'adherence' reinforce a paternalistic doctor-knows-best model of health care and implicitly devalue the views and experience of patients as users of medicines. Concordance seeks to redress this balance by acknowledging that patients and customers have a key role in the decision-making of whether or not to take their medicine.

The term adherence has been usefully split into those who are intentionally non-adherent and those who are unintentionally non-adherent. Unintentionally non-adherent patients are those who do not take their medicine because of a number of reasons, e.g. because they are unable to read the label due to poor eyesight, or forgot to take a tablet because a medicine regimen is complex and difficult to remember. Appropriate solutions to unintentional non-adherence are big print labels, improved medicines information, simplified medicine regimens or adherence aids, such as a Dosette box. Intentional non-adherence is where concordance can play a role; previous research has suggested that patients make reasoned decisions about whether or not to take their medicines. Patients may alter their medicine-taking behaviour for a number of reasons, e.g.:

- They have experienced side-effects
- Taking medicines interferes with their daily lives
- They have beliefs about the medicines or illness which conflict with medicine taking
- They are adjusting the medicine dose in response to symptoms.

Concordance has been called a partnership in medicine taking and has three important ingredients: (1) includes an explicit agreement between two people; (2) is based upon respect for each other's beliefs; and (3) gives the patient's view priority although they may choose to have the professional make all the decisions about treatment. This third ingredient recognizes that once the patient leaves the encounter with the healthcare professional, they will ultimately have the casting vote to decide whether or not to take that medicine.

Ethical considerations

The need to involve patients in decisions about their care is enshrined in 'principle 4' of the Standards of conduct, ethics and performance by the GPhC. This principle draws upon healthcare professionals' duty to obtain informed consent when initiating new medicines and the ethical principle of respect for patient autonomy. This recognizes that patients should be allowed to have control over their own lives and make decisions that affect their lives. In common with the concordance initiative, this principle advocates working in partnership with patients, to explain the options available and to help patients make informed decisions about different treatment options.

The concordance model

Concordance shares many characteristics with other models and themes currently prevalent in health care, most importantly those of shared decision-making and patient-centredness. There is a greater chance of a successfully concordant encounter when each participant knows what the other is thinking. For this reason, concordance shares many characteristics with shared decision-making, where both the doctor and patient share information with each other, when both take steps to participate in the decision-making process by expressing treatment preferences and they jointly agree on the treatment to implement. Shared decision-making may be considered part of the wider concept of patient-centredness. Patient-centredness has three themes: eliciting the patient's perspectives and understanding them within a psychosocial context; reaching a shared understanding of the patient's problem and treatment; and involving patients, to the extent they wish to be involved, in choices about their care. It is not a coincidence that the concept of concordance arose during the same time period that patient-centred care became dominant in healthcare policy. Concordance can be seen as part of the wider patient-centred political context but one which specifically focuses on medicine-taking behaviour. NICE has similarly produced guidance on medicines adherence which draws upon many of the themes relevant to concordance.

Concordance shares many features with the formative communication teaching guides, the Calgary–Cambridge guides as discussed in Chapter 17. Although designed as a formative aid in teaching medical students communication skills, the Calgary–Cambridge guides have a consultation structure which is readily adaptable to the

Box 18.1

A concordance model for pharmacy: involving patients in decisions about their medicines

New prescriptions	Repeat prescriptions

Reinforces prescriber's instructions and provides other important information

- Prioritizes key information: how to take the medicine, what it does, what it is for and important side-effects
- Gives information in manageable chunks so as not to overload patient

Explores patient's ideas, concerns and expectations	**Explores patient's ideas, concerns and expectations**
• Explores the patient's view on the possibility of having to take a medicine	• Explores previous experience with using the medicine
• Explores previous experience with medicines	• Explores patient concerns about taking the medicine(s)
• Explores patient concerns about taking the medicine(s)	

Develops rapport	**Develops rapport**
• Accepts legitimacy of patient's views	• Accepts legitimacy of patient's views
• Picks up on patient verbal and non-verbal cues	• Picks up on patient verbal and non-verbal cues
• Facilitates patient's responses	• Facilitates patient's responses

Provides additional information	**Provides additional information**
• Discusses the pros and cons of taking and not taking the medicine	• Finds out if the patient wants any other information
• Finds out if the patient wants any other information	• Gives information in manageable chunks
• Avoids jargon	• Avoids jargon
• Checks patient understanding	• Checks patient understanding

Deciding with the patient	**Deciding with the patient**
• Discusses other options or issues of importance to the patient	• Discusses other options or issues of importance to the patient
• Negotiates mutually acceptable plan	• Negotiates mutually acceptable plan
• 'Safety nets' so the patient knows where to go if they experience problems or have further questions and how to follow-up	• 'Safety nets' so the patient knows where to go if they experience problems or have further questions and how to follow-up

pharmacy setting. These guides assume a chronology to the consultation with distinct sections on initiating the consultation, gathering information, providing structure to the consultation, building a relationship, explanation and planning and closing the consultation. The Calgary–Cambridge guide has been adapted to reflect two common pharmacy consultation situations of (1) handing out a new prescription and (2) issuing a repeat prescription, as shown in Box 18.1. Sample phrases or 'catchphrases' useful in conducting a concordant consultation in pharmacy are shown in Box 18.2.

The Medicines Partnership at NICE has developed a competency framework for shared decision-making with patients, describing the skills and behaviours professionals need to reach a shared agreement about treatment. In this document, shared decision-making and concordance are used synonymously, highlighting the common approach underpinning these concepts. These eight competencies are shown in Box 18.3.

The evidence for concordance

Already presented has been the Haynes Cochrane review regarding the use of interventions to help patients take their medicines; that current methods

Box 18.2

Catchphrases useful in involving patients in decisions about their medicines: giving out medicines in a pharmacy

Eliciting the patient's view

- 'How do you feel about starting on a new medication?'
- 'Do you feel you will be able to take this medicine as suggested by your doctor?'
- 'What do you think about taking this medicine on a regular basis?'
- 'How have you been getting on with your medicines?' (repeats)
- 'What makes you think that [a particular problem] might be due to the medicine?'

Eliciting patient concerns

- 'Do you have any concerns about starting this medication?'
- 'How can I help you with this medicine?'
- 'Is there anything else you would like to know about?'
- 'Is there anything in particular that worries you?'

- 'Have you had any bad experiences with this kind of thing in the past?'
- 'Could you tell me a bit more about that?'

Giving patients the amount of information they want

- 'Can I give you some more information about that?'
- 'What do you know about it?'
- 'Would you like to know more?'
- 'What do you want to know about it?'
- 'Are there some more questions I can answer for you?'
- 'Would you like to go away and read this and think about it a bit more?'

Deciding with the patient

- 'You're quite right to worry about that kind of thing – it can happen with some medicines. How would you feel about giving this one a go for a month or so and see how you get on?'
- 'How do the good and bad effects of taking this medicine weigh up for you?'

Box 18.3

Competency framework for shared decision-making with patients: summary

Building a partnership

Listening

Listens actively to patients

Communicating

Helps the patient to interpret information in a way that is meaningful to them

Managing a shared consultation

Context

With the patient, defines and agrees the purpose of the consultation

Knowledge

Has up-to-date knowledge of area of practice and wider health services

Sharing a decision

Understanding	Exploring	Deciding	Monitoring
Recognizes that the patient is an individual	Discusses illness and treatment options, including no treatment	Decides with the patient the best management strategy	Agrees with the patient what happens next

After Clyne et al. 2007 with permission.

of improving adherence are complex and not very effective. Much of the information available about concordance relates to the doctor–patient consultation. As shown in Box 18.1, the concordant approach can be readily adapted to the pharmacy situation after a prescribing decision has been made. Examples are handing out new or repeat prescriptions, in repeat dispensing or in conducting a medicines use review. Yet pharmacists also have a role before treatment decisions about medicines are made: when giving over-the-counter advice or as pharmacist independent prescribers. The next sections will look at this evidence, drawing upon pharmacy literature where possible, as well as evidence from medicine. Medical literature may appear to be relevant only in the latter situation, i.e. before prescribing decisions are made. However, the evidence has resonance for the range of pharmacy consultations, both before and after treatment decisions have been made. These are grouped under four headings: eliciting the patient's view; developing rapport with the patient; providing information; and the therapeutic alliance.

Eliciting the patient's view

Previous research tells us that patients have beliefs about their medicines and illness, and that these beliefs can affect their medicine-taking behaviour. For example, individual patients will vary in their confidence in the medicine to help them. They may have doubts about a medicine and 'test' whether the medicine is having an effect by stopping it on occasions. Patients may believe that they will become 'immune' or addicted to a medicine if they take it long term. These beliefs can occur, even when we know these medicines are not associated with a true pharmacological dependence. Many people consider prescribed or over-the-counter medicines, particularly in comparison with herbal or homoeopathic products, to be unnatural, artificial and potentially harmful to their bodies. They might see themselves as being 'anti-drugs' people, where doing without a medicine is the preferred course of action, only resorting to medicine taking when it is absolutely necessary. Evidence also suggests that patients make complex judgements about their medicines, weighing up the benefits and drawbacks of taking a medicine within their individual patient experience. All of these patient beliefs have their own rationality when viewed from the patient's perspective of taking medicines within the context of their everyday life.

Research on doctor–patient consultations suggests that these beliefs are important because, if not elicited, they can lead to misunderstandings in consultations when prescribing decisions are made. Misunderstandings in consultations can be caused by non-disclosure of information from either the doctor or the patient, disagreement about causes of side-effects or failure of communication about a decision reached by the doctor. Misunderstandings arise when patients do not play an active role in the consultation by stating their views and beliefs about the medicine or illness under discussion. The consequence of consultation misunderstandings can be non-adherence to prescribed medication. While research has primarily focused on doctor–patient consultations, it can be hypothesized that eliciting the patient's views and beliefs on their medicine and medicine-taking behaviour is equally important in pharmacist–patient or pharmacist–customer interactions as well. However, this is an area pharmacists find particularly difficult to incorporate into their practice. Healthtalkonline is a website which gives videoclips of patients' experiences of health-related conditions and experiences. These videoclips may be useful when professionals want to gain insight into what it is like from a patient's perspective to experience an illness or face a specific health-related decision.

Developing rapport with the patient

Concordance is focused on a consultation process and, as such, is primarily concerned with professional–patient communication. Although we all tend to think of ourselves as good communicators, to participate in a concordant consultation is actually very difficult. If it seems easy, you are probably not doing it right! All of the 'generic' communication skills such as active listening, avoiding jargon, giving information 'in chunks' or a little bit at a time, using open questions, appropriate body language, encouraging the patient to ask questions, treating the patient as an equal and being non-judgemental are important. Checking patients' understanding and giving them explicit opportunities to ask questions are areas pharmacists find particularly difficult to include in their consultations. Other skills, such as presenting information in a way the patient is able to understand, without being patronizing, are essential. Both people in the consultation need to explore each other's viewpoint and confirm that they understand where the other person is coming from. While a patient may spontaneously volunteer their personal beliefs or views, if they do not, it is down to the skill of the professional to elicit the patient's view and ensure that the patient feels comfortable enough to discuss this information.

Empathy plays a key part in concordance. Empathy is distinct from sympathy. Empathy involves fully understanding an individual's emotions, while sympathy is simultaneously being affected by another's emotions. In interactions with patients, empathy allows for recognition and acknowledgement of the patient perspective. Professionals display their acceptance of the legitimacy of the patient's view by communicating their understanding of the patient's situation. Included within this are expressions of concern, a general willingness to help and an acknowledgement of the efforts the patient may have made thus far in terms of trying to manage their medicines and illness. It requires the professional to be able to deal sensitively with potentially embarrassing or unpleasant issues.

In a concordant consultation, it can be useful to overtly draw attention to the structure of the interaction and signpost when a different issue or change of subject will take place. This includes providing information in a logical sequence but may also consist of statements such as 'I would now like to move on to discussing potential options, is that okay with you?' or 'There are three ways in which this medicine can help you. First, …' or 'I'd now just like to summarize some of the things we've discussed'. Summarizing information at various points in the interaction, asking if the patient has any questions, as well as 'safety netting' – identifying appropriate follow-up or what to do if something changes or further questions arise – are important.

Providing information

Studies over the years have consistently shown that patients want information about their medicines (see Ch. 25). When patients are asked what they would like to know, they frequently respond that they want to know about side-effects, what the medication does, any lifestyle changes they might need to undertake and how to take the medication.

Surveys support the view that, while most patients have considerable confidence in their medicines, 30% also have concerns, particularly with regard to side-effects. Patients want to know information even when the information contains bad news or in terms of side-effects, no matter how rare. This may be impractical during a typically brief pharmacy encounter. Should the patient wish to have information beyond the more frequent and serious side-effects, this information can be provided in a written format. Nonetheless, it is not unusual for patients, when asked retrospectively about whether they would have liked more information about a prescribed medicine, to state that they would have liked more.

Information should be provided in a manner which takes account of what the patient may already know and what, and how much, information they would like to receive. Patients should be offered information on treatment options, to including non-pharmacological options or the choice to have no treatment. Addressing the 'no treatment' option is important, even when there is only one drug of choice or when the doctor has already prescribed the medicine. If the patient has reservations or concerns about a medicine that were not resolved before the medicine was prescribed, the patient will simply walk out of the pharmacy and not take it. This is the pharmacist's opportunity to provide information on both the benefits and risks of taking and not taking a medicine, which may influence the patient's decision-making process long after they have left the pharmacy. Throughout this process, it is important for both pharmacist and patient to communicate their thoughts, perceived dilemmas or uncertainties in treatment options, ideas and reactions to new pieces of information. Only through this process can a mutually agreeable treatment plan be devised.

Verbal information can be supported with written information, the most familiar written format being the patient information leaflet (PIL). European Union legislation requires a comprehensive medicines information leaflet to be provided in every medicines pack. There is strict guidance on the information to be included in this leaflet and, most recently, requirements on the readability of these leaflets. PILs often do not increase patient knowledge, nor do patients value them. This may, however, change as the development of PILs now includes a consultation process with the target patient groups to ensure the readability and usefulness. Findings from studies have indicated that patients would like information to be tailored to their particular illness and circumstances, to help with decision-making before prescribing occurs, and for it to contain a balance of benefit and harm information.

PILs are not the only way of communicating information. As well as verbal communication and information from PILs, other written information can include condition- or medicine-specific information guides, or use can be made of video, DVD or other interactive media. Information can also be presented in the form of a decision aid. Decision aids are patient decision support tools, which facilitate evidence-based patient choice. They normally have a number of informational elements. They provide information on available treatment options, consider the patient's values for benefits versus harm, and facilitate the patient's participation in treatment decisions. Like other educational materials, they can be provided as booklets, DVDs, videos or as interactive media. A systematic review of decision aids by O'Connor et al. (2003) has shown that they can increase patient knowledge, improve the proportion of patients with realistic perceptions of benefits and harms, reduce the proportion of patients who are undecided after counselling and decrease the proportion of patients who are passive in decision-making. There is a library of decision aids at the Ottawa Health Research Institute's website covering a broad range of clinical conditions and health issues (see Appendix 4). On this website library, each decision aid is rated using a series of internationally agreed quality criteria. Many of these decision aids are American but can be adapted to the UK setting. The Medicines and Prescribing Centre at NICE provides advice and support to underpin an evidence-based patient-choice approach.

A major issue for all types of written, computer-based, audio, video and interactive information is the quality of information available. Much of the information available is poor, particularly with regard to providing accurate and adequately detailed clinical information to assist patients in decision-making. Other issues exist, such as ensuring topics of relevance to patients are included and that uncertainties in treatment need to be clearly communicated. A number of tools have been developed to assess the quality of health information, such as the DISCERN tool and the International Patient Decision Aids Standards (IPDAS) instrument.

The tools use a range of criteria to judge the issue information, such as:

- Information accuracy, comprehensiveness and reliability
- Clarity of aims and target audience
- The comprehensibility and balance of information
- References to sources
- How up-to-date it is
- Support for shared decision-making
- Transparency of authorship and sponsorship (if any).

Pharmacists are not the only people who need to be able to judge the quality of health information. Patients are active information seekers and, although their most common source of health information is the doctor, other sources such as the internet are increasingly playing a part. The pharmacist is in an excellent position to act as the patient's 'internet guide': to provide advice on accessing and understanding web resources, to direct them to high-quality internet sites and to discuss with them any information affecting their decision to take, or not take, a medicine (see Ch. 16). This will show the pharmacist as a resource for accessing and discussing medicines information to which patients will be likely to return in the future.

Communicating risk

A key aspect of sharing information with patients is the ability to communicate risk: to provide information on the effectiveness of a medicine or the likelihood of a side-effect occurring. Pharmacists often use words such as 'rarely' or 'commonly' to indicate to patients how frequent a particular side-effect is likely to be experienced. In an effort to standardize the interpretation of these words, the European Union (EU) has issued a guideline banding the level of risk into five groups, from 'very common' to 'very rare' (Box 18.4). However, even this approach may not ensure consistency. Evidence suggests that the general public has a tendency to reliably overestimate the risk associated with these words in comparison with the risk frequency intended by the EU. Healthcare professionals also consistently overestimate the risk level associated with these words, although not to the same magnitude that the lay public does. The use of these verbal descriptors can lead to people perceiving there is a greater risk to their health than there actually

Box 18.4

EU recommended verbal descriptors and their frequency range

Verbal descriptor	EU assigned frequency level
Very common	>10%
Common	1–10%
Uncommon	0.1–1%
Rare	0.01–0.1%
Very rare	<0.01%

is, suggesting that they need to be used in combination with actual numbers in order to effectively communicate the intended risk level.

Expressing risks as natural frequencies (e.g. 3 out of 10 people will experience dizziness with this medicine) facilitates greater understanding of risk than presenting it as a probability statement (e.g. there is a 30% chance of dizziness with this medicine). As well as textual (or verbal) and numerical presentations of risk, other visual forms can be used, such as bar charts, icons (showing how many people in 100 are affected), pie charts, tables or survival curves. Graphical information may result in greater accuracy in determining the relative quantitative difference between risks, although icons have been found to be quite helpful to decision-making. Further research is needed on patient preferences and the benefits of alternative risk formats. It is also possible that different people may prefer different formats to aid their individual understanding of risk information. Verbal, textual, visual, graphical and numerical formats may all have a place and the key to communicating risk is a flexible approach. A greater desire for involvement in decision-making is associated with a preference for more complex risk information so the need for alternative risk formats, and flexibility in approach, is essential.

A number of factors have been shown to improve people's understanding of risk information, including both verbal or text information and numerical or graphical information on risks can aid understanding. Presentation of information which is both positive and negative provides a more balanced view of the benefits and risks of taking a particular medicine. Taking account of the starting or baseline risk levels can also improve the accuracy

of people's judgements about, for example, the benefit associated with introducing a new medication (e.g. reduction in stroke risk). This allows people to anchor their perception at their starting level of risk and extrapolate more accurately to the potential decrease in stroke risk with starting a new medication.

Finally, whether a risk is presented as an absolute-risk reduction or relative-risk reduction can also influence people's perception of risk. Absolute-risk reduction is the difference in risk between a control group and a treatment group. Relative-risk reduction is the absolute-risk reduction divided by the control group event rate. For example, if a new hypertensive drug decreases the risk of stroke from 0.004% (control group event rate) to 0.003% (intervention group event rate), the relative-risk reduction is 25%, although the absolute-risk reduction is only 0.001%. Relative-risk reduction sounds much more impressive and is more persuasive. Absolute-risk reduction is the preferred method for conveying accurate risk information and should be used on its own or in combination with the relative-risk reduction.

The therapeutic alliance

What are the benefits of a therapeutic alliance with patients? Once pharmacists have engaged with patients in a pharmacy consultation and a plan of action regarding medicines has been mutually agreed, what are the benefits of this process? Reviews have shown that good adherence to medication is associated with a decreased mortality. This includes adherence to placebo or beneficial drug therapy suggesting that there is a 'healthy adherer effect', where adherence to drug therapy may be a proxy for overall healthy behaviours. The question then becomes, does concordance improve adherence or affect other health outcomes? With concordance embracing a range of competences around the professional and patient sharing beliefs, preferences and information in a collaborative consultation process, the evidence for concordance affecting adherence depends upon how concordance has been defined. Patients rarely voice their concerns about medicines, unless encouraged to do so, and the issue of whether or not patients are taking their medicines is not always discussed in a consultation. Many of the elements perceived to be necessary for concordance (such as establishing whether or not both the professional and patient express their points of view, whether the professional respects the patient's perspective on their illness and medicine use, or whether both work together towards shared decisions) appear not to be taking place in practice, or only taking place to a limited extent. For these reasons, finding evidence that concordance improves adherence or other health outcomes is difficult.

There is evidence on specific aspects of communication which are relevant for concordance. When patients are given information about treatment options and coached to ask questions about their condition, they are more involved in the consultation and have better health outcomes. Improvement in health outcomes can, for example, include decreased blood pressure or blood glucose levels, an improved subjective evaluation of overall health or increased functionality in terms of activities of daily living. When professionals share treatment decision making with patients and focus on the patient as a person and not merely a disease state, patient satisfaction is likely to be increased. Effective communication involving activities such as encouraging the patient to ask questions, providing information and support and sharing the decision-making process has been shown, across a range of research studies, to improve emotional health, resolve symptoms, improve function and reduce pain.

Concerns about concordance

Concerns about concordance centre on four issues:
- *Time*. That a concordant consultation will take too long
- *Anxiety*. That providing information to patients makes them anxious and they will either experience the side-effects that have been described to them and/or stop taking their medication
- *Participation*. People do not want to participate in decisions about their medicines
- *Demands*. Concordance will lead to unreasonable patient demands for expensive medicines and health care.

Time is a concern for all healthcare professionals. Approaches such as concordance which have the potential to increase consultation times are an issue in any busy pharmacy setting. Research suggests that using a concordant approach with patients

may take longer initially, but as professionals gain experience and proficiency in this approach, consultation times will decrease. There is also some evidence that if professionals do not pick up on patient clues, defined as direct or indirect comments made by patients about personal aspects of their lives or emotions, then the consultation may be longer. It seems that if a patient has issues or ideas which they hint about during a consultation, it is best to address these issues openly. If not, the patient may feel obliged to continue seeking opportunities throughout the interaction to allude to these issues and this may ultimately prolong the consultation further.

It is also now possible to separate the provision of information about options from the consultation process. This has been facilitated through the use of decision aids and other interactive media. Patients can access the information outside of the consultation and have time to think about their options, discuss them with relevant others, make a list of questions to ask the healthcare professional and then participate as an informed patient in the consultation with their healthcare professional. This may be the best solution to deal with issues of time, i.e. de-couple the provision of information about options from the constraints on consultation length. Decision aids do not replace a consultation with a healthcare professional but may enhance informed discussion by giving patients the time to think about the issues of importance to them, having taken account of the clinical information in the decision aid.

There is a concern that telling patients about the side-effects of their medicines can lead to them experiencing these side-effects. This comes from the idea that humans are suggestible; that telling people about a side-effect makes them experience it. The research on whether forewarning of side-effects affects people's adherence can be conflicting. Yet the weight of research evidence indicates that provision of information about side-effects does not increase anxiety nor does it affect a patient's adherence. What does seem clear is that how this information is presented can affect adherence. So presenting information on both positive and negative effects of treatment, in a manner understandable (without being patronizing) to lay people, that links into lay theories of illness and treatment (see Ch. 3) and which promotes informed choice can avoid the potential negative consequences of information overload or 'information anxiety'.

Patients do not always want to be involved in decisions about what treatment is best for them. It is well known that there is a proportion of patients who want the doctor (most commonly) to decide what treatment is right for them. However, up to two-thirds of patients either want to decide for themselves, after the doctor has explained the options to them, or want to do so in partnership with a healthcare professional. While older people are less likely to want a more active role in decision-making than younger, more affluent people, half of those aged over 65 and those in lower social classes want to have a 'say' in decisions about their care. People need to be involved in decision-making to the extent that they want to be. The best way to do this is to ask them.

There is a view that if the patient's view takes priority in an interaction between healthcare professional and patient, the patient will simply demand expensive medicines or healthcare services at the expense of those who are less articulate but more in need of health care. Given the current emphasis on the need to ration scarce healthcare resources, this is a potentially valid concern. High-profile cases in the popular press with patients demanding expensive treatments reinforce this concern. Concordance is about both parties expressing their views and if a healthcare professional has reservations about a particular treatment option (e.g. that it is of uncertain benefit or the costs outweigh the benefits), they need to explain this rationale to the patient. A common cause of litigation is poor communication between professionals and patients, such as devaluing or failing to understand the patient's perspective. The alternative is not to inform patients of all options because one option may be particularly expensive. This can lead to patients seeking out this information on their own and raising a legitimate complaint that they were not informed about all options. Unreasonable demands may occur in a consultation but, provided both parties express their views and the rationale behind their views as part of a concordant consultation process, there is unlikely to be a basis for litigation against an individual practitioner. In the end, both parties may need to agree to differ.

Conclusion

Concordance is an opportunity for pharmacists to engage with patients on an equal level to understand their perspective on taking medicines. It argues for openness in the consultation where both professional and patient are able to express their views. Information is exchanged which may be clinical, personal, experiential and potentially worrying. Decisions are based on all types of information which are relevant for subsequent medicine taking. Ultimately, it is hoped that this will make the best use of medicines and, in situations where the patient has decided not to take a medicine, recognizes that an agreement to differ to include the open acknowledgement of the patient's perspective is preferable to the patient going away with concerns or issues which remain unaddressed.

KEY POINTS

- Concordance promotes the view that patients have a legitimate and valuable perspective on taking decisions about their health care
- The concept of concordance arose because of the need for innovative approaches to help patients with their medicines
- Non-adherence may be unintentional or intentional
- The Standards of conduct, ethics and performance state that pharmacists have a duty to encourage patients and the public to participate in decisions about their care
- The concordance model shares features with other models of effective communication
- Eliciting patient views is the first stage in establishing a concordant relationship
- Because concordance is concerned with the consultation, it is essential to have a good patient–pharmacist relationship
- Empathy plays a key role in concordance
- Patients want information and different techniques can be used, including the use of decision aids, PILs, the internet, medicine guides, video and DVDs
- When communicating risk to patients, pharmacists need to ensure that patients have understood the information fully and have received the breadth and depth of information they desire
- The ultimate aim of concordance is to establish a therapeutic alliance between patient and healthcare provider
- There are strategies for reducing concerns about concordance, particularly with respect to the time it involves

Pharmaceutical calculations

Arthur J. Winfield

STUDY POINTS

- Expressions of concentration
- Calculating quantities from master formulae
- Changing concentrations
- Small quantities (trituration)
- Solubility
- Calculations related to doses
- Reconstitution and rates of infusion

Introduction

Most pharmaceutical calculations are simple arithmetic. Calculating quantities in the dispensing process requires careful, methodical working which will minimize the risk of errors. Always try to relate the calculation to practice, visualize what you are doing and double-check everything.

How to minimize errors

As in all dispensing procedures, an organized, methodical approach is essential:

- Write out the calculation clearly – it is all too easy to end up reading from the wrong line
- If you are transferring data from a reference source, double-check what you have written down is correct
- Write down every step
- Do not take short cuts – you are more likely to make a mistake

- Try not to be totally dependent on your calculator – have an approximate idea of what the answer should be and then if you happen to hit the wrong button on the calculator you are more likely to be aware that an error has been made
- Finally, always double-check your calculation. There is frequently more than one way of doing a calculation, so if you get the same answer by two different methods the chances are that your answer will be correct. Alternatively, try working it in reverse and see if you get the starting numbers

Expressions of concentration

The metric system is the International System of Units (SI Units) for weight, volume and length. The basic unit for weight is the kilogram (kg), the basic unit for volume is the litre (L) and the basic unit of length is the metre (m). The prefix 'milli' indicates one-thousandth (10^{-3}) and 'micro' one-millionth (10^{-6}).

In some countries, the avoirdupois (or imperial) system (pounds and ounces) is still used in commerce and daily life. The imperial system of volume (pints and gallons) is still a common system for commerce and household measurement. Pharmacists need to know about these systems in order to avoid serious errors in interpretation of prescriptions. It is important to be able to change between the systems. Some conversion factors for the metric and avoirdupois systems are shown in Box 19.1 (see Examples 19.1–19.3).

Box 19.1

Weights and measures

- 1000 millilitres (mL) = 1 litre (L)
- 1000 micrograms (μL) = 1 milligram (mg)
- 1000 milligrams (mg) = 1 gram (g)
- 1000 grams (g) = 1 kilogram (kg)
- 1 kilogram (kg) = 2.2 pounds (lb)
- 1 teaspoonful (tsp) = 5 mL
- 1 tablespoonful = 15 mL (3 teaspoonfuls)
- 1 pint (pt) = 568 mL
- 1 fluid ounce (oz) = 29.57 mL (30 mL)

Example 19.1

A prescription is received for a dose of 125 mg of a drug. How many grams is the dose?

1 g = 1000 mg. Therefore:

125 mg = 125/1000 g = 0.125 g

Example 19.2

A 1-year-old child weighs 9 kg. What would this be in pounds (lb)?

1 kg = 2.2 lb. Therefore:

9 kg = 9 × 2.2 = 19.8 lb

Example 19.3

Gentamicin eye drops contain 200 drops in a 10 mL bottle. Calculate the volume of 1 drop.

200 drops = 10 mL. Therefore:

1 drop = 10/200 mL = 0.05 mL

Expressions of strength

Ratio is the relative magnitude of two like quantities. Thus:

$$1:10 = 1 \text{ part in } 10 \text{ parts or } 1 \text{ g in } 10 \text{ g}$$

Example 19.4

Express 0.1% w/w as a ratio strength:

0.1 g/100 g = 1 part/y parts.

$y = 100 × 1/0.1$

$y = 1000$

Therefore, the ratio strength = 1:1000

Example 19.5

Express 1:2500 as a percentage strength:

1 part/2500 parts = y parts/100 parts.

Thus, $y = 1 × 100/2500 = 0.04\%$

Example 19.6

Express 1 p.p.m. as a percentage strength:

1 p.p.m. = 1 part per million = 1:1 000 000

Let y be the percentage strength:

Thus, 1 part/1 000 000 = y parts/100 parts

$y = 1 × 100/1 000 000 = 0.0001\% = 1 × 10^{-4}\%$

Example 19.7

How many grams of a drug should be used to prepare 240 g of a 5% w/w solution?

Let y be the weight of the drug needed:

Thus, $y/240 = 5 \text{ g}/100 \text{ g}$

$y = 5 × 240/100 = 12 \text{ g}$

If 1 g of sucrose is in 10 g of solution, the ratio is 1:10. Therefore, 10 g of sucrose is in 100 g of solution. This can be expressed as a percentage, so it is equivalent to a 10% w/w (weight in weight) solution.

Ratio strength is the expression of a concentration by means of a ratio, e.g. 1:10. Percentage strength is a ratio of parts per hundred, e.g. 10% (see Examples 19.4–19.6).

Percentage weight in weight (w/w)

Percentage weight in weight (w/w) is the number of grams of an ingredient in 100 grams (solid or liquid) (Example 19.7).

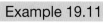

Example 19.8

If 5 g of iodine is in 250 mL of iodine tincture, calculate the percentage of iodine in the tincture.

Let y be the percentage of iodine in the tincture:

$y/100\,mL = 5\,g/250\,mL$

$y = 5 \times 100/250 = 2\%$ w/v

Example 19.9

If 15 mL of ethanol is mixed with water to make 60 mL of solution, what is the percentage of ethanol in the solution?

Let y be the percentage of ethanol in the solution:

$y/100\,mL = 15\,mL/60\,mL$

$y = 15 \times 100/60 = 25\%$ v/v

Example 19.10

Express 30 g of dextrose in 600 mL of solution as a percentage, indicating w/w, w/v or v/v.

Let y grams be the weight of dextrose in 100 mL:

$y/100\,mL = 30\,g/600\,mL$

$y = 30 \times 100/600\,mL = 5\%$ w/v

Percentage weight in volume (w/v)

Percentage weight in volume (w/v) is the number of grams of an ingredient in 100 mL of liquid (Example 19.8).

Percentage volume in volume (v/v)

Percentage volume in volume (v/v) indicates the number of millilitres (mL) of an ingredient in 100 mL of liquid (Example 19.9).

Miscellaneous examples

See Examples 19.10–19.13.

Moles and molarity

Concentrations can also be expressed in moles or millimoles (see Ch. 41). When a mixture contains the molecular weight of a drug in grams in

Example 19.11

What is the percentage of magnesium carbonate in the following syrup? Percentage is the number of grams of magnesium carbonate in 100 mL of syrup.

Magnesium carbonate	15 g
Sucrose	820 g
Water, q.s.	to 1000 mL

$y/100\,mL = 15\,g/1000\,mL$

$y = 15 \times 100/1000 = 1.5\%$ w/v (grams in 100 mL)

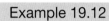

Example 19.12

Calculate the amount of drug in 5 mL of cough syrup if 100 mL contains 300 mg of drug.

By proportion,

$y\,mg/5\,mL = 300\,mg/100\,mL$

$y = 5 \times 300/100 = 15\,mg$

Example 19.13

Compute the percentage of the ingredients in the following ointment (to 2 decimal places):

Liquid paraffin	14 g
Soft paraffin	38 g
Hard paraffin	12 g

Total amount of ingredients

$= 14\,g + 38\,g + 12\,g = 64\,g$

To find the amounts of the ingredients in 100 g of ointment, each figure will be multiplied by 100/64:

Liquid paraffin $= (100/64) \times 14 = 21.88\%$ w/w

Soft paraffin $= (100/64) \times 38 = 59.38\%$ w/w

Hard paraffin $= (100/64) \times 12 = 18.75\%$ w/w

It is useful to double-check that these numbers add up to 100% (allowing for the rounding off to 2 decimal places).

1 litre of solution, the concentration is defined as a 1 molar solution (1 mol). It has a molarity of 1. Thus, for example, the molecular weight of potassium hydroxide (KOH) is the sum of the atomic weights of its elements, i.e. $KOH = 39 + 16 + 1 = 56$. Therefore a 1 molar solution (1 mol) of KOH contains 56 g of KOH in 1 litre of solution.

Example 19.14

Calculate the number of moles (molarity) of a solution if it contains 117 g of sodium chloride (NaCl) in 1 L of solution (atomic weights: Na=23, Cl=35.5):

Molecular weight of NaCl=23+35.5=58.5 g

Therefore, 58.5 g of NaCl in 1 litre is equivalent to 1 mole (1 mol) in solution.

Number of moles of NaCl=117 g/58.5 g=2 mol

Example 19.15

Calculate the number of milligrams of sodium hydroxide (NaOH) to be dissolved in 1 L of water to give a concentration of 10 mmol (atomic weights: H=1, O=16, Na=23):

Molecular weight of NaOH=23+16+1=40

1 mmol=40 mg in 1 L

Therefore, 10 mmol=400 mg in 1 L

Example 19.16

Express 111 mg of calcium chloride ($CaCl_2$) in 1 L of solution as millimoles (atomic weights: Ca=40, Cl=35.5):

Molecular weight of $CaCl_2$=Ca+(2×Cl)

=40+(2×35.5)=40+71=111 g

Therefore, 111 mg of $CaCl_2$=1 mmol in 1 L

A 1 millimole (mmol) solution of KOH contains one-thousandth of a mole in 1 litre=56 mg (see Examples 19.14–19.16).

Calculating quantities from a master formula

In extemporaneous dispensing, a list of the ingredients is provided on the prescription or is obtained from a reference source. It may be that this 'formula' is for the quantity requested, but more often, the quantities provided by the master formula have to be scaled up or down, depending on the quantity of the product required. This can be achieved using proportion or by deriving a 'multiplying

Example 19.17

Calculate the quantities to prepare the following prescription:

50 g Compound Benzoic Acid Ointment BPC.

The master formula is for 100 g, the prescription is for 50 g, therefore the multiplying factor is 50/100, i.e. each quantity in the master formula is multiplied by 50/100=0.5 to give the scaled quantity.

Ingredient	Master formula	Multiplying factor	Scaled quantity
Benzoic acid	6 g	0.5	3 g
Salicylic acid	3 g	0.5	1.5 g
Emulsifying ointment	91 g	0.5	45.5 g

Double-check: the quantities for the master formula add up to 100 g and the scaled quantities add up to 50 g.

Example 19.18

You are requested to dispense 200 mL of Ammonium Chloride Mixture BPC. The formula can be found in a variety of reference books such as *Martindale*. In this example, the master formula gives quantities sufficient for 10 mL. As the prescription is for 200 mL, the multiplying factor is 200/10. Thus the quantity of each ingredient in the master formula has to be multiplied by 20 to provide the required amount.

Ingredient	Master formula	Scaled quantity
Ammonium chloride	1 g	20 g
Aromatic solution of ammonia	0.5 mL	10 mL
Liquorice liquid extract	1 mL	20 mL
Water	to 10 mL	to 200 mL

Because this formula contains a mixture of volumes and weights it is not possible to calculate the exact quantity of water which is required. However, it is always good practice to have an idea of what the approximate quantity will be. The liquid ingredients of the preparation, other than the water, add up to 30 mL and there is 20 g of ammonium chloride. The volume of water required will therefore be between 150 mL and 170 mL.

factor'. The latter is the ratio of the required quantity divided by the formula quantity. The following examples illustrate this process (Examples 19.17 and 19.18).

In most formulae where a combination of weights and volumes is required, the formula will indicate that the preparation is to be made up to the required weight or volume with the designated vehicle. However, occasionally, as can be seen in the next example, a combination of stated weights and volumes is used and it is not possible to indicate what the exact final weight or volume of the preparation will be. In these instances an excess quantity is normally calculated for and the required amount measured (Example 19.19)

Example 19.19

Calculate the quantities required to produce 300 mL Turpentine Liniment BP 1988.

Ingredient	Master formula
Soft soap	75 g
Camphor	50 g
Turpentine oil	650 mL
Water	225 mL

When the total number of units is added up for this formula it comes to 1000. However, because it is a combination of solids and liquids, it will not produce 1000 mL. The prescription is for 300 mL and experience shows that calculating for 340 units will provide slightly more than 300 mL. The required amount can then be measured.

Ingredient	Master formula	Scaled quantity for 340 units
Soft soap	75 g	25.5 g
Camphor	50 g	17 g
Turpentine oil	650 mL	221 mL
Water	225 mL	76.5 mL

Calculations involving parts

In the following example the quantities are expressed as parts of the whole. The number of parts is added up and the quantity of each ingredient calculated by proportion or multiplying factor, to provide the correct amounts (Example 19.20).

There are some situations when extra care is necessary in reading the prescription (see Example 19.21).

Example 19.20

The quantity which is to be prepared of the following formula is 60 g.

Ingredient	Master formula	Quantity for 60 g
Zinc oxide	12.5 parts	7.5 g
Calamine	15 parts	9 g
Hydrous wool fat	25 parts	15 g
White soft paraffin	47.5 parts	28.5 g

The total number of parts adds up to 100, so the proportions of each ingredient will be 12.5/100 of zinc oxide, 15/100 of calamine and so on. The required quantity of each ingredient can then be calculated. Zinc oxide 12.5/100 of 60 g, calamine 15/100 of 60 g, etc. as indicated above.

Example 19.21

Two products are to be dispensed:

Betnovate® cream	1 part
Aqueous cream	to 4 parts

Prepare 50 g

Haelan® ointment	1 part
White soft paraffin	4 parts

Prepare 50 g

At first glance, these calculations look similar but the quantities required for each are different. In the Betnovate prescription the total number of parts is 4, i.e. 1 part of Betnovate and 3 parts of aqueous cream to produce a total of 4 parts. However, in the Haelan prescription the total number of parts is 5, i.e. 1 part of Haelan ointment and 4 parts of white soft paraffin.

The quantities required for the prescriptions are as follows:

Betnovate® cream	12.5 g
Aqueous cream	37.5 g
Haelan® ointment	10 g
White soft paraffin	40 g

Calculations involving percentages

There are conventions which apply when dealing with formulae which include percentages:

- A solid in a formula where the final quantity is stated as a weight is calculated as weight in weight (w/w)

- A solid in a formula where the final quantity is stated as a volume is calculated as weight in volume (w/v)
- A liquid in a formula where the final quantity is stated as a volume is calculated as volume in volume (v/v)
- A liquid in a formula where the final quantity is stated as a weight is calculated as weight in weight (w/w) (see Example 19.22).

In the following example, a liquid ingredient, the coal tar solution, is stated as a percentage and a weight in grams of final product is requested. The convention of % w/w is applied (Example 19.23).

When dealing with preparations where ingredients are expressed as a percentage concentration, it is important to check that the standard conventions apply because there are some situations where they do not apply. Two examples are given below:

1. Syrup BP is a liquid – a solution of sucrose and water. If the normal convention applied it would be w/v, i.e. a certain weight of sucrose in a final volume of syrup. However, in the BP formula the concentration of sucrose is quoted as w/w. Therefore Syrup BP is:

Sucrose 66.7% w/w
Water to 100%

This means that when preparing Syrup BP the appropriate weight of sucrose is weighed out and water is added to the required weight, not volume.

2. A gas in a solution is always calculated as w/w, unless specified otherwise. Formaldehyde Solution BP is a solution of 34–38% w/w formaldehyde in water.

Changing concentrations

Sometimes it is necessary to increase or decrease the concentration of a medicine by the addition of more drug or a diluent. On other occasions, instructions have to be provided to prepare a dilution for use. These problems can be solved by the dilution equation:

$$C_1V_1 = C_2V_2$$

where C_1 and V_1 are the initial concentration and initial volume respectively; and C_2 and V_2 are the final concentration and final quantity of the mixture, respectively.

When three terms of the equation are known, the fourth term can be made the subject of the formula, and solved (Examples 19.24–19.27).

Example 19.22

Prepare 500 g of the following ointment

Ingredient	Master formula	Quantity for 500 g
Sulphur 2%	0.2 g	10 g
Salicylic acid 1%	0.1 g	5 g
White soft paraffin to 10 g	to 10 g	485 g (to 500 g)

The master formula is for a total of 10 g. To calculate the quantities required for 500 g the multiplying factor for each ingredient is 500/10 = 50. Remember do not multiply the percentage figure. This always remains the same no matter how much is being prepared.

Example 19.23

The quantity to be made is 30 g.

Ingredient	Master formula	Quantity for 30 g
Coal tar solution 3%	3 g	0.9 g
Zinc oxide 5 g	5 g	1.5 g
Yellow soft paraffin to 100 g	92 g	27.6 g

Example 19.24

What is the final concentration if 60 mL of a 12% w/v chlorhexidine solution is diluted to 120 mL with water?

$C_1 = 12\%$, $V_1 = 60$ mL, $C_2 = y\%$, $V_2 = 120$ mL

$12 \times 60 = 120 \times y$

Therefore

$y = 12 \times 60/120 = 6\%$ w/v

Example 19.25

What concentration is produced when 400 mL of a 2.5% w/v solution is diluted to 1500 mL (answer to 2 decimal places)?

$C_1 = 2.5\%$, $V_1 = 400$ mL, $C_2 = y$, $V_2 = 1500$ mL

$2.5\% \times 400$ mL $= y \times 1500$ mL

Therefore

$y = 2.5 \times 400/1500 = 0.67\%$ w/v

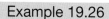

Example 19.26

What volume of 1% w/v solution can be made from 75 mL of 5% w/v solution?

$$1\% \times V_1 = 5\% \times 75\,mL$$
$$V_1 = 5/1 \times 75 = 375\,mL$$

Example 19.27

What percentage of atropine is produced when 200 mg of atropine powder is made up to 50 g with lactose as a diluent?

The atropine powder is a pure drug, so its concentration (C_1) is 100% w/w. The initial weight of the atropine powder (W_1) = 200 mg = 0.2 g. Therefore, we can modify the dilution equation to read:

$$C_1W_1 = C_2 W_2$$

where C_2 and W_2 are the final concentration and final weight respectively, of the diluted drug. The diluting medium is the lactose.

Thus, $100\% \times 0.2\,g = C_2 \times 50\,g$

Therefore $C_2 = 100 \times 0.2/50 = 0.4\%$ w/w

Example 19.28

Calculate the amounts of a 2% w/w metronidazole cream and of metronidazole powder required to produce 150 g of 6% w/w metronidazole cream (to 2 decimal places).

In alligation, the two starting material concentrations are placed above each other on the left hand side of the calculation. The target concentration is placed in the centre. The arithmetic difference between the starting material and the target is calculated and the answer recorded on the right hand end of the diagonal. The proportions of the two starting materials are then given by reading horizontally across the diagram.

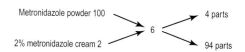

As shown above, the difference between the concentration of the pure drug powder (100%, recorded top left) and the desired concentration (6%) is 94 (recorded bottom right). This is equivalent to the number of parts of 2% cream required (read horizontally across the bottom). Similarly, the difference

between the concentration of 2% cream (recorded bottom left) and the desired concentration (6%) is 4 (recorded top right). This is equivalent to the number of parts of 100% drug (metronidazole powder) needed for the mixture (read horizontally across the top).

The total amount (4 parts + 94 parts = 98 parts) is 150 g

Thus, 1 part = 150/98 g

Therefore, the amount of 2% cream required = 94 parts × 150/98 g = 143.88 g

The amount of pure metronidazole (100%) required = 4 parts × 150/98 = 6.12 g

Example 19.29

Promazine oral syrup is available as 25 mg/5 mL and 50 mg/5 mL. Calculate the quantities used to prepare 150 mL of 40 mg/5 mL of the oral syrup.

Convert all the concentrations to percentages. Therefore, 25 mg/5 mL is equivalent to 0.025 g in 5 mL = 0.500 g in 100 mL = 0.5% w/v

Similarly, 50 mg/5 mL = 1% w/v; and 40 mg/5 mL = 0.8% w/v.

Using the alligation method:

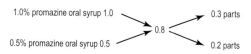

Total number of parts
= 0.3 part + 0.2 parts = 0.5 parts = 150 mL.

Amount of 50 mg/5 mL (1.0% w/v) oral syrup needed
= 0.3/0.5 × 150 mL = 90 mL

Amount of 25 mg/5 mL (0.5% w/v) oral syrup needed
= 0.2/0.5 × 150 mL = 60 mL.

Alligation

Alligation is a method for solving the number of parts of two or more components of known concentration to be mixed when the final desired concentration is known. When the relative amounts of components must be calculated for making a mixture of a desired concentration, the problem is most easily solved by alligation (Examples 19.28 and 19.29).

Calculations where quantity of ingredients is too small to weigh or measure accurately

When preparing medicines by extemporaneous dispensing, the quantity of active ingredient required may be too small to weigh or measure with the equipment available. In these situations, a measurable quantity has to be diluted with an inert diluent. The process is called 'trituration' (see Ch. 38).

Small quantities in powders

The method for preparing divided powders is described in Chapter 38 (see Example 19.30).

Example 19.30

Calculate the quantities required to make 10 powders each containing 200 micrograms (µg) of digoxin.

Assume that the balance available has a minimum weighable quantity of 100 mg. An inert diluent, in this case lactose, will be used for the trituration. The convenient weight of each divided powder is 120 mg.

The total weight of powder mixture required will be $10 \times 120 = 1200$ mg = 1.2 g.

Quantities for 10 powders:

Digoxin	2 mg
Lactose	1198 mg
Total	1200 mg

The weight of digoxin is too small to weigh. The minimum weighable quantity of 100 mg is weighed and used in the triturate. A 1 in 10 dilution is produced.

Trituration A

Digoxin	100 mg
Lactose	900 mg
Total	1000 mg

Each 100 mg of this mixture (A) contains 10 mg of digoxin.

Trituration B

Mixture A	100 mg (= 10 mg digoxin)
Lactose	900 mg
Total	1000 mg

Each 100 mg of this mixture (B) contains 1 mg of digoxin. This amount of digoxin is less than the required amount, so mixture B can be used to give the required quantity.

200 mg of mixture B provides the 2 mg digoxin required.

Final trituration (C)

Mixture B	200 mg (= 2 mg digoxin)
Lactose	(1200−200) = 1000 mg
Total	1200 mg

Each 120 mg of this mixture (C) will contain 200 µg (0.2 mg) of digoxin.

Small quantities in liquids

If the quantity of a solid to be incorporated into a solution is too small to weigh, again dilutions are used. In this case, a solution is prepared, so the solubility of the substance needs to be considered. Normally a 1 in 10 or 1 in 100 dilution is used (Example 19.31)

Solubilities

When preparing pharmaceutical products, the solubility of any solid ingredients should be checked. This will give useful information on how the product should be prepared. The objective of this section is to clarify the terminology used when solubilities are stated.

The solubility of a drug can be found in reference sources such as the drug monograph in *Martindale*. The method of stating solubilities is as follows:

> Sodium chloride is soluble 1 in 2.8 of water, 1 in 250 of alcohol and 1 in 10 of glycerol

This means that 1 g of sodium chloride requires 2.8 mL of water, 250 mL of alcohol or 10 mL of glycerol to dissolve it. An example of how knowledge of a substance's solubility can help in extemporaneous dispensing can be found in Chapter 30.

Example 19.31

Calculate the quantities required to prepare 100 mL of a solution containing 2.5 mg morphine hydrochloride/5 mL.

Quantities for 100 mL:

Morphine hydrochloride	50 mg
Chloroform water	to 100 mL

The solubility of morphine hydrochloride is 1 in 24 of water.

The minimum quantity of 100 mg of morphine hydrochloride is weighed and made up to 10 mL with chloroform water (this weight of morphine hydrochloride will dissolve in 2.4 mL).

5 mL of this solution (A) provides the 50 mg of morphine hydrochloride required. Take 5 mL of solution A and make up to 100 mL with chloroform water.

Calculations involving doses

A simple calculation which pharmacists sometimes have to make while dispensing, is to calculate the number of tablets or capsules or volume of a liquid medicine to be dispensed (Examples 19.32 and 19.33).

Calculating doses

An overdose of a drug, if given to a patient, can have very serious consequences and may be fatal. It is the responsibility of everyone involved in supplying or administering drugs to ensure that the accuracy and suitability of the dose are checked.

The standard way to check whether a drug dose is appropriate is to consult a recognized reference book. One of the commonest used for this purpose is the BNF. When first using any reference source it is important to be aware of the terminology used, to avoid misinterpreting the entries, especially where doses are quoted as '× milligrams daily, in divided doses'. An explanation of the terminology will usually be found in the introduction to the book (Example 19.34).

Calculations of children's doses

Children require different doses from those of adults. Ideally these should be arrived at as a result of extensive clinical studies, although this is often not possible. When this is the case, an estimate of the dose has to be made. This is best carried out using body weight (see next section), but where this is not available, there are three formulas which relate the child's dose to the adult dose.

Fried's rule for infants

Age (month) × adult dose/150 = dose for infant

Clark's rule

Weight (in kg) × adult dose/75 = dose for child

Body surface area (BSA) method

BSA of child (m^2) × adult dose/1.73 m^2

(average adult BSA) = approximate child's dose

Example 19.32

The doctor prescribes orphenadrine tablets, 100 mg to be taken every 8 hours for 28 days. Orphenadrine is available as 50 mg tablets. How many tablets should be supplied?

For each dose, 2 tablets are required. Every 8 hours, means 3 doses per day.
Therefore, the total number of tablets required is 2 × 3 × 28 = 168 tablets.

Example 19.33

The following prescription is received:

Sodium valproate oral solution:
100 mg to be given twice daily for 2 weeks.
Sodium valproate oral solution contains sodium valproate 200 mg/5 mL.
This prescription is therefore translated as:
2.5 mL to be given twice daily for 2 weeks.
The quantity to be dispensed will be:
2.5 × 2 × 14 = 70 mL.

Example 19.34

The following prescription is received:

Verapamil tablets 160 milligrams
Send 56
Take two tablets twice daily

There are a variety of doses quoted for verapamil in the BNF depending on the condition being treated. They are as follows for oral administration:

Supraventricular arrhythmias, 40–120 mg three times daily
Angina, 80–120 mg three times daily
Hypertension, 240–480 mg daily in 2–3 divided doses.

The dose given for hypertension is stated in a significantly different way. Whereas the other doses can be given three times daily, indicating a maximum of 360 mg in any one day, the hypertension dose is the total to be given in any one day and is divided up and given at the stated frequencies, i.e. a maximum of 240 mg, given twice daily or a maximum of 160 mg, given three times daily.

The prescription is for a dose higher than recommended, so consultation with the prescriber would be required. Be alert – variation in terminology and a lack of awareness could have very serious consequences.

Calculation of doses by weight and surface area

For some drugs the amount of drug has to be calculated accurately for the particular patient. This is normally carried out using either body weight or body surface area. When body weight is being used, the dose will be expressed as mg/kg. In countries which still use pounds, it will be necessary to convert the patient's weight in pounds into kilograms by dividing by 2.2. The total dose required is then obtained by multiplying the weight of the patient by the dose per kilogram.

Body surface area is a more accurate method for calculating doses and is used where extreme accuracy is required. This is necessary where there is a very narrow range of plasma concentration between the desired therapeutic effect and severe toxicity, such as with the drugs used to treat cancer. The body surface area can be calculated from body weight and height using the equation given below, but it is more usual to use a nomogram for its determination. The actual nomogram is published in many reference sources.

Body surface area (m^2)
$$= \text{weight (kg)}^{0.5378} \times \text{height (cm)}^{0.37} \times 0.024\,265$$

Reconstitution and infusion

Some drugs are not chemically stable in solution and so are supplied as dry powders for reconstitution just before use. Many of these are antibiotics, but there is also a range of chemotherapeutic agents used in cancer treatment. The antibiotics may be for oral use or for injection. An oral antibiotic for reconstitution comes as a powder in a bottle with sufficient space to add the water. Those for injection are sterile powders and are dissolved in sterile water aseptically (see Ch. 40). There are a number of calculations which may be required around the reconstitution processes (Example 19.35).

Sometimes, the doctor may request a more or less concentrated syrup to be produced which requires altering the amount of water added from that indicated by the manufacturer (Example 19.36).

However, this type of oral mixture is likely to have other ingredients – thickeners, colours, flavours, etc. – which will occupy some of the final volume.

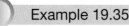

Example 19.35

What dose of antibiotic will be contained in a 5 mL spoonful when a bottle containing 5 g of penicillin V is reconstituted to give 200 mL of syrup?

For this type of calculation, the simple proportion equation can be used:

$\text{Wt}_1/\text{Wt}_2 = \text{Vol}_1/\text{Vol}_2$

$5\,\text{g} = 5000\,\text{mg}.$

Substituting we get:

$5000\,\text{mg}/y\,\text{mg} = 200\,\text{mL}/5\,\text{mL}$

$y = 125\,\text{mg}.$

Example 19.36

We have an ampicillin product for reconstitution. It contains 2.5 g of ampicillin to be made up to 100 mL. To what volume should it be made to give 100 mg per 5 mL dose?

The normal mixture will give a dose of:

$2500\,\text{mg}/y\,\text{mg} = 100\,\text{mL}/5\,\text{mL}$

$y = 125\,\text{mg per 5 mL}$

To calculate the amount of water to add, the same equation is used:

$2500\,\text{mg}/100\,\text{mg} = y\,\text{mL}/5\,\text{mL}$

$y = 125\,\text{mL}.$

Example 19.37

The label on an ampicillin bottle indicates that 78 mL of water must be added to produce 100 mL of final syrup. How much water must be added to give the 125 mL final volume?

Thus, the volume of powder in the final syrup is:

$100\,\text{mL} - 78\,\text{mL} = 22\,\text{mL}.$

Therefore, the volume to add to give 125 mL is:

$125\,\text{mL} - 22\,\text{mL} = 103\,\text{mL}.$

So this may not be correct and we need to be able to calculate exactly how much water to add (Examples 19.37 and 19.38).

Drugs for injection solutions do not normally contain ingredients other than the drug (or they make an insignificant contribution to the final volume). However, they are usually packed as a quantity of drug with the final volume left to be calculated by the pharmacist (Example 19.39).

Example 19.38

A child weighing 60 lb requires a dose of 8 mg/kg of ampicillin. Given that a 5 mL dose is to be given, what volume of water must be added when the powder is reconstituted? Instructions on the label indicate that dilution to 150 mL (by adding 111 mL) gives 250 mg ampicillin per 5 mL.

Conversion of weight to kg: 60/2.2 = 27.27 kg

Calculation of amount of ampicillin required:
27.27 × 8 = 218 mg.

Calculation of amount of ampicillin in container:
250 mg/y mg = 5 mL/150 mL,

therefore y = 7500 mg = 7.5 g

Calculation of amount of water (a) to add to give 218 mg per 5 mL: 218 mg/7500 mg = 5 mL/a mL,

therefore a = 172 mL

Volume occupied by powder: 150 mL–
111 mL = 39 mL

Therefore, volume to be added:

172 mL–39 mL = 133 mL.

Example 19.39

Calculate the amount of sterile water to be added to a vial containing 200 000 units of penicillin G in order to produce a solution containing 40 000 units per millilitre. Again, simple proportion is used:

40 000 units/200 000 units = 1 mL/y mL,
therefore y = 5 mL.

Example 19.40

An ampoule of flucloxacillin contains 250 mg of powder with instructions to dissolve it in 5 mL of water for injections. What volume of this solution should be added to 500 mL of saline infusion to provide a dose of 175 mg?

250 mg in 5 mL = 50 mg per mL

Therefore, we require: 175 mg/50 mg/mL = 3.5 mL.

Example 19.41

100 mg of phenylephrine hydrochloride are added to 500 mL of saline infusion. What should be the rate of infusion to give a dose of 1 mg per minute? How long will the infusion take?

Using simple proportion: 100 mg/1 mg = 500 mL/y mL

y = 5 mL and contains the required amount of drug

The infusion rate should be 5 mL per minute.

The total volume is 500 mL, therefore the time taken at 5 mL/min is:

500 mL/5 mL/min = 100 min.

Example 19.42

A doctor requires an infusion of 1000 mL of 5% dextrose to be administered over an 8 hour period. Using an IV giving set which delivers 10 drops/mL, how many drops per minute should be delivered to the patient?

First convert the time into minutes:

8 hour = 8 × 60 min = 480 min

Next calculate how many mL/min are required:

1000 mL/480 min = 2.1 mL/min

Then calculate the number of drops this requires:

2.1 mL/min × 10 drops/mL = 21 drops/min.

Calculation of infusion rates

Drugs may be given to patients intravenously by adding them to an intravenous (IV) infusion (see Ch. 41). Calculations involve working out how much drug solution should be added, working out how fast, in terms of mL/min, the infusion should be administered, and calculating what this means in terms of 'drops per minute' through the giving set. When an infusion pump is used, this can be set to deliver a specified number of mL/min (Example 19.40).

When administering intravenous infusions, the rate of administration is first calculated in terms of millilitres per minute (Example 19.41).

Most infusions are administered using a giving set with a dropping device on the tube Partial clamping of the tube can be used to adjust the rate of dropping. Depending on the drop size – that is the number of drops per millilitre – it is then possible to convert a rate of millilitres per minute into drops per minute which the nurse can adjust (Example 19.42).

Example 19.43

20 mL of a drug solution is added to a 500 mL infusion solution. It has to be administered to the patient over a 5 hour period. Using a set giving 15 drops per millilitre, how many drops per minute are required?

The total volume of infusion is:

20 mL + 500 mL = 520 mL

Then calculate the number of drops which will be administered in total:

520 mL × 15 drops = 7800 drops

The duration of the infusion is to be:

5 (hours) × 60 = 300 min

Calculate how many drops are required per minute:

7800 drops/300 min = 26 drops per min.

A variation on this is when the doctor wishes a drug solution to be added to the infusion (Example 19.43).

KEY POINTS

- Always work methodically and write down calculations clearly
- Check calculations, using a different method where possible
- Estimate the answer before you start
- Try to visualize the quantities you are using in the calculation
- Look carefully to see if a formula gives the quantities of all ingredients or uses 'to' for the vehicle
- Always check the units being used and be careful not to mix them during a calculation
- Be careful to read the wording; small changes in terminology can alter the calculation
- Triturates with solids and liquids normally use a 1 in 10 dilution per step
- Be very careful in checking doses, particularly with 'in divided doses' and 'mg/kg' statements in the reference books
- On completion of a calculation, ask yourself whether the answer is 'reasonable' given the numbers you are using

Section 4

Access to medicines and their selection

The prescribing process and evidence-based medicine

20

Jason Hall

STUDY POINTS

- Good prescribing ensures maximum benefit for the patient and value for money
- The stages involved in the prescribing process
- Evidence-based medicine

Introduction

The prescribing of medicines is the most common medical intervention in patient care and drug costs are a major component of NHS expenditure. Ensuring optimum benefits for patients and value for money for taxpayers and other individuals and organizations paying for health care are priorities and a model of 'good prescribing' has been proposed that has four aims. These aims are to:

- Maximize effectiveness
- Minimize risks
- Minimize costs
- Respect patient choice

Maximizing effectiveness is about selecting a drug therapy that will achieve its therapeutic objective in a suitable timescale.

Minimizing risks is recognizing that all drug treatments carry an element of risk of causing harm to the patient and that selection of the drug should be about managing these benefits and risks.

The cost of therapy should also be taken into account by the prescriber although such consideration should go beyond a simple review of the drug costs but also consider any costs of monitoring treatment such as blood tests, length of treatment and any additional items that could be required such as prescribing an additional drug to protect the gastrointestinal tract from adverse effects caused by the first.

Establishing the views of the patient is a vital part of the process of assessing the relative importance of the first three aims in this model. Patients may differ in their views regarding managing the symptoms of a condition, living with the consequences of a condition, exposing themselves to risks of harmful effects and the amount of money they would be willing or able to pay for treatment. In addition, patients may wish product selection to take their lifestyle into account such that the frequency and route of administration of the selected product fits in with their daily routine.

It is accepted that 'good prescribing' involves trade-offs between these four aims and that this often involves delicate balancing between each of the aims.

The prescribing process

The prescribing process will be considered under five headings although there is some overlap between these and their sequence may not be the same in all cases. The first is concerned with all the things that must be in place before a prescriber can start to prescribe; the second with collecting information; the third with analysing the information and making the prescribing decision and the fourth with making appropriate records and plans for monitoring the patients progress and the last with auditing and evaluating prescribing practice.

Prerequisites

Prescribing can only be carried out by healthcare professionals that have the appropriate prescribing qualifications and these will vary depending on the type of prescribing to be carried out. To prescribe prescription only medicines on the NHS or privately the prescriber, if not a medical prescriber, must have successfully completed the training to allow them to act as a supplementary or an independent prescriber. The training course consists of a taught element (around 26 days) and learning in practice (around 12 days), which includes prescribing under the supervision of a medical prescriber. To participate in a minor ailment scheme and prescribe pharmacy only medicines at NHS expense the pharmacist will likely have had to complete appropriate accreditation set by the local primary care organization.

Patients that are to receive their prescriptions from a supplementary prescriber must give informed consent. Patients do not need to sign this informed consent but is good practice to make a note in the patient's medical notes when informed consent was given. The exact nature of informed consent is difficult to define and it is likely that the input from the healthcare professional will vary between patients when obtaining consent. Observation of disputes between patients and physicians regarding whether informed consent was given show that simply handing the patient a leaflet does not discharge the physician from their obligation to obtain informed consent. In any legal dispute it is up to the courts to decide which party they believe but the disputes that found in favour of the physician tended to be those where the physician was able to demonstrate that they had given the information to the patient because they had documented the advice they gave in the patient's medical records.

Prior to the patient consultation, the prescriber should ensure that they are suitably prepared. Part of this preparation includes ensuring they have sufficient indemnity insurance that covers their prescribing and that their job description clearly shows that prescribing is part of their role. Another part of the preparation is acquiring the appropriate knowledge and skills (see Table 20.1).

Consulting with the patient

Where possible, prescribers should also familiarize themselves with the patient's medical history prior to the consultation. This however, would not be possible in minor ailment schemes, as patients are likely to arrive without an appointment and their medical notes will not usually be available to the community pharmacist.

During the consultation, prescribers must take a full history of the presenting condition and any other factors such as other conditions the patient have or any other medications including OTC medicines and complementary medicines that the patient may be taking. It may be necessary to carry out further investigations such as measuring the patient's blood pressure. This information must be recorded in the patient's medical notes.

Before any prescribing can take place a diagnosis must be made. If the pharmacist is acting as a supplementary prescriber the diagnosis will have been made by an independent prescriber but the pharmacist should interpret the information obtained before and during the consultation to check that patient's diagnosis remains valid. Independent prescribers must establish a working diagnosis based upon the information they have gathered on the patient. At this stage, it may be necessary to request laboratory tests such as urea and electrolytes, red blood cell count and haemoglobin tests to help confirm the working diagnosis.

With increasing complexity of health care and increasing specialization of the roles of healthcare professionals, there is a growing need for different professions to work together and pharmacists must ensure that they are aware of the different professions they could call on for support or to refer to patients (see Table 20.1).

Where patient care is shared between healthcare professionals there is an obvious need for clear communication links, especially around monitoring and reviewing the patient's therapy. Clear communication links are particularly crucial in supplementary prescribing where two different professionals can prescribe for a patient. There must be a clear description of the criteria that would require the supplementary prescriber having to refer the patient back to the independent prescriber. Examples of such referrals could be failure of the patient's condition to respond to the therapy outlined in the clinical management plan or suffering an adverse reaction to the prescribed medication. Both independent and supplementary prescribers must have access to a common medical record.

Table 20.1 Checklist for knowledge and skills required by pharmacist prescribers

Legal restrictions effecting which medicines can be prescribed	Independent pharmacist prescribers can prescribe any licensed or unlicensed medicine except diamorphine, dipipanone or cocaine for treating addiction but may prescribe those drugs when treating organic disease or injury. Supplementary prescribers can prescribe any licensed or unlicensed medicine including controlled drugs provided it has been specified in the clinical management plan.
Professional restrictions effecting which medicines can be prescribed	It is vital that each prescriber only prescribes within their own area of competence. Knowing one's own limitations is a key skill for a prescriber. In addition, they must also have an appropriate level of experience dealing with the condition and it might be appropriate to refer a patient presenting with a condition rarely experienced to another prescriber for assessment and any prescribing if required.
Administrative arrangements regarding payments for the service	The administrative arrangements regarding the prescribing process must be fully understood. In the case of minor ailments schemes these arrangements could include a description of records that should be kept and how payment for the service is to be made. For NHS prescribing the prescriber should be aware of the categories of patient that are exempt from NHS charges and what payments should be made by those that are not exempt.
Patient confidentiality	Pharmacist prescribers must maintain patient confidentiality and take steps to ensure that no unauthorized personnel can gain access to patient medication records by securely storing the data either via lock and key or via appropriate electronic security measures such as passwords for data stored electronically.
Ethics	Prescribers should be aware of the good practice guidance from the DH and the GPhC before they start to prescribe. The DH guidance addresses prescribers not prescribing for themselves, not normally prescribing for members of their family and also covers accepting gifts and hospitality for suppliers. Pharmacist prescribers must also comply with the GPhC Standards of conduct, ethics and performance.
Security	Prescribers must be aware of security issues surrounding prescribing and take steps to minimize the risks. Blank prescription forms could be used by drug misusers to try and obtain supplies of prescription medicines for abuse or to sell to others. Care must be taken to ensure that the forms are securely stored. Personal security must also be considered if the prescriber is visiting patients in their own homes or other locations in the community.
Therapeutic management of conditions	A pharmacist's knowledge and skills required for the management of a therapeutic area must be up to date and based upon the best evidence available at the time. The knowledge should extend to non-drug approaches to treatment as sometimes these could be the most appropriate intervention.
Other members of the healthcare team	Prescribers should be aware of other professionals they could refer patients to, e.g. general practitioner, the accident and emergency department in the hospital, dentists, the community nursing service (district nurses and health visitors) social services and self help groups.

Prescribing decision-making

Upon analysis and interpretation of the patient's signs, symptoms and laboratory test results, the prescriber must consider the treatment options including the option of offering no treatment to the patient. The consideration of therapy options must include concurrent diseases and concurrent medication, the patient's lifestyle (would the treatment regime fit in with the patient's schedule or would

side-effects of drugs affect their ability to perform their usual activities, e.g. driving).

A key component of this phase is involving the patient in the decision-making in order to achieve concordance (see Ch. 18). The prescriber must communicate the benefits and risks of the different treatment options to the patient or their carer. The principles of concordance dictate that patients should fully participate in the decision making process and a consultation style where patients are treated as equals and have the opportunity to ask questions and to raise any concerns or worries they might have helps to achieve this.

Following selection of the drug and formulation, the dosage regime must be determined. The dosage guidance in the summary of product characteristics, BNF or local and national clinical guidelines should be used to work out the dosage to be prescribed. In general it is recommended that dosage be started at the lower end of the dosing schedule and that the dose should be gradually increased until the required therapeutic benefits are seen and side effects are minimized. However, there are many exceptions to this such as prescribing a loading dose for certain antibiotics or prescribing drugs where the therapeutic benefits are not obvious such as drugs used in prophylaxis.

The prescriber must also indicate the quantity to be supplied on the prescription. The quantity to be supplied will depend upon whether the treatment is likely to be acute or chronic. If the treatment is acute then the quantity is likely to be enough for the recommended course of treatment. When determining the quantity to be supplied for a chronic condition the prescriber should bear in mind the frequency that they would wish to review the patient, whether the patient has to pay for the item, the patient's ability to pay the prescription levy and whether there are any dangers from accidental or deliberate overdose. In general, smaller quantities offer the opportunity to review patient's therapy more frequently and reduce waste if patients are unable to take their medicine through the occurrence of troublesome side effects or adverse drug reactions. However, smaller quantities can cause greater patient inconvenience as patients will to visit healthcare professional more frequently and greater expense if they have to pay for their medication, as well as increasing the prescriber's workload.

Recording and monitoring

It is important to realize that the responsibilities of the prescriber do not end with signing the prescription. The prescriber must make appropriate records of the medicine(s) prescribed and any advice given to the patient in the patient's medical notes. For paper held records the prescriber will obviously have to write the name of the prescribed item, the formulation, the strength, dosage instructions in the notes. In the case of electronic prescribing the details of what was prescribed, the date of prescribing and the directions will be stored automatically in the patient's records. However there may be a need to record additional information such as when the patient should next be reviewed and the monitoring that is recommended.

All prescribing should be followed-up with some monitoring although in some cases this may be left to the patient or carer to do themselves (see Ch. 51). Monitoring should address the anticipated benefits from therapy such as 'are the symptoms being controlled?' and harmful effects such as 'is the patient suffering from adverse effects?'. In many situations the patient or their carer will be given advice regarding what to do should the beneficial effects not materialize or if the harmful effects are troublesome, but there may be situations where these are not apparent such as monitoring blood cell counts following administration of a drug known to effect blood cell formation, and patients should be informed when they will next need to have their therapy reviewed.

Prescribers must appreciate any drug can cause an adverse drug reaction but that certain drugs are more likely to cause an ADR. Therefore, they must be aware of the action required if patients suffer from an adverse drug reaction. Minor ADRs that are known to occur with established medicines do not need reporting while serious suspected and actual ADRs for new and established medicines and all ADRs for new medicines should be reported via the yellow card reporting scheme.

Auditing prescribing practice

Prescribing audits involve reviewing prescribing activity against a set of explicit criteria such as a set of local or national clinical guidelines. For example, this could involve reviewing the prescribing for all patients registered with a practice that have a diagnosis of angina and comparing this with the guidance published by NICE. The audit should specify the standard of compliance with the guideline that is expected (e.g. 90% or 100%). If the audit reveals that expected standard of compliance has not been met then there should be a review of practice to identify why the standard has not been met. Prescribers should reflect upon the findings of the review and agree what action is required. The audit should then be repeated to determine whether the action has had an impact on the compliance with the standard. An audit cycle involves repeating the audit, review and action (see Ch. 12).

Evidence-based medicine

Evidence-based medicine (EBM) has been described as 'a means of closing the gap between research and everyday practice and ensuring that clinical decisions are based upon the best available scientific evidence'. It allows healthcare professionals to compare the evidence for different treatment options. This comparison may sound easy but unfortunately the available evidence is frequently of variable quality, which makes comparisons difficult.

The process of EBM involves four stages. The first involves identifying the question to be answered such as: Does treatment with drug X prevent more cardiovascular events than drug Y? The second stage involves searching the literature to find studies that have compared drug X with drug Y. The third stage is a critical appraisal of the studies that have been identified which involves making judgements about the quality of the studies, comparing the evidence supporting drug X with the evidence supporting drug Y and determining whether the balance of evidence favours one drug over the other. The final stage is about applying the evidence to clinical practice, which could involve recommending one drug be prescribed by clinicians rather than the other.

Assessing the quality of the evidence involves comparing the studies reported in the literature. There is a hierarchy of type of studies in terms of quality with meta-analysis of more than one randomized controlled trial at the top, then single randomized controlled trials, then controlled trials without randomization, then descriptive or case control studies and finally reports from expert committees (see Table 20.2 for a description of these terms). A key point to note concerning the method used in the study, is whether the study was double blind or not (double blind is where the researcher and the subjects did not know which treatments were given to the subjects).

The review of a study should also consider whether there is a potential for bias in the study by considering who funded the study and the affiliations of the authors.

It is important to review the doses of drugs used as some studies do not use equivalent doses of

Table 20.2 Descriptions of studies investigating health care

Type of study	Description
Meta-analysis	A statistical method of combining the results of more than one trial
Double blind randomized controlled trial (RCT)	A study where one group of subjects was randomly assigned to receive one treatment and the other group to receive an alternative treatment or placebo. Double blind is where neither the researchers nor the subjects are aware which group they have been assigned
RCT	A study where one group of subjects was randomly assigned to receive one treatment and the other group to receive an alternative treatment or placebo
Case–control studies	A study that compares one group of patients with another
Cohort studies	A study that follows the progress of a group of patients (a cohort) and compares their progress to the characteristics of the group members
Expert opinion	A report from an expert committee or opinions expressed by a respected group of experts

drugs particularly where one drug is compared with a competitor's drug. The reviewers should consider whether the study used healthy volunteers or patients suffering from the condition and whether the demographic profile of the subjects was similar to the general population. Generally, the larger the study in terms of the number of subjects included, the higher the quality of the study but the number of subjects needed to show an effect is dependent on the magnitude of the effect with larger numbers needed to demonstrate smaller differences between the different arms of the study.

The length of the study is another important consideration and this should be related to how the drug will be used in practice as the benefits reported in a study lasting 10 days would have more relevance to a drug used to treat acute short-term conditions compared with long-term chronic conditions, where the benefits could wear off after the study ends. The review should consider the endpoint reported in the study (what was measured in the study) and whether the endpoint was the same as the intended outcome (e.g. the intended outcome of a treatment in a study could be a reduction in the incidence of cardiovascular events but endpoint of the study might just address one risk factor for cardiovascular events).

Information sources

The evolution of modern medicines and appliances has resulted in a tremendous increase in the range of products available on prescription, and a corresponding increase in the amount of information available to support their use. This vast array of information originates from many sources including the pharmaceutical industry, academic institutions, professional bodies, government agencies and patient groups. Much of this information is aimed at prescribers and other professional groups, but with the increased availability of this information through advances in information technology and the upsurge of public demand, many patients also have greater access to information about medicines. With such a variety of sources all competing for the attention of the prescriber there is a danger that they could be overloaded with information of variable quality and which is potentially conflicting (see Ch. 16).

Reports of studies published in the literature can be obtained by using Medline, Embase or Pubmed, although it is likely that most searches will result in large numbers of hits and reviewing the quality of large number of papers will be very time consuming. Alternatively, there are several of sources of evidence based medicine reviews. The Cochrane Library is a collection of databases that contain evidence-based reviews and is available through the National Electronic Library for Health and University libraries. Clinical Evidence from the BMJ Publishing Group provides a summary of the evidence available for managing a wide variety of conditions and includes an assessment of the quality of the evidence.

Guidelines

There has been a recent proliferation in the number of guidelines produced in developed countries to assist practitioners in a wide variety of clinical roles. They have been defined as 'recommendations on the appropriate treatment and care of people with specific diseases and conditions'. However, it should be noted that foundations on which

guidelines are based range from guidance based on good quality evidence to those based upon expert opinion. The quality of guidelines can also vary and prescribers must decide whether a guideline is suitable for use in their practice. In addition, there are few if any guidelines that can provide guidance that is appropriate for 100% of patients and prescribers should not follow guidelines blindly but consider which situations the guideline should be used and those when it should not. If a prescriber decides to deliberately deviate from a guideline they should document their reasons for deviation in the patient's medical notes.

The National Institute for Health and Care Excellence (NICE) is an independent organization responsible for providing 'national guidance on the promotion of good health and the prevention and treatment of ill health'. NICE provides guidance to support the management of a wide range of clinical conditions. The Scottish Intercollegiate Guidelines Network (SIGN) produce evidence-based clinical guidelines for use by people working in the health service and for patients.

Computerized decision support

Software is available that can assist healthcare professionals with diagnosis and prescribing. Relevant patient information such as age, sex, symptoms, laboratory tests are entered into the computer and this software compares these with information held on a database, to suggest a diagnosis or further investigations that might be required. The NHS previously funded a service to help healthcare professionals make evidence-based decisions for their patients. This service, called Clinical Knowledge Summaries (CKS), is not currently being maintained by the NHS, although it is available through the NHS Evidence website (www.evidence.nhs.uk). CKS also provides a clinical summary of recommendations for managing the patient's condition and information to enable the writing of a prescription as well as providing access to patient information leaflets.

Formularies

Drug formularies are lists of medicines that prescribers use. These range from personal formularies from an individual prescriber to formularies used by one or more general practices or one or more hospital Trusts. It has been claimed that formularies can improve prescribing by improving prescriber familiarity with medicines as they only need knowledge of a limited range of medicines. Formularies that span different organizations have the potential to improve consistency of prescribing across the primary secondary care interface (see Ch. 23).

The process of producing a formulary can be very time consuming but it can be educational for those contributing to the process. It provides organizations with the opportunity to compare different medicines within a class on the grounds of effectiveness, safety, patient acceptability and cost and to consider which medicines they wish to see prescribed by prescribers in their organization. Deciding who to invite onto a formulary group to produce a new formulary is an important stage in the process. In small organizations such as a general practice, it is likely that all prescribers would be involved in the selection of drugs but care should be taken to include the views of those affected by the formulary such as the practice nurse, health visitors, district nurses and community pharmacists. In larger organizations it would not be feasible to include everybody in the formulary group but where possible, representatives from each section or department should be included to enable feedback to the rest of their section or department.

The methods used to inform prescribers regarding the formulary is another important step in the process especially in large organizations as prescribers could be unaware of its existence. The cost of printing and distributing paper copies of the formulary will depend upon the quantity involved and type of binding that is used ranging from a printed book to a ring binder with photocopied sheets. The formulary group should consider how often the formulary will be updated and how user friendly the format is to its prescribers, i.e. is it small enough to take of ward rounds or visit patients in their home. With computer generated prescribing the formulary medicines can often be highlighted or listed before non-formulary medicines.

In general, formulary groups should not expect 100% compliance with a formulary because there are always likely to be exceptional patients that do not respond to or have an ADR to certain drugs. The formulary group should therefore decide what level of compliance with the formulary they wish to see and also how they can monitor the actual compliance with the formulary. In some areas they will have no power to insist that formulary medicines are prescribed and they will have to persuade prescribers to consider formulary drugs first. If compliance with the formulary is particularly low then the formulary group should reflect on the suitability of the formulary (are the right drugs in the formulary?) and method of disseminating the formulary (are prescribers aware of the formulary and is it in a format they can use easily in their work?).

Competency framework

The National Prescribing Centre (NPC) was an NHS organization (now subsumed into NICE) that aimed 'to promote and support high quality, cost effective prescribing and medicines management across the NHS, to help improve patient care and service delivery'. The NPC has produced a competency framework which brings together the knowledge, skills, motives and personal traits that are considered to be required by a prescriber working effectively. This framework should be used as a checklist by prescribers preparing to prescribe for the first time and also by prescribers reviewing their own practice as part of their continuing professional development.

KEY POINTS

- The prescribing of medicines is the most common medical intervention
- Good prescribing has four elements: to maximize effectiveness, minimize risk and cost and to respect patient choice
- The prescribing process has five component stages
- Training requirements are laid out for non-medical prescribers
- Independent prescribers diagnose and prescribe
- Supplementary prescribers prescribe in response to the diagnosis of an independent prescriber
- Evidence-based medicine allows healthcare professionals to compare the evidence for different treatment options and make the best decisions for the patient

Prescribing for minor ailments

21

Paul Rutter

STUDY POINTS

- The growth of self-care and the increase in access to medicines
- Gaining information from patients who present at the pharmacy with symptoms or conditions
- Use of clinical reasoning to aid differential diagnosis and not an acronym-based approach
- Assessment of patient's symptoms in order to provide treatment and/or advice for minor ailments

Introduction

The community pharmacist plays an essential role in providing patient care. In most western countries, a network of pharmacies allows patients easy and direct access to a pharmacist without an appointment. Without pharmacists, general medical services would be unable to cope with patient demand. In effect, pharmacists perform a vital triage role for doctors by filtering those patients who can be managed with appropriate advice and medicines and referring cases which require further investigation. This has been a central role of community pharmacists for many decades, but over the last 20 years the role has taken on greater significance as there has been a shift in global healthcare policy to empower patients to exercise self-care. For pharmacists to safely, effectively and competently manage minor ailments requires considerable knowledge and skill. It involves having the underpinning knowledge on diseases and their clinical signs and symptoms, the ability to apply this knowledge to an individual patient and use problem solving to arrive at a working differential diagnosis. This has to be combined with good interpersonal skills such as picking up on non-verbal cues, asking appropriate questions and articulating clearly any advice which is given (see Ch. 25). This chapter attempts to provide the contextual framework behind the growing prominence of the pharmacist in managing minor ailments and the key skills required to maximize performance.

The concept and growth of self-care

The concept of self-care is not new. People have always treated themselves for common illnesses and pharmacists have always provided an avenue for people to practise self-care. Self-care does not mean individuals are left on their own and means more than just looking after themselves. It includes all the decisions and actions people take in respect of their health and covers recognizing symptoms, when to seek advice, treating the illness and making lifestyle changes to prevent ill health. The expertise and support provided by healthcare professionals, such as pharmacists, is crucial to making self-care work. The profile of self-care has dramatically increased in recent years and is largely government driven, consumer fuelled and professionally supported.

Government policy

The creation of national healthcare schemes, such as the NHS has encouraged the general population to become more reliant on institutional bodies to look after their health. This has led to increased demand on services provided by these bodies, including the management of minor illness. For example, more than one in three GP consultations are for minor illnesses and an estimated 20–40% of GP time could be saved if patients exercised self-care. Similar findings have been recorded for patients attending hospital emergency departments. This dependence by patients on bodies such as the NHS has led to government policies which encourage and facilitate self-care. In the UK, the government agenda for modernizing the NHS was spelt out in its White Paper-The NHS Plan (2000). Within this document, the government made its intention clear to make self-care an important part of NHS health care. It stated that the front line of health care was in the home. Since that time the government has published numerous papers detailing why and how maximizing self-care can be achieved.

NHS walk-in centres and telephone help lines

The UK government has been proactive in facilitating self-care, most obviously by the formation of NHS walk-in centres and the telephone help lines NHS Direct (England and Wales) and NHS 24 (Scotland). The aim of walk-in centres is to improve access to health care that supports other local NHS providers. The service is nurse led but some employ doctors to work at particular times. The first NHS walk-in centre opened in 2000 and there are now approximately 90 operating in England. The Department of Health states that over 5 million people have used a walk-in centre with the main users being young adults. NHS Direct is a 24-hour nurse-led service that receives over 500 000 calls per month. Although originally designed as a telephone help line service, NHS Direct now also offers an online service and direct interactive digital TV plus the publication of its self-help guide. In April 2013, NHS Direct was replaced by the NHS 111 service.

Deregulation of medicines

Less obvious, but arguably more important, has been the expansion of medicines available without prescription (Table 21.1). This has direct impact on community pharmacists and represents one of the major ways in which pharmacy can contribute to self-care. The switching of POMs to P status is now well established. Loperamide and ibuprofen were the first POMs to be switched in 1983. Between 1983 and 2012, over 80 POM to P and 50 P to GSL switches were made. Recent POM to P switches have seen new therapeutic classes deregulated (e.g. proton pump inhibitors, triptans, alpha-blockers) although the number of products switched has slowed. This is in contrast to P to GSL deregulation where the number of switches has steadily increased. This has led to the current situation where most medicines are now GSL and freely available from all retail outlets.

The pharmacists' role in facilitating patient self-care

Pharmacists play a vital role in acting as a custodian of medicines and being the gatekeeper between patient self-care and the necessity to see a GP. As pharmacists are able to provide an ever-increasing arsenal of medicines to treat a growing number of conditions their role as first-line healthcare professionals is taking on greater significance, which in turn has implications on patient safety. It is vital that pharmacists possess the right knowledge and diagnostic skills to make sound clinical decisions.

Arriving at a differential diagnosis

The aim of any patient consultation is to determine a diagnosis from the presenting signs and symptoms. In some instances, a specific diagnosis can be determined as the set of signs and symptoms the patient has point very clearly to only one cause. However, in many cases the exact cause can be hard to determine and a 'differential diagnosis' will be made. In other words there is a degree of uncertainty with the diagnosis and the practitioner will make a treatment plan based on what they think is the most likely cause. For example, someone who presents with acute cough is likely to have a viral self-limiting cough but it could possibly be bacterial in origin. Advice and treatment might well be the same but an exact diagnosis cannot be made.

Table 21.1 Chronological history charting prescription only medicine (POM) to pharmacy (P) and P to general sales list (GSL) deregulation

Year	POM to P	Examples	P to GSL	Examples
1983	3	Oral ibuprofen	0	
		Loperamide		
		Terfenadine[a]		
1984–86	0		0	
1987	3	Hydrocortisone	0	
1988	2		0	
1989	2		0	
1990	0		0	
1991	2	Nicotine gum	0	
1992	8	Vaginal imidazoles	0	
		Nicotine patches		
1993	5		0	
1994	17	H_2 antagonists, Minoxidil, Beclomethasone nasal spray	2	Effervescent aspirin and lidocaine
1995	7		2	Oral ibuprofen
1996	3		2	Clotrimazole
1997	3		8	Loperamide
1998	5		3	
1999	3		2	Nicotine gum
2000	4	Terbinafine	2	Famotidine
2001	5	Emergency hormonal contraceptives, Prochlorperazine	5	
2002	2		0	
2003	1		5	Minoxidil, Beclomethasone nasal spray
2004	3	Omeprazole, Simvastatin	3	Terbinafine
2005	2	Chloramphenicol	3	
2006	2	Sumatriptan, Amorolfine	1	
2007	5		5	
2008	3		7	
2009	3	Orlistat, Tamsulosin	3	
2010	1	Tranexamic acid	4	
2011	1		5	
2012 (up to July)	1		3	

[a]Terfenadine reverted back to POM control in 1997 following serious adverse events in America and was subsequently withdrawn by the manufacturers.

To be able to make sound and competent differential diagnoses pharmacists require the pre-requisite knowledge and good consultation skills.

Knowledge

The cornerstone of making any diagnosis is having a sound knowledge of the presentation of conditions, which are likely to be seen in a community pharmacy. Exact prevalence data is lacking for community pharmacy consultations but it does not seem unreasonable that patterns of presentation in a community pharmacy are not too dissimilar from a GP practice. Based on this assumption, it is simple to identify those conditions that are most likely to be seen by a community pharmacist. This should be the starting point from which to build subject specific knowledge. For example if we take red eye, prevalence data from general medical practice would show that:

- Most Likely – Bacterial or allergic conjunctivitis
- Likely – Viral conjunctivitis, sub-conjunctival haemorrhage
- Unlikely – Episcleritis, scleritis, keratitis, uveitis
- Very Unlikely – Acute closed angle glaucoma.

It would seem most prudent to have a thorough knowledge of the signs and symptoms of all types of conjunctivitis and sub-conjunctival haemorrhage as these will form the vast majority of red eye presentations seen by the community pharmacist. Of course this does not mean that other conditions that are seen less commonly by the pharmacist should be ignored. However, if basic information on common presentations is lacking then inappropriate referrals are more likely and signs or symptoms that might suggest more sinister pathology will be missed.

Gaining information

Observation, asking questions and physical examination should all be used, where appropriate, to elicit information from the patient. Most obvious is the need to ask questions (see below) to explore the presenting signs and symptoms. However, equally important is knowing who you are dealing with and the way in which they present in the pharmacy. Finally, in certain circumstances questioning and observation can be supplemented by performing a physical examination (see later).

Questioning

Pharmacists will rely heavily on asking questions to guide a differential diagnosis. Studies with doctors have shown that an accurate patient history (gained from asking questions alone) is a powerful diagnostic tool and will enable the practitioner to arrive at a right diagnosis in about 80% of cases. If a physical examination is conducted and/or diagnostic tests performed, then the probability of a correct diagnosis is increased by 10–15%.

The ability to ask appropriate questions to gain the necessary information is therefore critical. The choice of question asked is rooted in clinical reasoning (see below) but at a more basic level, the type of question and the way in which it is asked will dictate the level of response given.

Use of open and closed questions

There are two main types of questions: open and closed. A closed question requires the respondent to give a single word reply such as 'Yes' or 'No'. Closed questions often with words such as 'Are you', 'Have you' and 'Do you'. Examples of closed questions are:

- Are you taking any medicines from the doctor?
- Have you ever had this rash before?
- Do you suffer from hay fever?

Closed questions can be very useful when asking for specific information or to test a hypothesis. Over use of closed questions however should be avoided as the consultation can then feel more like an interrogation than a two-way conversation.

Open questions allow patients to respond in their own way. They do not set any 'limits' and generally will provide more detailed information. Open questions often start with words such as 'describe', 'what', 'where' and 'how'. Examples of open questions include:

- Describe your symptoms
- What does the pain feel like?
- Where is the pain?
- How does the pain affect you?

Open questions are not without their problems. Some patients when asked an open question will provide irrelevant information and it can be difficult to pick up on the important information that is mixed in with irrelevant facts. An active listening approach is required (see Chs 17 and 25).

In most consultations a mixture of closed and open questions will be needed.

Using observation and knowledge of epidemiology

Assessment of the patient begins the moment the patient enters the pharmacy. First impressions can provide 'cues' to their state of health. Most pharmacists will probably do this at a subconscious level but what is important is to bring this to the conscious level and build it into your consultations. Many visual cues will be apparent if they are actively looked for. It may give you an indication of severity, for example does the patient look well or poorly? Do they show any obvious signs of discomfort? This initial assessment will provide useful information which shapes your thinking and actions, and is the first step to reaching a differential diagnosis. It might transpire that they have a self-limiting condition such as viral cough that ordinarily you would not refer to the GP but because the person is elderly and has marked systemic upset, a referral is appropriate.

The key is to observe your patient. What is their physical appearance? Is the patient overweight or showing signs of being a smoker? Are there any signs of confusion, pain or systemic illness? Take time to assess what they look like, how they move and how they behave.

In tandem with observation, the pharmacist should draw on the epidemiology of conditions within a population. This will be very helpful in formulating early ideas about what the likely diagnosis will be.

Take headache as an example. The age and gender of the patient will affect diagnostic probability: migraine is three times more common in women than men, whereas cluster headache is eight times more common in men. Onset of migraine tends to occur in adolescents or young adults but is rare in people aged over 50 years old. Therefore, the age and sex of the patient asking for advice on headache symptoms will begin to shape your differential diagnosis even before you start to ask any questions. This principle can be applied to all consultations and can also be used while asking questions.

Take cough as an example. A question that pharmacists will ask is the symptom duration. Knowing how long the cough has lasted will again affect the most likely diagnosis. The longer the cough has been present, the more prevalent are conditions with sinister pathology. So for a patient with a cough of 3 days duration, the most likely cause will be a viral upper respiratory tract infection. At 3 weeks' duration, the chances of it being a viral cause are lessened but other conditions such as acute bronchitis become more likely. At 3 months' duration, then sinister causes of cough are much more likely, such as chronic bronchitis, TB and carcinoma.

The linking of epidemiological data of conditions to each patient consultation is an important aspect of clinical reasoning and should be an integral part of the process when making a differential diagnosis.

Physical examination

Within the confines of a community pharmacy, the type and extent of physical examination that can be performed is limited. Examples of physical assessments that are suitable within the pharmacy include eye and ear examinations, assessment of skin disease and general inspection of the oral cavity. These examinations require little training but will improve the odds of making a correct diagnosis. Before conducting any physical examination, it is important to explain to the patient what you would like to do and why. Informed consent must be received. Ideally, physical examinations should be conducted in a private area and consideration should be given to having a chaperone present.

Clinical reasoning

Clinical reasoning is a critical skill that all pharmacists should possess. It is central to the decision-making processes associated with clinical practice. It enables practitioners to act autonomously allowing them to make the best reasoned actions in a specific context. When attempting to make a diagnosis, pharmacists will often be faced with an ill-defined problem, working with limited information where outcomes are difficult to predict. By this very definition pharmacists have to use their professional judgement and make decisions where clinical uncertainty will exist.

Much has been written on clinical reasoning and the ways in which it can be taught. A number of models have been proposed to explain the process and include hypothetico-deductive reasoning, pattern recognition and knowledge reasoning integration.

Given that OTC patient consultations is akin to medical practice in terms of making a diagnosis, then pharmacists should learn from the medical approach to clinical reasoning when making a diagnosis.

Hypothetico-deductive reasoning

As stated previously, pharmacists will often be faced with limited information in the early stages of a clinical encounter. The 'art' of deciding what information must be collected, what areas need exploration and what information can be safely disregarded will form the basis of the consultation. Data collection can therefore be described as both sequential and selective, which allow inferences to be drawn about the underlying cause of the patient's signs and symptoms.

Research has shown doctors approach solving diagnostic problems by generating a small number of hypotheses early in a clinical encounter and based on limited information. The generation of these hypotheses then guides subsequent data collection. Each hypothesis can be used to predict what additional findings ought to be present if it were true and what further questions to ask in a guided search for these findings – a hypothetico-deductive approach. Hypothesis generation and testing involves both inductive (moving from a set of specific observations to a generalization) or deductive reasoning (moving from a generalization to a conclusion in relation to a specific case). Therefore, induction is used to generate hypotheses and deduction to test hypotheses.

An example may serve to illustrate this process:

A man in his early 60s (slightly overweight) wants something for his cough.

Step 1: Drawing on subject specific knowledge

A cornerstone of making rationale decisions will be the need to have a good subject specific knowledge on cough and understanding the epidemiology of conditions that cause cough. You should know that the causes of cough and their relative incidence in community pharmacy are:

- Most Likely – Viral infection (all ages)
- Likely – Upper airways cough syndrome (formerly known as postnasal drip and includes allergies), acute bronchitis
- Unlikely – Croup, chronic bronchitis, asthma, pneumonia, ACE inhibitor induced

- Very unlikely – Heart failure, bronchiectasis, tuberculosis, cancer, pneumothorax, lung abscess, nocardiosis, GORD

Step 2: Visual cues: age, sex and overweight

Before asking any questions, you are already using the visual cue information to start to generate hypotheses. If we consider his age and apply this to the prevalence of the above conditions, we can safely eliminate croup as a cause of cough and the diagnostic probability of other conditions is low; pneumothorax tends to occur in young people; heart failure and lung abscess tend to occur in the elderly; asthma (presenting as cough only) tends to occur in children.

We are now left with fewer possibilities as to the cause of cough, allowing us to generate hypotheses that do not (initially) consider those eliminated because of age. Early hypothesis generation may well centre on a viral cause of cough, as it is the most commonly encountered cause of cough in his age group. Other hypotheses will focus on those conditions deemed likely and to a lesser extent, those which are unlikely.

Step 3: Testing hypotheses

Questions now need to be asked to gain more information on the symptoms of the patient's cough. Consideration should be given to what questions are asked and why. All questions that are asked should have an underlying purpose or reason. At this stage, early in the clinical encounter, initial questions should enable hypothesis generation to be narrowed. Questions asked should enable this narrowing process. So, if we take length of time the patient has had the cough as an example, subject-specific knowledge means we know that a cough of duration of longer than 3 weeks suggests a non-acute cause. Establishing duration will therefore be discriminatory in terms of narrowing down the diagnostic possibilities left open to you:

- Acute causes
  - Acute bronchitis
  - Pneumonia
  - Upper airways cough syndrome
  - Medicines?
- Chronic causes
  - Chronic bronchitis
  - Bronchiectasis

○ TB

○ Medicines?

○ Cancer

○ Nocardiosis

○ Gastro-oesophogeal reflux disease (GORD).

Certain causes of cough do not become chronic in nature. Therefore, if a patient presents with a long-standing cough, you can eliminate acute causes and thus narrow down your diagnosis. At this point, you can reformulate your hypotheses and the next set of questions you ask will try to distinguish between those conditions which remain as a possibility.

Your next question may ask about sputum production. From the chronic causes listed above, a medicine cause and GORD will be eliminated if the patient states that they produce sputum, leaving five causes of cough that may be causing the patient's symptoms. From this point, you may need to ask specific (closed) discriminatory questions which allow you to hone your differential diagnosis still further. Some chronic cough conditions tend to show periodicity during the day, either being better or worse in the morning or evening. From our remaining conditions, we know that generally:

• Chronic bronchitis is worse in the morning
• Bronchiectasis is worse in the morning and evening
• Tuberculosis shows no variation
• Cancer shows no variation
• Nocardiosis shows no variation.

Our patient says that the cough is always worse after getting up in the morning. This therefore tends to point to a diagnosis of chronic bronchitis. Obviously, the diagnosis is very tentative and we can now ask supplementary questions that should support the differential diagnosis. For example, one hypothesis would be that the person is a smoker/ex-smoker (chronic bronchitis is closely associated with smokers or ex-smokers). To support our differential diagnosis, we would expect the patient to say he smoked or had smoked in the past. Again to support the differential diagnosis, we would expect to ask about the periodicity of cough in chronic bronchitis. Confirmation of this by the patient lends further support to your differential diagnosis. If the patient responds in a different way to that anticipated, then the differential diagnosis would need to be revised and hypotheses reconstructed to establish the cause of the cough. This example demonstrates that this model of clinical reasoning is sequential and selective.

Pattern recognition

What is pattern recognition? Simply, pattern recognition can be thought of as categorization or pattern interpretation. In the clinical context, it involves grouping similar patient presentations together. Each new case seen is stored in the practitioner's memory in the same category. A non-medical analogy would be that if a person sees a dog we categorize it as a dog, but not necessarily what breed of dog, however after seeing sufficient dogs that look the same, we further categorize these to the breed of dog. Thus, we draw on memory recall from previous experience to help us categorize each new dog seen. Therefore in clinical practice, we build up a stored memory of previously seen similar cases from which we can draw on to help inform our diagnosis. This can be applied to all patient presentations but is especially useful for dermatological presentations, as visualization of a skin rash is more helpful than a description provided by a patient. Certain dermatological conditions have very characteristic presentations. For example, once a pharmacist has seen several cases of impetigo, it is a relatively straightforward task to diagnose the next case by recalling the appearance of previous rashes seen. Therefore, much of daily practice will consist of seeing new cases that strongly resemble previous encounters.

Hypothetico-deductive reasoning versus pattern recognition

In reality, a combination of hypothetico-deduction and pattern recognition is used. Pattern recognition is often attributed to the practitioner exhibiting expertise in that situation and clinical context. Expertise in medicine is often associated with time and practice. However, time and practice in a community pharmacy context may be less relevant in differentiating between 'novice' and 'expert' behaviour. This is because pharmacists, regardless of their level of experience, use the default option of medical practitioner referral when clinical uncertainty exists. While undoubtedly this constitutes safe practice, it does not necessarily equate to improving an individual's ability at effective pattern recognition. As pattern recognition is rooted in memory recall by matching against similar previously seen cases, then the outcome is likely to be the same–referral. Pharmacists can therefore quickly reach a 'glass ceiling' of clinical competence unless they actively seek feedback from the medical practitioner (or patient) to either confirm or reject their original diagnosis.

Neither model provides an error-proof strategy and error rates of up to 15%, especially in difficult cases in internal medicine, have been reported in the medical literature. However, these models of 'responding to symptoms' are more likely to gain the correct diagnosis compared to using acronyms and the funnel method because acronyms and the funnel method tend to just gather information without having a hypothesis in mind.

Other approaches used in 'responding to symptoms'

In pharmacy education the use of acronyms has been widely taught at undergraduate level and subsequently adopted into community practice. A number of acronyms have been developed and include: ENCORE, ASMETHOD, SIT DOWN SIR and WWHAM. WWHAM (Who is the patient? 'What are the symptoms? How long have the symptoms been present? Action taken? Medication being taken?) is the most well known and most widely used, probably because of it being simple to remember. Acronyms will provide structure and consistency to patient consultation but the difficulty with using acronyms is that they are rigid and inflexible – a 'one size fits all' approach. Using an acronym is akin to strictly following a standard operating procedure. Questions may be asked because they are part of the acronym, but they may be of little diagnostic value or there might be no relevance or underpinning reasoning for asking the question.

The most commonly used acronym, WWHAM, is also the worst; this is because it is simple to remember and so provides the least information. In addition, not all questions are helpful in establishing a diagnosis; Action taken and Medication being taken are really questions designed to help with patient management rather than aiding a diagnosis. This means that if WWHAM is routinely used, then pharmacists are only asking three questions to determine the cause of the patients presenting signs and symptoms. Furthermore, the first question, 'Who is the patient', in the context in which

WWHAM is used is also diagnostically unhelpful. In the acronym, this question is only being used to identify the patient. It is not being asked to establish a link between presenting symptoms and prevalence of conditions – if it were, then the question would be much more useful.

A further major failing of WWHAM and other acronyms is they concentrate very much on the presenting symptoms. They tend not to consider past medical history of similar episodes, do not explore family history or consider social factors that might be causing or compounding the symptoms.

In short, pharmacists should not use acronyms. They are too simplistic, rigid, inflexible and are poor in allowing the pharmacist to arrive at a correct diagnosis. If we compare the example highlighting hypothetico-deductive technique versus an acronym, the difference between the methods is clear and obvious. If WWHAM was used, the nature of the cough would have been established, and if chronic in nature a referral probably made. However, the information gained would have been superficial, which would not establish a more precise cause and it would also ask irrelevant questions, such as who it was for (we already knew) and what medication they had tried. More fundamentally, with regard to pattern recognition, the practitioner would not be able to draw on this consultation to inform future thinking.

The funnelling technique

A funnelling technique can be used to allow direction and focusing of ideas on a specific topic. This involves initially asking background 'open' questions to provide basic information, then asking specific 'closed' questions to provide specific detail and clarify points. In these circumstances, it can be useful to paraphrase comments made, to ensure that the understanding of the information being obtained from the patient is accurate. This checking procedure allows the pharmacist to check understanding and minimizes misinterpretation. It is possible during any one conversation to use more than one 'funnel', e.g. establishing a patient's current medical condition, then going on to suggest appropriate action or medication available. In a pharmacy setting, where time can be a limiting factor, using the funnelling technique can be useful for directing and focusing a conversation to enable an end point to be achieved more quickly.

Outcomes from the consultation

The final step in prescribing for minor ailments is deciding what course of action is most appropriate. This could be a combination of referral to another healthcare professional, giving advice or supplying a product. It is important that you give the patient as much information as they want or need and this draws on your skills of counselling (see Ch. 25).

Conditional referrals

One of the key things a patient needs to know is: What is the best course of action to take. Obviously this will depend on a number of factors including the patient themselves, the differential diagnosis and the severity of the condition. As a general rule, all patients should be advised on a timescale, whether they return to the pharmacist or see another healthcare practitioner. This will have to be gauged on a person-to-person basis. For example, take two patients presenting with viral cough. Acute coughs can last up to 3 weeks, although the majority will have cleared in 14 days. Therefore, depending at which point each patient presented in the course of the condition will affect your conditional referral. If the first person presents after 10 days, then you might tell them to see the doctor in 5 days time if symptoms do not improve (beyond 14 days). The second patient has only had symptoms for 2 days, in which case you would tell them that symptoms may take another 12–14 days to fully resolve.

Treatment and advice

Once a full assessment of the symptoms has been made, and a decision made that the patient can be managed by the pharmacist, appropriate recommendations should be made. At this point, shared decision-making is recommended. The patient should be fully informed of the treatment options but be guided by the pharmacist to ensure the best option is agreed upon.

The pharmacist should take into account the efficacy, side-effects, interactions, cautions and contraindications of therapeutic options. With regard to efficacy, pharmacists should be aware that many OTC medicines have little or no evidence base. This does not necessarily mean they are not effective, but in today's climate of evidence-based health care, products with proven efficacy should constitute first-line treatment.

The difficulty in establishing efficacy has many explanations and includes: products that are available OTC predating clinical trials, a general lack of trial data or poorly conducted trials, the placebo effect seen with some OTC medicines and the

Table 21.2 Medicines to avoid during pregnancy

Medicine	Advice in pregnancy
Antihistamines – sedating	Some manufacturers advise avoidance, although chlorphenamine and triprolidine are classed by Briggs et al. as being compatible
Antihistamines – non-sedating	Manufacturers advise avoidance as limited human trial data, but animal data suggest low risk
Anaesthetics – local (benzocaine, lidocaine)	Avoid in 3rd trimester – possible respiratory depression
Bismuth	Manufacturers advise avoidance
Crotamiton (e.g. Eurax)	Manufacturers advise avoidance
Fluconazole	Avoid
Formaldehyde (e.g. Veracur)	Manufacturers advise avoidance
Ocular lubricants (e.g. hypromellose, carbomer)	Manufacturers advise avoidance as safety has not been established
H_2 antagonists	Avoid
Hyoscine	Manufacturers advise avoidance as possible risk of minor malformations
Migraleve (opioid component)	Avoid in 3rd trimester
Iodine preparations	Avoid
Midrid	Avoid
Minoxidil (e.g. Regaine)	Avoid
Selenium (e.g. Selsun)	Manufacturers advise avoidance
Systemic sympathomimetics	Avoid in 1st trimester as mild fetal malformations have been reported

Table 21.3 Interactions of OTC medicines with POMs that can be significant

Medicine	Possible interactions	Outcome
Antihistamines–sedating	Opioid analgesics, anxiolytics, hypnotics and antidepressants	Increased sedation
Antacids (containing calcium, magnesium and aluminium)	Tetracyclines, quinolones, imidazoles, phenytoin, penicillamine, bisphosphonates, ACE inhibitors, angiotensin II	Decreased absorption
Aspirin	NSAIDs and anticoagulants	Increased risk of GI bleeds
	Methotrexate	Reduced methotrexate excretion, toxicity
Bismuth	Quinolone antibiotics	Reduced plasma quinolone concentration
Chloroquine	Amiodarone, sotalol, antipsychotics	Increased risk of arrhythmias
Fluconazole	Anticoagulants	Enhanced anticoagulant effect
	Ciclosporin	Increased ciclosporin levels
	Carbamazepine and phenytoin	Increased levels of both antiepileptics
	Rifampicin	Decreases fluconazole levels
	Atorvastatin	Increased atorvastatin levels that can lead to muscle pain/myopathy
		Note: Seriousness of the possible outcome would mean it is good practice to avoid all statins with fluconazole
Hyoscine	TCAs, and other medicines with anticholinergic effects	Anticholinergic side-effects increased
Ibuprofen	Anticoagulants	Enhanced anticoagulant effect
	Lithium	Reduced lithium excretion
	Methotrexate	Reduced methotrexate
Opioid-containing products	Alcohol, opioid analgesics, anxiolytics, hypnotics and antidepressants	Increased sedation
Prochlorperazine	Alcohol, opioid analgesics, anxiolytics, hypnotics and antidepressants	Increased sedation
St John's wort	Anticoagulants	Reduced anticoagulant effect
	SSRIs	Potential serotonin syndrome
	Phenytoin, phenobarbital, carbamazepine	Reduced antiepileptic serum level
	Oral contraceptives	Reduced efficacy of contraceptive
	Antivirals, ciclosporin, digoxin	Reduced plasma concentrations
Systemic sympathomimetics, including isometheptene (ingredient in Midrid)	MAOIs and moclobemide Beta-blockers and TCAs	Risk of hypertensive crisis Antagonism of antihypertensive effect
Topical (nasal or ocular) sympathomimetics	MAOIs and moclobemide	Risk of hypertensive crisis
Iron salts	Tetracyclines, quinolones, penicillamine	Reduced absorption if taken at same time

ACE, angiotensin converting enzyme; GI, gastrointestinal; MAOI, monoamine oxidase inhibitor; NSAID, non-steroidal anti-inflammatory drug; SSRI, selective serotonin reuptake inhibitor; TCA, tricyclic antidepressant.

nature of self-limiting conditions–is it the medicine working or the symptoms resolving on their own? When selecting a product, the patient's needs should be borne in mind. Factors such as prior use, formulation and dosage regimens should be considered. Non-drug treatment should also be offered where appropriate. For example, providing medication for motion sickness can be supplemented with advice on how to reduce symptoms, for example focusing on distant objects, not overeating before travel or sitting in the front seat in car journeys will help to reduce symptoms.

Children and the elderly

Care is needed in assessing the severity of symptoms in children and the elderly, as both groups can suffer from complications. For example, the risk of dehydration is greater in children with fever or the elderly with diarrhoea. Invariably, lower doses are used in children, and because the elderly suffer from liver and renal impairment they frequently require lower doses than younger adults. Children should be offered sugar-free formulations to minimize dental decay and elderly people often have difficulty in swallowing solid dose formulations. It is also likely that the majority of elderly patients will be taking other medication for chronic disease and the possibility of OTC–POM interactions should be considered.

Pregnancy

The potential for OTC medicines to cause teratogenetic effects is real. The safest option is to avoid taking medication during pregnancy, especially in the 1st trimester. Many OTC medicines are not licensed for use in pregnancy and breast-feeding because the manufacturer has no safety data or it is a restriction on their availability OTC. Table 21.2 highlights those medicines where restrictions apply.

Interactions of OTC medicines with other drugs

Medicines that are available for sale to the public are relatively safe. However, there are some important drug–drug interactions to be aware of when recommending OTC medicines. These are listed in Table 21.3.

Conclusion

In conclusion, the pharmacist plays a pivotal role in helping patients exercise self-care and provides an effective screening mechanism for doctors. The continued deregulation of medicines to pharmacy control will mean that pharmacists over the coming years will be able to prescribe more medicines from more therapeutic classes. This necessitates that all pharmacists have up-to-date clinical knowledge and can competently perform the role. This might require many to acquire new skills (e.g. physical examinations) and take a much more active role in monitoring and following up the patient after advice and products have been given.

KEY POINTS

- Pharmacists have a traditional role in assisting patients with self-care
- Recent increases in patient self-care are government driven, consumer fuelled and professionally supported
- It is estimated that 20–40% of GP consultations are for conditions which are suitable for self-care
- Pharmacists require excellent consultation and communication skills in order to be effective in eliciting information from patients
- When prescribing, first-line treatment should have proven efficacy
- Special considerations apply to children, the elderly and women who are pregnant or breast-feeding

Drug evaluation and pharmacoeconomics

22

Janet Krska and Dyfrig A. Hughes

STUDY POINTS

- Safety, efficacy and economy
- Pre-marketing studies
- Post-marketing studies
- Pharmacoeconomic evaluation of medicines
- Drug utilization review and evaluation

Safety, efficacy and economy

The volume, complexity and costs of modern medicines are increasing. The need to compare the therapeutic efficacy (i.e. benefits) of medicines with their potential to cause harm (i.e. risks) and the economic implications of these is of paramount importance to the pharmaceutical industry, to healthcare providers and to society. Pharmacists play a major role in evaluating the safety, efficacy and economics of medicines use.

At a macro-level, the pharmaceutical industry decides which line of drug development would best serve its shareholders' interests. New chemical entities which show promise must be studied in clinical trials before they can be marketed as medicines (see Ch. 4). After products are licensed and marketed, society and its healthcare systems are then faced with difficult decisions about which specific patient populations to treat, or which new medicines to approve for use. Increasingly, decisions are based on economic evaluations, which attempt to calculate cost:benefit ratios for medicines in potential patient populations. In some countries, only medicines which have a clear cost-effective advantage over existing treatment are funded by government. In the UK, various organizations work in differing ways to examine this aspect of medicine evaluation. At a micro-level, clinicians (doctors, pharmacists or nurses) must then assess the relative harms and benefits of each medicine for individual patients. This involves consideration of factors which can affect drug disposition, efficacy and safety, such as concurrent disease states or other medicines, while also weighing up the risk of untreated disease and potential affordability. As pharmacists become more involved in selecting treatments, the importance of skills in evaluating all these factors to make individual clinical decisions increases. Furthermore, pharmacists are frequently required to evaluate the use of medicines in individual patients prescribed by others. This involves the further skills of drug use review and evaluation.

The techniques used in the evaluation of medicines for safety, efficacy and efficiency at pre- and post-marketing stages are summarized in Table 22.1.

Pre-marketing studies

In most countries, evidence of safety, efficacy and quality must be presented to government-appointed regulatory authorities before a new product can be marketed. Manufacturers wishing to market a product in the UK, can apply to the Medicines and Healthcare products Regulatory Agency (MHRA), or to the European Medicines Agency (EMA). Either body must be satisfied with the evidence provided before a marketing authorization (formerly called a product licence) can be

Table 22.1 Methods of evaluating medicines in humans

Method	Subjects	Outcome
Clinical trials		
Phase I	Usually healthy volunteers ($\leq$60 adults)	Pharmacokinetics of drug Tolerability and toxicity profile (SAFETY)
Phase II	Selected and limited target patient population	Optimal dosage range (EFFICACY) Balance between safety and efficacy (THERAPEUTIC RATIO)
Phase III	Larger numbers of target patients (1000–2000 patients)	Comparative safety and efficacy of medicine Identification of common adverse drug reactions (<1:250 incidence)
Post-marketing pharmacoepidemiological studies		
Post-marketing surveillance (Phase IV)	Up to 10 000 patients	Less common and unpredictable ADRs Identification of patients at risk
Pharmacoeconomic evaluations	Variable numbers of patients using the medicine in routine clinical practice	Comparative cost minimization, cost-effectiveness, cost-utility or cost-benefit
Drug utilization studies or reviews	Variable numbers of patients using the medicine in routine clinical practice	Quantitative studies→patterns of drug use Some qualitative studies→appropriateness of drug utilization
Drug utilization review programme or drug use evaluation or clinical audit	Variable numbers of patients using the medicine in routine clinical practice	Clinical, social and economic consequences of drug utilization

granted. The MHRA and EMA have responsibility for assuring the public that all medicines which reach the UK or European markets have been assessed for safety, efficacy and quality. Cost issues are not taken into consideration. Efficacy has to be balanced against toxicity for each product and, while the MHRA's evaluation includes the active ingredients of a product and its formulation, final decisions must also take into account the nature of the disease to be treated and the duration of the treatment. What is an acceptable benefit to risk ratio may differ for a medicine used to prolong survival in terminal conditions compared to a treatment for symptomatic relief of short-term symptoms.

Prior to clinical trials in humans, the pharmacokinetics and pharmacodynamics of any new drug are studied in animals to indicate therapeutic and possible toxic effects. However, because of substantial species differences in drug handling and response, new drugs must be screened in more than one animal species. Uncertainties in the relationship between the effects of drugs in animals and humans also mean that great caution is needed before progressing to 'first time in man' trials.

Phase I trials

These first trials are carried out in healthy adult volunteers, to determine the drug's toxicity profile and assess tolerability. A dosage range is tested initially with a stepwise increase in drug dose being given to successive volunteers. Subjects in Phase I trials are intensively monitored to determine the nature and severity of any predictable dose-related adverse effects. Pharmacokinetic data are usually generated from both single- and multiple-dose studies. These may be used to assist in deciding the best method of administration.

These trials provide only limited safety data, because the subjects are healthy adults and unlikely to have any compromised drug handling ability. Thus, the potential risks of using the drug in patients at extremes of age, or in those with poor hepatic or renal function, are not known. There are also few subjects (e.g. 50–60), so only very common ADRs are detected.

Phase II trials

They are carried out in relatively small groups of target patients, usually within hospital departments specializing in particular areas of medicine. Their main aims are to test for efficacy and to identify an effective dose in closely monitored and controlled conditions. Phase II studies give the first indication of the likely value of the drug in patients, i.e. its efficacy. There is less emphasis on safety assessments during this phase, but the results will enable a therapeutic ratio (i.e. the balance between efficacy and safety) to be determined. Double-blind randomized controlled trials use a control group with a matching placebo to further assess efficacy. Phase II studies also inform the design of Phase III studies which are more comprehensive. Phases II and III combined may study 1000–2000 patients. The regulatory authorities closely control Phase II and Phase III studies, for which clinical trial certificates or exemptions are required.

Phase III trials

These trials examine safety and efficacy. They are generally large-scale studies comparing a new medicine with other treatments or placebo. Where possible, they should have a randomized controlled design, which is generally accepted as the least biased method of conducting clinical research. Assigning each patient randomly to either the new treatment or control helps to prevent bias (see Ch. 20).

Phase III trials are the main source of the information included in the summary of product characteristics (SPC) for the product. The conduct of clinical trials is subject to guidelines which cover ethical issues, trial design, the roles of investigators and sponsoring company and the storage and analysis of data. For every clinical trial which takes place, approval must be obtained from a research ethics committee. This committee will scrutinize the design of the trial, the information given to patients and the procedures for obtaining consent and that adequate compensation and insurance are available.

Safety is assessed by close monitoring of clinical signs and symptoms during scheduled clinical examinations and consultations, complemented by relevant laboratory investigations. Baseline pre-treatment data are compared with data obtained during periods of treatment with the study medicine and the experiences of treated patients compared to controls. However, systematic assessment of symptoms experienced by the patients included in the trials is not always carried out and a systematic checklist for patients to complete has been suggested. Even with the numbers of patients involved in Phases II and III, these trials can only identify type A ADRs that affect 1 in ≥250 patients. Type B ADRs, which are not predictable from the drug's pharmacological profile and tend to be rare, are more likely to be detected in post-marketing surveillance studies.

Post-marketing studies

Once the licensing authority is satisfied that a product is safe, efficacious and of suitable quality, it grants a marketing authorization, which means that the product can then be promoted to prescribers. This usually results in a large increase in the numbers of patients using the product and it is important that its safety is continuously monitored. The MHRA operates a system of post-marketing surveillance which involves spontaneous reporting of suspected ADRs, similar to that in many other countries. It is known as the Yellow Card scheme (see Ch. 51) and anyone can report suspected ADRs to the MHRA. Such schemes provide early warning signals of potential problems and can lead to hypotheses about associations between a medicine and an effect. These can then be tested using retrospective (e.g. case–control studies) or prospective studies (e.g. cohort studies). The main problems with spontaneous reporting schemes are under-reporting, difficulty in identifying new ADRs and the fact that incidence cannot be calculated, since there is no information on the number of patients exposed to the medicine. The benefits of patients reporting their ADRs to the MHRA have been formally evaluated and it has been shown that patient reports add to the usefulness of data obtained through reports submitted by healthcare professionals. European legislation now requires all member states to develop systems enabling patients to report ADRs to the national medicines regulator.

Case–control studies retrospectively identify patients who have developed a particular ADR and determine their level of exposure to the suspected medicine. This is then compared to a control group of patients without the ADR of interest.

Case–control studies are smaller, much less expensive and generate results more quickly than cohort studies. They are used to investigate suspected ADRs identified by other means, e.g. cohort studies or spontaneous reporting and are particularly useful for confirming type B ADRs. They are capable of establishing whether an ADR is caused by a medicine, but cannot measure the incidence of ADRs.

Cohort studies measure the incidence of ADRs in a group of patients exposed to a medicine over a period of time and compare this with the incidence in a similar control group who were not exposed to the medicine. They are useful where a wide range of ADRs are associated with a single medicine, but are less useful for studying rare suspected ADRs. This is because large numbers of patients are required and must be followed-up for prolonged periods of time, which is very expensive and may result in patients being lost to follow-up.

Post-authorization safety studies (PASS)

Formal studies to evaluate the safety of medicines which are sponsored by the pharmaceutical industry are known as post-authorization safety studies PASS. A PASS is defined as any study relating to an authorized medicinal product conducted with the aim of identifying, characterizing or quantifying a safety hazard, confirming the safety profile of the medicinal product, or of measuring the effectiveness of risk management measures. The conduct of these studies is also subject to guidelines. A Code of Conduct requires investigators to register studies before they start and to publish all study findings irrespective of positive or negative results. Such studies use the standard methods of randomized clinical trials, case–control and cohort studies.

Further clinical trials against other drugs/treatments

Most products are marketed having been subject to clinical trials in relatively few patients, which may have excluded certain patient groups. Furthermore, trials may have been conducted against placebo to demonstrate efficacy, but there may be no data on the comparative efficacy of a new product versus an existing treatment for the same condition. Data available at the marketing stage will have demonstrated efficacy, but not the effectiveness of the treatment in practice. In addition, basic research may highlight new theories of how diseases may be treated which require older medicines to be tested for efficacy in conditions where they have not been used previously. Examples of this are the trials required to assess the efficacy of aspirin for prophylaxis against stroke and beta-adrenoceptor blockers in heart failure. As with any other clinical trial, the design is important and the randomized controlled design is considered the most appropriate.

Evaluation of medicines in children

While medicines used in adults must have undergone this rigorous testing before reaching the market and coming into widespread use, this is not generally the case for medicines used in children. Since there are many differences in both pharmacokinetic and pharmacodynamic aspects of medicines between children of different ages and adults, medicines to be used in children need to be tested in children. Information should also be available to prescribers, parents and carers about using medicines in children. Manufacturers are encouraged to develop specific formulations and information leaflets and European legislation requires them to provide and share data. This should ensure the increased availability of medicines which have been specifically developed, tested and licensed for use in children, as well as providing more relevant information about efficacy and toxicity.

Herbal and homoeopathic medicines

Most herbal remedies are not licensed medicinal products and therefore no evaluation is required before they are marketed, but manufacturers can apply to the MHRA for a marketing authorization. Currently around 500 herbal products hold a marketing authorization and so must have fulfilled the same criteria of safety, quality and efficacy (or effectiveness) as any other medicine and be accompanied by a patient information leaflet. Efficacy has not been demonstrated for most herbal medicinal products, therefore manufacturers can instead have the safety and quality formally assessed and recognized through the traditional herbal medicines registration scheme (see Ch. 24).

Homoeopathic remedies can be registered under a scheme which again only assesses quality and safety but does not allow indications to be specified. Alternatively, some homeopathic products may be registered under a different scheme which permits specification for treatment of minor conditions, but to gain such registration, manufacturers must demonstrate efficacy.

Pharmacoeconomic evaluation of medicines

Once a product is licensed, decisions must be made about whether it should be used. Local decisions may be made by drug and therapeutics committees (see Ch. 23). On a larger scale, decisions on whether new treatments should be available on the NHS in the UK are made by NICE, the Scottish Medicines Consortium and the All Wales Medicines Strategy Group. Pharmacoeconomic evaluations play a central role in informing NICE's decisions, so pharmacists may conduct economic evaluations and certainly need to understand them. It is important to appreciate how NICE's work differs from that of the MHRA, who decide whether products can be sold in the UK, by comparing benefits to risks. NICE considers whether medicines should be bought by the NHS, by comparing benefits to costs, i.e. whether they are cost-effective.

Estimates of cost-effectiveness are derived from economic evaluations, which are the comparative analysis of two or more alternative courses of action (interventions) in terms of their costs and consequences. Where the intervention is a medicine, the economic evaluation is called pharmacoeconomics. In an economic evaluation, cost refers to the sum product of the resources that are used and the unit cost of each item. Consequences are the health outcomes, for example the impact of therapy on mortality or quality of life (or both). An appreciation of the basic economic principles is necessary to understand the methods used and the basis for economic analyses.

Basic economic principles

Scarcity and choice

Resources such as land, labour and equipment are finite compared with their possible uses, which are infinite. Therefore, no person or organization is capable of achieving all the good things they desire and some hard choices must be made. These choices may concern the fundamental direction of a person's career or an organization's responsibilities. They may also be choices about how best to achieve a particular goal. For a person, their salary is one measure of the resources available to them. They might not be able to afford both a new car and an exotic holiday, but must choose which they would get the most pleasure from (economists refer to this as utility).

An organization, such as the NHS, a hospital or a primary care organization, has a budget to fund new and existing activities. The use of this budget should be reviewed to make sure that patients' health gains from the mix of activities are maximized. The purpose of economic evaluations is to inform decision-makers of the balance between costs and health gains in order that health outcomes are maximized at a population level.

Opportunity cost

When we make choices about personal or workplace activities, we usually spend money to engage appropriate resources. Considering only the amount of money spent as the 'cost' is a little narrow-minded. Economists would argue that the true cost (opportunity cost) of an activity is the utility from other activities that we can no longer afford. Thus, the opportunity cost of a person's car is not £10 000, but might be the pleasure of an expensive holiday which was not taken. Similarly, the opportunity costs of one coronary artery bypass graft might be two hip operations not performed. Acting to minimize opportunity cost, therefore, ensures that the utility we obtain from using resources in a particular way is maximized. We call this efficiency, which is of two types: technical and allocative:

- *Technical efficiency* is about achieving particular goals on a fixed scale in the most appropriate way (e.g. comparing a range of interventions, including medicines and lifestyle changes, within a programme to reduce blood pressure)
- *Allocative efficiency* is concerned with choosing the right goals in the first place (e.g. coronary heart disease prevention or treating lung cancer) and the most appropriate scale for a healthcare programme.

Few diseases are left completely untreated (because it would not be fair or equitable) but normally, efficiency demands that most of our scarce resources are used to maximize health gains for the greatest number of people. This philosophy is called utilitarianism. If people whose health status cannot be improved by health care are treated, there are fewer resources to help those who can benefit.

Supply and demand

Most people would not consciously consider 'minimizing opportunity cost' in their everyday lives. But they would usually try to get the most utility from the smallest amount of expenditure, which is the same thing expressed more simply. The price of goods and their availability are relied on as indicators of quality and desirability. The price mechanism for allocating resources works well if there are many buyers and sellers, each with similar accurate information about the goods and services on offer. However, the market for health care (unlike that for cars and package holidays) does not work very well. The reasons for this include:

- Health is demanded but cannot be directly provided
- The link between health care and improvements in health is uncertain
- We do not know when we will be ill
- Providers of health care have more information than consumers
- Insurance companies or governments usually pay for health care – not consumers.

When normal markets do not work well, economic evaluation can step in as a substitute for price to assist decision-makers. The costs measured and valued in economic evaluation are analogous to the costs of production for a normal good or service. The consequences measured and valued in economic evaluation are analogous to the utility consumers enjoy when using a normal good or service.

Methods of economic evaluation

The basic steps in all economic evaluations are to:

- Clarify the economic question, with particular regard to technical or allocative efficiency, the interventions that will be compared and the population of interest
- Obtain the best clinical and economic evidence
- Identify and carry out the appropriate form of evaluation to answer the economic question
- Identify the key variables that influence the results of the evaluation and test the influence of any assumptions
- Present the results clearly and in a form that decision-makers can easily interpret.

All the techniques of economic evaluation involve an explicit consideration and calculation of resource use, to ensure that healthcare expenditure has the maximum possible impact on health status. However, each method of evaluation handles consequences (or health effects) differently.

Principles of costing

The viewpoint (perspective) of an economic evaluation determines what should be included in measuring costs. Typical viewpoints are: a single healthcare organization, the whole healthcare system or society. For the same set of interventions, taking a different viewpoint can result in radically different economic conclusions. To give an example, the costs of drug therapy for attention deficit hyperactivity disorder from a health system perspective is very different to the cost from a societal perspective, which may also consider the impact of treatment on education, social problems and crime.

Resources used directly in healthcare interventions may include:

- Healthcare professionals' time, e.g. doctors, nurses and pharmacists
- Equipment, e.g. computers, medical scanners and beds
- Space in which to work, including heat, light and rent
- Consumables, e.g. medicines, diagnostic kits, syringes and dressings.

It is important to remember that it is not just the product acquisition cost that is used in economic evaluations, but the total costs related to treatment with that product, including for instance hospitalizations, blood tests, GP visits and so on.

Costs borne outside the healthcare system (e.g. by patients and carers, or in other sectors of the economy such as social care) may be less likely to have accepted and accessible market prices. Voluntary care costs, for example, might be valued using an average societal wage rate. Patients' public transport costs would be clear enough, but for car travel, an appropriate mileage rate needs to be agreed or calculated. The productivity of patients going back to work should normally be excluded from costings. This is because any gains or losses in productivity flow from health status changes, which will be valued separately.

When identifying costs for groups of interventions that will be compared, any costs that are identical for all interventions can be safely ignored. This is because economists are more interested in marginal costs (e.g. the cost of one additional day in hospital) than average costs. Note that these may be very different. For instance, if a hospital operates at normal capacity, the average daily cost of a hospital bed will be similar to the marginal cost. However, if increases in local hospital catchment population required that a new ward needed to be built, then the marginal cost for the first patient admitted to that ward is substantially higher than the average cost (as it includes the cost of building the ward). It is the costs of change and the differences between alternative interventions that are most relevant for practical and effective decision-making.

Healthcare interventions often incur costs over a number of years and the duration of two alternative interventions may be different. So timing is an important factor in many costings and is accounted for in a number of ways. First, all costs are counted in a base year, and are not inflated to account for price rises over the course of the interventions. This ensures that all costs reflect real resource use and not nominal monetary values. Second, capital costs (durable equipment) are apportioned over the lifetime of the equipment. This allows a fair comparison of interventions with different levels of up-front and recurring costs. Third, future costs are 'discounted' back to the base year. In general terms, this reflects a preference by people to put off costs rather than pay straightaway.

Whether consequences that occur in the future should be discounted in the same way as costs is open to debate. Without consistent discounting, it is particularly hard to fairly compare health promotion interventions (with up-front costs and far-off consequences) with normal clinical treatments. NICE's current practice is to discount both costs and benefits, at a rate of 3.5% per annum.

Economic analyses are useful for informing decisions on allocating scarce healthcare resources. Occasionally, decisions are very straightforward and do not require detailed economic analysis. These may include, for instance, examples where a new treatment is both more effective and less costly than existing therapy. Clearly in this situation, the new treatment is preferred, as this 'dominates' existing therapy. Conversely, a new treatment might be identified which is less effective, yet more expensive. This would be dominated by existing therapy (Fig. 22.1).

The two logical alternative scenarios, where additional benefits come at additional costs and where fewer benefits are generated at reduced cost, can be represented by the north-east and north-west quadrants of the cost-effectiveness plane, respectively (see Fig. 22.1). In the case of the former, the key question is whether the additional benefits justify the additional cost.

Types of economic evaluation

Cost-minimization analysis

Cost-minimization analysis (CMA) is only appropriate when there is robust evidence to show that two or more interventions have exactly the same health effects, i.e. are therapeutically equivalent in terms of health benefits and adverse effects. Interventions

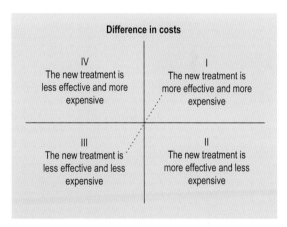

Figure 22.1 • Cost-effectiveness plane, illustrating where a new treatment is either less or more effective than current therapy (origin), and whether the costs associated with the new treatment are higher or lower. Decisions on treatments falling into the north-west and south-east quadrants are clear-cut. It is unlikely that treatments in the south-west will be adopted as they are less effective than available alternative therapy. Decisions on whether or not to approve treatments that are both more effective and more costly (north-east quadrant) require the use of economic evaluation, and a threshold cost-effectiveness ratio (represented by the diagonal line), below which treatments are deemed to be cost-effective.

to be assessed by CMA fall on the vertical axis of the cost-effectiveness plane (see Fig. 22.1).

This is a question of technical efficiency and the intervention that costs the least is usually preferred, because spare resources can be used to treat more patients or be reallocated to other programmes. Choosing a more expensive option must be justified because using additional resources to achieve the same outcome takes resources away from other programmes where they might achieve something positive.

An example of CMA is the comparison of different methods for providing domiciliary oxygen. The effectiveness of oxygen provided in cylinders or by concentrator is the same. Concentrators are cheaper for most patients, despite high purchase and maintenance costs.

CMA could also be used to compare branded and generic medicines, or different formulations of the same drug, but its practical applications are limited to cases where therapeutic equivalence has been demonstrated. It has been argued that a lack of significance in the effect differences between interventions in a clinical trial is insufficient grounds for conducting a CMA.

Cost-effectiveness analysis

Cost-effectiveness analysis (CEA) is appropriate when the health effects of two or more interventions are not identical, but are measured in the same units, e.g. life years gained or symptom-free days.

This is a question of technical efficiency and is often appropriate within a particular healthcare programme, for example different interventions which all reduce myocardial infarction and stroke. However, CEA can only deal with one dimension of outcome at a time. Some other examples include: accidents prevented, decrease in blood pressure, deaths averted and strokes avoided. These measures are often clinical indicators or intermediate outcomes, e.g. blood pressure reduction is a predictor of subsequent effects such as stroke and health-related quality of life (HRQoL). The use of clinical indicators can be problematical, not least because the choice of indicator critically affects the results of an evaluation. The most appropriate indicator or outcome should be chosen before a study commences. Examples of CEA are shown in Box 22.1.

Cost-utility analysis

Cost-utility analysis (CUA) is the most useful form of economic evaluation and is appropriate when the health effects of two or more alternatives can be measured in terms of overall impact on quality and quantity of life.

CUA is a special form of CEA in which the consequences are measured in terms of quality-adjusted life years (QALYs). QALYs are calculated by estimating the total life years gained from a treatment and weighing each year (or part thereof) with a quality of life (utility) score. The utility value is 0 for 'dead' and 1 for 'full health'. Various methods can be used to measure and quantify quality of life, to provide a single summary score. The method pharmacists are most likely to be familiar with is a questionnaire such as the EuroQol-5D.

Box 22.1

Examples of cost-effectiveness analyses

* An economic analysis of the Heart Protection Study compared simvastatin with placebo in over 20 000 adults with vascular disease or diabetes over 5 years. The authors estimated the costs of preventing a major vascular event with 40 mg simvastatin daily was £11 600. However, this ranged from £4500 among participants with a 42% 5-year major vascular event rate, to £31 100 among those with a 12% rate.
* Abacavir is a nucleoside-analogue reverse transcriptase inhibitor used in combination with other antiretroviral therapy for the management of HIV. Unfortunately, it causes severe hypersensitivity reactions in about 4–8% of patients; however, HLA B*5701 is a known genetic risk factor for hypersensitivity reactions. A cost-effectiveness analysis of testing patients for HLA B*5701 prior to initiation of abacavir therapy demonstrated that, depending on the choice of comparator, routine testing for HLA B*5701 ranged from being a dominant strategy (less expensive and more beneficial than not testing) to an incremental cost-effectiveness ratio (vs no testing) of €22 811 per hypersensitivity reaction avoided. This means that compared with some antiretroviral therapies, the use of the test costs an additional €22 811 to avoid one hypersensitivity reaction.

The advantage of the QALY is that it incorporates quality and quantity of life in a common currency that allows comparison of interventions from different clinical areas. So QALYs can be compared for very different interventions such as radiotherapy in advanced breast cancer, surgery for coronary artery bypass grafting and drugs for cardiovascular diseases. In contrast, a CEA measures consequences only in terms of quality or quantity: it is unidimensional. The advantage of CUA using QALYs is that it can answer questions of both technical efficiency and allocative efficiency in health care. For this reason, CUAs are the preferred form of economic evaluation for NICE appraisals.

Figure 22.2 presents a graphical representation of the impact of treatment, such as a medicine, on quality of life and life expectancy. The number of QALYs gained by one medicine over the other is the difference between the areas under the curves. In this figure, the disease is characterized by episodes of remission from symptoms, where quality of life is high, and relapses, where quality of life is low. Neither medicine A nor medicine B affects quality of life appreciably until the final stages of the disease, where it is clear that medicine B is superior – both in improving health-related quality of life and in increasing life expectancy. For each medicine, QALYs are calculated as the area under the curves, so the shaded area represents the number of QALY gains achieved with medicine B compared with medicine A.

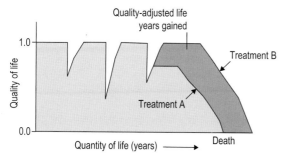

Figure 22.2 • A schematic representation of the impact of two treatments (A and B) on a chronic disease that is characterized by episodes of relapse and remissions. The area under the curves represents the total number of quality-adjusted life years (QALYs) associated with each treatment. The gain in QALYs is the shaded area between both curves.

Now imagine that this lifetime QALY gain is equal to 1.0 QALY and that the total lifetime costs to the healthcare system associated with medicine A are £10000 and with medicine B £20000, but remember that medicine B is more effective. The incremental cost utility ratio is calculated as the difference in costs divided by the difference in QALYs, which in this case equals £10000 divided by 1.0, which equals £10000 per QALY gained. The judgement as to whether this represents good value for money (and in which case whether it will be approved for use by the NHS) depends on whether or not £10000 per QALY gained is considered acceptable. In practice, treatments and healthcare interventions that cost less than £20000–£30000 per QALY gained are considered cost-effective, and are likely to be approved for use.

Table 22.2 lists a range of cost-utility estimates from a selection of appraisals conducted for NICE.

Cost-benefit analysis

Cost-benefit analysis (CBA) is the least common economic evaluation of health care because it is only appropriate when the benefits gained are expressed in monetary units. The term cost-benefit analysis is, however, sometimes used incorrectly in a general way to describe any form of economic evaluation.

In CBA, the monetary units used to assess consequences reflect the value of health status improvement and not the cost of health care. The treatment offering the largest net consequence (value of consequences minus costs) is preferred. This technique can answer questions concerning allocative efficiency across the whole economy. In principle at least, the largest net consequence rule can help us decide whether to build a new hospital or a new road.

There are three ways to place a monetary value on consequences: implied values, the human capital approach and willingness to pay. Implied values are taken from insurance companies, court awards for accidents or risk premiums we pay people to do dangerous jobs. For example, insurance companies may state how much they will pay for the loss of an eye or limb. These values could be applied to the consequences of ophthalmic and vascular surgery respectively. Although implied values are one way to put a publicly acceptable monetary value on health effects, they do not exist for all possible consequences, may not be adjusted regularly and may be unpredictable.

Table 22.2 A list of cost-utility ratios (cost per QALYs) for a range of interventions that were appraised by the National Institute for Health and Clinical Excellence (NICE)

Medicine and indication	Incremental cost-effectiveness ratio (cost per QALY gained)
Ticagrelor for the treatment of acute coronary syndromes	£7897 vs clopidogrel
Dabigatran etexilate for the prevention of stroke and systemic embolism in atrial fibrillation	£18 900 compared with warfarin
Botulinum toxin type A for the prevention of headaches in adults with chronic migraine	£18 900 compared to placebo
Fingolimod for the treatment of highly active relapsing–remitting multiple sclerosis	Between £25 000 to £35 000 vs β-interferon and best supportive care
Omalizumab for severe persistent allergic asthma	£34 300 as add-on therapy
Adalimumab for the treatment of adults with psoriasis	£36 700 vs intermittent etanercept; and dominating (greater effectiveness and lower costs for adalimumab) when compared with continuous etanercept
Abiraterone for castration-resistant metastatic prostate cancer previously treated with a docetaxel-containing regimen	£46 800 compared with prednisolone alone; and extendedly dominating when compared with prednisolone and mitoxantrone
Bevacizumab in combination with a taxane for the first-line treatment of metastatic breast cancer	Between £110 000 and £259 000 compared with weekly paclitaxel

The human capital approach places a value on human life that is equivalent to an individual's future income stream. This has the disadvantage of judging that the life of a managing director is worth more than that of a shop floor worker. This is unpalatable for most healthcare professionals and not widely applied. However, surveys do suggest that the general public values the lives of the very young and old less highly than the lives of productive workers with families. It has also been suggested that traditional societies tend to sacrifice weaker members first in times of hardship.

Willingness to pay (WTP) is the preferred way to place a monetary value on consequences. In a WTP survey, a description of the intervention and associated health effects is presented to disease sufferers or the general public. After reading the description, people are asked to place a monetary valuation on the scenario, which may incorporate preferences about the method of treatment, information provided by medical tests and actual clinical outcome. WTP may be related to income or ability to pay and this must be considered in any analysis.

Modelling and sensitivity analysis

More often than not, clinical trials do not capture all the data required for an economic analysis. Moreover, it is generally advisable to project the results of clinical trials beyond the time horizon of analysis, to capture lifetime costs and benefits. Economists use mathematical models to compile data from various sources, and to test the robustness of assumptions and uncertainties in the analysis. The most common forms of economic models are decision analyses (represented schematically as decision trees) and Markov models.

A decision tree maps out the alternatives being compared in as much detail as possible. Figure 22.3 shows the start of one possible tree, outlining various treatment options for use of a new medicine. The decision tree starts with a decision node (by convention a square). This is because most health care starts with a decision about whether one alternative or another is the most appropriate course of action. Subsequent probability nodes (by convention, circles) show the chances of each possible consequence occurring. At each probability node,

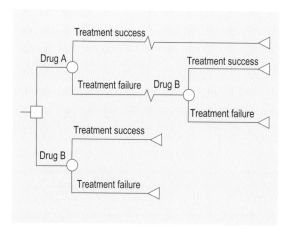

Figure 22.3 • An example of a decision tree as used in pharmacoeconomics.

the sum of probabilities is 1, that is, a 100% chance that something will happen.

A range of interventions and their possible consequences can be mapped out clearly in a decision tree. Once the options are clear, probabilities can be attached to them using either new trial data or information from the existing literature. For each option we may also identify and state costs. At the end of each route through the decision tree, there should also be a terminal node (by convention, a triangle) associated with a final outcome.

The expected costs and outcomes (e.g. QALY) for each initial decision can be calculated. For instance, if the probability of treatment success with medicine B (used first-line) is 60%, and the costs associated with treatment success and failure are £1000 and £2000, respectively, then the expected cost is $(60\% \times £1000) + (40\% \times £2000) = £1400$. This means that, on average, the costs associated with medicine B, if used as first-line therapy, is £1400. We can calculate the incremental cost-effectiveness ratio by performing the same calculation to the costs and benefits for all the branches of the tree. Computer software to help draw and analyse decision trees makes their use particularly attractive for the comparison of multiple interventions.

Sensitivity analysis is the act of changing assumptions about the value or probability of costs and consequences, to determine whether or not the results of an evaluation are sensitive to such changes. Even without the help of a decision tree

or computer software, evaluators should highlight any assumptions they make about costs and consequences and list the key variables that influence their recommendations.

Markov models are helpful for modelling the progression of chronic diseases. A disease is divided into health states (e.g. good health, bad health, death) and during a chosen period of time, a cohort of individuals is given a probability of moving from one state to another. Estimates of resource use and health effects are also attached to each state and transition. The model is then cycled to produce long-term estimates of cost-effectiveness in hypothetical patient cohorts.

Many healthcare professionals are distrustful of modelling and hypothetical data. However, in some cases, it is the best information we have. These techniques should not be rejected out of hand, but instead questions asked about the assumptions made to produce the model and the accuracy of typical clinical scenarios. Better information is better than nothing at all and modelling can be a great deal better than a badly designed trial.

Appraising economic evaluations

During the process of making decisions about whether to recommend drugs for use in the NHS, NICE and other similar bodies assess the quality of research which has been carried out, using standardized methods. The quality of published clinical studies and economic evaluations in the medical and pharmacy literature is variable. For both, methodological details must be critically appraised to ensure the validity of the results prior to decision-making. Examples of useful checklists can be found in SIGN Guideline 50: A Guideline Developer's Handbook (www.sign.ac.uk).

Drug utilization review and evaluation

As well as being involved in the evaluation of new medicines both before and after marketing, pharmacists play a large role in evaluating whether medicines are being used appropriately. Rational use of medicines increases the quality of patient care and promotes cost-effective health care. The techniques used for this are drug utilization review

(DUR), drug use evaluation (DUE) and clinical audit. (Audit is described in Ch. 12).

DUR is the assessment of patterns of drug use in a particular clinical context. DUE incorporates qualitative measures and emphasizes outcomes, including pharmacoeconomic assessment. DUE can identify problems in drug use, reduce ADRs, optimize drug therapy and minimize drug-related expenditure.

Selection of which drugs to study may be because of:

- High cost, e.g. pregabalin, dabigatran
- Wide usage or changes in usage, e.g. ulcer-healing drugs
- Known or suspected inappropriate use, e.g. clopidogrel
- Potential for improvements in patient care, e.g. bisphosphonates.

Some medicines will fall into more than one category, increasing the potential benefits of conducting DUR. Changes in legislation can result in changes in the way medicines are used and usage patterns may change when a new product is marketed. DUR can provide information on what these changes are and DUE can determine whether they are beneficial.

Drug utilization review

DUR was developed in the 1960s and focused on describing which medicines were being used and their costs. It can involve the development of standards for the use of each medicine or group of medicines, which can be used as criteria against which the actual use of the medicines can be measured. This form of DUR is therefore very similar to clinical audit (see Ch. 12). The general study of patterns of medicines use and their associated costs is an important activity for pharmacists. This activity is used to identify therapeutic areas where drug choice requires review, more cost-effective therapy can be substituted or there is unexplained variation in prescribing between groups of prescribers or between populations. The subsequent activities which are undertaken to address these issues also often involve pharmacists. These may include clinical medication review, MUR, prescription review, therapeutic switching programmes, clinical audit and DUE.

So that comparisons can be made between populations (such as those of different geographical areas or served by different prescribers), systems for classifying drugs and methods for quantifying their use are needed. The most widespread systems are the anatomical therapeutic chemical (ATC) system and the defined daily dose (DDD), recommended by the WHO for international use. In the UK, the BNF is more frequently used for therapeutic classification than the ATC, but DDDs are widely used to quantify medicines use. There is a DDD for every drug on the market, based on the average recommended daily maintenance dose for the drug when used for its most common indication in adults. It is expressed in g, mg, microgram (μg), mmol or units or as the number of tablets for combination products. The WHO sets the DDD for every drug.

While DDDs are used worldwide, other methods of measuring prescribing are also used in the UK primary care setting. The average daily quantity (ADQ) has been developed for a number of drugs to reflect typical prescribing in England. To make comparisons between populations, a denominator is required, often 1000 patients. For example, the DDD of diazepam is 10 mg. It may be found that diazepam is used with a DDD of 2000/1000 per year. This means that for every 1000 people, 2000 doses of diazepam were prescribed in a year, or 2 doses/person per year. By using DDDs, not only are quantities prescribed accounted for, but also an allowance is made for the frequency of administration. In order to enhance comparisons still further, a denominator which takes account of the differing needs of populations can be used. Examples of this are the ASTRO-PU (which accounts for the age, sex and temporary residential status of a population) and the STAR-PU which also accounts for variability within therapeutic groups.

Data can also be expressed in terms of cost, rather than quantity, again using this range of denominators. Thus it becomes possible to identify prescribing which is higher or lower than the norm for the actual population served in terms of either quantity or cost.

Drug use evaluation

Evaluating the use of medicines retrospectively, and relating them to patient outcomes can be a valuable learning experience, but prospective DUE is much more beneficial to both prescribers and patients. If changes in prescribing are found to be necessary, these can be implemented after or even during the evaluation. As with clinical audit, the involvement of relevant prescribers is essential, to ensure benefits.

There are various levels at which the use of medicines can be studied. These range from very broad measures with little detail, usually obtained from routinely collected data, to more expensive methods, in which a great deal of useful information is obtained on individual patients. DUR studies which use only drug supply, purchase or prescribing records cannot be used to determine medicines use in relation to indication and outcome. The information which they provide is incomplete and any suggestions of prescribing being inappropriate based solely on this type of data should be made cautiously. Prescribing advisers may use prescribing indicators as an indicative measure of the quality and cost of prescribing. They use the standard measures already described, but involve specific ways of combining data to enable more useful comparisons to be made. Some prescribing indicators are listed in Box 22.2. Their main purpose is to raise awareness of what is being prescribed and to highlight areas for more detailed methods of investigation, such as by examination of medical records.

Using purchasing records

The simplest level of information about which medicines are being used is obtained from purchasing records. Providing pharmacies use computerized systems for purchase, these data are readily available. This type of information allows comparison between pharmacies or over time, but does not show how the medicines are being used. It can point to potential areas which may need further investigation.

While DDDs can be used to measure purchases, other measures such as cost, number of containers and number of dosage units may be more readily available.

Using issue records

A more detailed record of use can be obtained from the medicines issued from pharmacies, to individual patients via prescriptions or to wards in hospitals. The units used are the same as those of purchase. Again, computerization allows these data to be obtained easily.

In the community, these data are captured when prescriptions are priced centrally. These data can then be used to enable prescribers to evaluate their prescribing. However, more commonly, pharmacists may undertake this evaluation, using the techniques described here. Central data are available, such as those by the Prescribing Support Unit of the NHS Information Centre, which enable comparison of an individual's or a group's prescribing to the national 'norm'.

In some hospitals, it is possible to link data from pharmacy issues to individual clinicians. This will increase as electronic prescribing becomes more widespread. Even if the data can only be applied at ward level, this can still be helpful in developing and monitoring ward-based policies on medicines use.

Using prescription records

More detailed information from prescriptions, which includes the actual dose prescribed and the concurrent medication, may be available in community pharmacies from PMRs. However, without patient registration and the recording of non-prescription medicines purchased, these are incomplete. In hospitals, this level of data is only easily obtainable with electronic prescribing. Prescription data however, allows evaluation of the appropriateness of doses used, the extent of polypharmacy, prescribing errors and drug interactions.

Using medical records and trained investigators

To examine decisions behind the use of particular medicines and their effectiveness in patients, it is necessary to examine medical records. This requires expertise and time and can often be frustrated by

Box 22.2

Examples of areas where prescribing indicators have been developed and are used to evaluate prescribing

- Proportion of generic prescribing (should be high)
- Benzodiazepine prescriptions measured as ADQ per STAR-PU (should be minimal)
- Prescribing rate of ACE inhibitors as a proportion of ACE inhibitors and angiotensin-2 receptor blockers (should be minimal)
- Prescribing rate of antibacterials measured as items per STAR-PU (should be minimal)

inadequate record-keeping. Some hospitals and many general practices have computerized patient records, which facilitate links between indications and drugs prescribed and possibly also to computerized laboratory data. Many systems, however, are either undeveloped or, as with PMRs, the records are often inaccurate or incomplete. Clearly, it is not possible to compensate for either a lack of data or inaccurate data. However, small studies undertaken manually can still be of considerable value in determining whether medicines are being used appropriately and effectively. These studies usually involve trained investigators, such as pharmacists, reviewing medical records.

Pharmacists can undertake prospective DUE, which avoids the problem of inadequate records, by allowing data to be recorded and questions to be asked at the time of prescribing. This may help to improve the use of medicines through changing prescribing behaviour. It can also involve the patient, so providing a full picture of medicines use, including outcomes and compliance. While more expensive than DUR using purchase, issue or prescribing data, this may be regarded as part of the routine practice of pharmacists. Increasingly, national and local clinical guidelines specify, among other things, the treatments to be given to patient populations, emphasizing the importance of both DUE and clinical audit. The labour-intensive nature of these activities will be reduced when complete and accurate computerized data are available in patient records which are shared between healthcare professionals.

Evaluation of non-prescription medicines

Published information on the epidemiology of self-limiting minor illnesses is limited. Similarly, data on the pharmacoepidemiology of the medicines used in self-treatment of these minor illnesses is limited. The number of such medicines which can be bought from pharmacies or other outlets is constantly increasing, with many former POMs being re-regulated to allow their purchase (see Ch. 4). Manufacturers of non-prescription medicines collect data on sales, which provide a global overview

of which medicines are being purchased. DUR requires similar methods to those used for prescription medicines, namely study of purchase or supply and data stored in community pharmacy PMRs. DUE of non-prescription medicines is increasing, through studies using patient questionnaires. Such studies show that use is often inappropriate, but usually only involve community pharmacies and not the use of medicines purchased from other outlets. As increasing numbers of potent medicines become widely available without prescription, the requirement for a practical yet scientifically robust method of evaluating both the use of and adverse reactions associated with these medicines increases.

KEY POINTS

- Pharmacists have an important role to play in evaluating the safety, efficiency and economy of medicines' use
- The MHRA or EMA require evidence of safety, efficacy and quality before granting a marketing authorization for a new drug
- Clinical trials take place in three phases: Phase I determines the basic toxicity and tolerability; Phase II tests for efficacy and identifies an effective dose; Phase III determines safety and efficacy on a larger sample using randomized controlled trials
- Post-marketing surveillance is required to establish many adverse reactions, particularly rarer ones
- Spontaneous reporting of ADRs to the MHRA is an important mechanism of post-marketing surveillance. Prescribers, pharmacists and patients can all report suspected ADRs
- Pharmacoeconomics applies the principles of economic evaluation to medicines
- Some of the basic economic concepts are scarcity, choice and opportunity cost
- The principles of costing may be straightforward but can be difficult to apply, especially when trying to identify all the cost consequences related to a given treatment
- Cost-minimization analysis (CMA) may be applied (with caution) when outcomes are the same and relative cost is the variation
- Cost-effectiveness analysis (CEA) is applied when both outcomes and cost can vary, but outcomes are measured in common units

- Cost-utility analysis (CUA) incorporates quality of life and quantity of life into a single index, and is the most useful form of economic evaluation to assist in informing resource allocation
- Cost-benefit analysis (CBA) is complex, and is not used frequently for evaluating healthcare interventions
- To accommodate decision-taking in health care, modelling and sensitivity analysis methods can be used

- Drug utilization review (DUR) is used to evaluate patterns of drug use within populations
- Drug use evaluation (DUE) relates drug use to patient outcome and along with clinical audit, can be used to evaluate whether drugs are used optimally in practice
- Data which can be used for DUR and DUE include drug purchase records, drug issue records, prescription records and medical records

Formularies in pharmacy practice

Janet Krska

STUDY POINTS

- Different types of formularies
- The benefits of using a formulary
- Developing a formulary
- Formulary management systems

Different types of formularies

Formularies were originally compilations of medicinal preparations, with the formulae for compounding them. The modern definition of a formulary is a list of drugs which are recommended or approved for use by a group of practitioners. It is compiled by members of the group and is regularly revised. Drugs are usually selected for inclusion on the basis of efficacy, safety, patient acceptability and cost. Drugs listed in a formulary should be available for use. Information on dosage, indications, side-effects, contraindications, formulations and costs may also be included. An introduction, giving information on how the drugs were selected, by whom and how to use the formulary, is usually provided.

The most common formulary in use in the UK is the BNF, which compiles details of all the drugs available for prescribing in the UK. It is produced through a collaboration between the British Medical Association and the RPS. It is revised every 6 months, is issued to all prescribers and registered pharmacies in both hospitals and the community and is available on-line with monthly updates. Formularies for dentists, the *Dental Practitioners' Formulary*, and for nurse prescribers, the *Nurse Prescribers' Formulary*, are also included

in the BNF. A separate BNF for children is also produced annually, in recognition of the need for different, more detailed information about prescribing in children.

Local formularies, or lists of recommended drugs, have been widely used in hospitals and in primary care throughout the UK for many years. Some are designed for small groups, such as one general medical practice; some are for all prescribers within a hospital; others may be intended for all prescribers within a large geographical area. The latter are often joint formularies, compiled by and intended for use by prescribers in both primary and secondary care. An NHS-funded minor ailments service delivered by community pharmacy is also widespread in the UK (see Ch. 21), which provides selected medicines free of charge to certain patients, requiring the development of formularies from which pharmacists can supply the recommended products. All of these are local formularies and are usually developed and maintained by an Area Drug and Therapeutics Committee (ADTC). These committees involve pharmacists, hospital doctors, general practitioners and nurses who practise within a locality, and often also include management, public health and financial expertise.

Worldwide, formularies as a concept are promoted by the WHO. The essential medicines list, which is recommended as necessary for basic health care in developing countries, is similar to a formulary. Any country can modify this list to meet its own particular needs and arrive at a 'national formulary'. The basis of any list is that the drugs it contains are of proven therapeutic efficacy, acceptable safety and satisfy the health needs of the populations they

Table 23.1 Examples of formularies

Purpose	Example formulary
General use	British National Formulary
Hospital formulary	University College London Hospitals NHS Trust Formulary
General practice	NHS Cambridgeshire Formulary
Joint formulary	Tayside Area Formulary
	Lothian Joint Formulary
Specialist formulary	Palliative Care Formulary
Developing countries	WHO Essential Drug List

serve. Some examples of formularies are given in Table 23.1.

A formulary may be thought of as a prescribing policy, because it lists which drugs are recommended. Prescribing policies should, however, be much more detailed than a formulary, giving details of drugs which should be selected for use in specific medical conditions. Examples of prescribing policies in common use are antibiotic policies, head lice eradication policies and malarial prophylaxis policies.

Clinical guidelines contain more detailed information than a formulary about how a service should be delivered or patients treated and do not always specify the drugs to be used. Many are developed nationally, by bodies such as NICE, Scottish Intercollegiate Guidelines Network (SIGN), British Thoracic Society, British Society for Haematology and so on. Local guidelines may be developed by ADTCs and are more likely to include recommendations which specify drugs included in the local formulary.

Benefits of formularies

Drug costs are a major component of the total cost of any health service, including the NHS and are constantly rising. As the resources of all healthcare systems are finite, it becomes increasingly necessary to contain the escalation in drug costs. Much evidence shows that drugs are not always prescribed appropriately. Therefore, improving prescribing could reduce expenditure on drugs. Local formularies which recommend specific drugs and exclude others are one means of achieving this. Prescribing

policies assist prescribers in using the drugs in a formulary and specific treatment protocols make them even more useful. Clinical guidelines help to ensure that the treatment of patients is based on evidence of best practice. Used together, formularies, clinical guidelines and treatment protocols can ensure that standards of prescribing are both uniform and high quality. All these are tools used to promote rational and cost-effective prescribing.

Rational prescribing

Prescribing, which is based on the four important factors of efficacy, safety, patient acceptability and cost, should be rational (see Ch. 20). While many drugs may be available to treat any particular condition, the process of selecting the most appropriate one for any individual patient should take account of all these factors, plus other patient factors, such as concurrent diseases, drugs, previous exposure and outcomes. The four factors can also be applied to selection of drugs to treat populations of patients and it is for this situation that formularies are developed. Providing drug selection is based on good quality evidence of efficacy, toxicity and cost-effectiveness, formularies then assist in making decisions regarding individual patients.

Cost-effective prescribing

Formularies often provide information on the cost of products to help users to become cost conscious. Local formularies usually include only a small proportion of the drugs listed in an extensive national formulary, such as the BNF. In general, only between 300 and 500 drugs are required to manage the majority of common conditions. If prescribers only use the drugs included in a local formulary, the range stocked by pharmacies can decrease, which reduces unnecessary outlay. Using a restricted range of drugs may allow pharmacists to buy these in bulk, further reducing costs. Formularies also encourage generic prescribing which may reduce costs even further. If fewer products are stocked, monitoring of expiry dates becomes easier and cash flow may improve. Any money saved by using a formulary may be used to benefit patients in other ways. For example, reducing the prescribing of drugs which have little evidence of therapeutic benefit, such as peripheral vasodilators, could enable more to be spent on lipid-lowering drugs. Formularies usually recommend using the most cost-effective option where there are a number of alternatives. In addition, as safety is also a key factor in drug selection, formularies may contribute to reducing the incidence of ADRs, which often carry a high cost.

Educational value

Compilation of a formulary involves researching the literature to gather evidence of efficacy and toxicity. This is highly demanding, but is of considerable educational benefit to those compiling the formulary. Formulary users also benefit. If prescribers use a restricted range of drugs frequently, they should know more about those drugs and their formulations. Ultimately, this should result in benefits for the patient, as prescribers' greater knowledge should reduce the risk of inappropriate prescribing and hence reduces the potential for adverse effects, interactions or lack of efficacy.

Continuous care

A joint local formulary covering both primary and secondary care encourages the same range of drugs to be prescribed, which makes continuing drug treatment across the interface easier. If patient packs are dispensed, patients are more likely to use their own medicines during a hospital stay. A joint formulary also helps, as there is less chance of drug therapy having to change to comply with a different formulary on admission to hospital.

Formulary development

Formularies can take a very long time to produce: several years is not uncommon. Obtaining everyone's opinions and discussing the drugs to be included are the main reasons for this. To be useful, formularies then need to be updated regularly, which is a further time commitment. There are two basic ways of producing a new formulary – either start from scratch or modify an existing one. Modifying another formulary to suit local needs is much less time-consuming than starting from scratch. Although much can be learned from looking at someone else's formulary, simply deciding to adopt it without any changes is not a good idea. Producing a formulary is an educational process,

during which all concerned learn from each other's experience and update their clinical pharmacology and therapeutics along the way. Producing a formulary also brings a sense of ownership, which encourages commitment to it and increases the chance of it being used. Local needs should also be addressed by a local formulary, so copying someone else's formulary exactly may not be satisfactory. On the other hand, there is little point in duplicating effort; therefore a balance is needed between accepting work done by others and adapting it for your needs.

A local ADTC is most likely to oversee the task of developing a formulary. Although the committee will include different healthcare professionals, pharmacists usually play a key role. Small subgroups of local experts may do most of the development work, but the opinions of potential users should also be sought. The people expected to use a formulary must have the opportunity to give their views on its content. If their opinions are not asked, they may feel that it does not apply to them and will be less likely to use it. Smaller formularies, such as for one general medical practice or ward, should be developed by all the prescribers working in that practice or ward together with a pharmacist. Such formularies may draw on the work of ADTCs and select even fewer drugs from the area formulary, but may add others. It is important that formularies reflect the needs of the population being treated. So obviously a formulary for a surgical ward will differ from that for a general practice, but both may be derived from the area formulary.

Content

The formulary should start with an introduction, giving the names of those who have compiled it, stating who is expected to use it and explaining its format. An example is shown in Figure 23.1A, from the NHS Tayside Area Formulary. It is important to state whether all the drugs included are recommended for all users, and if not, how different recommendations can be distinguished. The BNF, for example, lists drugs the Joint Formulary Committee considers less suitable for prescribing, in small type. The examples in Figures 23.1 and 23.2 illustrate how the recommended first choice drugs are highlighted. Local formularies may choose to place restrictions on some drugs, for use by specialists only, for certain indications only or in

(A)

Introduction to Pocket Guide

This pocket guide is designed to be a handy compact reference and includes the names of medicines recommended within the Tayside Area Prescribing Guide (TAPG). Where appropriate, medicines recommended as first choice are shaded in blue and those recommended for use in particular circumstances are in italics. First choice medicines are chosen on the grounds of efficacy, safety and cost-effectiveness and represent the best evidence-based and cost-effective choice for the majority of patients with a particular condition. Users should refer to the full document and the BNF for further detail and more specific information.

The most up to date version of the TAPG is maintained in electronic form at:
http://www.nhstaysideadtc.scot.nhs.uk/TAPG%20html/MAIN/Front%20page.htm

For enquiries contact: kharknesst.glet@nhs.net or clairejames@nhs.net
Tel: 01382 660111 ext 34374

Key

Drug name shaded blue: recommended first choice medicine
Drug name in italics: recommended only in particular circumstances (see full TAPG)

(B) **Extract from Pocket Guide**

3: Respiratory System

3.1 Bronchodilators
Beta₂-agonists
Short acting:
Salbutamol

Terbutaline

Beta₂-agonists: Long-acting
Indacaterol
Salmeterol

Antimuscarinic bronchodilators:
Short-acting:
Ipratropium

Antimuscarinic bronchodilators: Long-acting
Tiotropium
Glycopyrronium
Aclinidium

Theophylline – prescribe by brand name:
Uniphyllin®

Compound bronchodilator preparations:
Combivent®

3.2 Inhaled corticosteroids
Beclometasone

Budesonide

Fluticasone

Ciclesonide?

Compound preparations:
Seretide®

Symbicort®

3.3 Cromoglicate related therapy and leukotriene receptor antagonists
Cromoglicate and related therapy:
Sodium Cromoglicate

Leukotriene receptor antagonists:
Montelukast

3.4 Antihistamines and allergic emergencies

Non-sedative antihistamines:
Cetirizine

Loratadine

Fexofenadine

Sedative antihistamines:
Chlorphenamine

Alimemazine

Allergic emergencies:
Adrenaline/Epinephrine

3.7 Mucolytics
Carbocisteine

Figure 23.1 • Introduction and formulary recommendations for bronchodilators, illustrating presentation as a Pocket Guide. (Adapted from the TAPG Pocket Guide 2010, ©NHS Tayside Area Drug and Therapeutics Committee, with permission.)

(A)

Asthma: for management of asthma please refer to BTS/SIGN guideline No. 101 (revised May 2008) COPD: For COPD management please refer to NICE Clinical Guideline 12 (Feb 2004).

Although first choice drug have been indicated where possible, for any inhaled treatment, choosing the most suitable device for the patient is the most important factor for ensuring effective therapy (see guidance). In general, patients are best treated with single-ingredient preparations so that the dose of each drug can be individually adjusted.

3.1 Bronchodilators

See notes on Managing Chronic Asthma and COPD guidelines for further guidance.

Doses listed within this section are for adults and children over 12 years unless stated.

Beta₂ agonists
Short-acting

FIRST CHOICE: SALBUTAMOL

Salbutamol
Dose: (In asthma or COPD) By aerosol inhalation, 100-200micrograms (1-2 puffs), when required to relieve breathlessness. By inhalation of powder, 200-400micrograms when required to relieve breathlessness (Note: dose depending on inhaler device used – see BNF).

Terbutaline
Dose: (In asthma or COPD) By inhalation of powder using the Turbohaler® device, 500micrograms (1 inhalation), when required to relieve breathlessness.

Long-acting

FIRST CHOICE: INDACATEROL
▼

Dose: (In COPD) By inhalation of powder using the Onbrez Breezhaler® device, 150micrograms (one capsule) once per day increased to a maximum of 300micrograms (two capsules) once per day.

Salmeterol
Dose: (In asthma or COPD) By aerosol inhalation or inhalation of powder, 50micrograms (2 puffs or 1 blister) twice daily; up to 100micrograms (4 puffs or 2 blisters) twice daily in more severe airways obstruction.

☑**Long-acting inhaled beta-2 agonists should not be used without inhaled corticosteroids in asthma:** they should be added to existing inhaled corticosteroid therapy and not replace it.

Click here for advice on the place of long-acting beta-2 agonists in the management of chronic asthma. Where adequate asthma symptom control is not achieved at the above doses of long-acting beta-2 agonists please refer to algorithm click here and the BTS/SIGN asthma guidance for advice on maximising inhaled steroid therapy.

Antimuscarinic (Anticholinergic) bronchodilator
Short-acting

Ipratropium
Dose: (In COPD) By aerosol inhalation ▼, 20-40micrograms (1-2 puffs) 3-4 times daily.
(Ipratropium aerosol inhalation has had a black triangle status since it was changed to CFC-free).

Long-acting

(B)

FIRST CHOICE:
TIOTROPIUM

Dose: (In COPD) by inhalation of powder using the Spiriva HandiHaler® device, 18micrograms (one capsule) once per daily.

Glycopyrronium ▼ (2ⁿᵈ line)
Dose: (In COPD) by inhalation of powder using the Seebri Breezhaler® device, 44micrograms (one capsule) once per day.

Please note glycopyrronium should be used with caution in patients with severe renal impairment (eGFR<30ml/min), and should only be used if the expected benefit outweighs the potential risk.

Aclidinium ▼ (3ʳᵈ line)
Dose: (In COPD) by inhalation of powder using the Eklira Genuair® device, 322micrograms (one inhalation) twice per day. Note - Spiriva Respimat▼ has been removed from the core formulary and added to the respiratory specialist list due to safety concerns. Please see the MHRA Drug Safety Update NOV 2010 for more information.

See COPD therapeutic notes. Do not co-prescribe tiotropium with a short-acting antimuscarinic (anticholinergic) bronchodilator, including compound preparations.

Theophylline - prescribe by brand name

Uniphyllin® m/r tablets 200mg, 300mg, 400mg
Dose: 200mg every 12 hours, increased gradually according to response to 400mg every 12 hours.

Note: there are other oral theophylline brands available. However, there are differences in bioavailability between them and dosages are not equivalent. Patients should keep with the same brand if changes in dose are made. Oral theophyllines are weak bronchodilators with a high incidence of side-effects and are now less commonly used. Important interactions exist with other drugs: some may produce theophylline toxicity (e.g. clarithromycin, erythromycin, ciprofloxacin, and cimetidine); others may decrease plasma levels (e.g. anti-epileptics, rifampicin). See BNF for full interaction profile. Monitoring plasma levels of theophylline is not routinely necessary in stable patients but may be warranted in certain circumstances e.g. a change in clinical status, where toxicity is suspected or during concomitant use of interacting drugs. Note: smoking cessation may increase theophylline levels. Seek advice if unsure. See MHRA Drug Safety Update October 2008 for safety advice on theophylline containing medicines available over the counter from community pharmacists.

Compound bronchodilator preparations

In patients with severe COPD requiring regular nebulised bronchodilators, **salbutamol 2.5mg nebuliser solution** and **ipratropium 500microgram nebuliser solution** can be prescribed separately or as a combined product (**Combivent® nebuliser solution**).

Figure 23.2 • Formulary recommendations for bronchodilators, illustrating presentation as a detailed prescribing guide. (Reproduced with permission from NHS Tayside Area Drug and Therapeutics Committee. Extraction date: 11 February 2013.) http://www.nhstaysideadtc.scot.nhs.uk/TAPG%20html/MAIN/Front%20page.htm

certain locations only. These drugs should also be easily distinguishable from the others in the formulary; in Figure 23.1A, these are in italic. A list of contents and an index should be included to make the formulary easy to use.

Most UK formularies follow the BNF to classify medicines and may be designed to be used in conjunction with it. Users can be directed to the monographs there for information on dosage, indications, side-effects, contraindications and precautions. Some formularies include all this information, but only for the recommended drugs. Other important information which may be given in a local formulary is local drug costs and the reasons behind the selection.

Drug costs are one of the factors taken into account when compiling a formulary (see below). The price of a drug can be expressed in several different ways. While the easiest may be the price of different pack sizes, the cost of a period of treatment may be more useful if pack sizes of similar products differ and comparisons are being encouraged. A suitable period may be 1 day, 1 month (28 days) or a standard course of treatment (e.g. 5 days for antibiotics). Since the price of the drug usually varies with the pack size, this may not be as easy to calculate as it first appears. A further complicating factor is that prices may differ in hospital and community. If a formulary is designed to be used in hospital only, the hospital price may seem most relevant. However, patients may take the drug while living in the community for much longer than they take it in hospital. Therefore the price in primary care is also of relevance, especially in joint formularies.

When large numbers of prescribers are to use a formulary, it is unlikely that they will all have been consulted about its content. If that is the case, providing explanations of how drugs were selected for the formulary is of particular importance. Many formularies state the general basis of drug selection as being efficacy, safety, patient acceptability and cost, but sometimes additional information is given. The BNF gives this type of information in introductory paragraphs to each section. An example is the statement that 'other thiazide diuretics do not offer any significant advantage over bendroflumethiazide and chlortalidone'. It may be desirable to reference the formulary to give readers the opportunity to see the evidence on which statements such as these are based. It may also be useful to explain local preferences, particularly in the case of antibiotic selection, which should take local microbiological sensitivities into account.

Some or all of the formulary may be presented as prescribing policies or guidelines. If this approach is taken, details of which drugs are to be used in specific medical conditions should be given. It may be necessary to include alternatives and the particular occasions when they should be used. In a prescribing policy, details of the recommended dosage, route and method of administration and duration of therapy should also be included. The BNF includes a number of examples, such as a summary of antibacterial therapy for specific conditions, detailed guidance on the management of chronic and acute asthma (taken from the SIGN/BTS guideline) and extracts from NICE guidelines throughout.

A local formulary may have sections relating to prescribing in certain types of patients, such as the elderly, children, those with renal or hepatic impairment, or in pregnancy and breast-feeding. As there is little point in reproducing the BNF, these too should reflect local recommendations.

Presentation of a formulary

The appearance of a formulary is an indicator of the importance attached to it by those who have produced it. Poor presentation may result in those who are expected to use it having little respect for its contents, which may lead to poor adherence to its recommendations. It is therefore worth creating a document which is attractive and looks professional. It is also important to consider whether a paper or electronic format is desirable or whether both should be available.

Paper formats can be portable, making for ease of use in any clinical setting, from the hospital bedside to the patient's home. However, they are expensive to produce and still require regular updating. The size of the document is an important consideration. Ideally, it should be no bigger than pocket-sized, perhaps compatible in size with the BNF, to make it easy to use the two together. A simple list of formulary drugs is a useful option, such as that illustrated in Figure 23.1B, produced by NHS Tayside ADTC. This can be supplemented by a larger document in either paper or electronic form. If the formulary is only available as a large paper document which cannot be carried around, it is much less likely to be available when needed, which may mean its recommendations are ignored. Colour and a durable cover to withstand regular use can both add further to the appearance of a paper formulary, but also increase its cost.

Electronic formats are increasingly popular, but not all professionals use a computer when prescribing, so it may still be necessary to produce a paper version, even if this is only the list of drugs. A CD version is one option, but like a paper document, requires re-distribution whenever it is updated. Other options are to publish the formulary on a local intranet or to make it available as a locally downloadable application for smart phones. Linking the local formulary to electronic prescribing systems is perhaps the ideal option. Some prescribing systems incorporate decision support tools, which can include the formulary. Electronic versions may also make it easier to evaluate the formulary by examining prescribing adherence.

Ensuring that the formulary is up-to-date is extremely important and its presentation must allow for this. Loose-leaf binding will enable easy updating, but relies on everyone modifying their own copy. It is much easier to update an electronic version which is distributed via the Internet or intranet.

Whatever format is used, the formulary should be easy to use, to encourage prescribers to refer to it when necessary. This will be helped by a contents list, which for a paper version means the pages have to be numbered. Arranging the drugs in the same order as the BNF will also help to make the formulary easier to use, for prescribers who already use the BNF. Using different typefaces and print size can make a formulary easier to use. Highlighting the drug names can be useful, as often the name of the recommended drug may be all that someone is seeking (see Fig. 23.1B).

It may also be appropriate to provide access to the formulary for local patients. Increasingly, patients have access to clinical guidelines and are informed about what treatments are recommended for their medical problems. Providing a formulary has been developed using transparent methods and drugs selected on the basis of efficacy, safety, patient acceptability and cost, there is no reason to prevent patients from knowing of its existence. Access can be via the Internet, so need not add to publication costs.

Selection of products for inclusion

It is important to decide at the outset the range of indications which the formulary should cover. Some hospital formularies do not attempt to include drugs to treat all possible conditions. Some deliberately exclude certain drugs, such as those used in highly specialized areas such as cancer chemotherapy and anaesthetics. A formulary for use in primary care should aim to include enough drugs to treat between 80% and 90% of all commonly presenting conditions. It is also useful to have a separate list of emergency drugs, such as those which should be carried by GPs in their emergency bags. Clearly if a formulary includes many drugs and a lot of information about them, it will not only be bulky, but also will not have many of the advantages that a local formulary can provide. It should be possible to cover most needs, either in hospital or general practice, with about 300–500 drugs. In selecting drugs for inclusion in a formulary, it is important to remember that formularies are designed for treating the majority of the population. However, individual patients' needs and preferences should, where possible, be taken into account and there will be individuals for whom a specific formulary drug is not suitable. To provide for most commonly encountered situations, therefore, two drugs from the range available within a pharmacological class may be included, rather than one.

While the four important factors are efficacy, safety, patient acceptability and cost, other factors are also usually considered (Box 23.1). Formulary drugs must be effective for whatever indications they are to be used, with minimal toxicity. Evidence of efficacy should be based on well-conducted clinical trials rather than anecdotal reports. Generally,

---

Box 23.1

Factors influencing selection of drugs for inclusion in a formulary

- Efficacy for the indications to be included in the formulary
- Side-effect profiles and contraindications of individual drugs
- Interaction profile of individual drugs
- Pharmacokinetic profiles of individual drugs
- Acceptability to patients – taste, appearance, ease of administration
- Formulations available
- General availability, including generic availability
- Cost
- Usage patterns

Table 23.2 Example using beta-adrenoceptor antagonists of how factors can be used to select drugs for a formulary

Factor	Examples of information to be taken into account	Examples of possible selection
Licensed indications/ Evidence of efficacy	a. For hypertension, there are many to select from b. For arrhythmias, few are licensed c. For secondary prevention of myocardial infarction d. For heart failure	a. atenolol, propranolol, metoprolol, etc. b. sotalol, esmolol c. atenolol injection, metoprolol, propranolol d. bisoprolol, carvedilol
Toxicity	a. Water solubility results in fewer nightmares b. Intrinsic sympathomimetic activity causes less cold extremities	a. atenolol, sotalol b. oxprenolol, pindolol
Contraindications	Cardio-selectivity is preferable in asthma and diabetes	Atenolol, bisoprolol, metoprolol
Pharmacokinetic profile	Long-acting drugs/products require fewer doses	Atenolol, modified release propranolol
Generic availability	Usually reduces cost	Atenolol, propranolol, metoprolol
Acceptability to patients	Once daily doses, combination products may be useful	Atenolol, modified release propranolol with thiazide diuretics for hypertension
Cost	Cheapest preferable if all other factors equal	Atenolol, propranolol, metoprolol

prescribers' personal preferences are not a sound basis for selection of a particular drug or product as each may have their own preference. Occasionally, there may be a range of similar drugs from which to select, but not all are licensed for all the indications the formulary is to cover. An example is beta-adrenoceptor antagonists, some of which have a range of licensed indications (Table 23.2). In this situation, selection of the drugs which cover most indications may be appropriate. Alternatively, separate drugs could be selected and specified for use in different indications. This latter option makes it difficult to audit adherence, as it is impossible to tell from looking at prescribing data only whether the drug is prescribed in-line with the formulary recommendations.

If two drugs are equally efficacious, as is often the case within a group of pharmacologically similar drugs, the least toxic one is preferable. Any differences between the drugs in terms of their pharmacokinetics, contraindications, adverse effects and potential for interaction then become important.

Pharmacokinetic profiles of drugs are important in selecting drugs with an optimum half-life for their indications. It may also be possible to select drugs which are minimally affected by either liver or renal impairment. Among the benzodiazepine group, for example, those with short half-lives and which have no active metabolites are usually preferred as hypnotics, as they have no hangover effect. Differences in drug handling in children and the elderly may require different drugs to be recommended for use with these patients. Selection of drugs for use in pregnancy and breastfeeding will be influenced by their passage into the placenta and secretion into breast milk.

The range of contraindications, precautions and adverse effects may differ for drugs within a therapeutic class. While class effects are common, sometimes there are differences between individual drugs; again beta-adrenoceptor antagonists are a good example of this. Differences are most often found in the frequency and severity of adverse effects between drugs in a class. Where possible, formulary drugs should have the lowest frequency of, and least severe, adverse effects.

If drugs are similar in terms of efficacy and toxicity but have different potential for interaction, this could be a deciding factor. Drugs with fewer possibilities of interaction mean fewer problems in use.

Patient acceptability is an important factor, which will be affected by efficacy and toxicity. If drugs do not work, or if they cause side-effects, patients are less likely to take them. For orally administered drugs, palatability and ease of swallowing will contribute to acceptability. Other considerations may also be important, such as the extent to which a dispersible preparation actually disperses, or whether a modified-release tablet can be divided. Inhaled drugs are available in many different formulations and their selection will depend to an extent on what patients will or can use properly, to achieve maximum efficacy. For topical products, such as creams and ointments, patient acceptability is particularly important.

A local formulary may simply list drugs which are recommended or it may specify particular dosage forms of those drugs. Patient acceptability is likely to influence the different formulations selected for inclusion in a formulary more than the drug entities. However, the range of formulations available, which will in turn affect patients' acceptance of drug therapy, may be a factor in deciding which drugs to include. Drugs available in a wide range of formulations may be a better choice than those which have very few. It is simpler for a prescriber to remember one drug name within a particular therapeutic class, rather than several each in a different formulation.

Many formularies exclude all combination products which include two or more drugs in fixed ratio. This is because it is impossible to increase the dose of one drug without also increasing the dose of the other drug(s). Some patients may receive higher doses of one of the constituents than they require as a result. However, combination products are more favoured in primary care, where they are considered to improve patient compliance and also reduce prescription charges for the patient. Combination products may be useful if the pharmacokinetic characteristics of the components are compatible and it can be shown that patients require and obtain benefit from all the components individually, in the same ratio as the combination product. Unfortunately, very few combination products are used in this way. Their inclusion in a formulary will depend on local preferences and appropriate use will subsequently depend on individual prescribers.

Cost considerations are also important, but the aim of a formulary is to encourage rational and cost-effective prescribing, not primarily to save money. Cost-effective prescribing involves the use of the drug with the lowest costs which is also effective,

has minimal toxicity and is acceptable to patients. The cheapest drugs may not be the most acceptable, or of adequate efficacy. For some groups of drugs, prescribing costs may actually rise as a result of using a local formulary, since the optimum drugs may be the most expensive. However, where efficacy, toxicity and patient acceptability are equal, cost should be the deciding factor in drug selection. As described above, both hospital and community costs of drugs should be considered when selecting drugs for a hospital formulary, as the bulk of the cost is likely to be borne by primary care. The purchase price of a drug may not be the only factor to be taken into account when considering costs. Pharmacoeconomic evaluations, which take account of the costs of the consequences of treatments, may also be necessary (see Ch. 22).

All drugs included in a formulary should be easily available, so 'specials', drugs available in hospital only, or on a named patient basis, should be avoided. Generic availability is a bonus, as it usually means costs are lower than for drugs which are only available as branded formulations. Most formularies specify that prescribing should be generic, where appropriate. The use of computer systems for prescribing, which automatically change prescriptions to the appropriate generic name, increases the proportion of generic prescriptions considerably. This should also reduce costs.

As part of their role in formulary development, pharmacists frequently provide unbiased information about any differences in efficacy, toxicity and cost between drugs. Some useful sources of unbiased information are the NICE Medicines and Prescribing Centre and Drug and Therapeutics Bulletin.

Use of prescribing data

All the factors mentioned so far can also be applied to the selection of drugs for individual patients. A further factor which may be considered when selecting drugs for populations is current prescribing habits. The main reason for this is that it is much easier to encourage use of a formulary if it involves few changes of habit. However, if the commonly prescribed drugs are not efficacious, or have a high incidence or severity of toxicity, it is better not to include them. Frequent use does not necessarily imply appropriate selection. Information about current prescribing is increasingly obtainable for either hospital or primary care prescribers in many countries. Hospital prescribing data may be available from computerized pharmacy supply systems or electronic prescribing systems. In primary care, data can usually be obtained through the reimbursement system for prescriptions dispensed by pharmacists.

By looking at data on the frequency of prescribing of different products, it is usually possible to identify one or two drugs within each therapeutic class which account for the bulk of prescriptions. Providing these drugs are efficacious and have minimal toxicity, they should usually be considered for inclusion in a formulary, as little change in prescribing habits will be needed. It may be necessary for others to be included on a more restricted basis. If the commonly prescribed drugs are inappropriate on therapeutic grounds, alternatives may be required.

Formulary management systems

A formulary needs to be flexible and dynamic. A system must be devised which allows this. This is known as the formulary management system and it covers many other aspects of formularies.

Production, distribution and revision

Producing a formulary is a very time-consuming task which, although overseen by the ADTC, needs a driver to take responsibility for ensuring it is completed. Usually this is a pharmacist, who will be involved in collecting together the data on which the drug selection will be based (published evidence, prescribing data and expert or all group members' opinions), drafting material, reaching agreement on the format(s) and design to be used and seeing it through to production. The ADTC should consider who will need a copy, what format it should take and how it will be distributed.

Distribution of hard copies by mail with a covering letter may be easiest for large numbers of people, but hand delivery, with verbal explanation, may help to encourage interest and therefore adherence to a formulary's recommendations. Launching of a new formulary (or a revision) can usefully be accompanied by a meeting to explain its aims, describe how to use it and encourage discussion of its contents. Leaflets advertising the benefits of using the formulary and educational material may be usefully developed to encourage prescribers to learn about why they should consider using it.

Electronic versions can obviously be easily distributed within a health organization, but require just as much supplementary information to encourage their use. Specialist IT support to ensure that the formulary can be integrated with electronic prescribing systems is a key factor in their successful use.

After all the effort which goes into producing a new formulary has resulted in the final document, the thought of revising it is likely to be far from popular. However, because of the time taken to produce a new formulary, it will soon go out of date. If this is allowed to happen, respect for its content will decline. Adherence to its recommendations may follow suit. Revision should therefore be considered even before the formulary is finished. The printed BNF is revised every 6 months, but most local formularies cannot hope to achieve a similar frequency, because of the amount of work involved. Annual or biennial revision should be aimed at and specified at the launch. As new drugs are coming onto the market all the time, even 6-monthly revision will not be adequate to keep a formulary up-to-date. Some system, therefore, needs to be devised to allow new drugs to be considered for inclusion.

Responding to the needs of practice

Change is the norm in the world of drugs. New drugs are constantly becoming available; old drugs are removed from the market; new clinical trials provide evidence for efficacy of existing drugs in novel indications and post-marketing surveillance provides constantly changing data on adverse effect profiles. An awareness of all the facts this generates is essential, so that the formulary does not go out of date and can respond to the changes. In implementing a formulary, patients must not be deprived of the benefits of new information and drugs. There will also inevitably be an occasional need for patients to receive treatment out with a formulary's recommendations, since a formulary cannot be expected to cover all possible situations. Methods are therefore needed to allow drugs to be considered for inclusion in the formulary, to allow drugs to be removed from the formulary and to supply non-formulary drugs when these are appropriate.

A method for allowing drugs to be considered for inclusion in a formulary should not be restricted

Request for inclusion of a new drug in a formulary

Drug name _____ Manufacturer _____

Formulations available _____

Indication(s) for which request is made _____

Usual dose and duration of treatment _____

Type of inclusion requested

☐ recommendation for general use

☐ specialist use only

If specialist use, which specialist(s)?

_____

☐ restricted indication(s)

Reason for request   ☐ novel therapeutic advance

☐ benefits over existing drug

Will the new drug replace an existing drug?   Yes/No

If so, which? _____

Estimated number of patients per year who will receive drug _____

Estimated costs of treatment _____

Evidence provided in support of request:

☐ Summary of Product Characteristics

☐ Copies of RCTs, meta-analyses, review articles

☐ Pharmaco-economic evaluation

This request is supported by: (signatures required)

Consultant _____

Clinical Pharmacist _____

Trust Clinical Director _____

Figure 23.3 • Example of a form which could be used to request new drugs to be considered for inclusion in a formulary.

to newly available drugs. It must allow any user of the formulary to propose a drug for consideration and should be able to provide an evaluated response within a reasonable time. Evidence of any advantages the proposed drug has over drugs already included, in terms of efficacy, reduced toxicity or cost, will be needed. This must be based on well-designed published clinical trials, the same basis as that used in the initial formulary development. Many formulary management systems require a form to be completed; an example is given in Figure 23.3.

The person making the request must be informed whether the drug will be included and, if so, whether any restrictions will be placed on its prescribing. One option is to have an appraisal period, say 6 months, during which prescribers can gain experience with a newly recommended drug. After this period, the committee can then review the status of the drug.

If a drug is accepted onto an existing formulary between revisions, it is essential to inform all users of the change. One way of achieving this is to issue information bulletins, either by post or e-mail. A similar method can be used to inform users of any changes in the indications or doses of drugs, which may also occur during the life of a formulary. Similarly, if drugs are to be withdrawn from the formulary, users must be kept informed. Regular bulletins issued by the ADTC are therefore an important feature of formulary management.

Withdrawals may occur because of manufacturers ceasing production, product licences being withdrawn or changes in manufacturers' recommendations. However, it may also be useful to consider withdrawing drugs from the formulary if they have not been prescribed for a long time. Again, 6 months would be a suitable time to study the prescribing of most drugs, except those whose use is seasonal. This could be done on a regular basis between major revisions, but would require consultation with prescribers before the withdrawal was implemented. The advantage of a practice such as this is that it helps to keep the number of drugs in the formulary to a minimum.

As there will be situations when a non-formulary drug is requested for a patient, it may be necessary to have a method of ensuring that the request is dealt with promptly. In primary care, there should be no problem in supplying a non-formulary drug, although there may be a delay if it is not stocked by local pharmacies owing to rare use. In hospital, however, pharmacies tend to stock only a limited range of drugs. Formulary drugs should always be easily available, but non-formulary drugs may need to be purchased specially. This will lead to delays in treatment. Some formulary management systems, usually in hospitals, require completion of a form for every non-formulary drug which is prescribed. The purpose of this is two-fold: it acts as a deterrent to prescribing non-formulary drugs and also allows monitoring to see whether any drugs are frequently requested. Consideration may be given to including frequently requested drugs in the formulary. Usually forms require a senior medical staff signature, but there is a possibility that this requirement may be abused. Once a form with the appropriate signature is received, pharmacists should not simply assume that the request should be complied with. If this occurs, all that has been achieved is an elaborate ordering system. For the formulary system to operate effectively, all prescribers requesting a non-formulary drug should be questioned to determine the reasons why a formulary drug is not suitable.

One frequent reason for requesting a non-formulary drug in hospital is that the patient was taking the drug prior to admission and prescribers are reluctant to change it. This can be viewed as an opportunity to review the medication, ensuring that it is appropriate for the individual patient. If it proves to be so, it may be possible to use the patient's own supply of the drug, providing there are systems in place to ensure this is indeed required and fit for use. If this is not an option, a decision must be made on whether the requested drug will be supplied from the pharmacy. The systems in place must ensure that this is a rapid process, particularly if a special purchase is required.

The most common reason for using non-formulary drugs in primary care is also that patients are already taking them and either they or their GPs are reluctant to change the prescription. Pharmacists can use the opportunity of conducting medication reviews to consider the appropriateness of any non-formulary drugs prescribed. Pharmacists also undertake regular review of repeat prescribing in many practices, using the techniques of drug utilization review; drug use evaluation and audit (see Chs 12, 22). Non-formulary prescribing can be assessed through these mechanisms and therapeutic switching undertaken to address any changes which would be of benefit.

The promotional activities of drug manufacturers' representatives will need to be controlled to prevent them from undermining the principles of a local formulary. Many NHS trusts have policies on which staff representatives are allowed to see and what they are allowed to supply. Manufacturers can be an extremely useful source of information on their products, but the inclusion of a drug in a formulary must be evidence based and unbiased. Making constructive use of the visit from a pharmaceutical company's representative can be a beneficial educational exercise to staff involved in using a formulary.

Clearly a lot of effort goes into operating a formulary and there are many advantages of a good formulary management system. The measure of success of any formulary is in the extent to which it is used or adhered to and the demonstration that prescribing is more rational. It may be possible to show improvements in efficacy and reduced toxicity and also cost savings, but these may be more difficult to achieve and to demonstrate.

Changing practice

Developing local formularies and treatment protocols encourages good relationships between prescribers and pharmacists. Building on this relationship is important to enable the changes to practice to be made which will be necessary in implementing these. Changing prescribing habits can be extremely difficult. Some prescribers dislike losing the freedom to prescribe as they choose and may reject a formulary and its concept. Often prescribers have developed personal drug preferences over the years and, even if they have no objection in principle to prescribing a different drug, they may easily forget when actually writing prescriptions. Incorporating the formulary into electronic prescribing systems, which restrict choice or at least highlight formulary drugs as preferred, is therefore of great benefit. If agreement on what drugs should be used has been difficult to achieve, the resultant formulary may contain a large number of drugs. This can be more easily adhered to, but is less likely to achieve rational prescribing or to reduce drug costs. Conversely a formulary which is too restrictive is more likely to be difficult to adhere to.

When a formulary is first introduced, some patients will be receiving medicines which are not included and they, too, may be resistant to change. The doctors who prescribe for these patients may also be unhappy about changing individual patients' drugs. This is especially likely if the patient is well stabilized on a particular drug, with few adverse effects. As drugs included in a formulary will have been selected on a sound basis, it could be more suitable for a patient than their current drug. Change may therefore be of benefit. Education of prescribers and patients may be necessary to convince them of potential benefits and can be supported by educational packages, as already mentioned. Pharmacists are often those most actively involved in educating and persuading prescribers to carry out changes. They are also well placed to implement formulary recommendations themselves within their roles as prescribers. Even without changing individual patients' drug therapy, if the drugs recommended in a local formulary are used for all patients starting new therapy, most prescriptions will in time include formulary drugs.

Research has shown that for clinical guidelines, visits to prescribers to provide education, involving local opinion leaders in educational meetings and interactive educational workshops are successful methods of changing behaviour. The same is likely to apply to formularies. A strategy should be developed which ideally includes a mixture of methods, because the more frequent the reminder, the more likely it is that practice will change. Constant reminders may be necessary to maintain prescribing within the recommendations of a formulary. However, feedback on adherence to the formulary is another important mechanism for reminding prescribers about it.

Auditing performance

Providing feedback to prescribers on whether they follow formularies is essential. Because formularies encourage rational prescribing, the extent of their use can be used as one indicator of the quality of prescribing. For other types of prescribing indicators, see Chapter 22. The simplest way to gauge whether a formulary is being used is to analyze the same type of prescribing data used to help develop the formulary. Computerized prescribing data can easily be studied to assess whether formulary drugs are being prescribed. However, it provides no information about the patients for whom the drugs have been prescribed and cannot help to identify why patients have been prescribed non-formulary drugs. Nor can it be used to determine whether formulary drugs were prescribed appropriately or within local guidelines and treatment protocols. For this, drug utilization review or clinical audit is required (see Chs 12 and 22).

For data to be of any use, it must be easy to interpret, accurate, up to date and of direct relevance to the prescriber. Ideally data is compared either to earlier prescribing or to the prescribing of others. Comparing the prescribing of several doctors to each other is known as peer review. Comparison to a 'norm' of prescribing practice, or to the practices of others in the same peer group, often increases the desire of prescribers to conform to the 'norm' or the peer group. However, it is important to ensure that the 'norm' is desirable.

If hospital data generated by the pharmacy computerized stock control system refer to drugs issued to wards or directorates, care must be taken to determine whether this equates to drugs prescribed. Any drugs which were not issued through the computer system, such as patients' own drugs, may not show up in these data. Electronically incorporating the formulary into prescribing systems should make the measurement of formulary adherence relatively simple.

In primary care, the prescribing data available through reimbursement systems represent the number of prescriptions dispensed, excluding only prescriptions written which were never dispensed. Such systems cannot distinguish between formulary and non-formulary drugs. This must be done manually and a figure for adherence calculated, again taking the quantities of each drug into account. Another source of data in primary care is the computer used to generate prescriptions by the GP, which can again incorporate formulary drugs within its programs. However, if a practice does not generate or record all its prescriptions via the computer, the prescribing patterns obtained will not show the full picture. The number of prescriptions written usually differs from those dispensed, so a different picture of formulary adherence may be found depending on which data source is used.

When providing feedback to prescribers based on prescribing data, care should be taken to ensure that the quantities of the different drugs used are taken into account in some way. For example, if 180 tablets of a formulary drug and 20 tablets of a range of four other non-formulary drugs are used, adherence should be quantified as 90% (180 out of 200 tablets used in total). It could also be calculated that adherence was only 20% if the range of drugs were used (one out of a range of five), but this would not be a reasonable representation of the overall prescribing.

Another source of valuable data for the formulary pharmacist is the request forms for non-formulary drugs, if they are used. Review of these can indicate the extent of non-formulary prescribing. These should also explain the reasons why non-formulary drugs were used. Records of clinical pharmacists' interventions made during routine prescription review or medication review which relate to non-formulary prescribing can also be studied.

Regular provision of information on performance is an essential part of formulary management. Any data which are presented to prescribers as a means of informing them of adherence to formulary recommendations will need to be attractive and easy to use, just like the formulary itself. Graphics and colour can be used to highlight important points. Finally, evidence of cost savings, if they have been achieved, may help to encourage use of the formulary. This is probably best expressed as actual expenditure compared to expected expenditure had the formulary not been used. If formulary adherence is found to be low, then this is an important result, which needs to be investigated to determine whether the formulary best serves the needs of the population or requires revision.

All this feedback should be provided in the same variety of formats as the formulary – paper, electronic or both. It can be incorporated into regular published bulletins from the ADTC. This highlights the continuing importance of the formulary and should be an indication of the committee's willingness to update the formulary in the light of changing needs. Pharmacists can also use discussion of feedback information as another opportunity to market a formulary and gain the support of prescribers in its use.

KEY POINTS

- A formulary is a list of drugs which are recommended and available for prescribing
- A formulary may contain prescribing policies, which detail the use of drugs in specific medical conditions
- Local formularies are used in conjunction with clinical guidelines and treatment protocols to encourage rational and cost-effective prescribing
- Compiling a formulary is a valuable educational exercise
- Pharmacists should work with other health professionals to compile a formulary
- Drugs are selected for inclusion in a formulary on the basis of efficacy, toxicity, patient acceptability and cost
- Use of a formulary containing a restricted number of drugs may reduce the incidence of prescribing problems such as ADRs, interactions and lack of efficacy
- For a formulary to be accepted, there should be widespread consultation on its content
- A formulary should be easy to use, professionally presented in paper or electronic (or both) formats and revised at least every 2 years
- A formulary management system is required to provide systems for considering the inclusion of new drugs, deleting drugs and supplying non-formulary drugs
- Feedback information should be provided to prescribers on their adherence to a formulary to encourage its use
- Prescribing data can be useful in both developing a formulary and feeding back on performance
- Ideally a mixture of methods should be used to encourage use of a formulary

Complementary and alternative medicines

24

Brian Lockwood

STUDY POINTS

- Types of complementary medicines and complementary therapies
- Extent and reasons for use of complementary/alternative medicine (CAM)
- Regulation of CAM practitioners and complementary medicines
- The interrelationship between pharmacy and CAM

Introduction

Complementary/alternative medicine (CAM), originally referred to as 'fringe', 'holistic' or 'natural' medicine, was known as 'alternative' medicine in the 1970s and 1980s and, today, increasingly is called 'integrated' or 'integrative' medicine. Generally, it is referred to as complementary/alternative medicine, although the terms complementary medicine, alternative medicine and complementary therapies are used interchangeably. A definition of CAM, which has been adopted by the Cochrane Collaboration (see Ch. 20), is given in Box 24.1.

Historically, CAM was the main form of medicine available to the world's populations. In many parts of the world it still is today. The term CAM originates from the fact that what we now know as conventional or pharmaceutical medicine, did not exist, hence the modern usage of the term. With the advent and expansion of discovery and production of mainly synthetic medicines by pharmaceutical companies, usage of mainly plant-based traditional medicines declined. These medicines are what we now refer to as CAM.

CAM is an umbrella term for a collection of different approaches to diagnosis and treatment. Over 50 diverse complementary therapies have been listed, some involving use of medicinal substances, while others use a range of therapeutic techniques. These range from homoeopathy (which involves the use of infinitely dilute preparations) to herbal medicine (the use of chemically rich plant material), and from acupuncture (which involves the insertion of needles into specific points on the body) to therapeutic touch and spiritual healing (including 'distant' healing, which does not require the laying on of hands). In addition, there are many forms of complementary therapies available, which use a variety of techniques, but no medicinal products, some use

Box 24.1

Definition of complementary and alternative medicine

Complementary and alternative medicine (CAM) is a broad domain of healing resources that encompasses all health systems, modalities and practices and their accompanying theories and beliefs, other than those intrinsic to the politically dominant health system of a particular society or culture in a given historical period. CAM includes all such practices and ideas self-defined by their users as preventing or treating illness or promoting health and well-being. Boundaries within CAM and between the CAM domain and that of the dominant system are not always sharp or fixed.

(Zollman and Vickers 1999)

only medicinal products, and there are also those which involve both medicines and techniques.

Some of the most well known complementary therapies, including those using medicinal products, are described in Box 24.2.

Several complementary therapies, such as herbalism, homoeopathy, aromatherapy and others, involve the administration of remedies, often in recognizable pharmaceutical formulations, e.g. herbal medicines, homoeopathic remedies and essential oils. These are

---

 ## Box 24.2

Descriptions of complementary therapies common in the UK

Complementary medicines can be conveniently divided into three categories, those using only medicinal substances, those using a therapy without medicinal substances, and those using both.

Therapies using medicinal substances

Aromatherapy

The therapeutic use of aromatic substances, largely essential oils, which typically contain numerous chemical constituents, are extracted from plants.

Aromatherapists believe that essential oils can be used not only for the prevention and treatment of disease, but also for their effects on mood, emotion and well-being. Aromatherapy is claimed to be a holistic therapy in that practitioners will select an essential oil or combination of essential oils to suit each client's symptoms, personality and emotional state. The most common method used for application of essential oils is massage using a carrier oil; other methods include the addition of essential oils to baths and footbaths, inhalations, compresses and use in aromatherapy equipment, e.g. burners and vaporizers.

Flower remedies and essences

Developed in the UK by Dr Edward Bach, who believed that physical disease was the result of being at odds with one's spiritual purpose, i.e. negative states of mind induce illness. His approach to health focused only on the mental state of the patient. He identified 38 negative psychological states of mind (e.g. jealousy, guilt, hopelessness) and developed a remedy designed to be used for each of these emotional states. The Bach collection comprises 39 remedies, 38 of which originate from flowers/trees, and 'Rescue Remedy', a combination of five of the other 38 remedies. Flower remedies are extremely dilute preparations, but are not homoeopathic remedies.

Many other countries have their own collection of flower remedies/essences based on native plants/trees, e.g. Australian Bush Essences.

Herbalism

Traditional herbalism had an historical basis, party based on the galenical model of the four 'humours' and the belief that an excess of any of the humours leads to

disease. Today, treatment is aimed at 'restoring balance' and 'strengthening bodily systems'. Herbalists aim to treat patients in a holistic way by selecting a herb or combination of herbs to treat a particular person and his/her unique set of symptoms. One of the principal tenets is that the whole plant extract, and not an isolated constituent, is responsible for the clinical effect. It is claimed that herbal constituents, and even combinations of herbs, work synergistically to achieve benefit and reduce the possibility of adverse effects.

Rational phytotherapy/phytomedicine (science-based herbal medicine) has an entirely different approach to that of traditional herbalism. It involves the use of specific plant (or plant part) extracts standardized to specific constituents (where possible) with documented pharmacological activity for the treatment of specific clinical conditions. In this regard, phytotherapy has a similar approach to that of conventional medicine.

This involves preparations made from plants or plant parts. In some instances (e.g. use by herbalists), a crude drug (e.g. dried leaf) is used. Manufactured products use extracts of plants or plant parts, formulated as, e.g. tablets, capsules, creams and tinctures. They may contain a single or multiple herbal ingredients, obviously including numerous single chemical entities.

Homoeopathy

The use of highly dilute, succussed substances to stimulate the body's own healing activity (the 'vital force'). One of the key principles is 'like cures like' – a substance which in large doses causes a set of symptoms in a healthy person can be used to treat such symptoms in an ill person, e.g. homoeopathic preparations of coffee (Coffea) are used to treat insomnia. Treatment is holistic – two patients with the same set of symptoms may be given different remedies depending on their personal characteristics, physical appearance, mental and emotional state, etc. Although there are several hypotheses, there is not yet a plausible explanation for the mechanism of action of homoeopathy. Furthermore, on balance, rigorous clinical trials do not show an effect for homoeopathy over that of placebo.

This uses highly dilute preparations which may be of plant, animal, mineral, insect, biological, drug/chemical or other origin. Formulations include tablets, pilules, creams/ointments, liquids and injections.

(Continued)

Nutritional medicines

Nutraceuticals and food supplements are preparations of substances commonly found in the diet, such as fish oils, or occurring naturally in the body, e.g. co-enzyme Q_{10}. In the UK, many herbal products, e.g. garlic tablets, are sold as dietary/food supplements.

Traditional Chinese Medicine (TCM)

An ancient Chinese method of health care which coexists alongside orthodox medicine today. TCM includes a range of therapies, such as Chinese massage, but is best known for the practices of traditional Chinese acupuncture (see below) and traditional Chinese herbal medicine (CHM). The basic concepts of TCM ('yin-yang' and the 'five elements') apply to CHM. The fundamental principle of treatment is to restore 'balance and harmony'. Medicinal substances are classified as having particular attributes, e.g. hot, cold, tonifying, moistening and it is the consideration and combining of these attributes during therapy that is thought to bring about balance to patterns of clinical dysfunction. For example, 'cooling' herbs would be used to treat a patient whose pattern of illness is described as 'hot'. Usually, herbal formulae comprising around 4–12 different medicinal substances are used to treat specific clinical patterns. Substances used as part of traditional Chinese medicine may include animal as well as herbal material.

Therapies not using medicinal substances

Acupuncture

This involves insertion of needles into a specific point or set of points on the body for the treatment of specific conditions. Various forms exist, such as auriculoacupuncture (needling of specific points on the ear) and electroacupuncture (electrical stimulation of inserted needles). The two main types practised in the UK are described below.

Medical acupuncture: usually practised by doctors who have trained in acupuncture and who use the therapy alongside conventional medicine. Insertion of needles is given as far as possible according to the principles of neurophysiology and anatomy (i.e. directed at stimulating nerve endings).

Traditional Chinese acupuncture: part of the broader system of traditional Chinese medicine (TCM). Traditional Chinese acupuncturists aim to restore the balance of energy in the body by 'unblocking meridians' (pathways along which life energy is believed to flow) by inserting needles strategically in specific points along meridians.

Chiropractic

Chiropractors believe that misaligned or maladjusted vertebrae ('subluxations'), caused by accidents, strains, poor posture, innate skeletal distortions, etc., affect the spine and surrounding muscles, nerves and ligaments. This is believed to result in local or radiating pain, affecting joint movement, and causing swelling or weakening of muscle groups, thereby contributing to the disease process. There is, as yet, no clear explanation from current knowledge of spinal mechanics and neurophysiology how this might happen.

Chiropractic diagnosis includes physical examination, palpation of the vertebral column, assessment of posture, etc. and often the use of X-rays to examine bone alignment and to detect conditions such as osteoporosis which would contraindicate manipulative treatment. The principal technique used in chiropractic is a series of short sharp thrusts aimed at restoring normal joint motion, correcting subluxations, improving posture and/or removing painful stimulation to the nerves. Generally, chiropractors manipulate the neck and spine.

Healing

A transmission of 'therapeutic energy' between healer and patient, which may or may not be associated with particular religious beliefs. Can be performed at a distance ('distant healing') or by laying on of hands ('therapeutic touch').

Osteopathy

Osteopaths believe that a wide variety of disorders can be traced to disorders of the musculoskeletal system, particularly the spinal vertebrae, but also to dysfunction in certain muscle groups. Manipulative techniques are used to correct these joint and tissue disturbances to restore normal bodily function. Osteopaths use a detailed medical history, physical examination, assessment of posture, observation of patient movement, etc. and, occasionally, X-rays in diagnosis. Direct techniques (soft tissue and joint movement, and high-velocity thrusts) and indirect techniques (positioning-type techniques where the joints are moved without force) are used in treatment. Generally osteopaths use more rhythmical and gentler pressure on the whole body, including the spine, whereas chiropractors tend to use more sharp, short, thrusting pressure on the spine.

Reflexology (also known as reflex therapy)

A form of treatment and diagnosis which involves massage of specific points on the feet (mainly on the soles but also on the tops and sides – maps of the areas of the feet corresponding to different areas/organs of the body have been drawn up). It is based on the belief that there are reflexes in the feet for all parts of the body. Reflexologists claim to be able to identify sites of tenderness and 'lumps' or granules of crystalline material, which, in reflexology, are taken to represent remote organ disease. Manual stimulation of the reflex points is believed to break down the deposits so that they can be eliminated, and to increase the flow of 'healing energy' through 'channels'. At present, these theories are unsubstantiated.

(Continued)

Therapies using both medicinal substances and other treatment

Anthroposophical medicine

A philosophical vision of health and disease based on the work of Rudolf Steiner who explored how man's soul and spiritual nature relate to the health and function of the body. Steiner viewed each person as having four 'bodies' or 'forces': physical, etheric, astral, spiritual. Practitioners of anthroposophy aim to understand illness in terms of how these four elements interact; the aim of treatment is to stimulate the natural healing forces of the body. The anthroposophic approach is a holistic one; practitioners may use a range of therapies including diet, therapeutic movement (eurhythmy) and artistic therapies as well as anthroposophic medicines in an integrated therapeutic programme. The medicines are derived mainly from plant and mineral sources; many are combinations of herbal ingredients. Particular attention is paid to the source and methods of farming used in growing raw plant materials for preparing anthroposophic medicines (e.g. organic culture only).

Ayurvedic medicine

The traditional system of medicine of India. Its essence is to achieve and maintain balance between the 'elements' and 'energies'; illness is believed to result from imbalance. Ayurvedic diagnosis is based on physical observation and questioning. Treatment usually involves Ayurvedic herbal remedies, as well as dietary modifications, meditation, exercise, massage. The medicines are herbal/mineral preparations; heavy metals (e.g. lead, arsenic) are sometimes used in the manufacturing process.

collectively referred to as complementary (or 'alternative') medicines. As well as being used by some CAM practitioners in their practice, these types of products are widely available for purchase for self-treatment. Many of these are administered or recommended after consultation with therapists with varying range of abilities and qualifications, or simply bought by patients believing that they will be beneficial. In the UK, patients, the public, the media and many other groups consider the use of herbal medicines (whether prescribed by a herbalist or purchased over the counter), to be part of CAM. However, there is a view that herbal medicinal products with documented pharmacological activity and clinical efficacy lie alongside conventional medicines. Indeed, some herbal medicines, such as senna preparations, are conventional medicines.

This chapter discusses CAM, mainly from a UK perspective. In particular, the extent of use, and regulatory aspects of CAM are considered, as well as issues of importance to pharmacy and pharmacists. There is a particular emphasis on complementary medicines, as these are widely available in pharmacies, and especially on 'European' herbal medicines, as these are among the most widely used 'complementary medicines' in the UK. Also, from a biomedical perspective, herbal medicines (rather than, e.g. homeopathy) are likely to have the greatest potential in terms of both benefits and risks.

Extent of use of CAM

The use of CAM is a popular healthcare approach in developed countries, and there is evidence that use of complementary therapies and complementary medicines is increasing.

Over the last 10 years, a number of surveys of the use of CAM in patients suffering from serious disease states such as cancers, cardiovascular and inflammatory bowel diseases has shown that involvement in decision-making about the use of CAM and about changes in lifestyle health practices also appear to help survivor's emotional health related quality of life.

Market research by Mintel in 2009 estimated that retail sales of herbal medicines, would be worth £181 million by 2014, whereas sales of homoeopathic remedies would rise to £54 million, and aromatherapy oils to £47 million by 2014. Around 50% of sales of herbal medicines and homoeopathic remedies are made in pharmacies. Mintel have estimated that 12 million people in the UK population took CAM during 2009. Self-treatment using CAM remedies raises the issue of the cause of any beneficial effects, as many of these are practiced as holistic therapies, which is not the case when simply purchasing medicinal products.

The use of CAM is not limited to the private sector, in some cases, the NHS funds access. For example, there are now four NHS homoeopathic hospitals in the UK, to which GPs can refer their patients.

Table 24.1 Trends in homoeopathic prescribing on the NHS

Year	Number of items	Net cost (£)
1998	150 000	927 000
2004	94 500	661 400
2005	83 000	593 000
2007	49 300	321 300
2009	19 000	100 500
2011	15 500	130 600

Source: http://www.ic.nhs.uk/statistics-and-data-collections/primary-care/prescriptions.

Also, GPs can prescribe homoeopathic preparations on NHS prescriptions. In 1998, over 150 000 homoeopathic items were dispensed against NHS prescriptions; data from the Prescription Pricing Authority show that the net ingredient cost for these was £927 600. Since that year, there appears to have been a downward trend in NHS dispensing, dropping to 15 500 items in 2011, presumably as a result of increasing cost consciousness (see Table 24.1). Furthermore, a survey reported by Thomas et al. (2001) estimated that in 1998, there were over 2 million visits to complementary therapists funded by the NHS, and that the NHS expenditure on CAM was £50–55 million per year. However, it has been claimed that many people who might like to take advantage of a wide range of CAM, are prevented from doing so by lack of resources, as only 10% of CAM is currently provided by the NHS.

Reasons for use of CAM

Symptoms and conditions

Complementary medicines are used by the general public and by patients both for general health maintenance and for the relief of minor, self-limiting conditions. For example, studies involving pharmacists and customers have suggested that herbal products to help relieve stress and sleep problems are those most frequently requested by pharmacy customers and recommended by pharmacists to customers following consultations.

Use of complementary medicines is not necessarily limited to symptoms or conditions suitable for OTC treatment. Indeed, many patients use complementary medicines and complementary therapies for symptom relief in, or treatment of, serious chronic illnesses, such as cancer, HIV/AIDS, multiple sclerosis, rheumatological conditions, asthma, depression, gastroenterological disorders, skin conditions and so on. Use of CAM is usually (but not always) to supplement conventional health care, rather than to replace it. Special patient groups also use CAM, including the elderly and women who are pregnant or breast-feeding. It is also used by some parents/guardians for children in their care.

A number of surveys of CAM users have been carried out; frequently females have been shown to have higher use than males and usage tends to be greater between 35 and 64 years, and in higher social classes. One survey of the use of CAM, mainly herbal products and nutraceuticals, in over 60 000 elderly patients, revealed extensive use for a range of medical conditions, a number of which would normally be expected to be treated by conventional medicines (Table 24.2).

Beliefs, perceptions and attitudes

There are numerous reasons why people choose to use complementary medicines and therapies. They include dissatisfaction with conventional medicine in terms of effectiveness and/or safety; satisfaction with CAM, and the perception that it is 'safe'; as well as more complex reasons that are associated with cultural and personal beliefs, views on life and health, and experiences with conventional healthcare professionals and CAM practitioners.

An individual's choice to use CAM approaches is tied in with 'healthcare pluralism' – people may use any of several treatment options, such as taking advice from family and friends, consulting a CAM practitioner and consulting a pharmacist, GP or other healthcare professional. Related issues include whether individuals disclose CAM use to conventional healthcare professionals, and whether there is better compliance with CAM treatment regimens than with conventional drug regimens.

Table 24.2 Levels of use of a number of herbal and nutraceutical products for treating a range of medical conditions

Medical condition	Use among participants (%)	Herbal/ nutraceutical product
Prostate cancer	4.5	Saw palmetto
	1.2	Lycopene
	0.7	DHEA
Enlarged prostate	18.3	Saw palmetto
	1.6	Lycopene
	1.4	Cranberry
Osteoarthritis	28.7	Glucosamine
	19.9	Chondroitin
	6.2	MSM
Bladder infections	5.8	Cranberry
Neck, back, or joint pain	16.6	Glucosamine
	10.5	Chondroitin
	4.5	MSM
Depression	5.8	St John's wort
Lactose intolerance	0.9	Lycopene
Degenerative eye conditions	4.2	Lutein
Perimenopause	4.9	Black cohosh
	1.7	Dong quai
	6.7	Soy products
Stress	3.2	St John's wort
Memory loss	9.6	Ginkgo biloba
	7.1	Fish oil
	6.0	Coenzyme Q_{10}
Insomnia	3.6	Melatonin
Diabetes	0.2	Dong quai[a]
	0.3	Lycopene
High blood pressure	0.3	Dong quai[a]

Reprinted from the *Journal of the American Dietetic Association*, Gunther S, Patterson RE, Kristal AR, Stratton KL, White E. Demographic and health-related correlates of herbal and specialty supplement use. 2004; 104(1):27–34, with permission from the American Dietetic Association.
[a] *Angelica sinensis* root. MSM, methylsulfonylmethane.

Regulation of CAM

CAM practitioners

There are around 40 000 complementary practitioners in the UK. These practitioners are using either medicinal products, alternative techniques or both.

With the exception of osteopaths and chiropractors (who are regulated by the General Osteopathic Council and the General Chiropractic Council), CAM practitioners are not legally required to undertake any training before practising. While most CAM practitioners will have trained in their chosen therapy, others may not – or may have trained in one complementary therapy, but practise several. Furthermore, there is wide variation in the level of training and methods of assessment. For the major therapies such as acupuncture, homoeopathy, herbal medicine, osteopathy and chiropractic, training is generally highly developed, with many institutions having university affiliation and offering courses at degree level, although the validity of this has been widely questioned in the media. However, training for other complementary therapies is less intensive and more disparate.

The estimate of numbers of CAM practitioners is based on membership of CAM organizations, but cannot be precise, as some practitioners are registered with more than one organization and some are not registered at all. Generally, practitioners are members of a registering or accrediting body, although criteria for membership vary widely. Also, many complementary therapies have several registering organizations, although some disciplines are taking steps to become unified under one regulatory body.

The practice of complementary therapies is not limited to CAM practitioners – some conventional healthcare professionals including pharmacists practise CAM. Some institutions offer specialized courses for conventional healthcare professionals, and there are registering organizations which represent state-registered healthcare professionals who have undertaken training in and practise certain complementary therapies. For example, the British Medical Acupuncture Society represents medically qualified individuals with training in acupuncture.

Against this background, the House of Lords (2000) report on CAM included several recommendations regarding training and regulation of CAM practitioners, including conventional healthcare professionals who practise CAM. In summary, these recommendations were:

- Regulatory bodies of healthcare professionals should develop guidelines on competence and training in CAM
- Statutory regulation of CAM practitioners, particularly acupuncture and herbal medicine, and possibly non-medical homoeopathy; a Herbal Medicines Regulation Working Group has been set up to take the process forward for Herbal Medicines
- Training for CAM practitioners should be standardized, independently accredited and include basic biomedical science.

The issue of training also relates to staff employed in retail outlets, e.g. health-food stores, which sell a vast range of complementary medicines, who sell or advise on complementary medicines. A small study has suggested that information and advice given by health-food store staff may not always be appropriate or balanced.

Complementary medicines

The majority of complementary health products are not licensed as medicines and, therefore, evidence of their quality, efficacy and safety has not been assessed by the competent authority which, in the UK, is the Medicines and Healthcare Products Regulatory Agency (MHRA).

Herbal medicines

Herbal products are available on the UK market as licensed herbal medicines, herbal medicines exempt from licensing and unlicensed herbal products sold as food supplements. In several cases, the same herb is available in all three categories. Potentially hazardous plants are controlled as Prescription Only Medicines (POM) and certain others are subject to dose (but not duration of treatment) and route of administration restrictions, or can only be supplied via a pharmacy and by, or under the supervision of, a pharmacist.

Most licensed herbal products were initially granted a product licence of right (PLR) because they were already on the market when the licensing system was introduced in the 1970s. When PLRs were reviewed, manufacturers of herbal products

intended for use in minor self-limiting conditions were permitted to rely on bibliographical evidence to support efficacy and safety, rather than being required to carry out new controlled clinical trials, so, many licensed herbal medicinal products have not necessarily undergone stringent testing.

Herbal products exempt from licensing are those compounded and supplied by herbalists on their own recommendation, those consisting solely of dried, crushed or comminuted (fragmented) plants (i.e. they must not contain any non-herbal 'active' ingredients) sold under their botanical name and with no written recommendations for use, and those made by the holder of a specials manufacturing licence. This category was initially intended to give herbalists the flexibility to prepare remedies for their patients. However, manufacturers can legally sell products under this exemption. Furthermore, at present, there is no statutory regulation of herbalists in the UK, although this is under review.

The majority of herbal products are sold as food supplements without making medical claims and are regulated under food, not pharmaceutical, legislation. In the UK, the MHRA has the statutory power to decide whether a specific product satisfies the definition of a relevant 'medicinal product' and, therefore, is subject to the provisions of regulations relating to Medicines for Human Use Regulations. If a product is determined to be a relevant medicinal product, and if it does not meet criteria for exemption, then the manufacturer is required to submit an application for a full product licence and/or remove the product from the market. The procedure allows for the company to request a review of the decision. In this case, the views of an independent panel, the Independent Review Panel on Borderline Products, are taken into consideration.

Manufacturers of licensed medicines, including licensed herbal products, are required to satisfy the MHRA that their products are made according to the principles of good manufacturing practice (GMP), good agricultural practice (GAP) and good collection practice (GCP). While some established manufacturers of unlicensed herbal products also manufacture their products to GMP standards, others do not, and there is no guarantee that such products are of suitable pharmaceutical quality. The quality of plant raw materials can be affected by several factors and, therefore, it is important that finished (marketed) herbal products are of suitable quality. The *European Pharmacopoeia* 7th edn. (2010) contains over 232 monographs on herbal drugs, and examples are in preparation.

'Ethnic' medicines available in the UK include traditional Chinese medicines (TCM) and Ayurvedic medicines (see Box 24.2). Such products are subject to the same legislation as 'Western' complementary medicines. In the UK, there are further restrictions on certain toxic herbal ingredients, namely *Aristolochia* species, found in some TCM products, and on other herbal ingredients that may be confused with toxic herbal ingredients. In addition to containing non-herbal ingredients such as animal parts and/or minerals, some manufactured ('patent') TCM products have been found to contain conventional drugs as listed ingredients, some of which (e.g. glibenclamide) may have POM status in the UK. Non-herbal active ingredients of any type cannot legally be included in unlicensed herbal remedies, and inclusion of drugs with POM status represents an additional infringement of UK medicines legislation. For some ingredients, such as certain animal parts, restrictions under the Convention on International Trade in Endangered Species of Wild Fauna and Flora (CITES) also apply.

Prior to 2004, it was widely considered that the system of licensing for herbal medicines did not give consumers adequate protection against poor quality and unsafe unlicensed products, nor did it allow manufacturers to provide appropriate information to inform consumers' choice of products. Against this background, a new European Union (EU) directive (2004/24/EC) was proposed which aims to establish a harmonized legislative framework for authorizing the marketing of traditional herbal medicinal products. The directive requires EU member states to set up a specified simplified registration procedure for traditional herbal medicinal products which could not fulfil medicines licensing criteria. Under this EU directive, all manufactured traditional medicinal herbal products are required to be registered under the Traditional Herbal Medicines Registration Scheme (THMRS). This directive has been in force since October 2005, but there was a transition period of 5 years from that date for manufacturers to meet the requirements. This has now lapsed. Some of the main features of this are that manufacturers will be required to provide:

- Evidence that the herb has been used traditionally in the EU for at least 30 years (15 years' non-EU use will be taken into account)

- Bibliographic data on safety with an expert report
- Quality dossier demonstrating manufacture according to principles of good manufacturing practice (GMP).

Under this directive, it is not possible to make claims about the product's efficacy, but only regarding its traditional use. The new directive is not a route to licensing for herbal POMs or for traditional herbal medicines that can be licensed by the conventional route. As it stands, the proposed directive would accommodate ethnic medicines that have been used in the UK (or any other member state) for at least 15 years. This directive also lists problematic consequences of imported US products and restricted herbs.

EU Directive 2004/24/EC also gives guidance on permitted medicinal indications. Labelling may also be covered by the Joint Health Claims Initiative (JHCI), which restricts excessive claims.

Homoeopathic remedies

In the UK, homoeopathic remedies are subject to medicines legislation. A simplified registration scheme (Simplified Scheme) exists in the UK (and the rest of the EU) for homoeopathic medicinal products, which:

- Are intended for oral or external use
- Are sufficiently dilute (usually a minimum dilution of 1 in 10 000) and
- No medical claims are made.

Since 1 September 2006, new homeopathic products may be registered under The National Rules Scheme. For such products, manufacturers are required to demonstrate quality and safety, and evidence for their therapeutic applications derived from provings, together with appropriate product labelling and product literature. Manufacturers of homoeopathic medicinal products which are administered parenterally, are below the minimum dilution, or make efficacy claims are required to substantiate this in the same manner that is required for conventional drugs.

Other complementary medicines

Products marketed as food or dietary supplements include non-herbal substances, such as glucosamine, vitamins, minerals and fish oils. These products are sold under food legislation and are marketed without medical claims. Such products may be deemed to be a relevant medicinal product (see 'Herbal medicines', above). Some 'supplements' are subject to stringent restrictions on their use. Melatonin is a prescription-only medicine. However, in the USA, melatonin is sold as a food supplement. A new draft EU directive is aimed at harmonizing the marketing of food supplements in member states.

Gamma-linolenic acid (GLA), widely available as unfractionated evening primrose oil, was widely used as a supplement, principally for pre-menstrual syndrome, but later obtained a full product licence for two medicines, for psoriasis and mastalgia, although these were withdraw in 1995.

Essential oils used by aromatherapists in their practice for medicinal purposes are considered to be medicinal products, but are exempt from licensing provided they meet certain criteria (see 'Herbal medicines' above). Aromatherapy products sold through retail outlets are not subject to licensing regulations unless they are marketed as medicinal products. Some essential oils are available as licensed medicinal products, e.g. peppermint oil capsules, although such products are conventional medicines, not aromatherapy products. These examples highlight the possible confusion for both pharmacists and patients.

Pharmacy and provision of CAM

Pharmacies and pharmacists have several roles in the provision of CAM. Community pharmacies are a major source of complementary medicines for people who purchase and self-treat with these products, and pharmacists may be asked for information and advice on self-treatment with complementary medicines. In addition, community pharmacists may be presented with NHS prescriptions for homoeopathic medicines. Some independent pharmacies provide consulting rooms that are available for use on a sessional basis by CAM practitioners. Also, there are several community pharmacies which specialize in CAM, e.g. homoeopathic pharmacies which offer professional homoeopathic pharmaceutical services.

Pharmacists' involvement with CAM is not limited to the community. Pharmacists employed in NHS homoeopathic hospitals provide pharmaceutical services in the pharmacy and on the wards.

Pharmacists employed in conventional NHS hospitals may be involved with the supply of certain complementary medicines.

Pharmacists' training in CAM

In September 1999, the Science Committee of the RPS set-up a working group on complementary and alternative medicine to examine issues in this area of importance to pharmacy and pharmacists.

Pharmacists' involvement in the provision of CAM at any level raises several issues, particularly with regard to pharmacists' knowledge of and training in CAM, their professional accountability, and the quality, safety and efficacy of complementary medicines sold or supplied. The GPhC's Standards of conduct, ethics and performance states that pharmacists providing homoeopathic or herbal medicines or other complementary therapies have a professional responsibility:

- To ensure that stocks of homoeopathic or herbal medicines or other complementary therapies are obtained from a reputable source of supply
- Not to recommend any remedy where they have any reason to doubt its safety or quality
- Only to offer advice on homoeopathic or herbal medicines or other complementary therapies or medicines if they have undertaken suitable training or have specialized knowledge.

Almost all pharmacies sell complementary medicines, particularly herbal medicines and homoeopathic remedies, and the majority of pharmacists are asked for and 'recommend' specific complementary medicines. However, the extent of teaching on pharmacognosy (the scientific discipline which covers the chemistry, biological and clinical effects of natural products, particularly plants) and herbal and complementary medicines in the MPharm programme is limited. Furthermore, the majority of practising pharmacists have not undertaken training in areas of CAM.

Pharmacists' training in CAM should not be limited to complementary medicines. It should include an awareness of the background to, evidence for and safety concerns with regard to complementary therapies, such as acupuncture. This is because patients' use of such treatments may have implications for pharmaceutical care. For example, research involving community pharmacists in the USA has suggested that some patients with chronic conditions temporarily or permanently use complementary therapies instead of their prescribed medicines, and it has also been shown to have an effect during surgical operations. Another major problem of self-prescribed CAM is lack of professional diagnosis.

Pharmacists' professional practice

At present, pharmacists' professional practice with regard to complementary medicines is not optimal – many pharmacists do not routinely ask customers and patients specifically about their use of complementary medicines, nor record such use on patient medication records. Pharmacists are encouraged to apply principles of good professional practice with regard to complementary medicines, and to be aware that patients' use of complementary medicines may have implications for pharmaceutical care. For example, it is possible that patients may use complementary medicines in addition to, or instead of, conventional medicines, without telling their doctor or pharmacist. The concurrent use of complementary medicines, particularly herbal medicines, and conventional drugs is of concern, as there is a potential for interactions to occur. For example, important interactions have been documented between St John's wort and certain prescribed medicines, including warfarin, digoxin, theophylline, ciclosporin, HIV protease inhibitors, anticonvulsants and oral contraceptives. Many other examples have been reported.

The role of the pharmacist in reporting suspected adverse drug reactions (ADRs) associated with herbal medicines has been recognized by the MHRA. The MHRA Yellow Card scheme for ADR reporting includes reporting by all community and hospital pharmacists (see Ch. 51), and more recently members of the general public have been allowed to report. Community pharmacists are asked by the MHRA to concentrate on areas of limited reporting by doctors, namely conventional OTC medicines and herbal products. The Yellow Card scheme also applies to unlicensed herbal products and, while the MHRA do not formally request reports of suspected ADRs associated with other types of unlicensed products, it is unlikely that MHRA would ignore a genuine report of a serious suspected ADR associated with a non-herbal unlicensed product.

Efficacy and safety of CAM approaches

It is beyond the scope of this chapter to consider evidence for the efficacy and safety of individual complementary medicines and complementary therapies. Evidence from randomized controlled trials for the efficacy of complementary therapies for specific conditions is rare, but a search of the Cochrane Library database reveals varying evidence of efficacy for a range of CAM products.

This is not to say that such approaches are not efficacious, but that for many, rigorous research has not been carried out. There are several reasons for this, including a lack of research funding for and research infrastructure in CAM.

Similarly, CAM is often assumed to be 'safe', but this assumption is not based on appropriate studies. In fact, some complementary therapies have been associated with serious adverse effects. In addition, formal spontaneous reporting schemes (i.e. similar to the MHRA Yellow Card scheme for adverse drug reaction reporting) do not exist for 'manual' complementary therapies, such as acupuncture, chiropractice and osteopathy.

The relative lack of research in CAM means that there is also a lack of evidence-based information on which to base treatment decisions for specific patients. Nevertheless, there are several sources of information in CAM, including specialist databases and specialist fields within established databases, as well as several reference texts written by pharmacists which have summarized and critiqued the available evidence in areas of CAM (see Further reading, Appendix 4). The MHRA publishes a number of documents detailing herbal safety, such as lists of intrinsically toxic constituents of herbal ingredients, quality related issues, herb-drug interactions, and precautions in specific patient groups.

The future for complementary medicines

On the basis of current trends in market research data, it has been predicted that sales of complementary medicines will continue to increase. Longitudinal data on the utilization of complementary therapists are not available for the UK, although increasing numbers of such practitioners may suggest increasing public demand for holistic treatment with these therapies. In addition, the increasingly widespread marketing and sales of these products demonstrates the interest of large sections of the public to control their health by using these products.

With the EU directive on traditional herbal medicinal products, the future is set to bring improved quality standards for these preparations – manufacturers will need to meet standards for GMP, or remove their products from the market. Initiatives involving ethnic medicines are also aimed at improving quality standards for these preparations. However, as this sector is less developed in the UK, it is likely that improvements in the quality of ethnic medicines will be seen over a longer time period.

Improvements in quality standards, together with other requirements in the traditional herbal medicinal products directive, will put an increased emphasis on manufacturers to provide evidence supporting the safety of their products. At the same time, the increasing use of herbal medicines, particularly by patients using conventional drugs and those with serious chronic illness, may result in the emergence of new safety concerns, such as indications of uncommon ADRs, those occurring with long-term use and interactions with conventional medicines.

Against a background of widespread and increasing use of CAM, it is recognized that CAM practitioners need to be regulated, and that conventional healthcare professionals need to be knowledgeable about complementary medicines and therapies. The House of Lords' Select Committee on Science and Technology's report on CAM made several recommendations with regard to statutory regulation of those who practise CAM, and these recommendations were accepted by the government in 2001. Thus, it is now required that conventional healthcare professionals should have a basic knowledge of complementary medicines and therapies.

In its response to the House of Lords' report, the government stated that if a therapy gains a critical mass of evidence, the NHS and the medical profession should ensure that the public has access to that therapy. Thus, in addition to homoeopathic treatment, which is already available through the NHS, certain complementary therapies and licensed complementary medicines with a sound evidence base may also be available on NHS prescriptions.

In the long term, the future for complementary medicines, particularly herbal medicines and nutraceuticals, may lie with pharmacogenetics and pharmacogenomics. These relatively new fields of research are widely held to be central to the discovery of new drugs and to the future of therapeutics, yet the pharmacogenetics of ADRs, and optimizing treatment on the basis of a patient's genotype, has not been discussed in the context of herbal medicines. It is reasonable to assume that individuals with a different genetic profile will have different responses to complementary medicines as well as to conventional drugs.

The distrust of traditional CAM in the 1970s and 1980s has of course been followed by not only increased public awareness of their possible benefits, but also by major investigation by pharmaceutical companies, and government and institutional researchers. This has led to recent (in terms of the historical development of conventional medicine) development of single product plant medicines, such as galantamine (*Narcissus* cultivars), atracurium (intermediate from *Leontice leotopetalum*), artesunate and artemether (*Artemesia* spp.) and taxol (*Taxus* spp.), with the prospect of more chemical entities being derived from CAM.

KEY POINTS

- The use of complementary/alternative therapies, particularly herbal medicines, is widespread and appears to be increasing
- Most community pharmacies sell complementary medicines, particularly herbal medicines and nutraceuticals, and many pharmacists are asked for advice on such products
- Hospital pharmacists may also encounter patients who use complementary medicines
- The use of complementary medicines may have implications for pharmaceutical care, e.g. drug interactions can occur
- Most complementary medicines currently are sold as unlicensed products, so evidence of their quality, safety and efficacy has not been assessed by the MHRA
- Other than for osteopaths and chiropractors, there is at present no statutory regulation of practitioners of complementary therapies, including those using medicinal substances

Communication skills: advice and information on the selection of medicines

Judith A. Rees

- The rationale and need for giving information and advice
- Situations suitable for pharmaceutical information and advice
- Assessing the need for giving information and advice
- How to decide on the content and method of giving information and advice
- Aids to information and advice giving

Introduction

Pharmacists have always provided information and advice on the use of medicines. The Nuffield Report (1968) recognized that there were 'some categories of individuals who certainly will need advice, help and encouragement in the handling of their medicines' and that 'anyone who has to rely on a continuous drug regime, should be a candidate for additional support and help from pharmacies'. These statements highlight the traditional role of the pharmacist in the provision of advice to patients/customers.

The NHS Plan 2000 in the UK outlined the need for pharmacists to become more involved in helping patients to get the best from their medicines. The aim was to 'Give patients the confidence that they are getting good advice when they consult a pharmacist'. The introduction of MURs and the new medicine service (NMS), further develops the pharmacists role in advice and information giving. Other examples of advice giving by pharmacists include when handing out prescription medicines, selling OTC medicines, on hospital discharge and during medication reviews.

Medicines research has led to the production of new, effective drugs formulated in many specialised dosage forms, such as modified-release formulations, aerosols, patches, nail lacquers, etc. which utilize conventional and other absorption routes (e.g. percutaneous, nasal and vaginal) (see Ch. 29). Often these medicines are packaged in specialized containers, for example aerosols for rectal use, self-administration parenteral products, metered-dose nasal sprays. These developments mean that pharmacists are in an excellent position to provide advice to patients/consumers on how to correctly use/administer these medicines in as safe a manner as possible.

What is information and advice giving in pharmacy?

Patients and customers have a right to be involved in the decisions about their treatment and their use and choice of medicines (see Ch. 18). Thus, pharmacists require effective communication skills to be able to identify the individual needs of a patient/customer and to determine the type and amount of advice and level of explanation appropriate to provide at that particular time.

The BNF uses the term 'counselling' rather than advice in individual monographs to detail the type of advice to be given to a patient. Such advice is above that required on the label of a dispensed product and usually involves unusual/complicated methods or times of administration or the potential interaction with foods. For example, bulk-forming laxatives have the counselling statement, 'Preparations that swell in contact with liquid should always be carefully swallowed with water and should not be taken immediately before going to bed'.

The need for information and advice giving

It has been estimated that up to 50% of older people do not take their medicines as intended. Similarly, 50% of patients (not necessarily older people) with hypertension fail to take their medicines correctly. Thus, it has been suggested that advice by pharmacists could lead to better compliance and hence less therapeutic failure and possible death.

The aims of information and advice

Pharmacists in their patient-advising roles may adapt and make use of the problem-solving model of counselling developed by Egan (1990).

Thus the aims, in addition to the provision of advice, could be to:

- Encourage patients to identify any problems they perceive with medicines and also any solutions to these problems
- Encourage patients to develop their own action plan for taking/using medicines correctly
- Gain an understanding of the patient's perspective
- Respect the patient's beliefs and be non-judgemental of their use (or non-use) of medicines.

Opportunities for giving information and advice

The pharmacist is often the last healthcare professional whom a patient sees before starting drug therapy. It is at this stage that the pharmacist should identify the information and advice needs of the patient. Pharmacists should take a prominent and proactive role. The opportunities for giving information and advice to patients are many, but the main opportunity is at the end of the

dispensing process, the sale of a medicine, during a MUR or NMS opportunity (see Ch. 14).

No patient should receive a dispensed medicine without the pharmacist making an assessment of the needs of the patient. The availability of PMRs and the information contained within them will underpin the extent and type of information and advice provided to an individual patient.

The sale of medicines from a community pharmacy can be the result of: (a) a direct request for a named medicine by a customer and (b) a request for advice on the treatment of a symptom or minor ailment by a patient. The amount and content of the information and advice given to a patient will vary with the type of initial request, the medicine sold and the patient.

Thus, the opportunities for community pharmacists to become involved in patient advice are wide ranging. Other possible areas include:

- During domiciliary visiting
- Visits to care/residential/nursing homes
- Public health (see Ch. 13)
- Dietary advice
- Emergency supply of medicines
- Special weeks/days, e.g. Asthma Week, Breast Awareness Week, Stop Smoking Day
- Pet medicines (see Ch. 28).

Similarly, there are many opportunities for hospital pharmacists. Inpatients may require advice on their medicines during admission and should be made fully aware of any alterations in their medication on discharge. Outpatients will, also, require advice on newly prescribed medicines.

Pharmacists may be involved in providing medication to patients in long-term residential homes. In such situations it may be necessary to give information and advice to both the patient and/or their carers.

How to provide information and advice

Information and advice giving, wherever it occurs, should take place in a thoughtful, structured way. The pharmacist must possess not only a sound knowledge of the drugs and appliances being dispensed or sold, but also excellent communication skills. Pharmacists should be able to provide information and advice in a non-paternalistic way that allows the patient to ask questions in order to understand the information, so that they can make decisions about their own treatment and care. Pharmacists must have the ability to explain information clearly and unambiguously and in language the recipient can understand. They must know the right questions and how to ask them and, most importantly, they must know how to listen. For information and advice giving to be successful, it must be a two-way process. Rapport is built-up between the pharmacist and the patient and a much more meaningful dialogue can take place.

The Cambridge–Calgary model (see Chs 17 and 18) details how to provide explanations to patients. It is important to provide the correct amount and type of information:

- Chunks and checks. The information needs to be given in suitable bite-sized chunks. Observation of patient response should indicate whether the chunks are too small or too large and thus further chunks of information can be adjusted to suit the patient.
- Assess the patient's starting point. How much do they know? This should be assessed early on in the session.
- Ask patients what information would be helpful. For example, a patient may be more concerned about the immediate effects of the drug on their lifestyle rather than the long term.
- Give explanations at an appropriate time. Avoid giving advice or information prematurely.

To help the patient recall and understand the advice/information that you provide, the pharmacist should:

- Organize the explanation. Try to develop a logical sequences and discrete sections – do not combine information on side-effects with how to administer the medicine.
- Use signposting – in other words, if there are three points to get over, say so, and continue with first ..., second ..., etc.
- Use easily understood and concise language. Avoid using jargon, abbreviations and technical terms where possible.
- Use visual methods of explanation. Demonstration models of pharmaceutical packaging can be useful, e.g. aerosols.
- Check patient understanding at regular intervals. Ask the patient to explain to you or to demonstrate the use of a medicine.

What information to include

Each situation and each patient will have different information needs, but as a general summary, no patient who has been given medication should leave a community or hospital pharmacy without knowing:

- How to take or use the medicine
- When to take or use the medicine
- How much to take or use
- How long to continue to take or use
- What to expect, e.g. immediate relief, no effect for several days
- Why the medicine is being taken or used
- What to do if something goes wrong, e.g. if a dose is missed
- How to recognize side-effects and minimize their incidence
- Lifestyle changes which need to be made
- Dietary changes which need to be made
- How to obtain further supplies of the medication if appropriate.

Who to give advice and information to

Not every patient will require information and advice but it is important that pharmacists can correctly identify those who do by, first, considering the medication.

A multiple-item prescription may present problems to the patient in terms of different drugs, different dosage forms and regimens, etc. Additionally, the individual medicine on any prescription, because of its characteristics, e.g. complex dosage regimen, special delivery methods, novel packaging, etc., may require explanation to ensure the patient has a clear understanding of how to use it.

Other reasons for giving advice/information will be if the drug has:

- A narrow therapeutic index. The need for strict adherence to dosing should be emphasized. Drugs such as lithium or theophylline are common examples
- The potential for interaction with another drug. (See Appendix 1 in the BNF.)
- The potential to cause side-effects. The patient should be told not only how to recognize

the side-effects, but also how to reduce the incidence or severity of them and what to do if they occur (see Table 25.1). Select the side-effects which are most likely to occur and advise on them

- A cautionary and advisory label (BNF Appendix 3) should be attached to the medicine. The information on these labels should always be reinforced.

Second, consider the patient. The level and type of information given and how it is given will depend on a variety of factors:

- Is the patient known at the pharmacy and have they been identified previously as having problems with drug therapy?

Table 25.1 Some drugs and the type of side-effects that can occur

Drug	Side-effect	Precaution
Some drugs cause side-effects which can be minimized by good management		
Chlorpromazine	Photosensitivity	Use sunscreen
NSAIDs	GI disturbances	Take with food
Tamoxifen	Nausea	Take at bedtime
Bisphosphonates	Oesophageal erosion	Take with plenty of water and then stand or sit upright for 30 min
Some drugs have side-effects which require the patient to be warned for their benefit		
CNS drugs	Drowsiness	
Co-beneldopa	Colours urine	
Some drugs have side-effects that need monitoring		
Penicillamine	Blood and urine tests	
Chloroquine	Ocular tests	
Some drugs have side-effects that require immediate reporting to the prescriber		
Gold therapy	Sore throat, breathlessness, rashes	
Aminosalicylates	Bleeding, bruising	

- What information/advice has the patient previously received?
- What are the patient's comprehension levels?
- What level of support does the patient need or have?
- The age of the patient. In general, all patients who are elderly should be offered information and advice. If the prescription is for a child, the parent or guardian should be given advice.
- Is the patient pregnant or breast-feeding? Such patients may require reassurance that the therapy is safe to take. Similarly, a breast-feeding mother may require advice on when to take the medication so that it least affects the child.
- Does the patient have physical disabilities? These could include mobility problems, causing problems in opening containers, blindness or deafness.
- Does the patient have mental disabilities? These could include states of confusion, anxiety or forgetfulness. Limited intellectual capacity could lead to patients being unable to read labels, etc. or understanding instructions.
- Known poor compliance/concordance.

Other instances which should alert the pharmacist to the need for advice/information would be:

- The purchase by a patient of an OTC product, which is incompatible with the prescribed medication, e.g. a patient with hypertension who is taking atenolol and wishes to purchase pseudoephedrine for nasal congestion.
- A patient asking for an item not to be dispensed. This could indicate that the patient is non-compliant with that medication.
- A patient asking to buy an OTC medicine which is to relieve the side-effects of a prescribed medicine. An example of this would be when a patient who is being prescribed NSAIDs asks for an indigestion remedy. This should be investigated.

Stages in the information/ advice giving process

If information and advice giving is approached in a structured manner, then the time will be used efficiently and there will be a greater likelihood of success. The following stages have been adapted from the guidelines on Counselling and Advice on

Medicines and Appliances in Community Pharmacy Practice produced by the Scottish Office Clinical Research and Audit Group:

- Recognizing the need for counselling
- Assessing and prioritizing the needs
- Specifying the assessment methods to be used
- Implementation
- Assessing the success of the process.

Recognizing the need for information and advice

The pharmacist will need to consider the content of the prescription and the characteristics of the patient.

Has the medicine been prescribed before for the patient?

A patient medication record can be very useful.

Are the instructions clear?

It is the pharmacist's responsibility to make sure that the patient knows what instructions such as 'when necessary' or 'as directed', mean. In the UK, the Human Medicines Regulations 2012, allow a pharmacist to put detailed directions onto a label where the prescriber has written 'as directed' on the prescription.

Assessing and prioritizing the needs

Although all individuals should be considered for information and advice, there will be some for whom little or none is required. For example, a customer who asks for an OTC by name and has used it successfully on several previous occasions may require minimal information and advice. Giving information and advice is time-consuming and so pharmacists should concentrate their time and efforts on those patients requiring it. Also, the pharmacist may have to be selective in what advice is given to a patient. The average number of facts which can be retained at any one time by most individuals is three. Box 25.1 illustrates this point.

Specifying assessment methods

It cannot be assumed that because the information and advice has been given, that the patient understands or is able to adhere to that advice. It is, therefore, important that, before embarking on

---

Box 25.1

Example of a medicine requiring several additional cautionary labels

A prescription for metronidazole tablets is received. According to the BNF, metronidazole tablets should be labeled with five additional cautionary labels.

These are given, with reasons below:

'*Do not drink alcohol*'. This is because, when combined with alcohol, a disulfiram-like reaction occurs and the patient may suffer nausea and vomiting. Patients who are not aware of this interaction may think, incorrectly, that the drug does not agree with them and stop taking it.

'*Space the doses evenly throughout the day. Keep taking this medicine until the course is finished, unless you are told to stop*'. Because of the antimicrobial effect of metronidazole, blood levels must be maintained and therapy must be continued for a minimum time period to prevent bacterial resistance developing.

'*Take with or just after food, or a meal*'. Metronidazole can cause GI irritation and the presence of food in the stomach will reduce the likelihood of this.

'*Swallow this medicine whole. Do not chew or crush*'. Metronidazole tablets are film coated which gives a degree of protection to the GI tract. If the preparation is chewed the coating will be destroyed, the drug will come into contact with the stomach lining and GI irritation will occur.

'*Take with a full glass of water*'. The film coating on the tablets may become sticky and if not taken with a reasonable draught of water can stick in the oesophagus. The drug will be released and could cause irritation to this least protected area of the GI tract.

A pharmacist giving verbal advice about metronidazole would vary the advice depending on their knowledge about patient, e.g. Does the patient have difficulty swallowing? Do they like a beer every evening? Are they a bit forgetful?

any information advice giving process, the pharmacist has an idea how the success of the process can be measured.

This assessment could consist of checking that the patient can read the label, use an inhaler device or open a container with a child-resistant cap. Checking on understanding may require follow-up, such as an enquiry the next time the patient visits the pharmacy, to ensure that no problems have occurred and the response to the therapy is as expected.

Implementation

The appearance of the pharmacy and pharmacist are important and it should be apparent that information and advice are offered as a professional service.

Lack of time is a major barrier to good information and advice giving. Patients should be given an indication of why you wish to speak to them and you should always check that they have the time to listen. If the patient is unknown to the pharmacist, it is important at the beginning of the conversation to try to gauge not just the amount of information that is needed but also the patient's level of comprehension. Is the patient fluent in the language or are they hard of hearing? The information/advice giving process must not be a monologue by the pharmacist, giving a long list of information points. There should be ample opportunity for the patient to ask questions.

Assessing the success of the process

Having given the information, it is then of major importance to check if the process has been successful. What does the patient understand? Can he use his device? Does he have any problems? The ideal, where possible, is to assess compliance/concordance through follow-up.

During the information and advice giving process, the pharmacist should check if the patient understands the information imparted. Watching the patient's body language and maintaining eye contact can give useful clues as to whether the message is being understood and whether compliance/concordance is likely.

Aids to information and advice giving

Patient information leaflets (PIL), warning cards and placebo devices are all useful aids when giving advice to patients. All patient packs of medicines contain a PIL. These should be used where appropriate and important points highlighted. Placebo devices can be used to demonstrate a particular technique and also to check a patient's ability to use a device. Leaflets on how to use ear drops, eye drops, eye ointment, pessaries, suppositories, a nebulizer, malaria tablets and head louse lotions are available. These, along with warning cards for anticoagulant therapy, lithium, monoamine oxidase inhibitors and steroids should be available in all pharmacies. The use of Braille labels and pictograms should be considered for the vision impaired and illiterate, respectively.

An example

The following example illustrates the wide variety of issues which have to be dealt with by pharmacists. It is not intended to be comprehensive, as different situations and different patients will produce a variety of problems and issues.

Recognize the need for information and advice

Mrs Myrtle has not been prescribed the tablets before, therefore drug name and dose timings should be given.

> **Example 25.1**
>
> Mrs Myrtle, a woman of about 50 years of age, presents a prescription for diclofenac sodium 25 mg tablets. She has lived alone for 2 years. When she is signing the back of her prescription she has difficulty holding the pen and complains that her hands and fingers are rather sore and stiff and hopes that the prescription will help. This is the first time she has had these tablets.

NSAIDs can cause GI irritation if not taken with or after food. The warning label which indicates this will need to be reinforced.

Mrs Myrtle appears to have problems with her hands. Will she be able to open a bottle with a child-resistant cap? She lives alone, so does not have anyone to help her.

Has she been buying any OTC medication to try to alleviate the pain in her hands? Some of the OTC products available for relief of arthritic pain contain diclofenac or other NSAIDs.

Mrs Myrtle will need to be advised to swallow the tablets whole and not to chew them. Will she be able to swallow them whole? Other formulations of diclofenac are available and may need to be considered for this patient.

Assessing and prioritizing the information and advice needs

Compliance problems

It is important to ensure that Mrs Myrtle can open the container and that she will have no difficulty swallowing the tablets.

Side-effects

It is vitally important to alert Mrs Myrtle to the fact that the tablets may irritate her stomach and how she can avoid this.

OTC purchases

To avoid any duplication of drug therapy it is important to find out if Mrs Myrtle is taking any OTC medicines, what they are, and make sure they are not going to cause any problems.

Timing of doses and duration of treatment

Mrs Myrtle should be told that the NSAID tablets should give pain relief within 1 week and successful anti-inflammatory action should be seen within 3 weeks. The drug must be taken at regular intervals.

A simple demonstration with a child resistant container will identify if she needs a container with a plain cap fitted. If swallowing is identified as a problem, she can be reassured that alternative therapy is available in liquid or granular form. It may then be necessary to contact the prescriber to alert him to this.

Any potential OTC problems can be dealt with by simple questioning.

Mrs Myrtle should be invited to let you know how she is getting on with her tablets and to contact you if she has any queries.

Conclusion

Develop the habit of thinking about medicines from the patient's point of view. What do patients need to know? What are their concerns about taking the medicine? What can be done to help patients resolve their concerns? Identifying information and advice giving points from the information at your disposal is fundamental to good pharmacy practice. It is important to remember, however, that asking questions and listening carefully to the information provided by patients is critical to the success of the process.

KEY POINTS

- Advice/information giving is an important part of the role of the pharmacist
- The prescription is a useful guide to possible information and advice needs of the patient
- The extent to which patients should be told about side-effects will vary from one patient to another
- It may be necessary to limit the amount of information given to avoid confusion
- Checking is important in ensuring patient understanding
- Information and advice giving is not a lecture – patients must be given the opportunity to ask questions

Patient charges for medicines and their impact on access

26

Ellen Schafheutle

STUDY POINTS

- Know the reasons for charging patients for (part of) their prescribed medicines
- Define the different types of co-payments for medicines
- Understand the effect of patient charges on uptake of medicines
- Differentiate between essential and less essential medicines, and the differing effect of charges on them
- Define patient groups that are likely to be most susceptible/vulnerable to the impact of medication cost
- Describe strategies patients use to manage or reduce medication cost
- Describe strategies healthcare professionals, especially pharmacists, can use to help patients cope with medication cost sharing issues

Introduction

Healthcare expenditure has been rising steadily over the past decades, and with the ever evolving advent of new technologies and treatments, this trend is likely to continue. In the developed world, payment for health care is usually covered by third-party payment systems to which the population (or members) contributes in the form of regular insurance premiums or taxes. However, paying for health care and medicines through such third-party providers removes the price barrier to consumption, as healthcare services become – or rather appear – free to the patient on access. Getting patients to contribute something when accessing health care, is seen as the reintroduction of such a price barrier, with the aim of deterring unnecessary access and medicines use, and thus reducing potential waste. Such contributions or payments borne by patients are commonly referred to as cost sharing, as they make a contribution to the actual cost of treatment. Besides creating a cost barrier to (unnecessary) demand, cost sharing also creates another form of revenue to the healthcare provider.

Cost sharing can be levied on some or all types of health care. In some countries, patients have to pay when visiting a doctor. In the UK, for example, patients have to contribute considerably towards dental and optical care, but visits to family doctors and hospitals are free. One particular form of cost sharing that is relatively easily defined, identified and implemented, is on prescribed medicines. The impact of this cost has been widely studied and is of particular interest to pharmacists, which is why it is the focus of this chapter.

Types of cost sharing arrangements

Essentially, there are three types of cost sharing for medicines, i.e. the cost the patient has to pay themselves, out-of-pocket, in order to obtain prescribed medication. These are:

- A flat rate fixed fee
- Percentage co-payment system
- Deductible system.

A *flat rate fixed fee*, commonly called a prescription charge, is payable per item on a prescription or per prescription (containing one or more items).

Flat rate prescription charges are independent of actual drug cost and exist in Austria and the UK. They are used in combination with other forms of cost sharing in Finland, Germany and Iceland.

Percentage co-payment (also termed 'co-insurance') is probably the most common form of cost sharing and is based on a percentage payment of actual drug cost. The percentage amount that is payable by the patient can vary depending on the type of medicine and the seriousness of the underlying pathology. In France, for example, patients have to pay 35% of actual cost towards medicines that are classed as being of major therapeutic value, but have to contribute 65% for those where therapeutic value is judged as moderate or low. Certain drugs treating conditions that are considered as 'not usually of a serious nature' may need to be paid in full (100%). A number of other European countries (including Belgium, Finland, Iceland, Luxembourg, Portugal, Spain) have similar graded percentage co-payments.

In a *deductible system*, a patient has to pay 100% of the cost of their prescribed medication up to a set amount (the deductible), after which the cost is subsidized. This system is often combined with a percentage co-payment or prescription charge once the deductible has been reached.

Protection mechanisms and exemptions

In many countries, cost sharing arrangements are accompanied by mechanisms to protect vulnerable groups against undue or excessive expenses for drugs. Such protection mechanisms can take the form of reduced (i.e. subsidized) payments, exemptions, caps on expenditure or complementary insurance to cover all or part of out-of-pocket cost sharing. These protection mechanisms may be available to all (e.g. complementary insurance) or apply to particular types of drugs, e.g. essential drugs treating chronic or life-threatening conditions. They may also apply to particular groups in the population, who can access prescribed drugs at a reduced or no cost (i.e. exempt). Criteria that usually define vulnerable groups and qualify for exemption or subsidy include:

- *Clinical conditions* – commonly those defined as chronic or life-threatening and requiring essential medication, usually implemented as a

list of qualifying conditions or drugs. (In the UK, for example, patients requiring medication for type I or type II diabetes are exempt.)
- *Level of income* – where people on low incomes are protected against undue expense.
- *Age* – children are exempt in Austria, France, Germany, Italy, the Netherlands and the UK; older people are exempt or have reduced cost sharing arrangements in Austria, Italy, Japan, Portugal, Spain, the UK and Iceland. (Note: definitions for 'children' and 'older people' differ in the different countries, the latter being linked to retirement in some.)

Caps on co-payments

Only a few countries (e.g. New Zealand and Sweden) have reduced medication co-payments for high users, but many have some form of cap or ceiling, sometimes also referred to as out-of-pocket maximums. They define the maximum amount a patient should be asked to cost share. Caps can either apply per prescription or be annual ceilings. Caps per prescription exist, for example in Taiwan. Annual caps are probably more common and can either apply to the whole of the population (e.g. Norway, Sweden and Switzerland) or only to certain groups, such as the chronically ill (e.g. Denmark, Finland and Germany). Some countries also have systems where medication co-payments are tax deductible (e.g. Portugal).

Complementary insurance

Complementary insurance covering the cost of prescription co-payments is another form of protection mechanism; patients who have bought this type of insurance do not have to cost share or, if they are asked to pay an amount out-of-pocket, are subsequently reimbursed. Complementary insurance is widespread in France (*mutuelle*) but can also be found in a number of other countries. In England, a so-called pre-payment certificate (PPC) exists, which can be bought to cover the cost of any prescription charges over a 3- or 12-month period, thus providing a cap through advance payment. The problem with complementary insurance and PPCs is that they only alleviate the financial burden for those who can afford to purchase this cover, and those who can predict in advance that they are likely to benefit (so not ideal for episodic conditions, such as asthma).

Impact of cost sharing on drug use and health outcomes

Impact on drug consumption

A large body of international literature exists showing that cost sharing reduces access to health services in general (where cost sharing applies), and use of prescribed medication in particular. This is, of course, one of the aims of having such a policy in place, whereby patients respond to cost sharing by assessing whether a visit to their doctor, and the use of prescribed medication in particular, are seen as important enough to warrant the relevant out-of-pocket payment. For unnecessary visits or self-limiting conditions that patients may be able to treat themselves (e.g. either through self-care or the use of self-medication remedies), avoiding the use of formal healthcare may be the most appropriate action. This will save cost to the patient, as no cost sharing is incurred, or possibly a reduced amount is paid if OTC remedies are purchased. It further reduces resource use by the health service itself (third party payment), which is an aim of a cost sharing policy.

Differential effect on essential and less essential medication

Cost sharing should only affect patient demand that may not be entirely clinically necessary, so should only affect the use of less essential medication. The latter is defined as medication that provides symptomatic relief without having an affect on any underlying disease process (see Table 26.1 for a more detailed definition). Indeed, the negative effect of cost sharing on drug utilization has been found to be more pronounced for less essential drugs, but it does also reduce the use of essential medication (Austvoll-Dahlgren et al. 2008). As the terminology suggests, essential drugs are those whose withdrawal would have important effects on morbidity and mortality, and thus a cost-related reduction in essential medication is likely to have a negative effect on health outcomes.

Table 26.1 Definitions of essential and less essential medications (Tamblyn et al. 2001)

Drug category	Definition	Drugs included in categories
Essential drugs	'Medications that prevent deterioration in health or prolong life and would not likely be prescribed in the absence of a definitive diagnosis'	Insulin, anticoagulants, angiotensin converting enzyme inhibitors, lipid-reducing medication, antihypertensives, furosemide, β-blockers, antiarrhythmics, aspirin, antivirals, thyroid medication, neuroleptics, antidepressants, anticonvulsants, antiparkinson drugs, prednisone, β-agonists, inhaled steroids, ciclosporin
Less essential drugs	'Medications that may provide relief of symptoms but will likely have no effect on the underlying disease process'	

Effect on health outcomes

Even though there are not as many studies that show that a cost-related reduction in the use of essential medicines impacts negatively on health outcomes, convincing large-scale evidence does exist. Tamblyn and colleagues (2001) used interrupted time series analysis to examine the effect of the Quebec drug policy reform, where a 25% co-payment and income linked caps were introduced. Using a random sample of 93 950 elderly persons and 55 333 adult welfare recipients, the authors showed that the use of essential drugs decreased by 9.12% and 14.42% in the two groups; and the use of less essential drugs decreased by 15.14% and 22.39%, respectively. The authors further demonstrated an increase in emergency department visits and serious adverse events (defined as hospitalization, nursing home admission or mortality) in association with the decrease of essential drugs use, but not in association with the reduction in less essential drugs. They thus established a causal link between the reduction in drug use in response to cost sharing and a negative effect on health outcomes.

Furthermore, a number of literature reviews exist on the impact of prescription medicine fees on drug and health service use, as well as health status. They conclude that cost sharing leads to a decrease in essential drug use and a decline in health status in vulnerable populations (Austvoll-Dahlgren et al. 2008, Lexchin & Grootendorst 2004, Rice & Matsuoka 2004).

Negative effect on healthcare use and resources

If cost-related reduction in the use of essential medication leads to worse health outcomes, this will invariably lead to an increased use of healthcare services (such as increased numbers of visits, increased hospital admission and additional treatment and medication). This, in turn, will have an effect on resource use, as all such increased health service use will need to be funded. It is thus important to note that any savings in drug spend (due to a reduction in drug use because of cost sharing) may be offset by cost increases in other healthcare areas. However, very few studies exist that have demonstrated such a link. Soumerai and colleagues (1994) assessed the effect of a Medicaid imposed cap, allowing a maximum of three prescriptions a month, on 268 permanently disabled, non-institutionalized patients with schizophrenia. They demonstrated a decrease in the use of essential mental health drugs and a concomitant increase in the use of acute mental health services among low-income patients. They estimated that the average increase in mental healthcare costs per patient during the cap exceeded the savings in drug costs to Medicaid by a factor of 17. From a societal perspective, this runs counter to the aim of any cost sharing policy.

Effect of cost sharing on different population groups

Besides having differing effects on essential versus less essential drugs, cost sharing can also affect different groups in the population to differing extents. The elderly, people with disabilities (including mental health problems), those taking medication for chronic conditions and people on low incomes, are particularly vulnerable and susceptible. Essentially, these are the groups that are most likely to have high morbidity and high use of essential medication, while being least likely to be able to afford cost sharing. To protect them, many countries have exemptions and other protection mechanisms in place.

Impact of cost sharing on patients and healthcare professionals

The preceding sections have provided insight into the fact that medication cost sharing reduces drug utilization, and that certain groups of patients are more vulnerable or susceptible to this effect, particularly those on low incomes or regular medicine users. However, these studies provide little detail on how drug utilization is reduced, i.e. how individual patients cope with the cost of their medication. Rather than relying on the analysis of large insurance reimbursement or claims databases that provided much of the above evidence, studies that employed methodologies involving direct contact with patients have explored this. In-depth interviews and focus groups have provided some of the depth and detail on how patients cope with medication cost, and questionnaire surveys have allowed quantification of this information (Cox et al. 2001, Cox & Henderson 2002, Safran et al. 2005, Schafheutle et al. 2002, 2004, 2009).

Effect of cost sharing on patients – coping strategies

From these studies, we know that patients respond to cost sharing in complex ways. Furthermore, there are many factors that can impact on whether patients decide to adhere to their medication, and cost is just one of them. Indeed, medication cost is often not an overriding factor when patients decide whether to adhere to their prescribed medication regimen or not, but it can be at least a mediator. If patients perceive their condition as serious and the prescribed treatment as one providing an important health benefit, cost is less likely to have an effect. On the other hand, if a condition is judged to be less serious, and where treatment may be mainly symptomatic rather than curative, cost is more likely to impact. The actual amount of cost sharing is also important, and the higher it is the more likely it is to impact on patients' management behaviour (called 'price elasticity'). Patients' 'affordability factors' are also important, where patients on lower incomes and with competing demands on the resources they have available are more likely to be affected by cost sharing than patients on higher incomes, without affordability issues.

When cost sharing does affect patients' management behaviour, patients respond by using a variety and combination of strategies, which all aim to either make the cost manageable or reduce it. Their use is strongly influenced by patients' income and affordability, where people on below average incomes are significantly more likely to use these cost reduction strategies than those on above average incomes (Schafheutle et al. 2004).

In order to cope with cost sharing, patients may decide to:

- Not have their medication dispensed at all
- Take less of their medication to make it last longer
- Delay having their prescription dispensed until they have money available
- Borrow money to pay for their prescription
- Prioritize, i.e. get only some items dispensed if more than one has been prescribed.

In some cases, patients may also decide not to go to the doctor to avoid getting a prescription that would then need to be paid for; a strategy that will be particularly prominent in systems where cost sharing also exists for physician visits.

Patients in all types of cost sharing systems use many of the above strategies, as they reduce patients' out-of-pocket expense for prescription medicines, regardless of the type of cost sharing that is in place. However, some strategies are only used in certain systems, as their effectiveness in terms of cost reduction depends on the particular type of cost sharing system. A UK specific strategy, for example, would be to buy a pre-payment certificate, while the specific French strategy is to buy the complementary insurance 'mutuelle'. Strategies that are specific to patients who pay a proportional co-payment are to:

- Shop around at different pharmacies which may offer different discounts
- Purchase their prescribed medication cheaper in another country (e.g. Mexico if from USA)
- Apply to a pharmaceutical company's Prescription Drug Patient Assistance Program (USA).

Asking for cheaper generic drugs instead of more expensive brands is also a strategy likely to be used in countries with proportional co-payments.

Self-medication strategies

Patients may also respond to high medication cost sharing for prescribed medicines by opting to access cheaper OTC remedies, if they are available. This approach is only likely to work in systems with a flat prescription charge, where the cost of the charge is generally higher than the cost of many OTC products (such as in the UK). Buying OTC products will also be a strategy in countries where (some or all) OTC products are not prescribable (blacklisted) or are not covered (i.e. paid for) by the healthcare system (such as France, Germany and the Netherlands).

It is further interesting to note that patients are price sensitive when making self-medication choices. Especially if they experience affordability issues, patients consider the price of different OTC products and may choose a cheaper alternative. Conversely, in some cases, paying a prescription charge works out cheaper than buying one of the more expensive OTC products, which may make some patients more likely to visit the doctor rather than self-medicate. (This may be different in countries where patients have to pay out-of-pocket when they visit a doctor.)

Involving the prescriber

Prescribers also have a number of options available to them which allow them to, in effect, prescribe in a way that gives patients best 'value for money'. The types of strategies they can use, again, depend on the cost sharing system within which they operate. In a flat fee charge system (e.g. Austria, Germany or the UK), they can, for example, issue a prescription for a longer supply or a larger pack size, as this allows patients to obtain a larger supply for the same fixed charge. UK and German doctors may issue a private prescription for low cost drugs whose actual price is less than the flat fee prescription charge. In a proportional co-payment system, physicians can issue prescriptions for cheaper generic rather than branded items.

Physicians may try to prescribe more 'effectively' by issuing fewer items, provided this does not compromise the clinical effectiveness of their treatment. They may also prescribe a drug that may be more likely to be effective straight off and not require several attempts at finding a suitable drug, each requiring a further charge (one example being a prescription for a proton pump inhibitor for those that pay, rather than an H_2 antagonist, in the management of dyspepsia). UK doctors have further mentioned issuing samples that have been left by pharmaceutical industry representatives (thus avoiding any patient charge) (Weiss et al. 2001). Doctors also have a role to play in recommending money-saving options, such as the availability of pre-payment certificates (UK) or complementary insurance or suggesting cheaper OTC alternatives.

For prescribing doctors to be likely to use strategies that will help patients to afford their medication, doctors need to be aware that patients pay and that they do, in fact, experience affordability issues. However, patients are generally reluctant or embarrassed to raise issues of cost and affordability with their doctor, as they consider this to be their own problem rather than that of their doctor, whose role they see as choosing the clinically most appropriate treatment. Nevertheless, if cost sharing impacts negatively on patients' adherence to prescribed regimens, this can undermine their effectiveness, particularly if the medicines in questions are essential. In order for doctors to be able to find the best treatment for their patients, they need to know whether their patients adhere to their medication, and if not, why not.

The role of community pharmacies

In most countries, community pharmacies are the places where patients go to have their prescriptions dispensed. This is therefore also the place where patients have to pay the amount that is due for medication cost sharing, which makes it likely that patients will raise issues of cost and affordability there. Pharmacists and their staff thus have an important role to play in response to patients' cost and affordability issues, and the impact this may have on their decisions not to adhere to their prescribed medication regimen as intended. Pharmacists can support patients to make appropriate decisions, using some of the above mentioned patient strategies. They can, for example, raise awareness of complementary insurance programmes or pre-payment certificates (UK), recommend generic substitution or the purchase of a cheaper OTC product where available.

However, pharmacists will also be faced by patients delaying prescriptions, prioritizing certain items, i.e. getting only some dispensed, or choosing not to have any of their medication dispensed, because they cannot afford (or do not want) to pay the medication cost sharing amount that is due. In some cases, these requests will relate to essential medication where adherence is crucial to achieving full health benefit. In other words, cost-related non-adherence may lead to worse health outcomes for these patients. An example might be that a patient only wants to get his β-agonist inhaler dispensed when he also requires a steroid inhaler. Or patients may choose not to take medication for hypertension, as the effect of this medication is not immediately evident to them and any long-term benefits are intangible.

Pharmacists have an important role in advising patients about the action and benefits of their medication and the importance of adherence in order to fully achieve this benefit (see Chs 18 and 25). Nevertheless, this advice is unlikely to work for those patients who simply cannot afford to pay the cost sharing. In these cases, pharmacists may want to liaise with doctors and other members of the healthcare team to discuss options to support this patient's treatment. Pharmacists and their staff may also be able to inform patients about the availability of income-related systems for exemptions or subsidy and how to go about applying for them.

To ensure that issues of cost and affordability are raised where necessary, pharmacists could incorporate appropriate questioning into pharmaceutical care plans, or when conducting medication use reviews. They should also ensure that they communicate any relevant information to the prescribing doctor and any other relevant healthcare professionals, so that a therapeutic plan can be discussed and agreed, which meets the patient's clinical and other needs.

Conclusion

Cost sharing for medicines is a mechanism used in many healthcare systems with the aim of deterring unnecessary demand and thus containing healthcare and drug expenditure. Drug use is indeed reduced when cost sharing is implemented, but essential as well as less essential medicines are affected. This can have a negative impact on health outcomes, requiring additional healthcare services and treatment, leading to increased resource use.

Certain groups of patients are particularly susceptible or vulnerable to the negative impact of cost sharing, namely the elderly, people who take regular medication for chronic conditions and people on low incomes. These are, in effect, people who may experience problems affording prescribed medication, either due to regular and thus relatively large expenses for (sometimes multiple) chronic conditions or simply because they only have a limited income and thus limited resources available for payment. Many countries therefore have protective mechanisms in place which provide exemption or reduced payments. Caps and complementary insurance may also be available. The criteria that are used for such protection are usually based on clinical condition and/or need, income and age, thus aiming to protect those identified as most vulnerable.

Patients use many strategies to keep medication costs to a minimum. Some are appropriate but others jeopardize treatment with essential medicines where adherence is crucial to achieve the desired health benefit. Patients commonly do not communicate issues of cost and affordability or the strategies they use to cope with cost sharing, to their doctors. They are, however, more likely to raise these issues in community pharmacies as the places where money is exchanged when getting prescribed medication dispensed. This provides pharmacists and their staff with the important opportunity to explore cost issues and inform patients about the importance of adherence to essential medicines. They can also advise patients about options for managing cost sharing, such as exemptions and complementary insurance or PPCs. Pharmacists can also liaise with physicians and other healthcare professionals to inform and thus facilitate a jointly agreed treatment plan that takes account of cost sharing and affordability as much as possible.

KEY POINTS

- There are different types of cost sharing systems: flat fee prescription charges, proportional co-payments (co-insurance) and deductibles
- These systems are in place to deter unnecessary demand and thus avoid waste
- Many cost sharing programmes have protection mechanisms in place for vulnerable groups (elderly, chronically ill, low incomes)
- Medication cost sharing reduces drug consumption
- The reduction in drug use in response to cost sharing is more pronounced for less essential medicines than essential ones
- Patients use a variety of strategies to cope with medication costs, and these depend on the types of cost sharing within their country
- Healthcare professionals, including physicians and pharmacists, can advise on the importance of adherence and help with medication cost

The prescription

27

Ian Smith

STUDY POINTS

- The information required on a prescription
- The different types of prescriptions presented at a pharmacy
- The routine procedure for checking and dispensing prescriptions
- Information sources required for prescription dispensing

Introduction

A prescription is a paper or electronic document detailing the medicine or medicines to be dispensed for an individually named patient and issued by an authorized prescriber. A prescription item is one named medicine on a prescription, e.g. aspirin tablets. A prescription may contain more than one prescription item, e.g. aqueous cream, pholcodine linctus and aspirin tablets (three prescription items), in which case the prescription may be referred to as a 'multiple item' prescription. In addition to medicines, a prescription may contain other items or appliances required by the patient for their treatment, e.g. wound dressings, elastic hosiery, blood glucose monitoring equipment, needles and syringes, nutritionally complete feeds and gluten-free foods.

Although at present the majority of prescriptions are produced on paper, there will in future be a continued move towards electronic prescriptions in both the community and in hospitals. Electronic prescriptions have the same legal force as prescriptions signed in writing. The benefits of electronic prescriptions include patient convenience, easier ordering of repeat prescriptions and more complete information about prescribing. The production of electronic prescriptions might in the future mean an end to incomplete and illegible prescriptions. Although electronic prescriptions will become routine in the NHS, private prescriptions will, for the foreseeable future, remain as paper documents. The information contained on both paper and electronic prescriptions and the method of dispensing and recording is essentially the same.

Information required on a prescription

When producing a prescription, the prescriber is giving information and instructions to the person who will supply the medicine to the patient. A prescription is in effect three types of document in one, in that it is a clinical document, a legal document and an invoice. Laws may require some of the information on the prescription and some of the information is required to ensure the patient receives the correct medicine. The dispenser will also have to take payment for the medicine from the patient or send the prescription to the appropriate body for reimbursement; hence it is also an invoice.

Name and address of the prescriber

This identifies who the prescriber is and informs the pharmacist where to contact the prescriber should there be an issue related to the prescription. A telephone number on the prescription is helpful, but if the pharmacist suspects the prescription is a forgery, this number should not be used as there have been cases where the telephone number has been changed so the pharmacist has contacted someone who has then pretended to be the prescriber.

Date of the prescription

This identifies when the prescription was written. The law usually defines the length of time from being written that a prescription remains valid. In the UK, all NHS prescriptions should be dispensed within 6 months of the date on the prescription except for certain types of Controlled Drugs where the requirement is that they are dispensed within 28 days.

Name of the medicine (with strength and dosage form, if relevant)

The name of the medicine can be expressed as the generic or proprietary name.

Generic name

The generic name is also known as the approved name. All drugs are given an approved name, which is usually related to their chemical structure and the medical classification of the drug. This name is adopted by the World Health Organization and is known as the recommended international non-proprietary name (rINN). Prescribers in the UK are encouraged to use generic names for cost-saving reasons, as generic products are usually less expensive than the equivalent proprietary product (see below) and hence the generic name is the most commonly used name on prescriptions. If the prescription is written by the generic name, in the UK, any equivalent product can be supplied even if it also has a proprietary name. The person who dispensed the prescription may lose money if they supply a more expensive proprietary product when the prescription is written generically.

Proprietary name

This can also be referred to as the brand name, manufacturer's name or trade name. The company that first produces and markets a drug will give it a proprietary name. The company will apply for a trademark in respect of the proprietary name. The granting of a trademark means that no other company can use that name. Usually, proprietary names are short, distinct and easy to remember and write. They may reflect the name of the company or the condition the medication is being used to treat or the type of medication. After expiry of the patent (in the UK, 20 years from first date of discovery or, under a certificate of supplementary protection, 15 years from the date of first marketing) the drug may be produced by other companies using the approved (or generic) name. Drugs may be prescribed by their proprietary name. If the prescriber, in the UK, states the proprietary name or the manufacturer of the product, this product or the product manufactured by the stated manufacturer must be supplied.

Total amount to be dispensed or length of treatment time

This can be stated as the number of units or can be stated by indicating the dose and dosage regimen with a number of days' treatment. In the UK, the prescription has a number of days' treatment box, which can be used to indicate the quantity required.

Directions for use

Directions should be as specific as possible. Ideally, the amount to be used and the number of times a day that it should be taken should be stated. Vague directions – in particular 'Take as directed' – are of little value to the patient and should be avoided. In such situations, the pharmacist will have to ensure that the patient is clear about how to use or take their medication.

As well as the dose and dosage regimen, the prescriber may include additional information about the product. This can include how to use (e.g. spread thinly, dissolve in water), where to use (e.g. in the eye, in the ear, on the scalp), why they are using it (e.g. for pain, for sleeping). The prescriber may also indicate a maximum amount that should be taken, particularly if the medicine is dosed on a 'when required' basis.

Name and address of the patient

This identifies the patient who is to receive the medicine. The age of the patient would also be useful to enable the pharmacist to check the dose of the medicine, particularly if the person is very young or very old.

Prescriber's signature

This is usually a legal requirement of prescriptions.

The above details are not totally inclusive, depending on the prescription type and the legal requirements of the country. It is important that the person dispensing the product is aware of the information they require and is able to take the appropriate action to clarify and complete any missing or ambiguous information. A number of specific terms, for example 'dose', 'dosage regimen', etc. are used in the above list and are often confused. Example 27.1 demonstrates the terms using an extract from a prescription.

Types of prescription forms

In the UK, there are two providers of health care: the private sector and the NHS. Concomitantly, there are two categories of prescriptions: private prescriptions and NHS prescriptions. Additionally, prescriptions may be provided in both the primary

care sector (e.g. community) and the secondary care sector (e.g. hospitals). The format of prescriptions in these two sectors will be different.

Private prescription forms

Private prescriptions do not have a standard format and may just be a piece of paper containing all the required information. Normally some of the information, such as the name, the address and qualifications of the prescriber, are pre-printed on the paper. The symbol 'Rx' is often used on private prescription forms to indicate that the form is a prescription. Changes in the law relating to Controlled Drugs in the UK have led to the production of a standard form for private prescriptions for controlled drugs for human use. All veterinary prescriptions are private prescription.

NHS prescription forms

NHS prescriptions are only issued to NHS patients. There are a number of different types of NHS prescription forms available in the UK that may be dispensed at any community pharmacy. Each type of prescription form is given a different number and colour. They may have a different format depending on where in the UK they originate and the type of prescriber who generated the prescription.

Hospital prescription forms

There is no standard form for hospital prescribing for patients staying in hospital, and the actual format and design will depend on the individual hospital trust. Most hospitals have moved or are moving away from the paper-based system to an online electronic version. However, the forms usually contain much of the same information. They usually have space for the prescription details, as well as space for confirmation of the administration of the medicine by nursing or other staff. For convenience, most hospital forms are divided into three separate areas, namely medicines to be administered on a regular basis, medicines to be administered once only and medicines to be administered on an 'as required' basis. Some forms may also have an area for listed medicines that can be administered by nursing staff at their discretion. Such medicines may be simple analgesics, sore throat

---

Example 27.1

Examine the following details which have been abstracted from a prescription:

Brufen® tablets 200 mg

Two tablets to be taken three times a day

Send 84 tablets

Using the above prescription as an example, the dosage form, strength, dose, dosage regimen, total daily dose, total amount, proprietary name, generic name and length of treatment are:

Term	Example
Dosage form	Tablets
Strength	200 mg
Dose	400 mg (2 tablets of 200 mg)
Dosage regimen	400 mg three times a day
Total daily dose	1200 mg
Total amount	84 tablets
Proprietary name	Brufen®
Generic name	Ibuprofen
Length of treatment	14 days

lozenges, laxatives, etc. In addition, all hospital prescription forms will require space for identification of the patient and will also have room for important details about the patient, such as any allergies.

Routine procedure for dispensing prescriptions

The dispensing of prescriptions requires a logical and very thorough approach in order to ensure the patient gets the right product in the right form, at the right dose with the right advice. It is imperative that the pharmacist conducts a thorough check of the prescription to ensure that it is complete and clinically acceptable. The product should then be assembled and labelled in a manner that ensures the product and all the information is accurate and that it is professional in its appearance. All stages involved in the dispensing process should be covered by a standard operating procedure (SOP, see Ch. 11).

The stages involved in dispensing a prescription are:

- Receiving the prescription
- Clinical and legal checking of the prescription
- Assembly of the product and labelling
- Accuracy checking the product against the prescription
- Handover of the product to the patient with the appropriate advice about the product.

Receiving the prescription

It is important at this stage that the person receiving the prescription has checked the patient details so that:

- The appropriateness of the prescription for that patient can be assessed
- Any required records can be completed correctly
- The product can be labelled for that patient (Ch. 31)
- If necessary, the prescription can be delivered to the correct patient at the correct address
- The patient can be contacted, if necessary, even after the medicine has been dispensed and supplied to the patient.

The full name of the patient should be ascertained to ensure that the medicines reach the person for whom they are intended. The information should also include the sex of the patient, if it is not given elsewhere on the prescription. The sex of the patient may be necessary in the assessment of the appropriateness of the medicine for the patient (see Example 27.2).

The full address of the patient is also checked and completed if required. It may be possible that two patients have the same name and so the address will identify the patient. If two patients have the same address and name, then it is helpful if the age or date of birth of the patient is stated. The age or date of birth of the patient if they are under 12 years old is a legal requirement on prescriptions in the UK. Since the advent of computer-generated prescriptions and with electronic prescriptions, the date of birth of the patient is supplied on most prescriptions. On private prescriptions, the age of very young children may be expressed as a fraction. If the age is expressed in days, weeks or months, then the denominator is 7, 52 and 12, respectively. For example, an age of 3 days may be abbreviated to 3/7, an age of 3 weeks may be abbreviated to 3/52 and an age of 3 months to 3/12.

As well as checking patient details, the person taking the prescription in should also be able to check if the product is available in the pharmacy or whether it needs to be ordered and, if so, how long

---

Example 27.2

Examine the following details found on a prescription:

> Mrs Joyce Hind
> 2 High Street
> Mediton
> Hytrin tablets starter pack
> To be taken as directed
> Send 1 pack

Hytrin is the proprietary name for terazosin, an α-adrenoceptor blocking drug, which is used for the treatment of urinary retention in benign prostatic hyperplasia and for the treatment of mild to moderate hypertension. It is available as two starter packs, with different numbers of different strength tablets in them. In the above prescription, the patient is female and the drug is most likely to be prescribed for the treatment of hypertension. Thus, an indication of the sex of the patient is useful to the pharmacist in this case, since it would indicate that the patient should receive the starter pack for hypertension. However, it would still be important to check with the prescriber that this is the case.

it will take to arrive. This information is useful in advising the person collecting the prescription how long it will take before it is ready for collection.

The person taking in the prescription may also have to take payment for the prescription. They should understand how to calculate the cost of the prescription and may be required to understand the rules about who pays for their prescriptions and what checks may be required to ensure the patient is making a legitimate declaration of exemption.

Clinical and legal checking of the prescription

This is an essential role of the pharmacist to ensure that the prescription is legally complete and clinically correct for the patient. The pharmacist should check that all the information required to select and dispense the right product is available on the prescription. Any information which is missing or ambiguous will require the pharmacist to take some action before the prescription can go on to the next stage in the dispensing process. If information is not present, the pharmacist should ascertain this information and the prescription might have to be sent back to the prescriber for the prescription to be completed or altered. In the UK, if it is not possible to get the prescription back to the prescriber or the prescriber cannot be contacted, the pharmacist can add information relating to the dose, strength and quantity to be supplied using the endorsements 'prescriber contacted' and 'prescriber not contacted' as outlined in the BNF.

The pharmacist should also check that the prescription is appropriate for the patient and that it will be of benefit and not cause the patient harm. A number of court cases have identified that the pharmacist has a responsibility for what they have supplied under the directions of the prescriber. Therefore, in addition to ensuring the prescription is legal and complete, the pharmacist should be checking the clinical elements of the prescribing and contacting the prescriber to discuss any issues they have identified.

One suggested way to do this review is by using the mnemonic IDEAL CASE, as follows:

Interactions

Dose

Evidence of harm/benefit

Appropriate

Legal and complete (and here is where we make a CASE for the medication)

Cost-effective

Acceptable to the patient

Safe

Effective

Interactions

Does the drug interact with any other items the patient is taking or with the patient's condition? Many of the computer programmes which are used to produce labels and store a patient's medication record in the pharmacy have the functionality that will identify possible interactions. The information is normally highlighted on the computer screen in the pharmacy with an indication of the possible importance of the interaction. The pharmacist needs to be able to interpret this information and, using any other information they have, decide what action would be appropriate to ensure that no harm comes to the patient. The pharmacist also needs to remember that the patient medication record (PMR) may not be complete as the patient may use more than one pharmacy and OTC medicines may not be recorded on the PMR.

Dose

Is the dose and dosage regimen appropriate for the patient and their condition? (See Example 27.3). This is more significant when dealing with drugs that have a narrow therapeutic window (i.e. the dose difference between the therapeutic dose and the toxic dose is small) and when using medication in the very young or very old patient. Being able to calculate the appropriate dose for the patient is a key skill and will sometimes require knowledge about the weight of the patient. Doses should be checked against the maximum dosage information contained in the BNF in the UK. The BNF states maximum doses in a number of ways:

- A specific dose per day, e.g. 200 mg/day
- A specific dose per day for a specific time, e.g. 200 mg/day for 7 days
- A specific dose for a specific number of times per day, e.g. 200 mg three times daily
- A combination of the above, e.g. 200 mg/day, in divided doses, for 15 days

> ### Example 27.3
>
> Look at the following details which are written on a prescription:
>
> > Elizabeth Riley
> >
> > 2 Black Avenue
> >
> > Mediton
> >
> > Bendroflumethiazide tablets 5 mg
> >
> > 1 tablet to be taken at night
> >
> > Send 28 tablets
>
> On the above prescription there is no indication of the age of the patient. It cannot be assumed that the patient is an adult. If the patient is a child, then the dose may be inappropriate and the BNF for children would have to be consulted. Bendroflumethiazide is usually taken in the morning, not at night, but night workers may take the tablets at night. In this case it is essential to check with the patient and the prescriber for the correctness of the prescription. If the patient is taking the medication for hypertension then the normal dose would be 2.5 mg each morning and increasing the dose will have little enhanced effect, and this too may need to be discussed with the prescriber.

> ### Example 27.4
>
> Examine the following details which are written on a prescription:
>
> > Elizabeth Riley
> >
> > 2 Black Avenue
> >
> > Mediton
> >
> > Ibuprofen tablets 400 mg
> >
> > 1 three times a day
> >
> > Send 84
> >
> > Simvastatin tablets 40 mg
> >
> > 1 tablet to be taken at night
> >
> > Send 28 tablets
>
> With the above prescription you may find after talking to the patient that the ibuprofen is being prescribed to treat muscle pain. Muscle pain is a recognized adverse drug reaction (ADR) of a statin which the prescriber may have missed. You would then need to discuss with the prescriber the possibility that the symptoms may be due to an ADR to the statin. This would enable the prescriber to decide on an appropriate course of action to take which could mean undertaking further tests on the patient to establish if it is a true ADR.

- An initial dose, e.g. 200 mg initially, then …
- A dose per kg of body weight, e.g. 250 µg/kg
- A dose per square metre of body surface, e.g. 25 mg/metre squared
- A maximum dose, e.g. do not take more than 2 tablets at any one time; do not take more than 8 in 24 hours.

If the strength or dose and dosage regimen is missing or incorrect on the prescription, the pharmacist will have to calculate an appropriate strength, dose or dosage regimen. The pharmacist will then have to discuss this with the prescriber to ensure that this meets the patient's requirements.

The dose and dosage regimen of the medication may be affected by other medication on the prescription, or the conditions the patient may be suffering from. This is particularly true if they have any degree of kidney/liver failure, as these are the main routes of excretion of drugs from the body.

Evidence of benefit/harm

Is there any evidence the patient is benefiting from the treatment? Do they believe it is working and is there any evidence that their condition is improving? Could it be causing them any harm? Are they suffering from any adverse effects? Is another treatment on the prescription being used to treat these side-effects? (See Example 27.4.)

Appropriate

Is the product the most appropriate medication available for the patient and their condition? This leads into the use of the mnemonic 'CASE', which helps to look at the specifics of the drug in terms of its cost, its acceptability to the patient and its safety and efficacy.

Legal

Check the prescription complies with any laws related to the supply of medicines. The legal requirements are likely to require the prescription, at the very least, to be signed and dated by the prescriber. Clearly it is the responsibility of the pharmacist to check that the signature is genuine and the date correct.

Cost-effective

Is there a more cost-effective product? Does this treatment offer the most cost-effective option? This might be worth considering if a cheaper medication has the same evidence of safety and efficacy (e.g. comparing the use of simvastatin and atorvastatin). Sometimes the prescriber prescribes a dose of two 10 mg tablets when it would be cheaper to provide one 20 mg tablet.

Acceptable to the patient

Ask the patient if they can take or use the medication? Ask if they are able to take their medication as they are directed to take it? Try and find out if they take their medication all the time and investigate how concordant they are. If the patient does not or cannot take the medicine, there is little reason for it to be dispensed in the first place. Some of the considerations might be, for example, can they swallow tablets or would a liquid or soluble product be more acceptable? Or, can they use their inhaler correctly? If the patient cannot use the inhaler after effective counselling then they should be considered for an alternative device which they might find easier to use. Can they open child resistant containers? If not, could the medicine be supplied in a device that the patient can get into?

Safe

What do I have to do to ensure the product is safe for this patient? Which possible side-effects might they suffer? What should they do if they suffer from these side-effects? In some cases, this will mean that they have to return to the prescriber, but should they stop their treatment or keep taking it until they can see the prescriber? Do I need to tell them about any cautions when taking the medication? (This might be telling them about driving or operating machinery or taking alcohol when taking their medicine.) Does the treatment need to be monitored? If so, when, how often and how should it be monitored? When should the treatment be reviewed and stopped? When would I be justified in looking for a safer alternative treatment? If the patient is currently on a treatment dose, when can that be reduced to a maintenance dose or even stopped?

Evidence-based

Is the treatment the most effective treatment available? Is the treatment evidence-based? Does the treatment concur with any available guidelines or protocols? (See Chs 22 and 23).

The use of this mnemonic and considerations of the questions should help the pharmacist to clinically and legally review the prescription and thereby to ensure that the patient is being treated optimally. The pharmacist should then deal with any issue. Some issues will prevent the prescription from being dispensed, such as missing information, a potential overdose or a serious interaction. These will mean the pharmacist has to contact the prescriber before the prescription is sent on to the next stage in the dispensing process. Some issues can be raised with the prescriber after the prescription has been dispensed, such as issues about the cost-effectiveness of the treatment. Ensuring the patient gets adequate counselling when the medicine is delivered to the patient might be enough to satisfy some of the issues, particularly in relation to information about possible side-effects and cautions in using the medication.

Assembly of the product and labelling

This stage involves producing a label for the product, selecting the product from where it is stored in the pharmacy and doing any assembly work and putting the label onto the product. Usually trained pharmacy technicians carry out this stage in the process and some pharmacies have introduced dispensing robots to select the products. The assembly work can range from picking a patient pack from a shelf to making the product from its ingredients. Accuracy in this stage of the assembly process is paramount in ensuring that the patient gets the product ordered on the prescription. Picking the wrong strength or form, or even the wrong product, are errors that can occur at this stage. The dispenser needs to take great care in selecting the products because many drugs have similar names, as outlined in Box 27.1 or they may be in containers with a similar appearance (see Ch. 10).

At this stage of the process, the dispenser may be required to make records, either for legal purposes such as completion of a Controlled Drugs

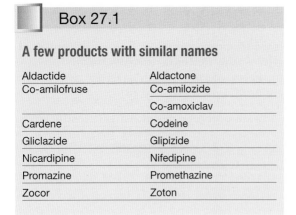

Box 27.1

A few products with similar names

Aldactide	Aldactone
Co-amilofruse	Co-amilozide
	Co-amoxiclav
Cardene	Codeine
Gliclazide	Glipizide
Nicardipine	Nifedipine
Promazine	Promethazine
Zocor	Zoton

Box 27.2

Some reference sources most frequently used in dispensing

British National Formulary (BNF)
Medicines, Ethics and Practice Guide (RPS)
Stockley's Drug Interactions
Drug and Therapeutics Bulletin
Drug Tariff
MeReC Bulletin
Effective Healthcare Bulletin
Prescribers' Journal
Pharmaceutical Codex
Drugs Safety Update
Martindale: the Extra Pharmacopoeia

register, or as good practice, such as adding information to a PMR. The prescription may need to be priced if it is a private prescription or endorsed if it is an NHS prescription.

Accuracy checking the product against the prescription

This final accuracy check is present to ensure that there has not been an error in the dispensing process. It is an important stage in minimizing risk to the patient. The person involved in carrying out this check needs to work in a structured and methodical manner without interruption to have the best chance of working effectively. Until recently, only pharmacists undertook the final check, but increasing numbers of accredited checking technicians are being trained to perform this task (Ch. 5).

Delivery of the product to the patient with the appropriate advice about the product

The final stage is to hand the product to the patient. This stage can be done by a pharmacist or can be delegated to another member of staff. It is important that whoever gives the medicine to the patient ensures the patient has all the advice they need. The pharmacist must be confident that the patient can take or use their medication correctly. The patient should be able to identify signs to tell if the medicine is having the desired effect or is

causing a problem and they should know what to do about it. Once the prescription has been handed to the patient, the prescription form will be filed or sent to the appropriate place so the pharmacy receives payment.

Information sources

When dealing with a prescription it is important that the pharmacist knows where to look for up-to-date information relating to different aspects involved in checking the prescription. Drugs are continually being introduced to the market and the indications for some drugs change, as do doses, dosage regimens and formulations. In addition, some drugs are removed from the market for a variety of reasons. Prescribers will need independent, accessible and unambiguous reviews of effective treatments when writing prescriptions, while pharmacists will require similar information to clinically check the prescription and advise the patient. In addition, the dispenser will also need information relating to the cost of the medication to the patient and any rules which they must apply to ensure appropriate remuneration and reimbursement, as well as information about the availability and where to order the products. Some of the most useful information sources in the UK are listed in Box 27.2 (see also Ch. 16).

The BNF is published and updated every 6 months and lists the products available for dispensing in the

UK. It is sent to all doctors, pharmacists and prescribing nurses in the NHS. The Nurse Prescribers' Formulary and Dental Practitioners' Formulary are included in the BNF and are also published as separate booklets. There is also a BNF for Children which has been produced to provide up-to-date information on the use of medicines for treating children. The BNF is the major source of easily available information on the characteristics of individual medicines, including proprietary and generic formulations, strengths, dose and dosage regimens, drug side-effects and drug interactions. The most recent copy should always be used. For more comprehensive information about medicines you should refer to *Martindale*.

The professional body in the UK produces the *Medicines, Ethics and Practice* guide. It outlines the legal requirements for the sale and supply of medicines.

The *Drug Tariff* is the resource which details the rules for the NHS remuneration and reimbursement for pharmacy contractors in the UK and contains information on what is or is not allowed on NHS prescriptions.

If the pharmacist cannot find the information that they require in the reference sources they have available, they can contact the local medicines information department which will be listed in the BNF, or the manufacturer of the product where appropriate.

KEY POINTS

- Prescriptions are paper or electronic documents issued by an authorized prescriber for an individual patient
- Prescriptions detail the medicinal treatment required for the patient and may be paper-based or electronic
- Prescriptions can be written by a number of people and may be private or NHS prescriptions
- Prescriptions can contain more than one prescription item
- Prescriptions must contain adequate information before they can be dispensed
- All prescriptions should be checked for clinical and patient appropriateness before assembly and dispensing
- Access to reference sources is often required.

Veterinary pharmacy

28

Sam Ingram and Jennie Watson

STUDY POINTS

- Differences in diagnosis, treatment, prescribing and supply of medicines between animals and humans
- Legislation and legal definitions that apply when dealing with medicines for animals
- Prescribing and the supply cascade
- Advice-giving for animal medicines
- Retail sale of veterinary medicines

Introduction

Veterinary medicines are not dealt with by every pharmacist on a day-to-day basis and some pharmacists may never supply a veterinary medicine during their whole career.

Some pharmacists however, choose to work more exclusively with animals and may undertake further training (e.g. a postgraduate diploma in veterinary pharmacy). Such pharmacists will often work in more rural areas and with food-producing animals (see Ch. 14).

The regulations relating to veterinary medicines are very different from those for human medicines and it is important that pharmacists understand the differences and where to access up-to-date information.

Animals, disease and medicines

It is unsafe to assume that the way a drug works in one animal species will be the same as the way it works in a human. This is also the case between different species of animals, and so in order to have a complete set of drugs available for every species of animal, very large sums of money would need to be invested in research and development. This does not happen and so anyone involved in treating animals may have to potentially prescribe medicines that have not been tested on that particular animal species. The other big difference between treating humans and animals is that humans are often in a position to describe symptoms, progression of symptoms and any contributing factors. When treating animals, a veterinary surgeon has to rely on physical examination and the owner's observation of the animal, thus making diagnosis more difficult.

It is also important to recognize that some animals are food-producing, either because some produce food, e.g. eggs, milk, or are eaten as meat. If they have been taking medicines in the period of time before they or their products enter the human food chain, then it is likely that humans could be consuming quantities of the medicine. These medicines may not have been tested in humans and so may cause adverse drugs reactions or interactions with other prescribed medications within the human. Pharmacists involved in supplying veterinary medicines need to be aware of these issues, as they influence the medicines supplied, records made and advice given.

Definitions

There are three additional definitions used when working with medicines and animals:

1. Classification of a veterinary medicine
   - For treating or preventing disease in animals, or for making a medical diagnosis, or to restore, correct or modify physiological functions

2. Classification of an 'animal'
- ○ 'Animal' means all animals other than man and includes birds, reptiles, fish, molluscs, crustacea and bees

3. Suitably qualified person (SQP)
- ○ This may include veterinary nurses, agricultural merchants, internet retailers and pet-shop staff. The list of SQPs is maintained by the Animal Medicines Training Regulatory Authority (AMTRA) and an individual can enter the list if they have undertaken an accredited training programme, have met the registration criteria and keep up-to-date. Registration allows the individual to supply certain legal classes of veterinary medicines.

Veterinary medicines directorate (VMD)

The VMD is the regulatory body for veterinary medicines. The vision of the VMD is the responsible, safe and effective use of veterinary medicinal products and in working towards this vision, the VMD aims to protect public health, animal health, the environment and promote animal welfare by assuring the safety, quality and efficacy of veterinary medicines.

Legal classifications

Each year, the VMD issues a new set of Veterinary Medicines Regulations (VMR), which are legally binding in the UK. These regulations displaced the Medicines Act in Great Britain and Northern Ireland. Other countries have similar regulations and there are also some European regulations.

There are four main legal classes of medicine and within these categories, there are also further classifications for controlled drugs (CDs).

POM-V (prescription only medicine – veterinarian)

May be sold or supplied by a pharmacist or a veterinary surgeon against a prescription which must be issued by a veterinary surgeon.

The prescription can be oral, i.e. not written down, unless it is being supplied elsewhere.

The veterinary surgeon must:

- carry out a clinical assessment
- ensure the animal is under the care of a veterinarian
- only prescribe the minimum amount of medicine required for treatment.

POM-VPS (prescription only medicine – veterinarian, pharmacist or SQP)

Must be both prescribed and supplied by a veterinary surgeon, pharmacist or SQP. The medicine must be supplied from registered premises.

The owner may request a written prescription if they do not want the prescriber to supply the medicine.

A clinical assessment of the animal is not required when prescribing this category of veterinary medicine.

NFA-VPS (non-food animal medicine – veterinarian, pharmacist, SQP)

Medicines in the NFA-VPS category are for companion animals (excluding horses). They must be supplied by a veterinary surgeon, pharmacist or SQP from registered premises.

A clinical assessment of the animal is not required for supply of this category of veterinary medicine.

AVM-GSL (authorized veterinary medicine – general sales list)

Medicines in the AVM-GSL category may be legally supplied by any retailer, to anyone, without restriction.

However, veterinary surgeons should take account of their professional duties in deciding when to supply all medicines, regardless of classification.

Prescribing and supply cascade

In-line with human medicines legislation, veterinary medicines regulations start from the principle that veterinary medicines must be authorized to protect the animal, user and the environment from untested or poor quality products. However, it is recognized that in some circumstances the benefits of supplying an unauthorized medicine will outweigh the risks and so veterinary surgeons have been given an exemption from the general rule under certain circumstances and this is known as the cascade.

The cascade tries to provide the balance between the need to use authorized products when available and the need for prescriber freedom when they are not. It is a way of increasing the range of products available to compensate for the lack of licensed products available for every condition in every animal species.

Any decision to supply a product under the cascade must take into account the following:

- The veterinary surgeon remains responsible for the treatment of the animal under their care and so should use clear clinical evidence to support their decision-making process
- If using a human medicine, the dose may seem appropriate but the formulation may mean it is not
- Safety information about human medicines cannot be assumed to be relevant to their use in animals
- Generic human medicines cannot be prescribed when a licensed veterinary product is available.

If there is no medicine authorized in the UK for a specific condition, the veterinary surgeon responsible for treating the animal(s) may, in order to avoid unacceptable suffering, treat the animal(s) in accordance with the following sequence:

1. A veterinary medicine authorized in the UK for use in another animal species or for a different condition in the same species
2. If there is no such medicine, use either a medicine authorized in the UK for human use or a veterinary medicine from another country
3. If there is no such medicine, a medicine prepared extemporaneously by a veterinary surgeon, pharmacist or a person holding an appropriate manufacturer's authorization.

After the decision to supply has been made, then a prescription will be produced. There are legal requirements about what needs to be on this prescription (see Box 28.1).

Supply under the cascade

Medicines prescribed by a veterinary surgeon in accordance with the cascade may be supplied against a written prescription by another veterinary surgeon, a pharmacist or a SQP, provided the medicine is of a classification and for a species for which the supplier would normally be permitted to supply it. For instance, a POM-VPS medicine authorized for dogs and horses, but prescribed under the cascade for cats could be prescribed by a veterinary surgeon and supplied against a written prescription by a SQP, but only if that SQP was qualified to supply companion animal medicines. Only veterinary surgeons and pharmacists may supply POM-V medicines.

The other conditions of supply must still be met. Other considerations when using the cascade:

- The legislation does not allow the cost of the medicine to be taken into account when deciding which medicine to use. For example, it is not permissible to use a human medicine because it is cheaper
- However, the cascade may be invoked in other appropriate circumstances, such as where microbiological tests show that a particular strain of an organism has developed resistance to all medicines whose labels contain indications against it.

Use of the cascade in food-producing animals

In food-producing animals, only authorized products may be administered or dispensed.

Food-producing animals also have a specified minimum withdrawal period, i.e. the minimum amount of time after administration of the medicine before food products can enter the human food chain. The withdrawal period is species specific:

- 7 days for eggs
- 7 days for milk
- 28 days for meat from poultry and mammals, including fat and offal
- 500-degree days for fish. The number of days of the withdrawal period is calculated by dividing 500 by the mean temperature of the water in degrees Celsius.

When the veterinary medicine is dispensed, there are requirements about the labelling of the product and these are listed in Box 28.2.

Box 28.1

Prescription requirements

- The name, address and telephone number of the person prescribing the product. It is considered good practice to include the registration number of the veterinary surgeon (MRCVS) or SQP writing the prescription
- The qualifications of the person writing the prescription
- The name and address of the owner or keeper of the animal
- The identification (including the species) of the animal or group of animals to be treated
- The premises at which the animal(s) is kept if this differs from the address of the owner or keeper
- The date that the prescription is written
- The signature of the person writing the prescription
- The name and amount of the medicine prescribed
- The dosage and administration instructions
- Any necessary warnings.
  Additional requirements for CD prescriptions – Schedule 2 or 3 (excluding temazepam):
- The address of the prescriber must be in the UK
- The total quantity of the drug must be written in words and numbers
- The form of the drug (e.g. injection, tablet) must be given
- The prescription must include a declaration that the animal(s) being treated is under the veterinary surgeon's care. It is a legal requirement to include the MRCVS registration number of the veterinary surgeon writing the prescription. The strength of the drug must also be included in the prescription if more than one is available
- The prescription no longer needs to be handwritten
- It is recommended that prescriptions should not be written for more than 30 days' supply
- Repeat prescriptions are not allowed for Schedule 2 or 3 drugs
- CD prescriptions for Schedule 2, 3 or 4 drugs are only valid for 28 days.

 Box 28.2

Labelling requirements for dispensed medicines

- The name and address of the pharmacy, veterinary surgery or approved premises supplying the veterinary medicine
- The name of the veterinary surgeon who has prescribed the medicine
- The name and address of the animal's owner
- The identification (including the species) of the animal or group of animals
- The date of supply
- The expiry date of the medicine (if applicable)
- The name or description of the medicine, which should include at least the name and quantity of the active ingredient(s)
- The dosage and administration instructions
- Any special storage precautions
- Any necessary warnings with reference to the user, target species, administration or disposal of the product
- The words 'Keep out of reach of children' and 'For animal treatment only'. Also the words 'For external use only' for topical preparations.

Box 28.3

Record-keeping

When supplying veterinary medicines (except AVM-GSL where record-keeping is good practice rather than a legal requirement), the following records should be kept:

- Date and nature of transaction
- Name of the veterinary medicine
- The batch number (in the case of a medicinal product for a non-food-producing animal, this need only be recorded either on the date the batch was received or the date the batch was first used or supplied)
- Quantity received or supplied
- Name and address of the supplier or recipient
- If there is a written prescription, the name and address of the person who wrote the prescription and a copy of the prescription.

Pharmacists need to also be aware of the requirements for record-keeping when involved in the supply of veterinary medicines and these are listed in Box 28.3.

Pharmacist advice-giving

If a pharmacist is involved in supplying a veterinary medicine from the following legal classes: POM-V, POM-VPS or NFA-VPS, then they must ensure that they:

- provide advice on how to safely administer the product
- provide advice about the warnings or contraindications that appear on the label or package leaflet
- be satisfied that the person receiving the product is competent to use it safely and intends to use it for authorized use.

When giving advice, it is also important to be aware of the requirements about advice and diagnosis in the Veterinary Surgeons Act 1966:

- That you cannot 'respond to symptoms' in animals as you would with a human
- That diagnosis and treatment are restricted to veterinary surgeons and owners
- That you cannot 'suggest' cures
- That pharmacists can only offer advice on the availability of medicines when asked
- That the final treatment choice has to be the owner's.

Retail sale

There are some opportunities for the retail sale of veterinary products to treat tick and flea infestations in cats and dogs. This is potentially a large market with the estimated numbers of 6 million dogs and 8 million cats living as domestic pets in the UK.

There are licensed products available as NFA-VPS containing the insecticide fipronil and these products can be sold by a pharmacist if the owner has diagnosed the condition or for prophylaxis.

Before a pharmacist begins selling these products, they should ensure they are competent by completing training that will enable the products to be sold appropriately with the correct advice and to ensure that the products are then used correctly, as they can be toxic to other species, especially fish.

Conclusion

While many pharmacists may never be involved in supplying veterinary medicines, all pharmacists should be aware that there are additional restrictions on the prescribing and supply of medicines to treat animals.

Pharmacists should be particularly aware of the restrictions placed on pharmacists that relate to them diagnosing animals and giving advice about veterinary medicines.

Treating animals with drugs can be more complex that treating humans, as there are fewer species-specific products available.

KEY POINTS

- Some pharmacists will specialize in veterinary medicines
- There are additional regulations that apply to the prescribing and supply of medicines for animals
- Animals are unable to describe their symptoms, so diagnosis is based on examination and observation only
- Medicines prescribed to animals that are food producing have additional safeguards to prevent these medicines entering the human food chain
- Medicines must be prescribed and supplied under a cascade system to ensure that the most appropriate product is supplied for a particular type of animal, to minimize harm
- Legal requirements for prescriptions, labelling and record-keeping for veterinary medicines
- Pharmacists are restricted in the advice they can give about animal health and veterinary medicines
- Retail sale of veterinary medicines

Section 5

Medicines and their preparation

Routes of administration and dosage forms

29

Arthur J. Winfield

STUDY POINTS

- The different routes of administration of drugs
- The advantages and disadvantages of each route
- The types and uses of dosage forms

Introduction

Following the administration of a medicine, the drug has to reach its site of action or receptor in order to produce an effect. How this is achieved is often a complex process affected by many factors. The first stage will be the release of the drug from the dosage form, to be followed by absorption into the body (unless it is for a surface effect at the site of administration). There is then a distribution process, usually in the blood, which will take the drug to the site of action. As soon as it is in the body, metabolic processes, especially in the liver, will start to change the drug and the elimination process will also commence. A detailed discussion of these processes is outside the scope of this book, although it does have a significant impact on the choice of both the route of administration and the actual dosage form. There is a growing awareness that the correct choices can have an important impact on therapeutic outcomes for the patient. This chapter will review the various routes of administration used for drug delivery and discuss some of their advantages and disadvantages. Brief details of a variety of dosage forms are also given. Figure 29.1 illustrates the principal routes of administration.

1 Buccal (inside mouth)
2 Oral (swallow)
3 Sublingual (under tongue)
4 Nasal
5 Rectal
6 Vaginal
7 Inhalation (to lungs)
8 Eye
9 Ear

10 Parenteral
　a Intravenous
　b Subcutaneous
　c Intramuscular
　d Intraspinal
Topical – skin (any site)

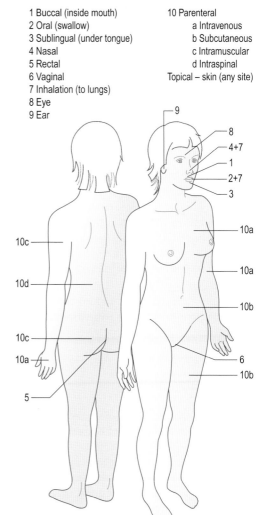

Figure 29.1 • Diagrammatic representation of the main routes of administration.

Routes of administration

The oral route

The oral route can produce either a systemic or a local effect. For a systemic effect, the drug, formulated in either a solid or a liquid form, is absorbed from the gastrointestinal tract (GIT). This is the most commonly used route for drug administration. There are several reasons for this:

- From a patient's point of view it is the simplest route
- Self-administration of drugs can be carried out
- If used properly, it is also the safest route.

However, there are disadvantages which should be borne in mind:

- The onset of action is relatively slow
- Absorption from the GIT may be irregular
- Some drugs are destroyed by enzymes and other secretions found in the GIT
- Because the blood supply from the GIT passes through the liver via the hepatic portal system, it is subject to hepatic metabolism before it enters the systemic circulation. This is called first pass or presystemic metabolism
- Drug solubility may be altered by the presence of other substances in the GIT, e.g. calcium
- Gastric emptying is very variable and can be influenced by factors such as food, drugs, disease state and posture. Not only does it affect the onset of action, but if it is extended it may cause a drug to be inactivated by gastric juices owing to prolonged contact
- It is an unsuitable route of administration in unconscious or vomiting patients and for immediate pre- or postoperative use.

The buccal routes

A drug is administered by these routes by being formulated as a tablet or spray and is absorbed from the buccal cavity. The highly vascular nature of the tongue and buccal cavity, and the presence of saliva, which can facilitate the dissolution of the drug, make this a highly effective and useful route for drug administration. It can also be used for a local action.

Two sites are used for absorption from the buccal cavity:

- For sublingual absorption, the area under the tongue is used. This gives a very fast onset of action of the drug but duration is usually short
- For buccal absorption, the buccal sulcus is used. This is the area between the upper lip and the gum. Tablets formulated for absorption from the buccal sulcus give a quick onset of action but will also give a longer duration of action than the sublingual route. This route can also administer drugs with a longer half-life for an extended duration of action.

It is important that patients are made aware of the difference between the two sites and they should be given full instructions on how to administer their tablets, to ensure maximum benefit. (For details of suitable patient instructions, see Ch. 39.)

The advantages of the buccal route:

- There is a relatively quick onset of action
- Drugs are absorbed into the systemic circulation, thereby avoiding the 'first pass' effect
- Drugs can be administered to unconscious patients
- Because the tablet is not swallowed, antiemetic drugs can be given by this route.

The rectal route

For administration by this route, drugs are formulated as liquids, solid dosage forms and semi-solids (see Ch. 37). The chosen preparation is inserted into the rectum from where the drug is released to give a local effect or it may be absorbed to give a systemic effect.

The rectum is supplied by three veins, namely the middle and inferior (lower) rectal veins, which drain directly into the systemic circulation and the upper rectal vein, which drains into the portal system, which flows into the liver. This means that, depending on the position within the rectum, only some of the drug absorbed from the rectum will be subject to the first pass effect. Bioavailability, therefore, may be less than 100% but may be better than that obtained from other parts of the GIT.

The amount of fluid present in the rectum is small, estimated at approximately 3 mL of mucus. This affects the rate of dissolution of the drug released from the suppository. However, there is also muscular movement which spreads the drug over a large area and promotes absorption.

The advantages and disadvantages of this route of administration are as follows.

Advantages

- Can be used when the oral route is unsuitable, e.g. severe vomiting, unconscious patient, with uncooperative patients such as children, elderly or mentally disturbed and patients with dysphagia
- Useful when the drug causes GIT irritation
- Can be used for local action.

Disadvantages

- Absorption can be irregular and unpredictable, giving rise to a variable effect
- Less convenient than the oral route
- There is low patient acceptability of this route in the UK. A wider acceptance is found in other parts of the world.

The vaginal route

For administration by this route, drugs may be formulated as pessaries, tablets, capsules, solutions, sprays, creams, ointments and foams which are inserted into the vagina. Most often this route is used for a local effect. However, drugs absorbed from the vagina are not subject to the first pass effect and can give systemic bioavailability better than with the oral route.

The inhalation route

Drugs are administered usually by inhalation through the nose or mouth to produce either local or systemic effects. This route is used predominantly for local administration to treat respiratory conditions such as asthma. For this, drugs are delivered directly to the site of action, i.e. the lungs. A variety of dosage forms are used, from simple inhalations consisting of volatile ingredients such as menthol to sophisticated inhaler devices (see Ch. 43). A major benefit of the inhaled route is that the drug dose required to produce the desired effect is much smaller than for the oral route, with a consequent reduction in side-effects. Because of the high blood flow to the lungs and their large surface area, drug absorption by this route is extremely rapid and can be used to give systemic action.

The nasal route

The nasal cavity has been traditionally used for producing local effects using solutions as drops or sprays. More recently it has been used for systemic action because of its good vascular supply, which avoids first pass metabolism (e.g. calcitonin), although it does have some local enzymic activity.

The topical route

In the topical route, the skin is used as the site of administration. This route is most commonly used for local effects using liquid and powder dosage forms in addition to the traditional ointments, creams and pastes (see Ch. 36). The skin has a natural barrier function, but specialized dosage forms have been developed which, when applied to the skin, allow the drug to pass through and produce a systemic effect. This avoids first pass effects and can produce close to zero-order kinetics over prolonged time intervals. (A more detailed discussion of this route of administration can be found in Ch. 36.)

The parenteral route

This is the term used to describe drug administration by injection. Within this general term, there is a variety of different routes. The main ones are:

- *Intravenous route*, where drugs are injected directly into the systemic circulation. This produces a very fast onset of action
- *Subcutaneous route*, where drugs are injected into the subcutaneous layer of the skin. This is the easiest and least painful type of injection to administer
- *Intramuscular route*, where drugs are injected into muscle layers. This method can be used to produce a fairly fast onset of action when the drug is formulated as an aqueous solution. A slower and more prolonged action will occur when the drug is presented as a suspension or in an oily vehicle.

These and other specialized types of injection are discussed more fully in Chapter 41.

Dosage forms

Drugs are presented in a wide variety of dosage forms. How a drug is formulated is dependent on a variety of factors and the same drugs may be presented in several different dosage forms. It is important for pharmacists to appreciate the different properties of the varying dosage forms in order that the most appropriate or most acceptable formulation is given to the patient. This section gives brief information on the different types of dosage forms. Additional, more detailed, information is found in the chapters dealing with specific formulations.

Aerosols

These consist of pressurized packs which contain the drug in solution or suspension and a suitable propellant. They are most commonly used for their local effect in the treatment of asthma. These devices are fitted with a metering valve which allows a known dose of drug to be delivered each time the device is fired. Some aerosols are for topical use, particularly in the treatment of muscle sprains and injuries. These may contain substances such as non-steroidal anti-inflammatory drugs or counter-irritants.

Applications

This is the name given to solutions, suspensions or emulsions which are for topical use. They contain substances such as ascaricides or antiseptics.

Capsules

These are solid dosage forms, generally for oral use. Some drugs formulated as capsules are intended to be inhaled. It is therefore important to inform the patient on their appropriate use. For both types of capsule, the drug is contained in a gelatin shell, usually as a powder or a liquid. Modified-release preparations are available where the drug is presented in the gelatin container as small pellets with different coatings.

Collodions

These are liquid preparations for external use. The liquid is painted on the skin, where it forms a flexible film. They contain substances such as salicylic acid, which is useful in the treatment of corns.

Creams

These are semi-solid emulsions for external use. Because of the water content they are susceptible to microbial contamination and either include a preservative or are given a short shelf-life. Creams are easier to apply and are less greasy than ointments, so patients often prefer them.

Dusting powders

These are finely divided powders for external use. Their main uses are as lubricants to prevent friction between skin surfaces and for disinfection and antisepsis in minor wounds.

Ear drops

These are used topically to treat a variety of ear problems. The drug, or mixture of drugs, is presented as a solution or suspension in a suitable vehicle such as water, glycerol, propylene glycol or alcohol. The drops are inserted into the ear, using a dropper. Some vehicles, such as alcohol, may cause a degree of stinging when applied to the ear. Ensure that the patient is aware of this and is assured that it is a normal sensation. If patients find the degree of stinging unacceptable they may have to be given ear drops with an aqueous vehicle. Oils such as almond or olive are often recommended for the alleviation of impacted earwax. It is usually suggested that such oils, before being dropped into the ear, should be warmed. This must be done very carefully and only minimal heat applied, i.e. the oil placed on a warm spoon. Excessive heat will have serious consequences for the integrity of the ear.

Elixirs

An elixir is a solution of one or more drugs for oral use. The vehicle generally contains a high proportion of sucrose or, increasingly nowadays, a 'sugar-free' vehicle such as sorbitol solution, which is less likely to cause dental caries. The therapeutic action of drugs presented as elixirs varies widely and includes antihistamines, antibiotics and decongestants.

Emulsions

These are mixtures of two immiscible liquids, usually oil and water. When the term 'emulsion' is used, this refers to a preparation for oral use.

Enemas

An enema is an oily or aqueous solution which is administered rectally. A number of drugs are formulated as enemas and are used to treat conditions such as constipation or ulcerative colitis. They are also used in X-ray examination of the lower bowel and for systemic effects, such as the use of diazepam in status epilepticus and febrile convulsions.

Eye drops and eye ointments

These are sterile preparations used to administer drugs to the eye.

Gargles

Gargles are aqueous solutions used to treat infections of the throat. They are often presented in a concentrated form with instructions to the patient for dilution. Gargles should not be swallowed but held in the throat while exhaling through the liquid. After a suitable time period, usually a minute or so, the patient should spit out the gargle.

Gels

Gels are semi-solid dosage forms for topical or other local use. They are usually transparent or translucent and have a variety of uses. Spermicides and lubricants are often presented in a gel form. Many patients prefer this formulation because it is non-greasy.

The term 'gel' is also used to describe colloidal suspensions of drugs such as aluminium and magnesium hydroxides.

Granules

This term is used to describe a drug which is presented in small irregularly-shaped particles. Granules may be packed in individual sachets containing a unit dose of medicament or may be provided in a bulk format, where the dose is measured using a 5 mL spoon. Some laxatives are among the drugs currently presented as granules.

Implants

This term refers to solid dosage forms which are inserted under the skin by a small surgical incision. They are most commonly used for hormone replacement therapy or as a contraceptive. Release of the drug from implants is generally slow and long-term therapy is achieved. In the case of the contraceptive implant, the effect continues for up to 3 years. A testosterone implant used in the treatment of male hypogonadism will maintain adequate hormone levels in the patient for 4–5 months. Implants must be sterile.

Inhalations

These are preparations which contain volatile medicaments, which may have a beneficial effect in upper respiratory tract disorders such as nasal congestion. Some inhalations contain substances that are volatile at room temperature and the patient can obtain a degree of relief by adding a few drops to a handkerchief or a pillowcase and breathing in the vapour. Other inhalations are added to hot water and the impregnated steam is then inhaled. Many users of the latter type of inhalation use boiling water. Pharmacists should advise against this, as the steam produced is too hot and can damage the delicate mucous membranes of the upper respiratory tract. Overuse of this type of preparation should also be avoided, as it may cause a chronic condition to develop. The use of these strong aromatic decongestants is not advised in the BNF in children under 3 months, owing to the risk of apnoea.

Injections

These are used parenterally and are sterile (see Ch. 41).

Irrigations

These are sterile solutions most commonly used in the treatment of infected bladders. Sterile solutions of sodium chloride 0.9% (physiological saline) are used to treat a wide range of common urinary tract pathogens. Antifungal drugs such as ampho-tericin and locally acting cytotoxics, e.g. doxo-rubicin and mitomycin, are introduced into the bladder, as irrigations, to treat mycotic infections and bladder tumours, respectively.

Linctuses

A linctus is a viscous liquid for oral use, the major-ity being for the relief of cough. The viscous nature of the preparation coats the throat and helps to alleviate the irritation which is causing the problem. Previously, many linctuses contained a high level of sucrose; however, many have been reformulated as 'sugar-free' products to reduce the risk of den-tal caries. Because the viscous nature of linctuses is beneficial, they should not be diluted prior to administration.

Liniments

These are liquids for external use. They are used to alleviate the discomfort of muscle strains and injuries. Because of the rubefacient nature of some of the ingredients, some sportsmen will use them prior to starting a sporting activity in an attempt to avoid any muscle damage. Examples of active ingre-dients found in liniments are turpentine oil and methyl salicylate. The BNF states that the evidence around topical rubefacients does not support their use in acute or chronic musculoskeletal pain.

Lotions

These are liquids for external use and may be solu-tions, suspensions or emulsions. They have a variety of uses, which include antiseptic, parasiticidal and soothing. Care should be taken when recommend-ing lotions for the treatment of head lice. Those which have an alcohol base should be avoided in asthmatics and young children, as the alcoholic fumes may cause breathing difficulties. Aqueous-based products should be advised.

Lozenges

These are large tablets designed to be sucked and remain in the mouth for up to 15 min. They do not contain a disintegrant and the active ingredient is normally incorporated into a sugar base, such as sucrose or glucose. The main use of lozenges is in the treatment of mouth and throat infections.

Mixtures

This is a generic term used for many liquid prepara-tions for oral use.

Mouthwashes

These are similar in formulation to gargles but are used specifically to treat conditions of the mouth. The active ingredients are usually antiseptics or bactericidal agents.

Nasal drops and sprays

These are isotonic solutions used to treat condi-tions of the nose. Locally acting decongestants are commonly presented as nose drops. The container includes a dropper device to allow the patient to deliver the appropriate dose into the affected nostril(s). Overuse of nose drops is common as patients find it difficult to judge the number of drops being delivered. Other preparations for both local and systemic use are presented as sprays (metered or pump).

Ointments

Ointments are semi-solids for topical use.

Paints

Paints are solutions for application to the skin. Those used on the skin are often formulated with a volatile vehicle. This evaporates on application and leaves a film of active ingredient on the skin surface.

Pastes

These are semi-solids for external use. They differ from creams and ointments in that they contain a high proportion of fine powder, such as starch. This makes them very stiff and means they do not spread readily over the skin's surface. Corrosive drugs such as dithranol are often formulated as pastes, so that paste applied to the psoriatic lesion will not spread onto healthy skin and cause irritation.

Pastilles

Pastilles are for oral use and, like lozenges, are designed to be sucked. They contain locally acting antiseptics, astringents or anaesthetics and are used to treat, or give symptomatic relief of, conditions affecting the mouth and throat. They have a jelly-like consistency produced by their basis of gelatin or acacia.

Pessaries

Pessaries are solid dosage forms for insertion into the vagina. They are used for both local and systemic action.

Pills

Pills are a moulded oral dosage form which has been superseded by tablets and capsules. The term is still used by the general public, incorrectly, to describe any solid oral dose form.

Powders (oral)

These occur as both bulk and divided powders. Bulk powders usually contain non-potent active ingredients such as antacids. The dose is measured using a 5 mL spoon.

Individual powders are used for more potent drugs, where accuracy of dosage is more important. An individual dose is packaged separately, either in a sheet of paper or in a sachet.

Suppositories

These are solid dosage forms for insertion into the rectum. They are used for both local and systemic actions.

Suspensions

Suspensions are liquid dose forms where the active ingredient is insoluble. Suspensions are available for both oral and external use.

Syrups

These are concentrated aqueous solutions of sugars such as sucrose. The term 'syrup' is frequently, but incorrectly, applied to certain sweetened liquids intended for oral use. The term 'syrup' should nowadays only be used to refer to flavouring vehicles. Sucrose is being replaced by sorbitol as the sweetening agent in many preparations to give 'sugar-free' syrups to reduce the risk of dental caries.

Tablets

This is the term used to describe compressed solid dosage forms generally intended for oral use, although some pessaries are tablets for vaginal use. As well as the standard tablet made by compression, there are many different types of tablet designed for specific uses, e.g. dispersible, gastro-resistant (enteric coated), modified release or buccal.

Transdermal delivery systems

This term is used to describe the adhesive patches which, when applied to the skin, deliver a controlled dose of drug over a specified time period to produce a systemic effect.

KEY POINTS

- The route can be chosen to give local or systemic effects, fast or slow onset, and is influenced by biopharmacy and pharmacokinetics
- The oral route is the most commonly used route
- Gastric emptying, stability and other materials present in the GIT may limit availability of the drug from the oral route
- Sublingual absorption gives a short, fast-onset activity
- Buccal absorption takes place between the gum and lip
- Buccal routes of administration can be used with unconscious patients and to avoid first pass metabolism
- Rectal absorption partially avoids first pass metabolism
- Rectal administration is useful for nil-by-mouth patients and in cases of gastric irritation. However, it is poorly accepted in the UK
- Vaginal administration can give systemic effects avoiding first pass metabolism
- Inhalation requires a much lower dose than the oral route, with a rapid onset

- Administration to the skin may be used for both local and systemic effects
- Injections can give the fastest onset of action but prolonged action is also possible using oily intramuscular injections

- A wide range of different dosage forms which have different properties and uses, has been devised
- The same drug may usefully be used in different formulations to assist different types of patients

Dispensing techniques (compounding and good practice)

30

Judith A. Rees

STUDY POINTS

- Practical aspects of dispensing
- The working environment and procedures
- Extemporaneous dispensing equipment and its correct use
- Manipulative techniques used in dispensing and compounding
- Ingredients and their selection
- Problem-solving in extemporaneous dispensing

Introduction

This chapter deals with some of the practical aspects of dispensing, concentrating on the small-scale manufacture of medicines from basic ingredients. This process is called compounding or extemporaneous dispensing. Additionally, good practice which applies to all aspects of dispensing will be considered.

Nowadays, most medicines are manufactured by the pharmaceutical industry under well-controlled conditions and packaged in suitable containers designed to maintain the stability of the product (e.g. sealed in an inert atmosphere). Extemporaneous dispensing, which cannot be as well-controlled, should only be used when a manufactured product is unavailable. Reasons for unavailability of products may include:

- Non-licensed products
- Products no longer on the market or unavailable from the manufacturer
- Products requiring an individualized dose, e.g. for paediatric or geriatric patients
- Products requiring an individualized formulation for a patient, e.g. the removal of colouring agents
- Veterinary products, e.g. formulations for different species.

The pharmacist undertaking extemporaneous dispensing has a responsibility to maintain equipment in working order, to ensure that the formula and dose are safe and appropriate and that all materials are sourced from recognized pharmaceutical manufacturers. There are also requirements concerning calculations, maintaining good records and labelling. Any staff involved in the process should be adequately trained. These requirements should all be incorporated within standard operating procedures (SOPs, see Ch. 11).

In any dispensing process, the end-product will be used or taken by a person or an animal. Therefore, it is important that the medicine produced is of the highest achievable quality. This, in turn, means that the highest standards must be applied during the preparation process.

The working environment and procedures

Organization

The working environment needs to be organized, with well trained, efficient staff. A safe system of working is essential for a dispensary and the development and use of SOPs should be followed. Additionally, health and safety regulations must be applied in the dispensary.

Cleanliness and hygiene

The dispensing bench, the equipment, utensils and the container which is to hold the final product must all be clean. Lack of cleanliness can cause contamination of the preparation with other ingredients. For example, a spatula which has been used to remove an ingredient from one container will adulterate subsequent containers if not washed before being used again. Cleanliness will also minimize microbial contamination.

Dispensing staff should have a high standard of hygiene and hand-washing facilities should be readily available. A clean overall should be worn, hair tied back and, preferably, be covered with a disposable hat/cap and any skin lesions covered with a dressing. Disposable gloves should be worn during preparative work and discarded afterwards. Consideration should be given to the use of masks if volatile substances or fine powders are to be handled.

Documenting procedures and results

Keeping comprehensive records is an essential part of the dispensing process. Records must be kept for a minimum of 2 years (ideally 5 years) and include the formula and any calculations, the ingredients and quantities used, their sources, batch numbers and expiry date. All calculations or weights/volumes should be checked by two people and recorded. Any substances requiring special handling techniques or hazardous substances should be recorded with the precautions taken. The record for a prescribed item should also include the patient and prescription details and date of dispensing. A record must be kept of the personnel involved, including the responsible pharmacist. Any deviations from a SOP should be recorded.

Equipment

Not only is the selection of the correct equipment for the job essential, but the equipment must be used in the correct way and maintained in good order.

Weighing equipment

Weighing equipment can be divided into non-automatic and automatic weighing equipment.

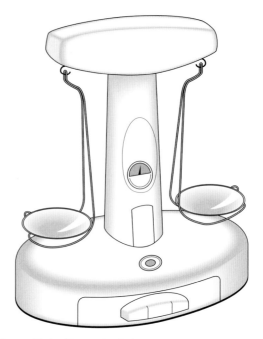

Figure 30.1 • Dispensing balance.

Non-automatic weighing equipment requires an operator to place and/or remove the items from the balance pan. Such weighing equipment can be a mechanical beam balance, which has a pan on one end of the beam for weights and a pan on the other end of the beam for the material to be weighed (Fig. 30.1) or it can be an electronic top-pan balance, in which case the substance to be weighed is placed on the pan and an electronic display gives the weight. Automatic weighing equipment is designed to automatically fill a package to the required weight without the intervention of an operator. Such equipment is used in the pharmaceutical industry, and nowadays for extemporaneous dispensing. Whichever type of weighing equipment is used, it must be suitable for its intended use and be sufficiently accurate. In the UK, weighing equipment must be calibrated in metric units and must be marked with maximum and minimum weights that can be weighed.

General rules for the use and maintenance of weighing equipment

The following points are important to ensure accurate weighing:

- Balances must be placed on a level surface; most will incorporate a level indicator device to allow adjustment for a non-level surface

- Balances' readings must indicate zero, before use. If zero is not indicated, then incorrect readings, and hence weights, may be obtained
- Strong draughts, caused by air conditioning or a breeze, can affect some balances and make a correct reading impossible. Therefore always site a balance in a draught-free area
- Always keep the balance pan clean and free from debris
- Regular checks with stamped weights should be made to ensure the balance is working correctly
- If possible keep a record of when, and by whom, the check was carried out, as well as the result
- Never weigh less than the declared minimum weight or more than the maximum weight declared on the balance
- Do not weigh ingredients on a piece of paper, as this introduces a potential inaccuracy. The exception is when weighing greasy or semi-solid materials, e.g. white soft paraffin, when a counterbalanced piece of paper should be used
- Always read the manufacturer's instructions before using an electronic balance
- Use tweezers to handle weights, if used. Never handle weights, as this will affect their accuracy and risks contamination.

Measuring liquids

Liquid measures

All measures for liquids must comply with current weights and measures regulations and should be stamped accordingly. Traditionally, conical measures (Fig. 30.2) have been used in dispensing.

When using a measure always ensure the following:

- The level of liquid is read to the bottom of the meniscus at eye level
- The measure is vertical when reading the meniscus. If this is not done, considerable errors in quantities can occur
- The measure is thoroughly drained to deliver the correct volume
- Always select the smallest measure which will hold the desired volume because this gives the greatest accuracy
- If the substance being measured is so viscous that it would be very difficult to drain the

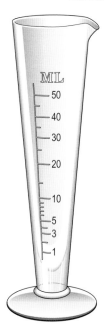

Figure 30.2 • Conical dispensing measure.

measure effectively, then the volume should be measured by difference. This is done by pouring an excess into the measure and then pouring off the liquid until only the excess volume remains.

Measuring small volumes

Graduated pipettes can be used for small volumes from 5 mL down to 0.1 mL. For volumes smaller than this, a dilution should be made. The viscosity of the substance being measured should also be considered.

Correct use of pipettes

Pipettes can be either the 'drainage' or 'blowout' variety. A rubber bulb or teat should be used. Never use mouth suction.

- A bulb or teat should be placed over the mouth of the pipette
- Only a short length of the pipette should be immersed in the liquid
- The correct amount of liquid should be drawn up the pipette
- The measured liquid is then released into the desired container.

Nowadays, semi-automatic pipettes can be used for dispensing.

Mixing and grinding

Mortar and pestle

The mortar (bowl) and pestle (pounding device) are used to reduce the size of powders, mix powders, mix together powders and liquids and to make emulsions. Two types, each available in a range of sizes, are used.

Glass mortar and pestle

These are generally small. The smooth surface of the glass reduces the friction which can be generated, so they are only suitable for size reduction of friable materials (such as crystals). Glass mortars and pestles are useful for mixing small quantities of fine powders and for the mixing of substances such as dyes which are absorbed by and stain composition or porcelain mortars.

Porcelain or composition mortars and pestles

These mortars have a rough surface. They are ideal for size reduction of solids and for mixing solids and liquids, as in the preparation of suspensions and emulsions.

Size reduction using a mortar and pestle

Selection of the correct type of mortar and pestle is vital for this operation. A flat-bottomed mortar and a pestle with a flat head should be chosen.

Using a mortar and pestle for mixing powders

Adequate mixing will only be achieved if there is sufficient space. Overfilling of the mortar should be avoided. The pestle should be rotated in both right and left directions to ensure thorough mixing. Undue pressure should not be used, as this will cause impaction of the powder on the bottom of the mortar.

Filters

There are occasions when clarification of a liquid is required. Where filtration is required, filter paper or membrane filters should be used. Filter paper and membrane filters come in different grades and selection of the correct grade is determined by the size of the particles to be removed. Filter paper has the disadvantages of introducing fibres into the filtrate and may also absorb significant amounts of active ingredient. This is less likely with membrane filters.

Heat sources

In the dispensing process it may be necessary to heat ingredients, e.g. melt semi-solids in the preparation of ointments/creams, warm liquids to aid dissolution of solids.

Nowadays, water baths or electrically heated hot plates are used for heating.

Manipulative techniques

Selection of the correct equipment and using it appropriately is fundamental to good compounding. Several basic manipulative techniques may require practice.

Mixing

The goal of any mixing operation should be to ensure even distribution of all the ingredients has occurred. If a sample is removed from any part of the final preparation, it should be identical to a sample taken from any other part of the container.

Mixing of liquids

Simple stirring or shaking is usually all that is required to mix two or more liquids. The degree of stirring or shaking will be dependent on the viscosities of the liquids.

Mixing solids with liquids

Particle size reduction will either speed up the dissolution process or improve the uniform distribution of the solid throughout the liquid. When a solution is being made, a stirring rod will be adequate. However, a suspension will require a mortar and pestle.

Mixing solids with solids

Where the quantity of material to be mixed is small and the proportions are approximately the same, the materials can be added to an appropriately sized mortar and effectively mixed. Where a small quantity of powder has to be mixed with a large quantity, in order to achieve effective mixing, it must be done in stages:

- The ingredient with the smallest bulk is placed in the mortar

- A quantity of the second ingredient, approximately equal in volume to the first, is added and carefully mixed, using the pestle
- A further quantity of the second ingredient, approximately equal in volume to the mixture in the mortar, is now added
- This process, known as 'doubling-up', is continued until all the powder has been added (see Ch. 38).

Mixing semi-solids

If all the ingredients are semi-solids or liquids, they can be mixed together by rubbing them down on an ointment slab, using a spatula. If there is a significant difference in the quantities of the ingredients, a 'doubling-up' process should be used. An alternative method is the fusion method.

The fusion method

- Place the bases in an evaporating basin and gently heat until they have just melted. Excess heat should not be used, as overheating may cause physical or chemical changes in some materials
- The basin is then removed from the heat and the contents are stirred continuously, but gently, until the mixture has cooled and set. Stirring at this stage is of vital importance as otherwise the components may segregate on cooling. Rapid stirring should be avoided as it will introduce air bubbles into the mixture.

When using the fusion method, do not be tempted to add any solid active ingredients to the basin before the bases have set. Addition of any further ingredients is best done by rubbing down on an ointment slab. (Further details of methods used in the preparation of ointments can be found in Ch. 36.)

Tared containers

Liquid preparations should, as far as possible, be made up to volume in a measure. There are, however, instances when accurate transfer of the preparation to the final container is difficult, e.g. with some suspensions it can be almost impossible to remove all the insoluble ingredients when pouring from one container to another. Emulsions and viscous preparations can also be difficult to transfer accurately. In these cases, a tared container should be used.

To tare a bottle

A volume of potable water identical to the volume of the product being dispensed is accurately measured. This is then poured into the chosen medicine container and the meniscus marked with the upper edge of a small adhesive label, effectively making the bottle into a single-point measure. The container is then emptied and allowed to drain thoroughly. The preparation is then poured into the container and made up to volume, using the tare mark as the guide. Remove the tare label.

Ingredients

All ingredients must be sourced and obtained from reputable suppliers and be of a quality suitable for the preparation and dispensing of pharmaceutical products. Additionally, ingredients must be suitably stored to preserve stability and integrity. For example, regular checks on expiry dates of stored products should be made and any ingredient outside its expiry date should be discarded. Some ingredients may require special storage conditions and these should be provided. Many pharmaceutical ingredients and products require storage in a refrigerator, which should be fitted with a maximum/minimum thermometer and both maximum and minimum temperatures checked and recorded on a daily basis.

Selection

When dispensing, selection of the correct product is vital. The label on each container must be read carefully and checked to ensure that it contains the required product. There are many examples of drugs and preparations where names may be misread if care is not taken; examples include folic acid and folinic acid, cefuroxime and cefotaxime. (Further examples are given in Ch. 27.)

Variety of forms

Some ingredients of extemporaneously dispensed medicines may occur in a variety of forms or a synonym is used. Coal tar, for example, is available as coal tar solution, strong coal tar solution and coal tar. Some other materials where confusion can occur are listed in Table 30.1. This list is not meant to be comprehensive and only contains common exemplars. To reduce the risk of errors you need to read the container label carefully and have it checked by a second person.

Problem-solving in extemporaneous dispensing

For extemporaneous dispensing, it is helpful if a method detailing how to prepare the product is available. Methods for 'official' preparations can sometimes be found in reference sources such as the *Pharmaceutical Codex*. However, on many occasions, no method is available. In such a situation, it may be helpful to consider similar formulas in reference sources. Additionally, the application of simple scientific knowledge, especially of physical properties, is often all that is needed. The following gives an example of how this is done.

Table 30.1 Some substances which occur in a variety of forms	
Substance/form	**Use**
Light magnesium carbonate	Because of its lightness and diffusible properties, it is used in suspensions
Heavy magnesium carbonate	Normally used in bulk or individual powders
Light kaolin	Used in suspensions
Heavy kaolin	Used in the preparation of kaolin poultice
Precipitated sulfur	This has a smaller particle size than sublimed sulfur and is preferred in preparations for external use, e.g. suspensions, creams and ointments
Sublimed sulfur	Slightly gritty powder, which does not produce such elegant preparations as precipitated sulfur
Yellow soft paraffin	Used as an ointment base
White soft paraffin	Bleached yellow soft paraffin, normally used when the other ingredients are not strongly coloured

Putting theory into practice

Solubility

Always check the solubility of any solid materials. If they are soluble in the main vehicles, then a solution is likely to be produced. If solubility is limited to one liquid, this will assist in achieving uniform dose distribution. Solution will be achieved more quickly if the particle size is small and so size reduction should be considered for any soluble ingredients which are presented in a lumpy or granular form. It is also necessary to add less soluble solids before more soluble solids. If the substance is not soluble, then a suspension will need to be produced. Whether a suspending agent will be required should be considered (see Ch. 34). Where one material is an oil and another aqueous, it is likely that an emulsifying agent will be required to produce an emulsion (see Ch. 35).

Volatile ingredients

If an ingredient is volatile then it should be added near the end of the dispensing process and often directly into the final container. If it is added too early, much may be lost due to evaporation.

Viscosity

The viscosity of a liquid will have a bearing on how it is measured, i.e. is a pipette or measure suitable, or should it be measured by difference, and how will it be incorporated?

Expiry date

All extemporaneously prepared products should be labelled with an expiry date. Ideally, stability studies should be undertaken in order to predict an accurate shelf-life for all products. This is not usually possible for 'one-off' preparations and most hospital pharmacies have guidelines based on previous stability studies. If in doubt, use the shortest possible expiry date, e.g. 3 days, and be prepared to produce the medicine in small quantities every 3 days.

Conclusion

Developing good practice in dispensing takes time and requires attention to detail.

KEY POINTS

- Extemporaneous dispensing should only be used when manufactured medicines are not available
- Accurate dispensing requires clean and methodical work
- Always comply with SOPs
- Comprehensive records of extemporaneous dispensing are required to be kept for at least 2 years
- Always use all equipment correctly
- Ensure that liquid measures comply with the weights and measures regulations
- Always use the bottom of the meniscus when measuring liquids
- Viscous liquids should be measured 'by difference'
- Select the smallest measure or pipette for the volume of liquid to be measured
- A glass mortar and pestle can be used for size reduction of friable materials and mixing small quantities of fine powder
- A porcelain mortar and pestle is used for larger quantities, for mixing solids and liquids, making emulsions and for size reduction
- Confusion can arise with different forms of the same material and the use of synonyms
- Simple problem-solving techniques can produce a satisfactory method of dispensing a product

31

Labelling of dispensed medicines

Judith A. Rees

STUDY POINTS

- Reasons for labelling dispensed products
- Requirements for labels
- Standard details required on labels
- Additional labels
- Specific UK legal requirements
- Patient-specific labels

Introduction

All dispensed medicines, whether extemporaneously prepared, repackaged from a manufacturer's pack or a manufacturer's patient pack, should be individually labelled for the patient. The label on a dispensed medicine has several main functions:

- To identify the contents of the container
- To provide clear and concise information which will enable the patient to take or use their medicine in the most effective and appropriate way
- To identify clearly the patient for whom the medicine is dispensed
- To satisfy legal requirements.

Most countries have both legal and professional requirements for the labelling of dispensed medicines. It is the pharmacist's responsibility to ensure that these requirements are satisfied and that all labelling is accurate and comprehensible. Normally, there are standard details which must appear on every label. However, some medicines may require additional details. The provision of an adequate label, however, does not remove the need to give advice and counselling to the patient (see Ch. 25).

Standard requirements for labelling dispensed medicines

All labels should be in printed form and so the information should be legible. However, it is good professional practice to check each label for legibility (including size of print) before handing the product to the patient.

The details which should appear on the label of a dispensed medicine are:

- Name of the preparation, strength and form (if more than one available)
- Quantity
- Instructions for use
- Precautions relating to the use of the product
- Patient's name
- Date of dispensing
- Name and address of the pharmacy
- 'Keep out of reach of children' or similar
- The phrase 'For external use only' for certain formulations.

Additional labelling requirements

- Warning or advisory labels should be attached to the container, where appropriate
- A batch number should be indicated if the preparation has been prepared extemporaneously

- An expiry date should be indicated if the preparation has been prepared extemporaneously or the shelf-life has been shortened, e.g. a diluted preparation
- Additional legal requirements, e.g. 'For animal treatment only' on veterinary prescriptions
- Storage conditions.

The name of the preparation, strength and form

The name which appears on the label must be the same as the one which appears on the prescription. The preparation may be prescribed generically but only be available as a proprietary or branded product; however, the prescribed name must be used. The reason for this is to avoid the patient becoming confused with a variety of names.

The name may be omitted only when the product is prepared to a prescriber's own formula and contains several active ingredients and has no official name. In these instances, it may be difficult to list all the ingredients on the label and so the pharmaceutical form is used, e.g. 'the ointment', 'the mixture'.

If the preparation is available in more than one strength, e.g. amoxicillin 250 mg and 500 mg capsules, the strength must be included on the label. Such information clearly identifies the medicine.

Similarly, the form of the medicines should be included on the label. This is especially important if the product is available in more than one form (e.g. capsules, syrup, suspension, sachets, injection). The inclusion of the form identifies the medicine and may give an indication of how it is to be used/taken (e.g. suppositories, inhalations, enemas).

Quantity and multiple packs

Normally, the quantity which appears on the label will be the quantity which has been prescribed. Nowadays, many medicines are supplied in the manufacturer's patient packs, which will be labelled according to the legal requirements. If the quantity on the prescription requires more than one of these patient packs to be dispensed, e.g. two patient packs each containing 28 tablets of the same medicinal product (a total of 56 tablets), then the quantity on the label should be the amount in each container. One of the packs should be labelled

as '1 of 2' and the other pack labelled '2 of 2'. The patient should be directed to use the pack labelled 1 of 2 and when the contents have been used, the patient should use the pack labelled 2 of 2.

Instructions for use

No patient should leave a pharmacy without knowing how much, how often and how to use/take his or her medication (see Ch. 25). Although the label should be seen as a back-up to the verbal counselling and advice given by the pharmacist, it is still essential to ensure that the wording on the label is clear, concise and comprehensible to the patient. If the prescriber's instructions are missing or incomplete on the prescription, it is the pharmacist's professional duty to obtain instructions from the prescriber or use professional discretion to interpret BNF statements.

The way in which instructions are worded is very important and will greatly influence how easily a patient understands the message. Pharmacists should therefore give serious consideration to the wording on medicine labels.

The Royal Pharmaceutical Society Working Party Report (1990) on 'The Labelling of Dispensed Medicines' made several recommendations. The use of active verbs is preferred, e.g. 'take' instead of 'to be taken'; 'apply' instead of 'to be applied'. The reason is that research has shown that active verbs are more easily understood and remembered than passive verbs. It is bad practice to have two numbers appearing together in instructions, e.g. 'take two three times daily'. It is easy for a patient to mentally transpose the position of the numbers so that the previous instruction becomes 'three twice daily' in the patient's mind. To avoid this, the numbers should always be separated by using the formulation name, e.g. 'take two tablets', 'two capsules', 'two powders three times daily'. Other recommendations in the report can be seen in Table 31.1.

Numbers which are part of an instruction must always be written as words, except in the case of, e.g. 5 mL, when referring to a 5 mL spoonful, or oral syringe quantities, e.g. a 2.5 mL dose using the oral syringe provided.

Many manufacturers' packs of medicines contain a patient information leaflet. These normally give detailed instructions (with illustrations) of how to use a medicine, along with other details about

Table 31.1 Recommended wording for directions

Recommended wording	Wording to be replaced
Do not swallow	Not to be taken
Put two drops in the affected eye	Instil two drops into the affected eye
For creams or ointments: Spread thinly	Use sparingly
For pessaries or suppositories: Gently put one into the vagina/rectum	Insert one into the vagina/rectum

the medicine. Patients should be told to read the patient information leaflet before using the medicine. This is a back-up to the label.

Precautions relating to the use of the product

Labelling the product with precautions relating to its use, is for safety reasons. Such labels will be specific to the product and can include: 'Caution flammable: keep away from fire or flames' or 'Not to be consumed by mouth'.

The patient's name

It is a legal requirement that the name of the patient for whom the medication has been prescribed must appear on the label of all dispensed medicines. If possible, the status of the patient, i.e. Mr, Mrs, Miss, Master, Child or Baby, should be included in order to clearly differentiate from other members of a household, where there may be other persons with the same name. For the same reason, a full first name should also be included if possible, rather than an initial, e.g. Mr James Burnett instead of J. Burnett.

The date and name and address of the pharmacy

The majority of pharmacies use computer systems for prescription labelling and this information will normally appear automatically, with the date being re-set daily. This information is a legal requirement, and enables the source of the medicine and date of dispensing to be traced, if necessary. For example, in the case of possible overdose or poisoning, the label would assist any investigation.

'Keep out of reach of children'

In order to prevent accidental ingestion of medicines by children, all dispensed medicines are required to carry the label 'Keep out of reach of children' or similar wording.

Additional labelling requirements

In addition to the standard details required on all dispensed medicines, there are several extra details which are required in certain circumstances. Some information may be specific to a particular type of formulation.

Storage

General information for different types of preparation can be found in the relevant chapters in this book. Some formulations require special storage and this information should be attached to the label, e.g. transdermal patches should be stored in a cool place. Other labels relating to storage include: 'protect from light' and 'store in a fridge'. Any specific pharmaceutical precautions relating to storage should always be indicated, e.g. glyceryl trinitrate tablets should be labelled with 'Store the tablets in this bottle with the cap tightly closed. Get a new supply 8 weeks after opening'.

The *British Pharmacopoeia* (and other pharmacopoeias) uses the terms 'freshly prepared' and 'recently prepared' for extemporaneously prepared products with a short keeping time. 'Freshly prepared' is defined as having been made no more than 24 h before issue for use, but there is no indication of when it should be discarded. In this case, it is usual to give a 1 week discard date. The term 'recently prepared' is used for products which should be discarded 4 weeks after issue when stored at 15–25°C.

Information on proprietary medicines can be accessed in the Association of British Pharmaceutical Industries' (ABPI) *Medicines Compendium*.

Warnings for patients

Many drugs cause side-effects about which the patient should be informed. It is a professional requirement, subject to the pharmacist's discretion, that if indicated, these special warnings should be affixed to the container. The BNF contains a list of Cautionary and Advisory labels for dispensed medicines. Nowadays, most computer systems will automatically print these warnings when a label for a particular drug is being produced. However, there are instances when use of this information is inappropriate and professional discretion should be used. For example, the antihistamine, chlorphenamine, requires the warning: 'Warning. This medicine may make you sleepy. If this happens do not drive or use tools or machines. Do not drink alcohol'. Young children may be prescribed a drug such as this but this warning would be inappropriate. Obviously, it is important to draw attention to the problem of sedation and in this case, a more suitable warning, e.g. 'Warning. This medicine may make you sleepy', could be used.

A batch number

When a product has been prepared extemporaneously it is good practice to award it a batch number and incorporate this onto the label. When preparing an extemporaneous product, details of the ingredients used should be recorded (see Ch. 30). The batch number allows referral back to this information.

Expiry date

It is not normally necessary to put an expiry date on the label of a dispensed medicine, although with the increasing dispensing of manufacturers' original packs, this information will be part of the patient pack labelling. Manufacturers' expiry dates relate to ideal storage conditions but, unfortunately, when a product has been dispensed and given to the patient there is no longer any control over how it is stored. For this reason, under current legislation, when a product is repackaged for dispensing, no expiry date is stated. Patients should be encouraged to complete the course of medication or, if for any reason a supply is not finished and is no longer required, to bring any remainder back to the pharmacy.

There are, however, specific occasions when an expiry date must be added to the label:

- An expiry date should always be put onto any extemporaneously prepared item
- An expiry date should always be used when a product has been diluted, thereby affecting its stability and shelf-life
- An expiry date should always be indicated when the preparation is sterile, e.g. eye drops. Once opened the product is no longer sterile and if used beyond a certain timescale, there is a serious risk of infection. It is therefore recommended that eye drops and eye ointment, unless otherwise specified by the manufacturer, should be discarded 4 weeks after opening. This instruction should be indicated on the label (see Ch. 42 for further details).

Although the majority of patients will understand what 'expiry date' means, it is important to express the information in a clear and unambiguous way. 'Any unused … to be discarded on … (date)' or 'Do not use after … (date)' are preferred methods of expressing expiry dates.

Legal requirements in certain circumstances

Veterinary dispensed products

The words 'For animal use only' or similar, must always be added to the label of a dispensed veterinary product. Instead of the patient's name, the name of the animal's owner should appear, along with the owner's address or address where the animal is kept (see Ch. 28).

Emergency supply

When a preparation is dispensed using the emergency supply procedures, the words 'Emergency supply' must appear on the label.

Private prescriptions

A label for a medicine dispensed from a private prescription must bear a reference number. This reference number will relate to the entry in the private prescription register.

Labels for vulnerable patients

Some patients may have difficulty in reading the normal print size of a label due to failing eyesight or blindness. In such cases, consideration should be given to providing additional support to these patients, in the form of large print size on labels or the provision of large print size copies of the labels. In all cases, the medicinal products should be labelled. Additionally, consideration should be given to providing Braille labels for those patients able to read Braille.

Some patients may not be able to read the language on the label due to either illiteracy or being a non-native language reader. It may be possible to provide such a patient with a picture or series of pictures to illustrate the instructions. Many pictograms (a symbol representing a concept, object, activity, place or event by an illustration) have been developed for labelling medicines with instructions on how often and how to take medicines. Similarly, many toxic chemicals are labelled with pictograms to avoid harm to the public. The Risk-benefit Assessment of Drugs-analysis and Response (RAD-AR) Council of Japan, FIP and the USP all have websites showing pictograms for use on pharmaceutical packaging.

Clearly any patient with difficulty reading or understanding a label on a dispensed medicine should be given advice and counselling by the pharmacist before leaving the pharmacy.

Errors in labelling

The potential for making errors when producing a label is considerable and it is important that constant checking is carried out. Practice procedures should be such that the chances of errors occurring are minimized.

KEY POINTS

- A label is used to identify and instruct on the use of a medicine, so simple language should be used
- All labels must be typewritten or computer-generated
- All labels must state the name and quantity of the preparation, patient's name and instructions, name and address of pharmacy, date of dispensing and 'Keep out of reach of children' or similar wording
- Warning labels may also be required
- Active verbs should be used on the label
- Adjacent numbers should be separated by the formulation name (e.g. 'take two tablets three …') on a label
- As full a name of the patient as possible should be included on the label
- The BNF contains details of side-effect warnings which should be used, unless there is a good reason not to do so
- Some warning labels may require verbal explanation
- It is good practice to give an extemporaneous preparation a batch number
- Expiry dates are required on the label when dispensing diluted, sterile and extemporaneous preparations

Packaging

Derek G. Chapman

STUDY POINTS

- Definition of a container
- Considerations made in selecting a container
- The difference between primary and secondary packaging
- The materials used for packaging, including glass, plastics, metal and paper
- Types of container in common use
- Child-resistant closures and tamper-evident seals
- Patient pack dispensing

Introduction

Pharmaceutical formulations must be suitably contained, protected and labelled from the time of manufacture until the patient uses them. Throughout this period, the container must maintain the quality, safety and stability of the medicine and protect the product against physical, climatic, chemical and biological hazards. The *British Pharmacopoeia* identifies the closure as part of the container.

To promote good patient compliance, the container must be user-friendly. Thus, containers should be easy to open and reclose, most notably for elderly or arthritic patients. Other factors must also be considered in the selection of the container used to package a pharmaceutical formulation, including the cost and the need for both child-resistant closures and tamper-evident seals.

Repackaging may be performed for dispensing purposes in the community and hospital pharmacies and in specialized production facilities (see Chs 30, 39).

Bulk medicines are repackaged into smaller quantities in dispensing containers for distribution to hospital wards, clinics and general practitioners for direct supply to patients. This is mostly carried out with tablets and capsules that are transferred from bulk quantities into smaller amounts that are more suitable for patient use. In the UK, this process is performed in the hospital pharmacy where the MHRA allows the repackaging of small batches of up to 25 containers. Larger batches must be packed in licensed manufacturing premises. The facilities used for these repackaging operations are designed to maintain the quality of the medicine.

The composition of containers and closures used for the repackaging of bulk medicines must be carefully selected and must be of a quality as good as the original container. Both glass and plastic containers are used for repackaging but glass containers are often preferred due to the more inert qualities of glass.

Primary containers used for repackaging must not:

- Allow product leakage
- Chemically react with the product
- Release components
- Absorb or adsorb the product components.

The container used in the repackaging process must protect the product from:

- Physical damage
- Chemical and microbial contamination
- Light, moisture and oxygen as appropriate.

As the medicine has been transferred into a new container, the expiry date of the repackaged medicine must not exceed 12 months, unless the stability of the repackaged product justifies a longer shelf-life. The details of these repackaging processes must be recorded.

Each container of the repackaged batch is labelled with the:

- Identity and quantity of the medicine
- Batch number
- Appropriate storage instructions
- Product expiry date
- Requirements for handling and storage.

There are some situations where the repackaging is limited, such as with glyceryl trinitrate tablets, owing to the potential loss of the volatile drug (see Ch. 39). Sterile products cannot easily be repackaged and require effective closure systems to minimize the risk of microbial contamination of the contents within the container. In addition, the pack itself must withstand sterilization procedures. Consequently, care must be applied to the selection of the container and its closure for the packaging of sterile products (see also Chs 40, 41, 44, 46).

Primary and secondary packaging

Primary packaging materials are in direct contact with the product. This also applies to the closure, which is also part of the primary pack. It is important that this container must not interact with the medicine. It must protect the medicine from damage and from extraneous chemical and microbial contamination. In addition, the primary packaging should support the use of the product by the patient. Secondary packages are additional packaging materials that improve the appearance of the product and include outer wrappers or labels that do not make direct contact with the product (Table 32.1). Secondary packages can also supply information about the product and its use. They should provide evidence of tampering with the medicine.

The following terms are used to describe containers:

Single-dose containers hold the medicine that is intended for single use. For example, a glass ampoule

Multidose containers hold a quantity of the material that will be used as two or more doses. For example, a multiple dose vial or a plastic tablet bottle

Table 32.1 Types of primary and secondary packaging materials and their use

Material	Type	Examples of use
Glass	Primary	Metric medical bottle, ampoule, vial
Plastic	Primary	Ampoule, vial, container, infusion fluid dropper bottle
Plastic	Secondary	Wrapper to contain primary pack
Board	Secondary	Box to contain primary pack
Paper	Secondary	Labels, patient information leaflet

Well-closed containers protect the product from contamination with unwanted foreign materials and from loss of contents during use

Airtight containers are impermeable to solids, liquids and gases during normal storage and use. If the container is to be opened on more than one occasion it must remain airtight after reclosure

Sealed containers such as glass ampoules are closed by fusion of the container material

Tamper-evident containers are closed containers fitted with a device that irreversibly indicates if the container has been opened

Light-resistant containers protect the contents from the effect of radiation at a wavelength between 290 nm and 450 nm

Child-resistant containers, commonly referred to as CRCs, are designed to prevent children accessing the potentially hazardous product

Strip packs have at least one sealed pocket of material with each pocket containing a single dose of the product. The pack is made of two layers of film or laminate material. The nature and the level of protection that is required by the contained product will affect the composition of these layers

Blister packs are composed of a base layer, with cavities that contain the pharmaceutical product, and a lid. This lid is sealed to the base layer by heat, pressure or both. They are more rigid than strip packs and are not used for powders or semi-solids. Blister packs can be printed with day and week identifiers to produce calendar packs. These identifiers will support patient compliance

Tropicalized packs are blister packs with an additional aluminium membrane to provide greater protection against high humidity

Pressurized packs expel the product through a valve. The pressure for the expulsion of the product is provided by the positive pressure of the propellant that is often a compressed or liquefied gas (see Ch. 43)

Original packs are pharmaceutical packs that are commercially produced and intended for finite treatment periods. These packs are dispensed directly to the patient in their original form. Manufacturer's information is contained on the pack but the pharmacist must attach a dispensing label.

An important consideration when selecting the packaging for any product is that its main objective is that the package must contribute to delivering a drug to a specific site of effective activity in the patient.

The selection of packaging for a pharmaceutical product is dependent on the following factors:

- The nature of the product itself: its chemical activity, sensitivity to moisture and oxygen, compatibility with packaging materials
- The type of patient: is it to be used by an elderly or arthritic patient or by a child?
- The dosage form
- Method of administering the medication
- Required shelf-ife
- Product use.

Packaging materials

Glass

Historically, glass has been widely used as a drug packaging material. It continues to be the preferred packaging material for many pharmaceutical products.

Glass does have several advantages:

- It is inert to most medicinal products
- It is impervious to air and moisture
- It allows easy inspection of the container's contents
- It can be coloured to protect contents from harmful wavelengths of light
- It is easy to clean and sterilize by heat
- It is available in variously shaped containers.

The disadvantages of glass include:

- It is fragile: glass fragments can be released into the product during transport or contaminants can penetrate the product by way of cracks in the container
- Certain types of glass release alkali into the container contents
- It is expensive when compared with the price of plastic
- It is heavy, resulting in increased transport costs.

The chemical stability of glass for pharmaceutical use is given by the resistance of the glass to the release of soluble minerals into water contacting the glass. This is known as the hydrolytic resistance. Details are given in the *British Pharmacopoeia* (2012) for three types of glass.

Type I glass

This is also known as neutral glass or borosilicate glass. It possesses a high hydrolytic resistance due to the chemical composition of the glass. It is the most inert type of pharmaceutical glass with the lowest coefficient of thermal expansion. As a result, it is unlikely to crack on exposure to rapid temperature changes. Type I glass is suitable for packing all pharmaceutical preparations. However, it is expensive and this restricts its applications. It is widely used as glass ampoules and vials to package fluids for injection. In addition, it is used to package solutions that could dissolve basic oxides in the glass. This would increase the pH of the formulation and could affect the drug stability and potency.

Type II glass

This is made of soda-lime-silica glass with a high hydrolytic resistance due to surface treatment of the glass. Type II glass is used to package aqueous preparations. In general, it is not used by manufacturers to package parenteral formulations with a pH <7. It is the glass used to produce containers for eye preparations and other dropper bottles.

Type III glass

This is made of a soda-lime-silica glass. It has a similar composition to Type II glass but contains more leachable oxides. It is commonly used to produce dispensary metric medical bottles. It is also suitable for packaging non-aqueous parenteral products and powders for injection.

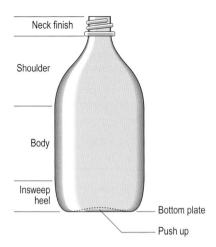

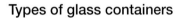

Figure 32.1 • Metric medicine bottle.

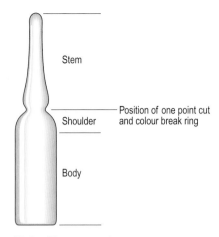

Figure 32.2 • Glass ampoule.

Types of glass containers

Bottles

These are commonly used in the dispensary as amber metric medical bottles and are available in sizes from 50 mL to 500 mL supplied with a screw closure.

Amber metric medical bottles have a smooth curved side and a flat side (Fig. 32.1).

Dropper bottles

Eye drop and dropper bottles for ear and nasal use are hexagonal-shaped amber glass containers fluted on three sides. They are fitted with a cap, rubber teat and dropper as the closure. The bottles are used at a capacity of 10 mL or 20 mL. The label is attached to the plain sides of the bottle.

Jars

Powders and semi-solid preparations are generally packed in wide-mouthed cylindrical jars made of clear or amber glass. The capacity of these jars varies from 15 mL to 500 mL. Ointment jars are used for packing extemporaneously prepared ointments and pastes. They are also used to repackage commercial products where microbial contamination by the patient's fingers is not detrimental to the product.

Containers for parenteral products

Small-volume parenteral products, such as subcutaneous injections, are typically packaged in various containers made of Type I glass. Glass ampoules (Fig. 32.2) are used to package parenteral solutions intended for single use.

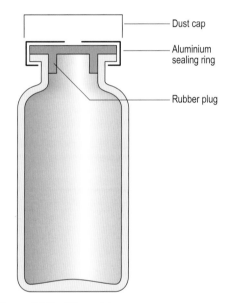

Figure 32.3 • Glass vial.

Multiple-dose vials (Fig. 32.3) are used to package parenteral formulations that will be used on more than one occasion. Large-volume parenteral fluids have been packaged in 500 mL glass containers but these have been largely superseded by plastic bags.

Plastics

Plastics have been widely used for several years as containers for the product and as secondary packaging in the form of a carton. In more recent times, plastic has been developed for the packaging of

Table 32.2 The application of thermoplastic polymers for the packaging of pharmaceutical products

Polymer	Examples of application
High-density polyethylene	Solid dosage form containers
Low-density polyethylene	Flexible eye drop bottles
Linear low-density polyethylene	Heat-sealable containers
Polypropylene	Container closures, intravenous solution bottles
Polyvinyl chloride	Laminate for blister packs, intravenous bags
Polystyrene	Containers for oils and creams and solid dosage forms

parenteral products, including infusion fluids and small-volume injections.

Two classes of plastics are used in the packaging of pharmaceutical products. These are known as thermosets and thermoplastics. The thermosets are used for making screw caps for glass and metal containers. Thermoplastic polymers are used in the manufacture of a wide variety of pharmaceutical packages, as detailed in Table 32.2.

The advantages of plastics for packaging are that they:

• release few particles into the product
• are flexible and not easily broken
• are of low density and thus light in weight
• can be heat-sealed
• are easily moulded into various shapes
• are suitable for use as container, closure and as secondary packaging
• are cheap.

The disadvantages of plastics are that:

• They are not as chemically inert as Type I glass
• Some plastics undergo stress cracking and distortion from contact with some chemicals
• Some plastics are very heat sensitive
• They are not as impermeable to gas and vapour as glass
• They may possess an electrostatic charge which will attract particles
• Additives in the plastic are easily leached into the product
• Substances such as the active drug and preservatives may be taken up from the product.

Plastic pharmaceutical containers are made of at least one polymer together with additives. The additives used will depend on the composition of the polymer and the production methods used.

Additives used in plastic containers include:

• Plasticizers
• Resins
• Stabilizers
• Lubricants
• Antistatic agents
• Mould-release agents.

Plastic containers

These are used for many types of pack, including rigid bottles for tablets and capsules, squeezable bottles for eye drops and nasal sprays, jars, flexible tubes, strip and blister packs. The composition and the physical shape of the containers vary widely to suit the application.

The principal plastic materials used in pharmaceutical packaging

Polyethylene

This is used as high- and low-density polyethylene, both of which are compatible with a wide range of drugs and are extensively used for the packaging of various pharmacy products. Of these two forms of polyethylene, low-density polyethylene (LDPE) is softer, more flexible and more easily stretched than high-density polyethylene (HDPE). Consequently, LDPE is usually the preferred plastic for squeeze bottles. By contrast, HDPE is stronger, stiffer, less clear, less permeable to gases and more resistant to oils, chemicals and solvents. It is commonly pigmented or printed white to block light transmission and improve label clarity. HDPE is widely used in bottles for solid dosage forms.

Disadvantages of LDPE and HDPE for packaging are that they:

• are softened by flavouring and aromatic oils
• are unsuitable for packing oxygen-sensitive products owing to high gas permeability
• adsorb antimicrobial preservative agents
• crack on contact with organic solvents.

Polyvinyl chloride (PVC)

This is extensively used as rigid packaging material and as the main component of intravenous bags.

Polypropylene

This is a strong, stiff plastic polymer with good resistance to cracking when flexed. As a result it is particularly suitable for use in closures with hinges which must resist repeated flexing. In addition, polypropylene has been used as tablet containers and intravenous bottles.

Polystyrene

This is a clear, hard, brittle material with low impact resistance. Its use in drug packaging is limited due to its high permeability to water vapour. However, it has been used for tubes and amber-tinted bottles where clarity and stiffness are important and high gas permeability is not a drawback. It is also used for jars for ointments and creams with low water content.

Closures

Any closure system should provide an effective seal to retain the container contents and exclude external contaminants. Child-resistant containers (CRCs) commonly consist of a glass or plastic vial or bottle with a specially designed closure. These CRCs are a professional requirement for dispensing of solid and liquid dosage forms in the UK and are ultimately a compromise between child resistance and ease of opening. They are not an absolute barrier to children accessing medicine containers, therefore the containers should be stored in a safe place. Several designs of CRCs are currently used for pharmaceutical packaging, including cap–bottle alignment systems, push down and turn caps and, less commonly, squeeze and turn caps.

The closures in common use with dispensed medicines are the Snap-safe® alignment closure (Fig. 32.4) and the push down and turn Clic-loc® closure (Fig. 32.5). The Clic-loc® child-resistant closures are based on the assumption that young children are unable to coordinate two separate and dissimilar actions; that is, applying pressure and rotating the closure top. The Clic-loc® closure has a two-piece mechanism with springs between the inner and the outer parts. As a result of this design, the closure produces an audible clicking noise when the cap is turned without first being depressed. The inner cap is composed of polypropylene while the outer overcap is made of HDPE.

Contamination of the screw thread with crystallized sugar arising from syrups can increase the

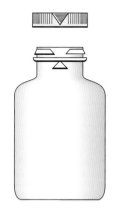

Figure 32.4 • Snap-safe® closure.

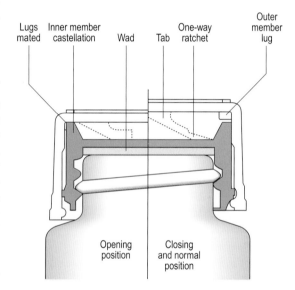

Figure 32.5 • Clic-loc® closure.

torque necessary to open these Clic-loc® closures. This type of problem can restrict their suitability for use. Owing to opening difficulties experienced by some adults, these closures should not be used on containers supplied to elderly or disabled patients with poor manual dexterity. They should not be used when a request is made that the product is not dispensed with a CRC fitted. A Clic-loc® closure must only be dispensed on one occasion as continued use increases the penetration of moisture vapour into the container and decreases the child-resistant properties of the closure.

In recent years, greater awareness of the vulnerability of products has led to the development of tamper-evident closures. The closures indicate if unlawful access to the container contents

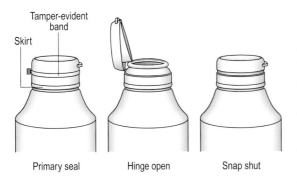

Figure 32.6 • Tamper-evident closure.

Primary seal Hinge open Snap shut

Tamper-evident band

Skirt

has occurred and are currently available in various designs suitable for different containers and closures. Dispensary stock containers are frequently fitted with a Jaycap® type of tamper-evident closure. These closures are made of either white polypropylene or LDPE. With this closure design the tamper-evident closures snap over a security bead on the neck of the container. The closures cannot be opened until the tamper-evident band connecting the cap to the skirt is torn away (Fig. 32.6). Clic-loc® closures are available with this design, whereby an external tamper-evident coloured band must be removed before the closure can be turned. Tamper-evident inner seals are positioned within the closure and are attached to the rim of the opening to the container isolating its contents. The seal must be torn or removed from the container to gain access to the packaged product. These seals are commonly made of a combination of paper, plastic and foil.

Collapsible tubes

These are flexible containers for the storage and dispensing of creams and ointments. Tubes made of tin are used to package certain sterile formulations. Typically, the formulation is aseptically filled into the pre-sterilized tubes. However, the most common metal tubes in current use are made of aluminium with an internal lacquered surface. With this package the tube remains collapsed as the product is removed. These tubes are frequently sealed at both ends and the nozzle must be punctured to access the product. An alternative seal that can be used with these packages is a heat seal band between the closure and the container. This band must be torn to gain access to the container contents.

Plastic tubes made from a variety of materials are superseding metal tubes. For example, the tube sleeve may be made of LDPE with either a LDPE or HDPE head or the entire tube may be made of polypropylene.

Unit-dose packaging

This term usually means that a single item such as a tablet or capsule or a specific dose is enclosed within its own disposable packaging. The most commonly used methods for unit-dose packaging are blister packs and strip packs.

Blister packs

These are used for packaging unit doses of tablets and capsules and can act as an aid for patient compliance. The medication is placed in a compartment in a base material made of paper, board, plastic or metal foil or a combination of these. The blister is generally composed of a thermoformed plastic sheet such as PVC. The protection given by the plastic blister depends on its composition, design and the method used to form it. Perforations in the base material allow individual sections of the package to be broken off. Blister packages are rigid, unlike strip packs that are flexible.

Strip packaging

With strip packaging, two webs of material sandwich various types of medicine such as tablets, capsules, suppositories or pessaries. Each of these dosage forms is contained within its own compartment. The composition of the two webs can be selected to meet the necessary protective requirements for the medicine. Aluminium foil is commonly used to manufacture strip packs and provides a good barrier against moisture penetration. The foil is used as a laminate in which the other components add strength to the fragile aluminium foil. They also block small holes, which can occur in the thinner foil layer.

Paper

Paper is used more than any other material in packaging. Although it has an insignificant role in primary packaging, it remains the predominant secondary and tertiary packaging material. In this role, it is used as the carton which contains the primary package and, in the form of board, is the corrugated shipping container which contains both.

Patient pack dispensing

A patient pack consists of a course of medication, together with a patient information leaflet in a ready to dispense pack. Liquid formulations are supplied in a standard pack. Solid dose forms are supplied as a strip or blister pack. The size of the sealed patient pack is based on a 28, 30 or 56 dose unit appropriate to the medicine. It is supplied in this amount unless a doctor prescribes that a different quantity of medicine is to be dispensed. The patient pack is designed as a balance between the need for child resistance and the need for ease of opening. If requested by the patient, the pack contents can be repackaged in a more suitable container.

Advantages of patient packs

- They contain product information such as product and manufacturer identification and the batch number
- More efficient dispensing results in greater opportunity for patient counselling
- More information is supplied to the patient about the product.

Disadvantages of patient packs

- Increased storage space is required
- Elderly and debilitated patients may experience difficulty in opening the pack.

KEY POINTS

- Containers should preserve the quality of a medicine for its stated shelf-life
- Glass has both advantages and disadvantages in use, but remains the preferred material in many situations
- The types of glass have different uses
- Plastics may be thermosets or thermoplastics
- A variety of additives to plastics may enter medicines with which they are in contact
- CRCs may have alignment closures (Snap-safe®) or push and turn (Clic-loc®)
- Use of CRCs is a professional requirement for dispensed medicines unless requested otherwise
- Tamper-evident closures indicate that there has been no unlawful access to the medicine
- Aluminium is being replaced by plastics for collapsible tubes
- Unit dosage packaging may be either blister or strip packaging
- The main use for paper is for cartons and boxes
- A patient pack consists of the medicine and patient information leaflet in a ready to dispense outer pack

Solutions

33

Arthur J. Winfield

Introduction

Solutions are homogeneous mixtures of two or more components. They contain one or more solutes dissolved in one or more solvents, usually solids dissolved in liquids. The solvent is often aqueous but can be oily, alcoholic or some other solvent.

There are many types of pharmaceutical solutions. Solutions may be used as oral dosage forms, mouthwashes, gargles, nasal drops and ear drops and externally as lotions, liniments, paints, etc. Solutions may also be used in injections and ophthalmic preparations (see Chs 41, 42).

Solutions for oral dosage

Oral solutions are usually formulated so that the patient receives the usual dose of the medication in a conveniently administered volume, 5 mL or a multiple thereof, given to the patient using a 5 mL medicine spoon.

Advantages of solutions for oral use over a solid dosage form are that liquids are much easier to swallow than tablets or capsules and the medicament is readily absorbed from the gastrointestinal tract. Ease of taking is especially useful for children, elderly patients or those with chronic conditions such as Parkinson's disease, who may have difficulty swallowing a solid oral dosage form. An advantage of solutions over suspensions is that the medicament is dispersed homogeneously throughout the preparation, without the need to shake the bottle. This makes the preparation easier for the patient to use and should ensure consistent dosage. Sometimes substances with a low aqueous solubility may be made into solution by the addition of another solvent rather than formulate the medicine as a suspension.

Disadvantages of solutions are that they are bulky, not convenient to carry around and less microbiologically and chemically stable than their solid counterparts. Oral solutions may have an unpleasant taste. The accuracy of oral dosage is dependent on the patient measuring the dose carefully.

The different forms of oral solutions are:

- *Syrups*, which are aqueous solutions that contain sugar. An example is Epilim® syrup (sodium valproate)

- *Elixirs*, which are clear, flavoured liquids containing a high proportion of sucrose or a suitable polyhydric alcohol and sometimes ethanol. Examples are phenobarbital elixir and chloral elixir (see Example 33.5)
- *Linctuses*, which are viscous liquids used in the treatment of cough. They usually contain a high proportion of sucrose, other sugars or a suitable polyhydric alcohol or alcohols. Examples are Simple Linctus BP and diamorphine linctus (see Example 33.4)
- *Mixtures* is a term often used to describe pharmaceutical oral solutions and suspensions. Examples are chloral hydrate mixture and ammonium and ipecacuanha mixture BP (see Example 33.3)
- *Oral drops* are oral solutions or suspensions which are administered in small volumes, using a suitable measuring device. A proprietary example is Abidec® vitamin drops.

Containers for dispensed solutions for oral use

Plain, amber medicine bottles should be used, with a reclosable child-resistant closure. Exceptions to this are: if the medicine is in an original pack or patient pack, if there are no suitable child-resistant containers for a particular liquid preparation or if the patient requests it, e.g. if they have severe arthritis in their hands. Advice to store away from children should then be given. A 5 mL medicine spoon or an appropriate oral syringe should be supplied to the patient.

Special labels and advice for dispensed oral solutions

An expiry date should appear on the label for extemporaneously prepared solutions. Most 'official' mixtures and some oral solutions are freshly or recently prepared. 'Official' elixirs and linctuses and manufactured products are generally more stable, unless diluted. Diluted products generally have a shorter shelf-life than the undiluted preparation. Linctuses should be sipped and swallowed slowly, without the addition of water.

Solutions for other pharmaceutical uses

Topical solutions for external use are considered in Chapter 36. Some topical solutions are designed for use in body cavities, such as the nose, mouth and ear.

Mouthwashes and gargles

Gargles are used to relieve or treat sore throats and mouthwashes are used on the mucous membranes of the oral cavity, rather than the throat, to refresh and mechanically clean the mouth. Both are concentrated solutions, although gargles tend to contain higher concentrations of active ingredients than mouthwashes. Both are usually diluted with warm water before use. They may contain antiseptics, analgesics or weak astringents. The liquid is usually not intended for swallowing. Examples are Phenol Gargle BPC and Compound Sodium Chloride Mouthwash BP (see Example 33.7). Proprietary examples are chlorhexidine (Corsodyl®) mouthwash and povidone-iodine (Betadine®) mouthwash.

Containers for mouthwashes and gargles

An amber medicine bottle should be used for these extemporaneously prepared solutions.

Special labels and advice for mouthwashes and gargles

Directions for diluting the preparations should be given to the patient. If the preparation is not intended for swallowing, the following label is appropriate: 'Not to be swallowed in large amounts'.

Nasal solutions

Most nasal preparations are solutions, administered as nose drops or sprays. They are usually formulated to be isotonic to nasal secretions (equivalent to 0.9% normal saline) and buffered to the normal pH range of nasal fluids (pH5.5–6.5) to prevent damage to ciliary transport in the nose. The most frequent use of nose drops is as a decongestant for the common cold or to administer local steroids for the treatment of allergic rhinitis. Examples are normal saline nose drops and ephedrine nose drops, 0.5% or 1%. Overuse of topical decongestants can lead to oedema of the nasal mucosa and they should only be used for short periods of time (about 4 days) to avoid rebound congestion, called rhinitis medicamentosa. The nasal route may also be useful for new biologically active peptides and polypeptides which need to avoid the first pass metabolism and destruction by the gastrointestinal fluids. The nasal mucosa rapidly absorbs applied medicaments to give a systemic effect. There are some products utilizing nasal delivery currently available on the market, e.g. desmopressin (e.g. Desmospray®, DDAVP®), used in the treatment of pituitary diabetes insipidus. Accurate dosage is achieved using metered spray devices.

Ear drops

Ear drops are solutions of one or more active ingredient which exert a local effect in the ear, e.g. by softening earwax or treating infection or inflammation. They may also be referred to as otic or aural preparations. Propylene glycol, oils, glycerol (to increase viscosity) and water may be used as vehicles. Examples are aluminium acetate ear drops, almond oil ear drops and Sodium Bicarbonate Ear Drops BP (see Example 33.8).

Containers for nasal and aural preparations

Nose and ear drops that are prepared extemporaneously should be packed in an amber, ribbed hexagonal glass bottle which is fitted with a teat and dropper. Manufactured nasal solutions may be packed in flexible plastic bottles which deliver a fine spray to the nose when squeezed, or in a plain glass bottle with a pump spray or dropper. Manufactured ear drops are usually packed in small glass or plastic containers with a dropper.

Special labels and advice for nasal and aural preparations

Patients should be advised not to share nasal sprays or nose and ear drops in order to minimize contamination and infection. Manufactured nasal sprays and nose and ear drops will usually contain instructions for administration. Patients should be given advice on how to administer extemporaneously prepared nose and ear drops, accompanied by written information if possible (Fig. 33.1). For

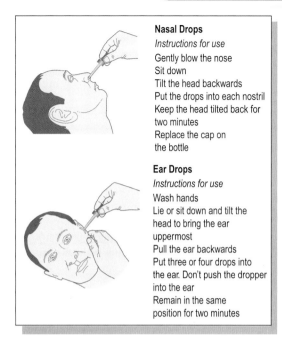

Nasal Drops
Instructions for use
Gently blow the nose
Sit down
Tilt the head backwards
Put the drops into each nostril
Keep the head tilted back for two minutes
Replace the cap on the bottle

Ear Drops
Instructions for use
Wash hands
Lie or sit down and tilt the head to bring the ear uppermost
Pull the ear backwards
Put three or four drops into the ear. Don't push the dropper into the ear
Remain in the same position for two minutes

Figure 33.1 • Patient instruction leaflets for use of nose and ear drops.

nose drops, it may be easier if the patient is lying flat with the head tilted back as far as comfortable, preferably over the edge of a bed. The patient should remain in this position for a few minutes after the drops have been administered to allow the medication to spread in the nose.

For ear drops, it may be easier for someone other than the patient to administer the drops. If desired, the drops can be warmed by holding the bottle in the hands before putting them in, but they must not be overheated. The ear lobe should be held up and back in adults, down and back in children, to allow the medication to run in deeper. They may cause some transient stinging. If the drops are intended to soften earwax, then the ears should be syringed after several days of use.

Extemporaneous preparations should be labelled with the appropriate expiry date following the official monographs. 'For external use' is not an appropriate label and so 'Not to be taken' is advised.

Enemas

Enemas are oily or aqueous solutions that are administered rectally. They are usually anti-inflammatory, purgative, sedative or given to allow X-ray examination of the lower bowel. Examples are arachis oil enema and magnesium sulphate enema. Retention enemas are administered to give either a local action of the drug, e.g. prednisolone, or for systemic absorption, e.g. diazepam. They are used after defecation. The patient lies on one side during administration and remains there for 30 min to allow distribution of the medicament. Microenemas are single-dose, small-volume solutions. Examples are solutions of sodium phosphate, sodium citrate or docusate sodium. They are packaged in plastic containers with a nozzle for insertion into the rectum. Large-volume (0.5–1 L) enemas should be warmed to body temperature before administration.

Enemas are packed in amber, glass bottles. Manufactured enemas will usually be packed in disposable polythene or polyvinyl chloride bags sealed to a rectal nozzle.

Special labels and advice for enemas

Patients should be advised on how to use the enema if they are self-administering and the time that the product will take to work. The label 'For rectal use only' should be used.

Expression of concentration

Strengths of pharmaceutical solutions can be expressed in a number of ways. The two most commonly used are in terms of amount of drug contained in 5 mL of vehicle or percentage strength (see Ch. 19).

Formulation of solutions

Solutions comprise the medicinal agent in a solvent as well as any additional agents. These additional agents are usually included to provide colour, flavour, sweetness or stability to the formulation. Most solutions are now manufactured on a large scale although it may be occasionally required to make up a solution extemporaneously. When compounding a solution, information on solubility and stability of each of the solutes must be taken into account.

Chemical and physical interactions that may take place between constituents must also be taken into account, as these will affect the preparation's stability or potency. For example, esters of *p*-hydroxybenzoic acid, which can be used as preservatives in oral solutions, have a tendency to partition into certain flavouring oils. This could reduce the effective concentration of the preservative agent in the aqueous vehicle of the preparation to a level lower than that required for preservative action.

Solubility

The saturation solubility of a chemical in a solvent is the maximum concentration of a solution, which may be prepared at a given temperature. For convenience, this is usually simply called solubility. Solubilities for medicinal agents in a given solvent are given in the *British Pharmacopoeia* (BP) and *Martindale* and other reference sources. Solubilities are usually stated as the number of parts of solvent (by volume) that will dissolve one part (by weight or volume) of the substance. In other situations, words are used to describe the solubility (see Examples 33.1 and 33.2). Using this information, it is often possible to calculate whether a solution can be prepared. Most solutions for pharmaceutical use are not saturated with solute.

Example 33.1

Potassium chloride is soluble in 2.8–3 parts of water.
This means that 1 g of potassium chloride will dissolve in 2.8–3 mL of water at a temperature of 20°C (taken as normal room temperature).

Example 33.2

Diazepam is described as being 'very slightly soluble' in water (which means 1 in 1000 to 1 in 10 000), 'soluble' in alcohol (which means 1 in 10 to 1 in 30) and 'freely soluble' in chloroform (which means 1 in 1 to 1 in 10).
This means that 1 g of diazepam will dissolve in between 10 and 30 mL of alcohol, but would need 1000–10 000 mL of water to dissolve, at a temperature of 20°C.

Vehicles

In pharmacy, the medium which contains the ingredients of a medicine is called the vehicle. In solutions, this is the solvent. The choice of a vehicle depends on the intended use of the preparation and on the nature and physicochemical properties of the active ingredients.

Water as a vehicle

Water is the vehicle used for most pharmaceutical preparations. It is widely available, relatively inexpensive, palatable and non-toxic for oral use and non-irritant for external use. It is also a good solvent for many ionizable drugs. Different types of water are available as outlined below:

- *Potable water* is drinking water, drawn freshly from a mains supply. It should be palatable and safe for drinking. Its chemical composition may include mineral impurities, which could react with drugs, e.g. the presence of calcium carbonate in hard water
- *Purified water* is prepared from suitable potable water by distillation, by treatment with ion-exchange materials or by any other suitable treatment method such as reverse osmosis. Distilled water is purified water that has been prepared by distillation
- *Water for preparations* is potable or freshly boiled and cooled purified water, which can be used in oral or external preparations which are not intended to be sterile. The boiling removes dissolved oxygen and carbon dioxide from solution in the water. Any stored water, for example drawn from a local storage tank, should not be used because of the risk of contamination with microorganisms
- *Water for injections* is pyrogen-free distilled water, sterilized immediately after collection and used for parenteral products (for further details, see Ch. 41).
- *Aromatic waters* are near-saturated aqueous solutions of volatile oils or other aromatic or volatile substances, and are often used as a vehicle in oral solutions. Some have a mild carminative action, e.g. dill. Aromatic waters are usually prepared from a concentrated ethanolic solution, in a dilution of 1 part of concentrated water with 39 parts of water. Chloroform water is used as an antimicrobial preservative and also adds sweetness to preparations

Other vehicles used in pharmaceutical solutions

- *Syrup BP* is a solution of 66.7% sucrose in water. It will promote dental decay and is unsuitable for diabetic patients. Hydrogenated glucose syrup, mannitol, sorbitol, xylitol, etc. can replace the sucrose to give 'sugar-free' solvents
- *Alcohol (ethyl alcohol, ethanol)*. This is rarely used for internal preparations but is a useful solvent for external preparations
- *Glycerol (glycerin)* may be used alone as a vehicle in some external preparations. It is viscous and miscible both with water and alcohol. It may be added as a stabilizer and sweetener in internal preparations. In concentrations above 20% v/v, it acts as a preservative
- *Propylene glycol* is a less viscous liquid and a better solvent than glycerol
- *Oils*. Bland oils such as fractionated coconut oil and arachis oil may be used for fat-soluble compounds, e.g. Calciferol Oral Solution BP. Care is required when using nut oils due to hypersensitivity reactions
- *Acetone* is used as a co-solvent in external preparations
- *Solvent ether* can be used as a co-solvent in external preparations for preoperative skin preparation. The extreme volatility of ether and risk of fire and explosion limit its usefulness.

Factors affecting solubility

Compounds that are predominantly non-polar tend to be more soluble in non-polar solvents, such as chloroform or a vegetable oil. Polar compounds tend to be more soluble in polar solvents, such as water and ethanol. The pH will also affect solubility, as many drugs are weak acids or bases. The ionized form of a compound will be the most water soluble, therefore a weakly basic drug will be most soluble in an aqueous solution that is acidic. Acid or alkali may therefore be added to manipulate solubility. Most compounds are more soluble at higher temperatures. Particle size reduction will increase the rate of solution.

Increasing the solution of compounds with low solubility

Co-solvency

The addition of co-solvents, such as ethanol, glycerol, propylene glycol or sorbitol, can increase the solubility of weak electrolytes and non-polar molecules in water.

Solubilization

Surfactants may be used as solubilizing agents. Above the critical micelle concentration (CMC), they form micelles which are used to help dissolve poorly soluble compounds. The dissolved compound may be in the centre of the micelle, adsorbed onto the micelle surface, or sit at some intermediate point, depending on the polarity of the compound. Examples of surfactants used in oral solutions are polysorbates, while soaps are used to solubilize phenolic disinfectants for external use.

Preservation of solutions

Most water-containing pharmaceutical solutions will support microbial growth unless this is prevented. Contamination may come from raw materials or be introduced during extemporaneous dispensing.

Preservatives may be added to the formulation to reduce or prevent microbial growth. Chloroform is the most widely used in oral extemporaneous preparations, although there are disadvantages to its use, including its high volatility and reported carcinogenicity in animals. Use in the UK is limited to a chloroform content of 0.5% (w/w or w/v). For oral solutions, chloroform at a strength of 0.25% v/v will usually be incorporated as Chloroform Water BP. Alternatively, double strength chloroform water may be included in pharmaceutical formulae as half the total volume of the solution, to effectively give single strength chloroform water in the finished medicine (see Example 33.3). Benzoic acid at a strength of 0.1% w/v is also suitable for oral administration, as are ethanol, sorbic acid, the hydroxybenzoate esters and syrup. Some of the alternative preservatives have pH-dependent activity.

Syrups can be preserved by the maintenance of a high concentration of sucrose as part of the formulation. Concentrations of sucrose greater than 65% w/w will usually protect an oral liquid from growth of most microorganisms by its osmotic effects. A problem with their use occurs when other ingredients are added to the syrup, as this dilutes the syrup. This may cause a loss in the preservative action of the sucrose. Accidental dilution by, for example, using a damp bottle, may have a similar effect.

Preservatives used in external solutions include chlorocresol (0.1% w/v), chlorbutanol (0.5% w/v) and the parahydroxybenzoates (parabens).

Additional ingredients

Solutions that are intended for oral use may contain excipients such as flavouring, sweetening and, sometimes, colouring agents. These are added to improve the palatability and appearance of a solution for the patient. Stabilizing and viscosity enhancing agents may also be used.

Flavouring agents

Flavours added to solutions can make a medicine more acceptable to take, especially if the drug has an unpleasant taste. Selection of flavours is a complex process in the pharmaceutical industry. Flavours should be chosen to mask particular taste types, e.g. a fruit flavour helps to disguise an acid taste. The age of the patient should be taken into account when selecting a flavour, as children will tend to enjoy fruit or sweet flavours. Some flavours are associated with particular uses, e.g. peppermint is associated with antacid preparations. The flavour and colour should also complement each other. Extemporaneous medicines tend to use natural flavours added as juices (raspberry), extracts (liquorice), spirits (lemon and orange), syrups (blackcurrant), tinctures (ginger) and aromatic waters (anise and cinnamon). Some synthetic flavours are used in manufactured medicines.

Sweetening agents

Many oral solutions are sweetened with sugars, including glucose and sucrose. Sucrose enhances the viscosity of liquids and also gives a pleasant texture in the mouth. Prolonged use of liquid medicines containing sugar will lead to an increased incidence of dental caries, particularly in children. Attempts should be made to formulate oral solutions without sugar as a sweetening agent, using sorbitol, mannitol, xylitol, saccharin and aspartame as alternatives. Oral liquid preparations that do not contain fructose, glucose or sucrose are labelled 'sugar free' in the *British National Formulary* (BNF). These alternatives should be used where possible.

Colouring agents

Colouring agents are added to pharmaceutical preparations to enhance the appearance of a preparation or to increase the acceptability of a preparation to the patient. Colours are often matched to the flavour of a preparation, e.g. a yellow colour for a banana-flavoured preparation. Colour is also useful to give a consistent appearance where there is natural variation between batches. Colours can give distinctive appearances to some medicines, e.g. the green colour of the *Drug Tariff* formula of methadone mixture.

Colouring agents should be non-toxic and free of any therapeutic activity themselves. Natural colourants are most likely to meet this criterion and include materials derived from plants and animals, e.g. carotenoids, chlorophylls, saffron, red beetroot extract, caramel and cochineal. As with all natural agents, the disadvantage is that batches may vary in quality. Synthetic organic dyes such as the azo compounds are alternatives for colouring pharmaceutical solutions as they give a wide range of bright, stable colours. Colours appear in pharmaceutical formulae less often now, especially in children's medicines. Some consumers see their use as unnecessary and some colouring agents, e.g. tartrazine, have been implicated in allergic reactions and hyperactivity of children. Additionally, coloured dyes in medicines can lead to confusion when diagnosing diseases, e.g. a red dye appearing in vomit could be wrongly assumed to be blood. In the European Union, colours are selected from a list permitted for medicinal products, with designated 'E' numbers between 100 and 180.

Stabilizers

Antioxidants may be used where ingredients are liable to degradation by oxidation, e.g. in oils. Those which are added to oral preparations include ascorbic acid, citric acid, sodium metabisulphite and sodium sulphite. These are odourless, tasteless and non-toxic.

Viscosity-enhancing agents

Syrups may be added to increase the viscosity of an oral liquid. They also improve palatability and ease pourability. Other thickening agents may also be used (see Ch. 34).

Shelf-life of solutions

There may be individual variations, but most solutions which are prepared extemporaneously should be freshly or recently prepared. The data sheets should be consulted for information about particular manufactured solutions and for storage conditions.

Oral syringes

If fractional doses are prescribed for oral liquids, they should not be diluted, but an oral syringe should be supplied with the dispensed oral liquid. The standard 5 mL or 10 mL capacity oral syringe is marked in 0.2 mL divisions to measure fractional doses. An adapter fits into the neck of all common sizes of the medicine bottle. Instructions should be supplied with the oral syringe: 'Shake the bottle and then remove the lid and insert the adapter firmly into the top of the bottle. Push the tip of the oral syringe into the hole in the adapter and turn the bottle upside down. Pull the syringe plunger to draw liquid to the appropriate volume. It may be desirable to indicate this on the syringe. Turn the bottle right way up and carefully remove the syringe, holding the barrel. Gently put the tip into the child's mouth to be inside the cheek. Slowly and gently push the plunger in and allow the child to swallow the medicine before removing the syringe. Do not squirt the liquid or direct it towards the throat. After completing the process, remove the adapter and replace the cap on the bottle. The adapter and syringe should be rinsed and left to dry'. Patient information leaflets are available to accompany the oral syringe.

Diluents

If a prescriber insists that a manufactured solution is diluted, then a suitable diluent must be selected. Information sources to obtain this information are the *Medicines Compendium* or the National Pharmaceutical Association (NPA) *Diluent Directory*. An indication of the expiry date for the diluted preparation is also given in these references. The dilution should be freshly prepared.

A short shelf-life for a diluted solution may require patients to return to the pharmacy to collect the balance of their medication. This may happen, for instance, where an oral sodium chloride solution has been prescribed for 1 month. The solution has a 2-week expiry, and must therefore be supplied in two instalments. The patient, or their representative, should be issued with an owing slip, or some similar documentation. This should state the name of the patient, the pharmacy, the item and quantity of medicine owed and the date of issue. A record should also be kept in the pharmacy. Most computer labelling systems have the facility to handle 'owings'.

Example 33.3

Prepare 100 mL of Ammonium and Ipecacuanha Mixture BP.

	Master formula	For 100 mL
Ammonium bicarbonate	200 mg	2 g
Liquorice liquid extract	0.5 mL	5 mL
Ipecacuanha tincture	0.3 mL	3 mL
Concentrated camphor water	0.1 mL	1 mL
Concentrated anise water	0.05 mL	0.5 mL
Double strength chloroform water	5 mL	50 mL
Water	to 10 mL	to 100 mL

Traditionally used as an expectorant cough preparation but no longer recommended.

Formulation notes. Ammonium bicarbonate, ipecacuanha and camphor water are mild expectorants. Anise water acts as a mild expectorant and a flavouring agent. Liquid liquorice extract is used as a mild expectorant, flavouring and sweetening agent. Chloroform water acts as a sweetener and a preservative. Ammonium bicarbonate is soluble 1 in 5 of water, so will dissolve to give a solution. All other ingredients are liquids.

Method of preparation. Weigh the ammonium bicarbonate on a suitable balance and dissolve in approximately 15 mL water, in a 100 mL conical measure. Add the double strength chloroform water to this solution. Measure the other liquid ingredients and add to the solution. Make up to volume with water in the conical measure. Pack into an amber medicine bottle with a child-resistant closure. Polish the bottle and label, and provide a 5 mL spoon.

Shelf-life and storage. Store in a cool, dry place. It is recently prepared, therefore a shelf-life of 2–3 weeks is applicable.

Advice and labelling. 'Shake well before use'. While this is not strictly required, it is good practice to include it.

Example 33.4

Prepare 200 mL of Diamorphine linctus.

	Master formula	For 200 mL
Diamorphine hydrochloride	3 mg	120 mg
Oxymel	1.25 mL	50 mL
Glycerol	1.25 mL	50 mL
Compound tartrazine solution	0.06 mL	2.4 mL
Syrup	to 5 mL	to 200 mL

Traditionally used as a cough suppressant in terminal care, no longer recommended.

Formulation notes. Oxymel is a solution of acetic acid, water and purified honey, used as a demulcent and sweetening agent in linctuses. Glycerol is also a demulcent and sweetener. Compound tartrazine solution is a colouring agent and syrup is a demulcent vehicle. Diamorphine is soluble 1 in 1.6 of water and 1 in 12 of alcohol, so a solution will be produced.

Method of preparation. Weigh 120 mg diamorphine on an appropriate balance. Transfer to a 200 mL measuring cylinder. Dissolve the diamorphine in the oxymel and glycerol. Add about 50 mL of syrup, then add the compound tartrazine solution. Transfer to a previously tared amber medicine bottle (see Ch. 32). Make up to volume with the syrup in the tared bottle in order to overcome difficulties in draining all the viscous mixture from a measure. Close with a child-resistant closure, polish and label the bottle and give a 5 mL medicine spoon or oral syringe with the medicine (depending on the dosage prescribed).

Shelf-life and storage. Store in a cool, dry place. It is recently prepared, therefore a shelf-life of 2–3 weeks is applicable.

Advice and labelling. 'Shake well before use'. The linctus should be sipped and swallowed slowly, undiluted. 'Warning. This medicine may make you sleepy. If this happens, do not drive or use tools or machines. Do not drink alcohol' (BNF Label 2). Since this patient is terminally ill, they are unlikely to be driving or operating machinery so this part of the advisory label can be omitted. Alcohol should be avoided, as this will increase the sedative effect.

Example 33.5

Prepare 50 mL of Chloral elixir, paediatric.

	Master formula	For 50 mL
Chloral hydrate	200 mg	2 g
Water	0.1 mL	1 mL
Blackcurrant syrup	1 mL	10 mL
Syrup	to 5 mL	to 50 mL

Action and uses. Traditionally used for short-term use in insomnia.

Formulation notes. Chloral hydrate is soluble 1 in 0.3 of water and has an unpleasant taste. Blackcurrant syrup is used as a flavouring agent to mask this.

Method of preparation. Weigh 2 g chloral hydrate on a suitable balance. Transfer it to a 50 mL measuring cylinder and dissolve it in water. Add the blackcurrant syrup. Add some of the syrup (rinsing the measure used for the blackcurrant syrup). Transfer the mixture to a tared, 50 mL amber medicine bottle and make up to volume, to avoid loss of the viscous product in the measures. Polish and label the bottle and give a 5 mL medicine spoon or oral syringe with the medicine.

Shelf-life and storage. Store in a cool, dry place. Chloral hydrate is volatile and sensitive to light. It is recently prepared and a shelf life of 2–3 weeks is appropriate.

Advice and labelling. 'Shake well before use' and BNF Labels 1 and 27. An appropriate dose for a child up to 1 year is one 5 mL spoonful to be given, well diluted with water, at bedtime. The parent should be advised that this might make the child drowsy.

Example 33.6

Prepare 200 mL of Potassium Citrate Mixture BP.

	Master formula	For 200 mL
Potassium citrate	3 g	60 g
Citric acid monohydrate	500 mg	10 g
Syrup	2.5 mL	50 mL
Quillaia tincture	0.1 mL	2 mL
Lemon spirit	0.05 mL	1 mL
Double strength chloroform water	3 mL	60 mL
Water	to 10 mL	to 200 mL

Traditionally used for the alkalinization of urine to relieve discomfort in mild urinary tract infections or cystitis.

Formulation notes. Citric acid and potassium citrate are the active ingredients; both are soluble 1 in 1 of water. Lemon spirit, which is lemon oil in alcoholic solution, is a flavouring agent. The oil tends to be displaced from solution in an aqueous medium, especially in the presence of a high concentration of salts. The quillaia tincture is a surfactant used to emulsify any displaced lemon oil. Syrup is a sweetening agent.

Method of preparation. The solids should be size reduced, weighed and dissolved in the double strength chloroform water and syrup. The quillaia tincture should be added before the lemon spirit is added with stirring, so that immediate emulsification of the oil will be achieved if required. Make up to volume with water. Pack in an amber medicine bottle with a child-resistant closure. Polish and label the bottle and give a 5 mL medicine spoon with the medicine.

Shelf-life and storage. Store in a cool, dry place. It is recently prepared, therefore a shelf-life of 2–3 weeks is applicable.

Advice and labelling. 'Shake well before use'. The medicine should be diluted with plenty of water (BNF Label 27).

Example 33.7

Prepare 500 mL of Compound Sodium Chloride Mouthwash BP.

	Master formula	For 500 mL
Sodium chloride	1.5 g	7.5 g
Sodium bicarbonate	1 g	5 g
Concentrated peppermint emulsion	2.5 mL	12.5 mL
Double strength chloroform water	50 mL	250 mL
Water	to 100 mL	to 500 mL

Action and uses. Mechanically cleans and freshens the mouth.

Formulation notes. Concentrated peppermint emulsion is used as a flavouring and the chloroform water is a sweetener and preservative. Sodium chloride is soluble 1 in 3 of water and sodium bicarbonate is soluble 1 in 11 of water.

Method of preparation. The solids are weighed on a suitable balance and dissolved in a 500 mL conical measure in approximately 100 mL of water. Add the double strength chloroform water and the concentrated peppermint emulsion. Make up to volume with water. Pack in an amber bottle with a child-resistant closure. Polish and label the bottle.

Shelf-life and storage. Store in a cool, dry place. It is recently prepared, therefore a shelf-life of 2–3 weeks is applicable.

Advice and labelling. 'Shake well before use'. The patient should be directed to use about 15 mL diluted in an equal volume of warm water, usually morning and night, unless otherwise directed. The solution should be used as a mouthwash and should not be swallowed, although reassure the patient that it is not harmful to swallow small amounts of the mouthwash.

Example 33.8

Prepare 10 mL of Sodium Bicarbonate Ear Drops BP.

	Master formula	For 10 mL
Sodium bicarbonate	5 g	500 mg
Glycerol	30 mL	3 mL
Water	to 100 mL	to 10 mL

Action and uses. For the softening and removal of earwax (usually prior to syringing with warm water).

Formulation notes. Sodium bicarbonate is soluble 1 in 11 of water. Glycerol is a viscous liquid used to thicken the drops, but presents problems in measuring the volume accurately.

Method of preparation. Weigh 500 mg sodium bicarbonate and dissolve in 6 mL of water, using a 10 mL conical measure. Carefully make up to 7 mL using water. Carefully add glycerol up to the 10 mL mark (this will result in 3 mL of glycerol being added to the solution). Pack in a 10 mL hexagonal, amber, ribbed bottle with a dropper. Polish and label the bottle on the three smooth sides.

Shelf-life and storage. Store in a cool, dry place. The drops are recently prepared, therefore a shelf-life of 2–3 weeks is applicable.

Advice and labelling. 'Shake well before use' and 'Not to be taken'. The bottle may be warmed in the hands before placing drops in the ears. A patient information leaflet should be used to describe how to use the drops (see Fig. 33.1).

KEY POINTS

- Pharmaceutical solutions are given different names depending on their nature and use
- There are both advantages and disadvantages in the use of oral solutions
- Solutions may also be used for mouthwashes, gargles, nasal drops and sprays, ear drops and enemas
- Many different vehicles may be used in pharmaceutical solutions, but water is the most common
- Saturation solubility of a drug in a solvent is affected by polarity of both drug and solvent
- Saturation solubility can be increased by techniques such as co-solvency and solubilization
- Antimicrobial preservation is required for most aqueous solutions
- Various additives such as flavours, sweeteners and colours may be added to improve the palatability of oral solutions
- Oral syringes will be required for doses of less than 5 mL and its use explained

Suspensions

Arthur J. Winfield

STUDY POINTS

- The nature of suspensions
- The pharmaceutical uses of suspensions
- The properties of an ideal suspension
- Formulating a suspension
- Ingredients which may be added to suspensions
- The dispensing of suspensions for internal and external use

Introduction

Suspensions contain one or more insoluble medicaments in a vehicle, with other additives such as preservatives, flavours, colours, buffers and stabilizers. Most pharmaceutical suspensions are aqueous, but an oily vehicle is sometimes used. Suspensions may be used for oral administration, inhalation, topical application, as ophthalmic preparations, for parenteral administration and as aerosols.

A pharmaceutical suspension may be defined as a disperse system in which one substance (the disperse phase) is distributed in particulate form throughout another (the continuous phase). Most are classified as a coarse suspension, which is a dispersion of particles with a mean diameter >1 μm. A colloidal suspension is a dispersion of particles with a mean diameter <1 μm. Suspended solids slowly separate on standing, but redispersion may be difficult if they form a compacted sediment.

Pharmaceutical applications of suspensions

Suspensions may be used pharmaceutically for a number of reasons. Some are given below:

- Drugs with low solubility in the continuous phase can be formulated as suspensions
- Patient acceptability – a liquid form rather than a solid dosage form
- Drugs that have an unpleasant taste in their soluble form can be made into insoluble derivatives, and formulated as a suspension, which will be more palatable, e.g. chloramphenicol (soluble) and chloramphenicol palmitate (insoluble)
- In oral suspensions, the drug is delivered in finely divided form, therefore optimal dissolution occurs in the gastrointestinal (GI) fluids and hence the rate of absorption is increased
- Insoluble forms of drugs may prolong the action of a drug by preventing rapid degradation in the continuous phase
- If the drug is unstable when in contact with the vehicle, suspensions should be prepared immediately prior to handing out to the patient in order to reduce the amount of time that the drug particles are in contact with the dispersion medium. For example, in ampicillin suspension, water is added to powder or granules prior to giving out to the patient. A 14-day expiry date is given, if the product is to be kept in the fridge

- Drugs which degrade in aqueous solution may be suspended in a non-aqueous phase, e.g. tetracycline hydrochloride has been suspended in a fractionated coconut oil for ophthalmic use
- Bulky, insoluble powders can be formulated as a suspension so that they are easier to take, e.g. kaolin, chalk and magnesium trisilicate (see Examples 34.1 and 34.2)
- Intramuscular, intra-articular or subcutaneous injections are often formulated as suspensions to prolong the release of the drug
- Lotions containing insoluble solids are formulated to leave a thin coating of medicament on the skin. As the vehicle evaporates, it gives a cooling effect and leaves the solid behind. Examples are Calamine Lotion BP (see Example 34.3) and Sulphur Lotion Compound BPC (see Ch. 36).

Properties of a good pharmaceutical suspension

In preparing a pharmaceutically elegant product, several desirable properties are sought:

- There is ready redispersion of any sediment which accumulates on storage
- After gentle shaking, the medicament stays in suspension long enough for a dose to be accurately measured
- The suspension is pourable
- Particles in suspension are small and relatively uniform in size, so that the product is free from a gritty texture.

Formulation of suspensions

The three steps that can be taken to ensure formulation of an elegant pharmaceutical suspension are:

1. Control particle size. On a small scale, this can be done using a mortar and pestle, to grind down ingredients to a fine powder
2. Use a thickening agent to increase viscosity of the vehicle, by using suspending or viscosity-increasing agents
3. Use a wetting agent.

Some of the theoretical and practical aspects of these will be considered in the context of extemporaneous dispensing.

The insoluble medicament may be a diffusible solid or an indiffusible solid:

Diffusible solids (dispersible solids). These are insoluble solids that are light and easily wetted by water. They mix readily with water, and stay dispersed long enough for an adequate dose to be measured. After settling, they redisperse easily. Examples include magnesium trisilicate; light magnesium carbonate; bismuth carbonate and light kaolin (see Example 34.1).

Indiffusible solids. Most insoluble solids are not easily wetted, and may form large porous clumps in the liquid. These solids will not remain evenly distributed in the vehicle long enough for an adequate dose to be measured. They may not redisperse easily. Examples for internal use include phenobarbital and chalk (see Example 34.2), and for external use calamine, hydrocortisone, sulphur and zinc oxide.

Problems encountered when formulating insoluble solids into a suspension

Various factors need to be considered when formulating insoluble solids into a suspension.

Sedimentation

The factors affecting the rate of sedimentation of a particle are described in Stokes' equation:

$$y = \frac{2gr^2(\rho_1 - \rho_2)}{9\eta}$$

where y = velocity of a spherical particle of radius r, and density ρ_1, in a liquid of density ρ_2, and viscosity η, and where g is the acceleration due to gravity.

The basic consequences of this equation are that the rate of fall of a suspended particle in a vehicle of a given density is greater for larger particles than it is for smaller particles. Also, the greater the difference in density between the particles and vehicle, the greater will be the rate of descent. Increasing the viscosity of the dispersion medium, within limits, so that the suspension is still pourable, will reduce the rate of sedimentation of a solid drug. Thus, a decrease in settling rate in a suspension may be achieved by reducing the size of the particles and by increasing the density and the viscosity of the continuous phase.

Flocculation

The natural tendency of particles towards aggregation will determine the properties of a suspension. In a deflocculated suspension, the dispersed solid particles remain separate and settle slowly. However, the sediment that eventually forms is hard to redisperse and is described as a 'cake' or 'clay'. In a flocculated suspension, individual particles aggregate into clumps or floccules in suspension. Because these flocs are larger than individual particles, sedimentation is more rapid, but the sediment is loose and easily redispersible. Excess flocculation may prevent 'pourability' due to its effect on rheological properties.

The ideal is to use either a deflocculated system with a sufficiently high viscosity to prevent sedimentation, or controlled flocculation with a suitable combination of rate of sedimentation, type of sediment and pourability.

Wetting

Air may be trapped in the particles of poorly wetted solids, which causes them to float to the surface of the preparation and prevents them from being readily dispersed throughout the vehicle. Wetting of the particles can be encouraged by reducing the interfacial tension between the solid and the vehicle, so that adsorbed air is displaced from solid surfaces by liquid. Suitable wetting agents have this effect, but decrease interparticular forces, thereby affecting flocculation.

Hydrophilic colloids such as acacia and tragacanth can act as wetting agents. However, care should be taken when using these agents, as they can promote deflocculation. Intermediate HLB (hydrophilic–lipophilic balance) surfactants (see Ch. 35) such as polysorbates and sorbitan esters are used for internal preparations. Solvents such as ethanol, glycerol and the glycols also facilitate wetting. Sodium lauryl sulphate and quillaia tincture are used in external preparations.

Suspending agents

Suspending agents increase the viscosity of the vehicle, thereby slowing down sedimentation. Most agents can form thixotropic gels which are semi-solid on standing, but flow readily after shaking. Care must be taken when selecting a suspending agent for oral preparations, as the acid environment of the stomach may alter the physical characteristics of the suspension, and therefore the rate of release of the drug from suspension. Some suspending agents may also bind to certain medicaments, making them less bioavailable.

Suspending agents can be divided into five broad categories: natural polysaccharides, semi-synthetic polysaccharides, clays, synthetic thickeners and miscellaneous compounds.

Natural polysaccharides

The main problem with these agents is their natural variability between batches and microbial contamination. Tragacanth is a widely used suspending agent and is less viscous at pH4-7.5. As a rule of thumb, 0.2g Tragacanth Powder is added per 100mL suspension or 2g Compound Tragacanth Powder per 100mL suspension. Tragacanth Powder requires to be dispersed with the insoluble powders before water is added to prevent clumping (see Example 34.2). Compound Tragacanth Powder BP 1980 contains tragacanth, acacia, starch and sucrose and so is easier to use. Other examples include acacia gum, starch, agar, guar gum, carrageenan and sodium alginate. These materials should not be used externally as they leave a sticky feel on the skin.

Semi-synthetic polysaccharides

These are derived from the naturally occurring polysaccharide cellulose. Examples include methylcellulose (Cologel®, Celacol®), hydroxyethylcellulose (Natrosol 250®), sodium carboxymethylcellulose (Carmellose sodium) and microcrystalline cellulose (Avicel®).

Clays

These are naturally occurring inorganic materials, which are mainly hydrated silicates. Examples include bentonite and magnesium aluminium silicate (Veegum®).

Synthetic thickeners

These were introduced to overcome the variable quality of natural products. Examples include carbomer (Carboxyvinyl polymer, Carbopol®), colloidal silicon dioxide (Aerosil®, Cab-o-sil®) and polyvinyl alcohol.

Miscellaneous compounds

Gelatin is used as a suspending and viscosity-increasing agent.

Preservation of suspensions

Water is the most common source of microbial contamination. All pharmaceutical preparations that contain water are therefore susceptible to microbial growth. Also the naturally occurring additives such as acacia and tragacanth may be sources of microbes and spores. Preservative action may be diminished because of adsorption of the preservative onto solid particles of drug, or interaction with suspending agents. Useful preservatives in extemporaneous preparations include chloroform water, benzoic acid and hydroxybenzoates.

The dispensing of suspensions

The method of dispensing suspensions is the same for most, with some differences for specific ingredients.

- Crystalline and granular solids are finely powdered in the mortar. The suspending agent should then be added and mixed thoroughly in the mortar. Do not apply too much pressure, otherwise gumming or caking of the suspending agent will occur and heat of friction will make it sticky.
- Add a little of the liquid vehicle to make a paste and mix well until smooth and free of lumps. Continue with gradual additions until the mixture can be poured into a tared bottle. Further liquid is used to rinse all the powder into the bottle, where it is made up to volume.

Variations

- If wetting agents are included in the formulation, add them before forming the paste
- If syrup and/or glycerol are in the formulation, use this rather than water to form the initial paste
- If soluble solids are being used, dissolve them in the vehicle before or after making the paste
- Leave addition of volatile components, colourings or concentrated flavouring tinctures such as chloroform spirit, liquid liquorice extract and compound tartrazine solution until near the end.

Most 'official' suspensions will be prepared from the constituent ingredients. There may be some occasions where an oral solid dosage form, such as a tablet or capsule, will have to be reformulated by the pharmacist into an oral suspension, e.g. where the medicine is for a child (see Example 34.4). It is important to obtain as much information (physical, chemical and microbiological) as possible about the manufactured drug and its excipients. Typically, the tablet will be crushed or capsule contents emptied into the mortar and a suspending agent added. A paste is formed with the vehicle and then diluted to a suitable volume, with the addition of any other desired ingredients such as preservative or flavour. A short expiry of no more than 7 days should be given owing to the lack of knowledge about the stability of the formulation.

Containers for suspensions

Suspensions should be packed in amber bottles. There should be adequate air space above the liquid to allow shaking and ease of pouring.

Special labels and advice for suspensions

The most important additional label for suspensions is 'Shake well before use', as some sedimentation of medicament would normally be expected. Shaking the bottle will redisperse the medicament and ensure that the patient can measure an accurate dose.

'Store in a cool place'. Stability of suspensions may be adversely affected by both extremes and variations of temperature. Some suspensions, such as those made by reconstituting dry powders, may need to be stored in a refrigerator.

Extemporaneously prepared and reconstituted suspensions will have a relatively short shelf-life. They are usually required to be recently or freshly prepared, with a 1–4-week expiry date. Some official formulae state an expiry date, but many do not. The pharmacist may have to make judgements about the expiry date for a particular preparation, based on its constituents and likely storage conditions. The manufacturer's literature for reconstituted products will give recommended storage conditions.

Inhalations

Suspensions are useful formulations for inhalations. The volatile components are adsorbed onto the surface of a diffusible solid to ensure uniform dispersion throughout the liquid. When hot water is added, the oils vaporize. Where quantities are not stated, 1 g of light magnesium carbonate is used for each 2 mL of oil (such as eucalyptus oil) or 2 g of volatile solid (such as menthol). An example of a traditional inhalation is menthol and eucalyptus inhalation.

Example 34.1

Prepare 150 mL Kaolin and Morphine Mixture BP.

	Master formula	For 150 mL
Light kaolin	2 g	30 g
Sodium bicarbonate	500 mg	7.5 g
Chloroform and morphine tincture	0.4 mL	6 mL
Water	to 10 mL	to 150 mL

Traditionally used, but no longer recommended, for the treatment of acute diarrhoea.

Formulation notes. Light kaolin is a diffusible solid; therefore no suspending agent is required.

Method of preparation. Weigh the light kaolin and place in the mortar. Dissolve the sodium bicarbonate in about 100 mL of water. Gradually add this to the light kaolin in the mortar with mixing to disperse the solid. Add the chloroform and morphine tincture. Wash the mixture into a tared, amber medicine bottle, and make up to volume with water.

Example 34.2

Prepare 100 mL of Chalk Mixture, Paediatric BP.

	Master formula	For 100 mL
Chalk	100 mg	2 g
Tragacanth	10 mg	200 mg
Syrup	0.5 mL	10 mL
Concentrated cinnamon water	0.02 mL	0.4 mL
Double strength chloroform water	2.5 mL	50 mL
Water	to 5 mL	to 100 mL

Traditionally used, but no longer recommended, as an antidiarrhoeal mixture for children.

Formulation notes. Chalk is practically insoluble in water and is an indiffusible solid, which requires a suspending agent. Tragacanth Powder is used in this formulation. The concentrated cinnamon water is a flavouring agent and the syrup increases the viscosity as well as acting as a sweetener. Chloroform water is the preservative.

Method of preparation. The chalk and tragacanth should be weighed and lightly mixed in a mortar and pestle. Add the syrup and mix to make a paste. The double strength chloroform water should be gradually added, with mixing, followed by the concentrated cinnamon water. The mixture should be rinsed into a previously tared 100 mL amber medicine bottle and made up to volume with water. Seal the bottle and shake the suspension well.

Example 34.3

Prepare 200 mL Calamine Lotion BP.

	Master formula	For 200 mL
Calamine	15 g	30 g
Zinc oxide	5 g	10 g
Bentonite	3 g	6 g
Sodium citrate	500 mg	1 g
Liquefied phenol	0.5 mL	1 mL
Glycerol	5 mL	10 mL
Water	to 100 mL	to 200 mL

Action and uses. As a cooling lotion for sunburn or skin irritation and pruritus.

Formulation notes. Calamine is a coloured zinc carbonate and is practically insoluble in water, as is zinc oxide. Both are indiffusible solids. Sodium citrate is added to control the flocculation of calamine. Bentonite is a thickening agent and glycerol will thicken the product and help powder adherence to the skin. Liquefied phenol acts as a preservative and antiseptic.

Method of preparation. The dry powders should be weighed and mixed in a mortar so that the bentonite is well distributed. Add the glycerol to the powders and mix. The sodium citrate is dissolved in about 140 mL of water, and gradually added to the mixture in the mortar, so that a smooth paste is produced. Add the liquefied phenol, taking care not to splash, as it is caustic. Transfer the mixture to a tared, amber ribbed glass bottle, adding washings from the mortar, and make up to volume. Seal with a child-resistant closure.

Shelf-life and storage. Store in a cool, dry place. It is recently prepared; therefore, a shelf-life of 2–3 weeks is applicable.

Advice and labelling. 'For external use only', 'Shake well before use' and 'Do not apply to broken skin'. The lotion should be applied to the affected areas when required and allowed to dry.

Example 34.4

Prepare Spironolactone suspension 15 mg/5 mL.
   Label: 5 mL three times a day. Send 100 mL. For a 4-year-old child.

	Master formula	For 100 mL
Spironolactone	q.s.[a]	300 mg
Compound orange spirit	0.2%	0.2 mL
Cologel	20%	20 mL
Water	to 100%	100 mL

[a]q.s. means sufficient.

Action and uses. A potassium-sparing diuretic used in oedema of heart failure and nephrotic syndrome.

Formulation notes. Spironolactone is practically insoluble in water. Cologel® (methylcellulose) acts as the suspending agent. Compound orange spirit is a flavouring agent.

Method of preparation. Tablets may be used, and sufficient crushed in a mortar and pestle to give 300 mg spironolactone (e.g. 6×50 mg tablets). Alternatively, weigh the powder and transfer to a mortar and pestle. Add the Cologel® and mix to a paste. Gradually add some of the water. Add the compound orange spirit. Rinse the suspension into a tared, amber medicine bottle and make up to volume with water. Shake the bottle well and seal with a child-resistant closure. Polish and label the bottle and give a 5 mL medicine spoon with the medicine.

Shelf-life and storage. It is recently prepared with a shelf-life of 4 weeks when stored in a refrigerator. Spironolactone should be protected from light.

Advice and labelling. 'Shake well before use' and 'Give one 5 mL spoonful three times a day'. BNF Label 21 should be used. Reinforce the storage conditions.

KEY POINTS

- Suspensions can be used to administer an insoluble solid by the oral route
- Suspensions may be used to replace tablets, to improve dissolution rate, to prolong action and to mask a bad taste
- Solids may be diffusible or indiffusible and require different dispensing techniques
- Stokes' equation can be applied when formulating a suspension to help ensure accurate dosage of the drug
- Flocculated particles settle quickly and redisperse easily, while deflocculated particles settle slowly but tend to cake
- Hydrophobic solids may require wetting agents
- Suspending agents are added to slow down the rate of settling of the solid
- Suspending agents may be natural polysaccharides, semi-synthetic polysaccharides, clays or synthetic polymers
- Some suspensions are made by adding water to reconstitute manufactured powders when stability is a problem
- 'Shake well before use' and 'Store in a cool place' should be part of the labels on a suspension
- Inhalations are suspensions of a volatile material adsorbed onto a diffusible solid

Emulsions

Arthur J. Winfield

STUDY POINTS

- The uses of pharmaceutical emulsions
- The different types of emulsion and their identification
- The formulation of emulsions
- Selection of emulsifying agents and other ingredients
- The dispensing processes for emulsions

Introduction

An emulsion consists of two immiscible liquids, one of which is uniformly dispersed throughout the other as fine droplets normally of diameter 0.1–100 μm. To prepare a stable emulsion, a third ingredient, an emulsifying agent, is required. Oral emulsions are stabilized oil-in-water dispersions that may contain one or more active ingredients. They are a useful way of presenting oils and fats in a palatable form. Emulsions for external use are known as lotions, applications or liniments if liquid, or creams if semi-solid in nature. Some parenteral products may also be formulated as emulsions. Most important of these is total parenteral nutrition (see Ch. 44). Pharmaceutically, the term 'emulsion', when no other qualification is used, is taken to mean an oil-in-water preparation for internal use.

Pharmaceutical applications of emulsions

Emulsions have a wide range of uses, including:

- Oral, rectal and topical administration of oils and oil-soluble drugs

- Formulation of oil- and water-soluble drugs together
- To enhance palatability of oils when given orally by disguising both taste and oiliness
- Increasing absorption of oils and oil-soluble drugs through intestinal walls
- Intramuscular injections of some water-soluble vaccines: these provide slow release and therefore a greater antibody response and longer-lasting immunity
- Total parenteral nutrition (see Ch. 44).

Examples of traditionally used emulsions for oral use are cod liver oil emulsion (see Example 35.1), Liquid Paraffin Oral Emulsion BP (see Example 35.2). An example of emulsion for external use is Oily Calamine Lotion BP (see Example 35.3).

Emulsion types

Emulsions may be oil-in-water (o/w) emulsions, where oil is the disperse phase in a continuous phase of water, or water-in-oil (w/o) emulsions, where water is the disperse phase in a continuous phase of oil. It is also possible to form a multiple emulsion, e.g. a water droplet enclosed in an oil droplet, which is itself dispersed in water–a w/o/w emulsion. Multiple emulsions are increasingly used in manufactured pharmaceutical products and are used for delayed action drug delivery systems.

If the emulsion is for oral or intravenous administration it will always be oil-in-water. Intramuscular injections may be water-in-oil for depot therapy. When selecting emulsion type for preparations for external use, the therapeutic use, texture and patient acceptability will be taken into account. Oil-in-water emulsions are less greasy, easily washed off the skin and more cosmetically acceptable than water-in-oil emulsions. They have an occlusive effect, which hydrates the upper layers of the skin (called an emollient, see Ch. 36). Water-in-oil emulsions rub in more easily.

Identification of emulsion type

There is a range of tests available to identify the emulsion type. Some of the tests that can be used are outlined below.

Miscibility test. An emulsion will only mix with a liquid that is miscible with its continuous phase. Therefore an o/w emulsion is miscible with water, a w/o emulsion with an oil.

Conductivity measurement. Systems with an aqueous continuous phase will conduct electricity, while systems with an oily continuous phase will not.

Staining test. A dry filter paper impregnated with cobalt chloride turns from blue to pink on exposure to stable o/w emulsions.

Dye test. If an oil-soluble dye is used, o/w emulsions are paler in colour than w/o emulsions. If examined microscopically, an o/w emulsion will appear as coloured globules on a colourless background while a w/o emulsion will appear as colourless globules against a coloured background.

Formulation of emulsions

An ideal emulsion has globules of disperse phase that retain their initial character, that is the mean globule size does not change and the globules remain evenly distributed. The formulation of emulsions involves the prevention of coalescence of the disperse phase (often called 'cracking') and reducing the rate of creaming.

Emulsifying agents

Emulsifying agents help the production of a stable emulsion by reducing interfacial tension and then maintaining the separation of the droplets by forming a barrier at the interface. Most emulsifying agents are surface-active agents. Emulsion type is determined mainly by the solubility of the emulsifying agent. If the emulsifying agent is more

soluble in water (i.e. hydrophilic), then water will be the continuous phase and an o/w emulsion will be formed. If the emulsifying agent is more soluble in oil (i.e. lipophilic), oil will be the continuous phase and a w/o emulsion will be formed. If a substance is added which alters the solubility of the emulsifying agent, this balance may be altered and the emulsion may change type. The process is called phase inversion. The ideal emulsifying agent is colourless, odourless, tasteless, non-toxic, non-irritant and able to produce stable emulsions at low concentrations.

Emulsifying agents can be classed into three groups: naturally occurring, synthetic surfactants and finely divided solids.

Naturally occurring emulsifying agents

These agents come from vegetable or animal sources. Therefore, the quality may vary from batch to batch and they are susceptible to microbial contamination and degradation.

Polysaccharides. Acacia is the best emulsifying agent for extemporaneously prepared oral emulsions as it forms a thick film at the oil–water interface to act as a barrier to coalescence. It is too sticky for external use. Tragacanth is used to increase the viscosity of an emulsion and prevent creaming. Other polysaccharides, such as starch, pectin and carrageenan, are used to stabilize an emulsion.

Semi-synthetic polysaccharides. Low-viscosity grades of methylcellulose (see Example 35.2) and carboxymethylcellulose will form o/w emulsions.

Sterol-containing substances. These agents act as water-in-oil emulsifying agents. Examples include beeswax, wool fat and wool alcohols (see Ch. 36).

Synthetic surfactants

These agents are classified according to their ionic characteristics as anionic, cationic, non-ionic and ampholytic. The latter are used in detergents and soaps but are not widely used in pharmacy.

Anionic surfactants. These are organic salts which, in water, have a surface-active anion. They are incompatible with some organic and inorganic cations and with large organic cations such as cetrimide. They are widely used in external preparations as o/w emulsifying agents. They must be in their ionized form to be effective and emulsions made with anionic surfactants are generally stable at more alkaline pH.

Some pharmaceutical examples of anionic surfactants include:

- Alkali metal and ammonium soaps such as sodium stearate (o/w)
- Soaps of divalent and trivalent metals such as calcium oleate (w/o) (see Example 35.3)
- Amine soaps such as triethanolamine oleate (o/w)
- Alkyl sulphates such as sodium lauryl sulphate (o/w).

Cationic surfactants. These are usually quaternary ammonium compounds which have a surface-active cation and so are sensitive to anionic surfactants and drugs. They are used in the preparation of o/w emulsions for external use and must be in their ionized form to be effective. Emulsions formed by a cationic surfactant are generally stable at acidic pH. The cationic surfactants also have antimicrobial activity. Examples include cetrimide and benzalkonium chloride.

Non-ionic surfactants. These are synthetic materials and make up the largest group of surfactants. They are used to produce either o/w or w/o emulsions for both external and internal use. The non-ionic surfactants are compatible with both anionic and cationic substances and are highly resistant to pH change. The type of emulsion formed depends on the balance between hydrophilic and lipophilic groups which is expressed as the HLB (hydrophilic–lipophilic balance) number (see below). Examples of the main types include glycol and glycerol esters, macrogol ethers and esters, sorbitan esters and polysorbates.

The HLB (hydrophilic–lipophilic balance) system. An HLB number, usually between 1 and 20, is allocated to an emulsifying agent and represents the relative proportions of the lipophilic and hydrophilic parts of the molecule. The lower the number, the more oil soluble the emulsifying agent. Higher numbers (8–18) indicate a hydrophilic molecule which produces an o/w emulsion. Low numbers (3–6) indicate a lipophilic molecule which produces a w/o emulsion. Oils and waxy materials have a 'required HLB number' which helps in the selection of appropriate emulsifying agents when formulating emulsions. Liquid paraffin, for example, has a required HLB value of 4 to obtain a w/o emulsion and 12 for an o/w emulsion. Two or more surfactants can be combined to achieve a suitable HLB value and often give better results than one surfactant alone. HLB values of some commonly used emulsifying agents are given in Table 35.1.

Table 35.1 HLB values of emulsifying agents

Emulsifying agent	HLB value
Acacia	8.0
Sorbitan laurate (Span 20®)	8.6
Sorbitan stearate (Span 60®)	4.7
Polysorbate 20 (Tween 20®)	16.7
Polysorbate 80 (Tween 80®)	15.0
Sodium lauryl sulphate	40.0
Sodium oleate	18.0
Tragacanth	13.2
Triethanolamine oleate	12.0

Finely divided solids

Finely divided solids can be adsorbed at the oil–water interface to form a coherent film that prevents coalescence of the dispersed globules. If the solid particles are preferentially wetted by oil, a w/o emulsion is formed. Conversely, if the particles are preferentially wetted by water, an o/w emulsion is formed. They form emulsions with good stability which are less prone to microbial contamination than those formed with other naturally derived agents. Examples are bentonite, aluminium magnesium silicate and colloidal silicon dioxide. Colloidal aluminium and magnesium hydroxides are used for internal preparations. For example liquid paraffin and magnesium hydroxide oral emulsion is stabilized by the magnesium hydroxide.

Choosing an emulsifying agent

The active ingredients that are to be emulsified and the intended use of the product will determine the choice of emulsifying agent. The natural polysaccharides (acacia) and non-ionic emulsifying agents are useful for internal emulsions because they are non-toxic and non-irritant. Quillaia can be used in low concentrations, but soap emulsions irritate the gastrointestinal tract and have a laxative effect. The taste should be bland and palatable, for example, natural polysaccharides. Polysorbates have a disagreeable taste, therefore flavouring ingredients are necessary. Only certain non-ionic emulsifying agents are suitable for parenteral use including leci-thin, polysorbate 80, methylcellulose, gelatin and serum albumin. A wider range of emulsifying agents can be used externally, although the polysaccharides are normally considered too sticky.

Antioxidants

Some oils are liable to degradation by oxidation and therefore antioxidants may be added to the formulation. They should be preferentially soluble in the oily phase.

Antimicrobial preservatives

Emulsions contain water, which will support microbial growth. Microbes produce unpleasant odours, colour changes and gases. In addition they may affect the emulsifying agent, possibly causing the breakdown of the emulsion. Other ingredients in emulsions can provide a growth medium for microbes. Examples include arachis oil which supports *Aspergillus* species and liquid paraffin which supports *Penicillium* species. Contamination may be introduced from a variety of sources including:

- Natural emulsifying agents, e.g. starch and acacia
- Water, if not properly stored
- Carelessly cleaned equipment
- Poor closures on containers.

Antimicrobial preservative agents should be free from toxic effects, odour, taste (for internal use) and colour. They should be bactericidal rather than bacteriostatic, have a rapid action and wide antibacterial spectrum over a range of temperatures and pH. Additionally emulsion ingredients should not affect their activity and they should be resistant to attack by microorganisms. The effect of the partition coefficient is also important. Microbial growth normally occurs in the aqueous phase of an emulsion; therefore it is important that a sufficient concentration of preservative is present in the aqueous phase. A preservative with a low oil/water partition coefficient will have a higher concentration in the aqueous phase. A combination of preservatives may give the best preservative cover for an emulsion system. The ratio of the disperse phase volume to the total volume is known as the phase volume or phase volume ratio. If, for example, a preservative is soluble in the oil and if the proportion of oil is increased, the concentration of preservative in the

aqueous phase decreases. This could reduce the concentration in the aqueous phase below an effective concentration.

Some preservatives in use are listed below:

- Benzoic acid: effective at a concentration of 0.1% at a pH below 5
- Esters of parahydroxybenzoic acid such as methyl paraben (0.01–0.3%)
- Chloroform, as chloroform water (0.25% v/v)
- Chlorocresol (0.05–0.2%)
- Phenoxyethanol (0.5–1.0%)
- Benzyl alcohol (0.1–3%)
- Quaternary ammonium compounds, e.g. cetrimide, which can be used as a primary emulsifying agent but can also be used as a preservative
- Organic mercurial compounds such as phenyl mercuric nitrate and acetate (0.001–0.002%).

Colours and flavourings

Colour is rarely needed in an emulsion, as most have a white colour and thick texture. Emulsions for oral use will usually contain some flavouring agent.

Stability of emulsions

Phase inversion

This is the process in which an emulsion changes from one type to another, say o/w to w/o. The most stable range of disperse phase concentration is 30–60%. As the amount of disperse phase approaches or exceeds a theoretical maximum of 74% of the total volume, so the tendency for phase inversion to occur increases. Addition of substances which alter the solubility of an emulsifying agent may also cause phase inversion. The process is irreversible.

Creaming

The term 'creaming' is used to describe the aggregation of globules of the disperse phase at the top or bottom of the emulsion, similar to cream on milk. The process is reversible and gentle shaking redistributes the droplets throughout the continuous phase. Creaming is undesirable because it is inelegant, and inaccurate dosing is possible if shaking is not thorough. Additionally, creaming increases the likelihood of coalescence of globules and therefore the breakdown of the emulsion due to cracking.

Cracking

Cracking is the coalescence of dispersed globules and separation of the disperse phase as a separate layer. It is an irreversible process and redispersion cannot be achieved by shaking.

Causes and prevention of cracking or creaming

- *Globule size.* Stable emulsions require a maximal number of small sized (1–3 μm) globules and as few as possible larger (>15 μm) diameter globules. A homogenizer will efficiently reduce droplet size and may additionally increase the viscosity if more than 30% of disperse phase is present. Homogenizers force the emulsion through a small aperture to reduce the size of the globules
- *Storage temperature.* Extremes of temperature can lead to an emulsion cracking. When water freezes it expands, so undue pressure is exerted on dispersed globules and especially the emulsifying agent film, which may lead to cracking. Conversely, an increased temperature decreases the viscosity of the continuous phase and disrupts the integrity of the interfacial film. An increasing number of collisions between droplets will also occur, leading to increased creaming and cracking
- *Potential for globule coalescence.* Increasing the viscosity of the continuous phase will reduce the potential for globule coalescence as this reduces the movement of globules. Emulsion stabilizers, which increase the viscosity of the continuous phase, may be used in o/w emulsions, e.g. tragacanth, sodium alginate and methylcellulose
- *Changes which affect the interfacial film.* These may be chemical, physical or biological effects: microbiological contamination may destroy the emulsifying agent, especially if a polysaccharide emulsifying agent is being used, addition of a common solvent, addition of an emulsifying agent of opposite charge, for instance cationic to anionic
- Incorporation of excess disperse phase, as discussed above.

Dispensing emulsions

Emulsions can be extemporaneously prepared on a small scale using a mortar and pestle. Electric mixers can also be used, although incorporation of excess air may be a problem. All equipment used must be thoroughly clean and dry. All oil-soluble and water-soluble components of the emulsion are separately dissolved in the appropriate phase. A suitable emulsifying agent must then be used.

Emulsions for oral use

Acacia gum is usually used when making extemporaneous o/w emulsions for oral use, unless otherwise specified. A primary emulsion should be prepared first. This is a thick, stable emulsion prepared using optimal proportions of the ingredients. These vary with the nature of the oil.

Calculating quantities for primary emulsions

Proportions or 'parts' for preparation of primary emulsions are given in Table 35.2. These refer to parts by volume for the different types of oil and water and weight for the acacia gum. If more than one oil is to be incorporated, the quantity of acacia for each is calculated separately and the sum of the quantities used.

Variations to primary emulsion calculations

If the proportion of oil is too small, modifications must be made. Acacia emulsions containing less

Table 35.2 Quantities for primary emulsions

Type of oil	Examples	Oil	Water	Gum
Fixed	Almond, arachis, cod-liver, castor	4	2	1
Mineral (hydrocarbon)	Liquid paraffin	3	2	1
Volatile	Turpentine, cinnamon, peppermint	2	2	1
Oleo-resin	Male fern extract	1	2	1

than 20% oil tend to cream readily. A bland, inert oil, such as sesame, cottonseed or maize oil, should be added to increase the amount of oil.

Methods of preparation of extemporaneous emulsions

There are two possible methods, the dry gum method being the more popular.

Dry gum method of preparation

* Measure the oil accurately in a dry measure. It is important that the measure is dry
* Allow measure to drain into a dry mortar with a large, flat bottom
* Weigh acacia gum
* Measure the water for the primary emulsion in a clean measure
* Add acacia to the oil and mix lightly to disperse lumps. Do not over-mix, and keep the suspension in the bottom of the mortar
* Immediately add all of the water (aim to do this within 10–15 s of adding the acacia to the oil) and stir continuously and vigorously until the mixture thickens and the primary emulsion is formed. The mixture thickening, becoming white and producing a 'clicking' sound, characterizes this
* Continue mixing for a further 2–3 min to produce the white stable emulsion. The whiter the product, the smaller the globules
* Gradually dilute the primary emulsion with small volumes of the vehicle, ensuring complete mixing between additions
* Gradually add any other ingredients, transfer to a measure and make up to final volume with the vehicle.

Wet gum method of preparation

Water is added to the acacia gum and quickly triturated until the gum has dissolved to make a mucilage. Oil is added to this mucilage in small portions, triturating the mixture thoroughly after each addition until a thick primary emulsion is obtained. The primary emulsion should be stabilized by mixing for several minutes and then completed in the same way as for the dry gum method.

Problems when producing the primary emulsion

The primary emulsion may not form and a thin oily liquid is formed instead. Possible causes are:

* Phase inversion has occurred
* Incorrect quantities of oil or water were used
* There was cross-contamination of water and oil
* A wet mortar was used
* The mortar was too small and curved, or the pestle head was too round, giving insufficient shear
* Excessive mixing of oil and gum before adding water (dry gum method)
* Diluting the primary emulsion too soon
* Too rapid dilution of primary emulsion
* Poor-quality acacia.

Emulsions for external use

Liquid or semi-liquid emulsions may be used as applications, liniments and lotions (see Ch. 36). The extemporaneous preparation of emulsions for external use does not require the preparation of a primary emulsion. Soaps are commonly used as the emulsifying agent and some are prepared 'in situ' by mixing the oily phase containing a fatty acid and the aqueous phase containing the alkali. Alternatively the emulsifying agent can be dissolved in the oily or aqueous phase and the disperse phase added to the continuous phase, either gradually or in one portion.

Creams are semi-solid emulsions which may be o/w (e.g. aqueous cream) or w/o (e.g. oily cream). (These are considered in more detail in Ch. 36.)

Shelf-life and storage

Emulsions should be stored at room temperature and will either be recently or freshly prepared. Some official preparations will have specific expiry dates. They should not be frozen.

Containers

An amber medicine bottle is used with an airtight child-resistant closure.

Special labelling and advice for emulsions

- 'Shake well before use'
- 'Store in a cool place'. This is to protect the emulsion against extremes of temperature which will adversely affect its stability
- Expiry date
- 'For external use only', for external emulsions.

Worked Examples

Example 35.1

Prepare 200 mL cod liver oil emulsion to the following formula:

Cod-liver oil	60 mL
Chloroform	0.4 mL
Cinnamon water	to 200 mL

Formulation notes. Cod-liver oil is a fixed oil that requires the addition of acacia gum as an emulsifying agent. The proportions are: 4 oil; 2 water; 1 gum. Therefore 60 mL cod-liver oil, 30 mL of cinnamon water and 15 g of acacia gum will be used to prepare the primary emulsion. Cinnamon water acts as a flavouring agent and vehicle. It may need to be prepared from concentrated cinnamon water, at a dilution of 1 part to 39 parts of water. Since 60 mL of the emulsion is the cod-liver oil, it is not necessary to prepare 200 mL of cinnamon water, so 160 mL is adequate. Therefore, 4 mL of concentrated cinnamon water will be diluted to 160 mL with water. Chloroform is dense and only slowly soluble and acts as a preservative.

Method of preparation. Use the dry gum method. Weigh 15 g of acacia, measure 60 mL of cod-liver oil and 30 mL of cinnamon water, which will be used to create the primary emulsion. Place the cod-liver oil in a dry, flat-bottomed mortar. Add the acacia and mix very lightly and briefly. Immediately add the cinnamon water, mixing vigorously until a clicking sound is heard and a white primary emulsion is formed. Continue mixing for a few minutes to stabilize the primary emulsion. Scrape the mortar and pestle with a spatula to ensure that all the oil is incorporated. Add the chloroform by pipette and mix thoroughly. Gradually add most of the remainder of the cinnamon water to the emulsion in the mortar, stirring well between additions. Transfer the emulsion to a 200 mL measure, rinsing the mortar with cinnamon water, adding these washings to the measure. Make up to volume with cinnamon water and pack in an amber medicine bottle with a child-resistant closure.

Storage. Store in a cool, dry place.

Example 35.2

Prepare 100 mL Liquid Paraffin Oral Emulsion BP 1968.

Liquid paraffin	50 mL
Vanillin	50 mg
Chloroform	0.25 mL
Benzoic acid solution	2 mL
Methylcellulose 20	2 g
Saccharin sodium	5 mg
Water	to 100 mL

Formulation notes. Methylcellulose 20 at a concentration of 2% acts as an emulsifying agent for the mineral oil, liquid paraffin. A primary emulsion is not required. Benzoic acid and chloroform act as preservatives and vanillin and saccharin sodium act as flavouring and sweetening agent respectively. The amount of saccharin sodium is not weighable on a dispensing balance and will be obtained by trituration using water as the diluent (since this is the vehicle for the emulsion).

Trituration for saccharin sodium:

Saccharin sodium	100 mg
Water	to 100 mL
5 mL of water will contain	5 mg of saccharin sodium.

Method of preparation. First, prepare a mucilage by mixing the methylcellulose 20 with about six times its weight of boiling water and allow to stand for 30 min to hydrate. Add an equal weight (about 15 g) of ice and stir mechanically until the mucilage is homogeneous. Dissolve the vanillin in the benzoic acid solution and chloroform. Add this mixture to the mucilage and stir for 5 min. Make up the saccharin sodium trituration and stir in the appropriate volume of solution to the mucilage. Make the volume of the mucilage up to 50 mL, taking care to ensure that there is no entrapped air in the mucilage. Make the emulsion by mixing together 50 mL of liquid paraffin and 50 mL of prepared mucilage with constant stirring. The emulsion is more stable if passed through a hand homogenizer. Pack in an amber medicine bottle with a child-resistant closure. Shake well to ensure that the emulsion is thoroughly mixed. Polish and label the bottle and give a 5 mL medicine spoon with the medicine.

Storage. Store in a cool, dry place.

Example 35.3

Prepare 100 mL Oily Calamine Lotion BP 1980.

Calamine	5 g
Wool fat	1 g
Oleic acid	0.5 mL
Arachis oil	50 mL
Calcium hydroxide solution	to 100 mL

Formulation notes. The emulsifying agent for the arachis oil is the soap calcium oleate produced from the calcium hydroxide and oleic acid when they are shaken together. Wool fat is included as an emulsion stabilizer. This is a w/o emulsion.

Method of preparation. The wool fat, oleic acid and arachis oil should be warmed gently together in an evaporating basin (using a water bath or heating block) until melted. Mix them thoroughly. The calamine should be sieved and weighed and placed on a warm ointment tile. Add a little of the oily mixture and rub in with a large spatula until smooth. Gradually add more of the oily mixture until it is fluid. Transfer back to the evaporating basin and stir to evenly distribute the calamine powder. Pour into a previously tared, amber ribbed bottle and add the calcium hydroxide solution to the bottle in small amounts, shaking well between additions. Make up to volume and seal with a child-resistant closure. Polish and label the bottle.

Storage. Store in a cool, dry place.

KEY POINTS

- Emulsions may be oil-in-water (o/w) or water-in-oil (w/o)
- Emulsions may be used orally, externally or by intramuscular and intravenous injection
- Oral emulsions are always o/w
- The type of emulsion may be determined by miscibility, conductivity, staining and dye tests
- Emulsifying agents are required to reduce the interfacial tension and act as a barrier between the oil and water phases
- Naturally occurring emulsifying agents include polysaccharides (acacia), semi-synthetic polysaccharides (methylcellulose) and sterols (wool fat)
- Synthetic surfactants can be used and are selected using the HLB number
- Care is required to avoid anion–cation incompatibilities
- Some finely divided solids will stabilize emulsions
- Emulsions require antimicrobial preservation
- Phase inversion, creaming and cracking are instabilities of emulsions which must be avoided
- A primary emulsion is prepared when making an emulsion using acacia as the emulsifying agent using either the 'dry gum' or 'wet gum' method
- The ratio of oil:water:acacia used for the primary emulsion will vary with the type of oil in the formulation
- Liquid emulsions should have 'Shake well before use' and 'Store in a cool place' labels and should not be frozen

External preparations

36

Arthur J. Winfield

STUDY POINTS

- Skin structure and sites of action of drugs
- The types and functions of solid, liquid and semi-solid skin preparations
- The ingredients used in skin preparations
- Dispensing preparations for use on the skin
- Transdermal drug delivery for systemic activity

Introduction

Skin is the largest organ in the body and has three distinct regions. The hypodermis is the innermost and is often called subcutaneous fat. The dermis is the bulk of the thickness of the skin and contains blood vessels, nerve fibres, sweat glands and hair follicles. The outermost region is the epidermis, which is made up of several layers. One of these layers is the stratum basale, in which cells divide and as they move towards the surface, they change appearance and function. The outermost layer, the stratum corneum, acts as the skin barrier. It is made up of about 20 layers of dead keratinized cells. The hair follicles and sweat ducts pass through the stratum corneum to reach the surface. A simplified diagram showing the main skin structures is given in Figure 36.1.

There are a large number of diseases which may affect different regions of the skin. Any drug used will need to reach the site of the disease in order to act. Unless it is for a surface effect only, the drug must either pass through the stratum corneum or go through hair follicles or sweat ducts. Examples of drugs applied to the skin and their sites of action are shown in Figure 36.1. Once in the skin, a lipid-soluble drug will tend to accumulate in lipid regions, while more water-soluble drugs will tend to enter the blood capillaries and be removed from the skin. There are also many metabolic enzymes in the skin which can deactivate drugs.

Effective formulation makes it possible to achieve adequate and reproducible percutaneous absorption, which is close to zero order kinetics. As a consequence, absorption through the skin from toxic materials is possible and so gloves should always be worn when preparing external preparations.

There are an increasing number of drugs that are effective against skin diseases, but drugs are not the only way of treating skin conditions. Creating physiological changes in the skin can also be beneficial. The main change is to control the moisture content of the skin. Normal skin has 10–25% moisture in the stratum corneum. This level may be reduced in, for example, eczema, or increased, as in skin maceration between the toes. By using an occlusive product (that is, an oily product), water leaving the body through the skin will be trapped and the moisture content will increase. These products are called emollients. An excess of moisture may be removed using an astringent, a hygroscopic material or, to a lesser extent, a dusting powder. Where an oily vehicle is needed, but moisture must not increase, adding solid particles to the vehicle will allow water to escape. Lubrication of sensitive skin is achieved by using finely divided solids, applied either as a powder or, more efficiently, as a suspension. Cooling the skin relieves inflammation and eases discomfort. It is achieved by evaporating a solvent, usually water or a water and alcohol

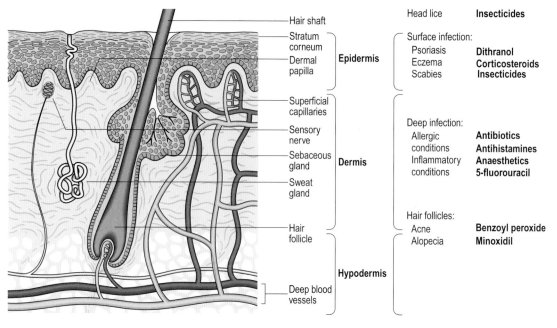

Figure 36.1 • Diagrammatic representation of the skin showing the main structures, location of diseases and the sites of action of drugs.

mixture. Volatile solvents sprayed on the skin give intense cooling.

Types of skin preparation

There are a large number of different types of external medicine, ranging from dry powders through semi-solids to liquids. The names are often traditional making classification difficult. Figure 36.2 illustrates the formulation of the main types of preparation used on the skin.

Solids

Dusting powders are applied to the skin for a surface effect such as drying or lubricating, or an antibacterial action. They are made of a fine-particle-size powder, which may be a drug alone or together with excipients.

Liquids

Soaks have an active ingredient dissolved in an aqueous solvent and are often used as astringents,

for cooling or to leave a film of solid on the skin. Oily vehicles can be used in bath additives to leave an emollient film on the skin surface.

Lotions are aqueous solutions, suspensions (see Example 36.1) or emulsions that cool inflamed skin and deposit a protective layer of solid.

Liniments are alcoholic or oily solutions or emulsions (see Example 36.2) designed to be rubbed into the skin. The medicament is usually a rubefacient.

Applications are solutions or emulsions that frequently contain parasiticides (see Example 36.3).

Paints and *tinctures* are concentrated aqueous or alcoholic antimicrobial solutions.

Collodions are organic solvents containing a polymer and drug.

There are also many other liquid products including shampoos and foot washes.

Semi-solids

Ointments are usually oily vehicles that may contain a surfactant to allow them to be washed off easily (barrier creams). They are used as emollients, or for drug delivery either to the surface or for deeper penetration.

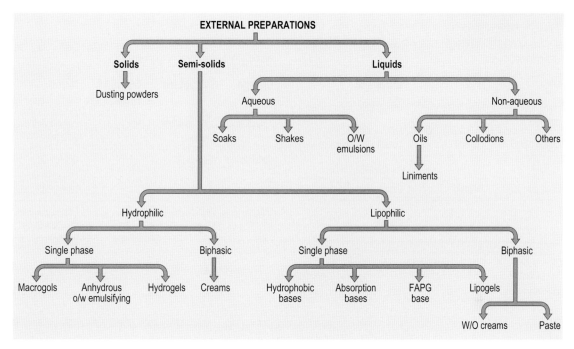

Figure 36.2 • Schematic representation of types of external medicines.

Creams are traditionally oil-in-water (o/w) emulsions while *oily creams* are water-in-oil (w/o) emulsions. However, there are also 'creams' that are not emulsions. Emulsified creams usually give cooling, are less greasy than ointments and can be used for drug delivery onto or into the skin. They require antimicrobial preservatives.

Pastes are vehicles (aqueous or oily) with a high concentration of added solid. This makes them thick so they do not spread and so localizes drug delivery (e.g. Dithranol in Lassar's Paste, see Example 36.9). They can also be used for sun blocks.

Gels are usually aqueous gels used for lubrication or applying a drug to the skin. Oily gels are also available where occlusion is required.

Ingredients used in skin preparations

Water-miscible vehicles

These include water, alcohol and the macrogols. Alcohol, usually industrial denatured alcohol, is often added to water to increase the rate of evaporation and produce a more intense cooling effect. The macrogols (polyethylene glycols) are available with a range of molecular weights. As chain length increases, so the properties change from liquid, through semi-solid to waxy solid. They have good solvent properties for a wide range of drugs and can be blended to produce intermediate consistencies. They tend to dry the skin, inactivate some antimicrobials, interact with some plastics and can give poor release of drugs.

Oily vehicles

Oils used in external preparations come from one of three sources.

Mineral oils (paraffins) are the most widely used. They are complex mixtures of mainly saturated hydrocarbons, which are available in different fractions. Different names are used in different pharmacopoeias (Table 36.1).

Light liquid paraffin is not normally used in external medicines. Soft paraffin is the main ingredient in many products, with liquid or hard paraffin being used to thin or thicken them respectively. There are two forms of soft paraffin: yellow and white. The latter has been bleached, residues of

Table 36.1 Paraffins used in external preparations: the names used are different in the UK, USA and European pharmacopoeias

UK	USA	European
Light liquid paraffin	Light mineral oil	Paraffinium perliquidum
Liquid paraffin	Mineral oil	Paraffinium liquidum
Soft paraffin	Petrolatum	Paraffinium molle
Hard paraffin	Paraffin	Paraffinium durum

Table 36.2 The ingredients used in the emulsifying waxes described in the *British Pharmacopoeia* (BP) and *British Pharmaceutical Codex* (BPC)

Charge	Surfactant	CSA:SAA ratio	Name
Anionic	Sodium lauryl sulphate	9:1	Emulsifying Wax BP
Cationic	Cetrimide	9:1	Cetrimide Emulsifying Wax BPC
Non-ionic	Cetomacrogol 1000	8:2	Cetomacrogol Emulsifying Wax BPC

CSA, cetostearyl alcohol; SAA, surface active agent.

which may remain. As a general rule, white is used with white or pale coloured ingredients, while yellow is used for darker ingredients. The paraffins are occlusive and chemically inert, but do not give good skin penetration.

Vegetable oils come from plant sources such as castor, olive, peanut and coconut. The latter two would be rarely used because of severe reactions in patients with nut allergies.

Synthetic oils, such as the silicone oils (Dimethicone BP), are used as water repellents and occlusives because they are very hydrophobic. The semi-synthetic isopropylmyristate is similar to vegetable oil in its properties and use.

Emulsifying agents

Liquid and semi-solid emulsions, both o/w and w/o, are used externally and require the addition of emulsifying agents. The latter may also be added to an oil without water as in Emulsifying Ointment BP. The presence of a surfactant usually increases the skin penetration of any drug. A wide range of materials can be used as surfactants, either alone or in combinations. Selection is made in view of the type of emulsion required (o/w or w/o) and the charge on the other ingredients (anionic, cationic or non-ionic).

Emulsifiers – w/o

Hypoallergenic commercial wool fat is a complex mixture of fatty acid esters of cholesterol and other sterols and alcohols. Wool alcohol, a solid, is richer in cholesterol and lanosterol and has fewer impurities. Both it and wool fat increase the 'water-holding' capacity of greasy bases. Hydrous wool fat is 7 parts

wool fat and 3 parts water and is a softer material. Beeswax is a traditional w/o emulsifier which is occasionally used.

Emulsifiers – o/w

Emulsifying waxes each contain two ingredients: cetostearyl alcohol and a surface-active agent, as shown in Table 36.2. All three bases are waxy solids that mix with oily materials. Addition of water produces an o/w emulsion – a cream. Both the non-aqueous blends and the creams are easily washed off the skin. Varying the amount of bodying agent, usually cetostearyl alcohol, can control consistency. The ratio of oil to water will also alter the consistency of a cream.

Other emulsifiers

Calcium soaps and soft soap have traditionally been used to make o/w emulsions.

Synthetic surface-active agents are used particularly in commercial products. Low HLB (hydrophilic–lipophilic balance) materials will produce w/o emulsions, while higher HLB surfactants give o/w emulsions.

Suspending agents

These materials can be used for suspending solids in lotions, or to produce gels, depending on the concentration used. Examples are the clays, of which there are many forms, including bentonite, atta-pulgite, montmorillonite and Veegum® (aluminium magnesium silicate). They leave a lubricant layer of powder on the skin. They are unsuitable for use below pH 3.5 and their consistency may be affected by alcohol and electrolytes (see Example 34.5).

Gelling agents can be used to produce a wide range of consistency from slightly thickened (as in artificial tears), through lubricants and semi-solids for the delivery of drugs to very thick bases used to immobilize the skin. For aqueous gels the materials used include tragacanth, alginates, pectin, gelatin, methylcelluloses, carbomer, polyvinyl alcohol and clays. Oils may be thickened using cetostearyl alcohol, hard paraffin, beeswax, wool alcohols and polyvalent soaps such as magnesium stearate. The latter, when heated with an oil, produces a clear 'lipogel'.

Other ingredients

Wetting agents are required for hydrophobic solids. Tincture of quillaia is the traditional material (see Example 36.1), but alcohol alone may be effective. Synthetic materials, such as Manoxol OT, can also be used.

Humectants are materials added to reduce the rate of water loss from creams and gels. They are all hygroscopic materials and include glycerol, propylene glycol, PEG 300 and sorbitol syrup, typically used at concentrations of 5–15%.

Solids may be added to semi-solid occlusive bases. They provide channels for the migration of water from the skin surface and so reduce the occlusiveness. Solids used include zinc oxide, talc, starch and Aerosil®. Some, such as talc, must be sterilized to kill bacterial spores.

Whenever there is a danger of microbial growth, antimicrobial preservation is required.

Preparation of external preparations

A wide range of dispensing techniques are used in compounding external medicines, some of which have been reviewed in other chapters (see Chs 30, 33, 34, 35, 38). In the section that follows, only those types of product which require different dispensing techniques are described in detail.

Dusting powders

A simple mixing in a mortar and pestle using 'doubling-up' is used (see Ch. 38). Sieving may be necessary to disperse aggregates of cohesive powders. A 180 μm sieve should be used. Powders such as starch, which contains a lot of moisture, may need drying to ensure optimum flow properties. With coloured materials, considerable working with the pestle is required before proceeding to 'doubling-up', otherwise a speckled product may result. A liquid may be added by pipette to a small quantity of the powder and be worked in before further mixing. A worked example of a dusting powder is given in Example 38.3.

Liquid preparations

These include solutions, suspensions and emulsion. Most liquid preparations are used unsterilized, but if they are intended for application to broken skin, eyes or body cavities, they should be sterilized. They should be labelled 'For external use only', and carry a 'Shake the bottle' label if they are emulsions or suspensions. Worked examples are given, of a lotion in Example 34.3 and of an oily lotion in Example 35.3.

Example 36.1

Prepare 100 mL Compound Sulfur Lotion BPC.

	Master formula	For 100 mL
Precipitated sulfur	40 g	4 g
Quillaia tincture	5 mL	0.5 mL
Glycerol	20 mL	2 mL
Industrial denatured alcohol	60 mL	6 mL
Calcium hydroxide solution	to 1000 mL	to 100 mL

Formulation notes. This an example of a 'shake' lotion, an aqueous suspension prepared without a suspending agent, but including a wetting agent for the hydrophobic sulfur.

Method of preparation. Sieve the precipitated sulfur. Weigh out 4 g and place in a glass mortar. Using a 1 mL pipette, add 0.5 mL quillaia tincture and work well into the sulfur using a pestle. Add 6 mL of industrial methylated spirits followed by 2 mL glycerol, working in after each addition (thus achieving maximum wetting before water is added). Add 20–30 mL calcium hydroxide solution to produce a pourable suspension. Transfer to a tared bottle. Rinse the mortar with calcium hydroxide solution, adding it to the bottle, before making up to volume.

Shelf-life and storage. There are no special requirements for storage. An expiry date of 4 weeks is suitable.

Example 36.2

Prepare 100 mL Methyl Salicylate Liniment BP.

	Master formula	For 100 mL
Methyl salicylate	250 mL	25 mL
Arachis oil	to 1000 mL	to 100 mL

Formulation notes. The methyl salicylate requires to penetrate the skin. The vegetable oil, arachis oil, is used as the solvent to assist in the penetration of the skin by methyl salicylate. Other similar fixed oils can be used.

Method of preparation. Measure 25 mL of methyl salicylate in a 100 mL measure and add arachis oil to make up to volume. Transfer to a dry 100 mL amber ribbed bottle.

Shelf-life and storage. This liniment should be kept in a well-closed container in a cool place. An expiry date of 4 weeks is appropriate.

Example 36.3

Prepare 100 mL of Benzyl Benzoate Application BP.

	Master formula	For 100 mL
Benzyl benzoate	250 g	25 g
Emulsifying wax	20 g	2 g
Purified water, freshly boiled and cooled	to 1000 mL	to 100 mL

Formulation notes. Benzyl benzoate is water immiscible and is being emulsified using the anionic Emulsifying Wax BP. The application is an o/w emulsion.

Method of preparation. Weigh the emulsifying wax and place it in an evaporating basin on a water bath or hot plate to melt. Add the benzyl benzoate and mix and warm. Warm about 75 mL of the water to the same temperature. Add about half of this to the evaporating basin and mix very gently. Transfer the mixture, again very gently to avoid frothing, to a tared bottle. Add warmed water to volume. Close the bottle and shake vigorously. Care is required to avoid frothing when water is present, because it will be very difficult to make up to the tare mark when froth has formed. Shake frequently during cooling.

Shelf-life and storage. The application should be kept in a cool place, but not be allowed to freeze. An expiry date of 4 weeks is appropriate.

Semi-solid preparations

Mixing by fusion

The compounding of many semi-solid preparations includes the blending together of oily materials, some of which are solids at room temperature. The process called 'mixing by fusion' achieves this. As the name implies, it involves melting the ingredients together (see Example 36.4). The process is carried out in an evaporating basin on a water bath or hot plate. It should be noted that a high temperature is not required so 60–70°C is usually adequate. Waxy solids should be grated before weighing and should be added first, so that melting can start while other ingredients are being measured. When all the ingredients are melted, remove the basin from the water bath and gently stir until cold. Mixing, which should be gentle to avoid air bubbles, is necessary to avoid lumps forming. This could happen because the higher melting point ingredients in the eutectic system may precipitate out. Any medicament may be added at different stages of preparation depending on its properties. If soluble and stable, it can be added when the base is molten. If it is less stable, or insoluble but easy to disperse, it can be added during cooling. However, if it is unstable or if dispersion is difficult, it should be added when cold using mixing by trituration.

When evaporating basins are being used, recovery of all the product is not possible. Thus, in order to be able to pack the prescribed amount, it is necessary to make an excess of about 10%.

Example 36.4

Prepare 50 g of Simple Ointment BP.

	Master formula	For 60 g
Wool fat	50 g	3 g
Hard paraffin	50 g	3 g
Cetostearyl alcohol	50 g	3 g
Yellow or white soft paraffin	850 g	51 g

Formulation notes. This is a simple blend of solid and semi-solid oily ingredients made by fusion. Yellow or white soft paraffin is chosen according to the colour of the finished product. In this case, since there is nothing else to be added, white soft paraffin should be used; 60 g is made to allow 50 g to be dispensed.

Method of preparation. Grate the hard paraffin and cetostearyl alcohol. Weigh 3 g of each and place in an evaporating basin on a water bath or hot plate. Weigh the wool fat, using a piece of paper to allow full recovery of the material, and add it to the evaporating basin, followed by the soft paraffin (also weighed on paper). Stir gently until fully melted. Remove from the heat and continue to stir gently until cold. Weigh 50 g of base into a tared ointment jar. If an ointment jar is used, a greaseproof paper disc should be placed on the surface of the ointment to protect the liner of the lid from the greasiness.

Shelf-life and storage. Store in a cool place. An expiry date of 4 weeks is appropriate.

Mixing by trituration

Insoluble solids or liquids are incorporated into bases using the technique called 'mixing by trituration'. Any powders should be passed through a 180 μm sieve before weighing to avoid grittiness in the finished product. Mixing by trituration is carried out on an ointment slab or tile, which may be made of glass or glazed porcelain. A flexible spatula is used to work the materials together. Powders are placed on the tile and incorporated into the base using 'doubling-up' as it is worked in. However, it is usually necessary to have two to three times the volume of base to powder, otherwise it will 'crumble'. Liquids, if present, are usually present in small amounts. To incorporate a liquid, a portion of the base is placed on the slab and a recess made to hold the liquid which is then worked in gently. Larger quantities of liquid should be added a little

at a time using the same method. In theory it is possible to recover all material from the slab, but it is normal to allow up to 10% excess for losses. These processes can be carried out in a mortar with a flat base using a pestle with a flat head. However, because recovery of the product is difficult, this is usually reserved for larger-scale batches.

Example 36.5

Prepare 50 g of Sulfur Ointment BP.

	Master formula	For 50 g	For 55 g
Precipitated sulfur, finely sifted	100 g	5 g	5.5 g
Simple ointment	900 g	45 g	49.5 g

Formulation notes. The BP directs that the simple ointment be prepared with white soft paraffin. If simple ointment is available, the trituration can be carried out on a slab and all the product recovered. However, if simple ointment is also being made, 50 g should be adequate to ensure that 45 g are available. Precipitated sulfur, while of smaller particle size than sublimed sulphur, can give a gritty feel unless it is passed through a 180 μm sieve.

Method of preparation. Sieve and then weigh out the precipitated sulfur and place it on the slab. Weigh out the simple ointment (using a piece of paper to prevent it sticking to the balance), and place it on a different part of the slab. Take a portion of the sulfur and a portion of the base of about three times the volume of the sulfur and work them together vigorously until there is no sign of any particles of sulfur. Spreading a thin layer on the slab helps check this. Gradually add the remaining sulfur and base. Collect the ointment together on the slab using the spatula and pack 50 g.

Shelf-life and storage. Store in a cool place. An expiry date of 4 weeks is appropriate.

Example 36.6

Prepare 30 g of Methyl Salicylate Ointment BP.

	Master formula	For 35 g
Methyl salicylate	500 g	17.5 g
White beeswax	250 g	8.75 g
Hydrous wool fat	250 g	8.75 g

Formulation notes. Methyl salicylate is a liquid. With the high proportion present, the product would be runny without the addition of the beeswax as a thickening agent. The base ingredients require to be blended by fusion.

Method of preparation. Grate and weigh the beeswax. Melt it with the hydrous wool fat (weighed on a piece of paper) in an evaporating basin on a water bath or hot plate. Remove from the heat and stir until almost cold before adding the methyl salicylate (it is volatile). Continue stirring until cold. Pack 30 g in a glass ointment jar (plastic should be avoided with methyl salicylate).

Shelf-life and storage. Store in a cool place. An expiry date of 4 weeks is appropriate.

Creams

Creams are emulsified preparations containing water. They are susceptible to microorganisms which may cause spoilage of the cream or disease in the patient. While preservatives are included, they are usually inadequate to cope with a heavy microbial contamination and growth so the possibility of microbial contamination during preparation should be minimized. Ideally aseptic techniques should be used, but this is not normally possible in extemporaneous dispensing and so thorough cleanliness is employed. As a minimum, all apparatus and final containers should be thoroughly cleaned and rinsed with freshly boiled and cooled purified water, then dried just prior to use. Swabbing of working surfaces, spatulas and other equipment with ethanol will also reduce the possibility of microbial contamination.

The basic method of making an emulsified cream is to warm both the oily phase and aqueous phase separately to a temperature of about 60°C, mix the phases and stir until cold. It is important that the temperatures of the two phases are within a few degrees of each other and it is advisable to use a thermometer to check this. Rapid cooling will cause the separation of high melting point materials, and excessive aeration as a result of vigorous stirring will produce a granular appearance in the product. Medicaments may, if they are stable, be dissolved in the appropriate phase before emulsification, or can be added by trituration when cold.

Example 36.7

Prepare 50 g of Aqueous Cream BP.

	Master formula	For 55 g
Emulsifying ointment	300 g	16.5 g
Phenoxyethanol	10 g	0.55 g
Purified water, freshly boiled and cooled	690 g	37.95 g

Formulation notes. This is an o/w cream made using an anionic emulsifying agent. To reduce the risk of microbial contamination, all equipment should be washed before use. Phenoxyethanol is present as an antimicrobial preservative. It is a liquid, so has to be weighed, or, if its density is obtained, it could be measured by pipette. If the emulsifying ointment has to be made, exactly 16.5 g can be made because the emulsification can be carried out in the same evaporating basin.

Method of preparation. The phenoxyethanol is dissolved in the water warmed to 60°C. Weigh the emulsifying ointment (using a piece of paper to prevent it sticking) and melt it in an evaporating basin on a water bath or hot plate. Ensure that both phases are close to 60°C, then add the aqueous phase to the melted ointment. Remove from the heat and stir continuously until cold, taking care not to incorporate too much air. Weigh 50 g and pack in an ointment jar.

Shelf-life and storage. The preparation should be stored in a cool place, but not allowed to freeze. A shelf-life of 2–3 weeks is appropriate because the preparation has not been made in the cleanest conditions.

Example 36.8

Prepare 50 g of Hydrous Ointment BP (also known as Oily Cream).

	Master formula	For 60 g
Wool alcohols ointment	500 g	30 g
Phenoxyethanol	10 g	0.6 g
Dried magnesium sulphate	5 g	0.3 g
Purified water, freshly boiled and cooled	485 g	29.1 g

Formulation notes. This is a w/o cream prepared using wool alcohols as the emulsifying agent. Phenoxyethanol is present as preservative, but all equipment should be washed before use. Phenoxyethanol is a liquid and so must be weighed, or, if its density is obtained, it can be measured by pipette. Quantities for 55 g produce amounts that cannot be weighed on a dispensing balance, so 60 g is made. If the wool alcohols ointment is also to be made, exactly 30 g is adequate, because it does not have to be removed from the evaporating basin.

Method of preparation. All equipment should be thoroughly cleaned before use. Dissolve the magnesium sulphate and phenoxyethanol in the water and warm to 60°C on a water bath or hot plate. Weigh the wool alcohols ointment, using a piece of paper, and melt it in an evaporating basin at 60°C. Check that the two temperatures are the same. Add the water, little by little, to the ointment, stirring constantly until a smooth creamy mixture is produced, while maintaining the temperature at 60°C. When all the water is added, remove from the heat and stir gently until the cream is at room temperature. Pack 50 g in an ointment jar.

Shelf-life and storage. Store in a cool place but do not allow to freeze. If liquid separates on storage, stirring may reincorporate it. An expiry date of 4 weeks is appropriate.

Dilution of creams

It is sometimes necessary to prepare a dilution of a commercially produced cream, although the practice is undesirable. Choice of diluent is crucial, since the diluent may impair the preservative system in the cream, may affect the bioavailability of the medicament, or be incompatible with other ingredients. The process of dilution also increases the risk of microbial contamination. Thus, dilutions should only be made with the diluent(s) specified in the manufacturer's data sheet and heat must be avoided. All diluted creams should be freshly prepared and be given a 2-week shelf-life.

Pastes

Pastes are dispersions of high concentrations of solid in either an aqueous or oily vehicle. They can be used to treat infections by making use of their high osmotic pressure, or as very thick materials to prevent irritant drugs spreading over the skin surface. Incorporation of the solid is by mixing on an ointment slab.

Example 36.9

Prepare 100 g of Dithranol Paste BP.

	Master formula	For 100 g
Dithranol	1 g	0.1 g
Lassar's paste	999 g	99.9 g
Lassar's paste	**Master formula**	**For 110 g**
Zinc oxide	240 g	26.4 g
Salicylic acid	20 g	2.2 g
Starch	240 g	26.4 g
White soft paraffin	500 g	55 g

Formulation notes. The Lassar's paste has to be made first before incorporating the dithranol. Dithranol is prone to oxidation, so contact with metal should be avoided. Gloves should be worn during preparation.

Method of preparation. Sieve the zinc oxide and salicylic acid through a 180 μm sieve before weighing. Weigh the soft paraffin (on a piece of paper) and melt in an evaporating basin on a water bath. Take some of the powder and stir into the melted base. Continue until all the powder is added, then stir gently until cold. Weigh out the Lassar's paste (using paper to avoid sticking). Only when the Lassar's paste has been completed, weigh out the dithranol. Care is required because it is very irritant to skin. Place it on a slab and incorporate it in a small portion of the paste using a plastic spatula, ensuring that a smooth, even product is produced. Dilute gradually with the remainder of the paste. Pack in a brown ointment jar, with a circle of greaseproof paper and a tight-fitting closure.

Shelf-life and storage. The product should be kept in a cool place, protected from light. An expiry date of 2 weeks is appropriate because of chemical instability.

Transdermal delivery systems

Transdermal drug delivery systems aim to provide continuous drug release over a period of time which can be from a few hours to 7 days.

The principle of this dosage form is that, by optimization of physicochemical factors, the drug is absorbed through the skin into the systemic circulation. Absorption through the skin is variable so the rate of release of the drug must be controlled to a slower rate than the skin can absorb it. This may be achieved either by using a matrix system or a rate-limiting membrane. These devices are commonly known as 'patches'. Drugs available as transdermal therapeutic systems include Glyceryl trinitrate, Oestradiol, Nicotine, Hyoscine, Testosterone, Fentanyl, Rivastigmine. Transdermal therapeutic systems are always produced by pharmaceutical manufacturers because of the technology involved.

Advantages

- Continuous drug delivery, producing steady-state plasma levels
- No drug deactivation in the gastrointestinal tract
- No first pass effect, as the liver is bypassed (although there is metabolism in the skin)
- Cessation of treatment by removing the patch. (This is not immediate because of a reservoir effect which will continue to deliver drug from the skin for several hours.)

Although these are benefits, various problems are associated with this type of dosage form. For these reasons, few drugs so far have been formulated in this way.

Disadvantages

- Only potent drugs, i.e. those with a small therapeutic dose, are suitable to be incorporated into a patch. Skin permeability is inadequate to allow larger doses from an acceptable size of patch
- Because the drug is being absorbed through the skin, lipid-soluble drugs are most likely to be effective
- Drugs with long half-lives are not suitable for this type of formulation
- There have been reports of local skin reactions due to irritancy by drugs To minimize possible skin reactions, new patches should be placed on fresh skin each time, the same site being not used for at least 7 days
- In some instances the steady-state blood levels have produced tolerance, e.g. glyceryl trinitrate. This has led to the practice of patients being given a 'nitrate-free' period which prevents tolerance occurring
- Steady-state blood levels of nicotine have caused central nervous system disturbance; in particular, patients have reported suffering nightmares.

Normally, nicotine levels in a smoker will fall during the hours of sleep as no cigarette smoking occurs. No such fall will occur when 24-h nicotine patches are used. For this reason, manufacturers have developed patches which are applied for 16 h then removed. A new one is applied 8 h later.

Method of use

It is important that patients are informed how to use patches correctly. All patients who purchase or are prescribed patches should be given the following information about their use:

- To ensure adequate adhesion, the patch must be applied to a clean, dry area of skin
- The old patch must always be removed before applying a new one
- When a patch is replaced with a new one it must be applied to a different area of skin. The area of skin from which a patch has just been removed will be soft and possibly moist. This alters the permeability of the skin. In order to maintain the same level of drug absorption, a different, intact area of skin must be used
- The patch must be disposed of carefully. It should be folded together to prevent it being stuck on to another person's skin. Particular care should be taken to keep patches away from children.

KEY POINTS

- Drugs applied to the skin are usually for a local effect, although systemic action is possible
- Skin preparations may be solids, liquids or semi-solids
- For liquids and semi-solids, the vehicles may be water based, water miscible, oily or emulsified
- A wide range of emulsifying agents may be used to produce either o/w or w/o emulsions
- Suspending agents used on the skin are usually clays
- Other ingredients include wetting agents, humectants and finely divided solids
- All skin preparations should carry the label 'For external use only'
- Dusting powders are simple mixtures made by 'doubling-up'

- Lotions are aqueous solutions, suspensions or emulsions
- Liniments are oily solutions or emulsions
- Mixing by fusion is the process of melting together the ingredients of ointment bases followed by stirring until cold
- Mixing by trituration is the incorporation of solids or liquids into semi-solid vehicles on an ointment slab

- Cleanliness is essential when making creams to avoid excessive microbial contamination
- Transdermal delivery systems (skin patches) are used to give prolonged constant plasma concentrations for a number of drugs
- Patients must be carefully counselled on the use of skin patches

Suppositories and pessaries

Arthur J. Winfield

STUDY POINTS

- Ideal suppository bases
- Types of base
- Suppository moulds and mould calibration
- Displacement values
- Methods of preparation of suppositories and pessaries
- Containers, labelling and patient advice for suppositories and pessaries

Introduction

Drug administration by the rectum can be used for local or systemic action. Dosage forms used include suppositories, rectal tablets, capsules, ointments and enemas. Vaginal administration can be for both local and systemic action, using pessaries and vaginal formulations of tablets, capsules, solutions, sprays, creams, ointments and foams. This chapter gives details of how suppositories and pessaries are prepared extemporaneously, the substances and equipment used in their preparation, the calculations involved and patient advice.

Suppositories and pessaries are drug delivery systems where the drug is incorporated into an inert vehicle; base. Suppositories are formed by melting the base, incorporating the drug and then allowing them to set in a suitable metal or plastic mould.

Suppository bases

A number of criteria can be identified as desirable in an ideal base, including:

- Melt at, or just below, body temperature or dissolve in body fluids
- Solidify quickly after melting
- Easily moulded and removed from the mould
- Chemically stable even when molten
- Release the active ingredient readily
- Easy to handle
- Bland, i.e. non-toxic and non-irritant.

No base meets all these requirements, so a compromise is required. There are two groups of materials, the fatty bases and the water-soluble or water-miscible bases.

The fatty bases

Theobroma oil

Theobroma oil, a naturally occurring oil, has a melting point range of 30–36°C and so readily melts in the body. It liquefies easily on heating but sets rapidly when cooled. It is also bland, therefore no irritation occurs. The main technical difficulty is the ease with which lower melting point polymorphic forms of theobroma oil are formed. The stable β-form has a melting point of 34.5°C and forms after melting at 36°C and slowly cooling. If it is overheated, the unstable α-form (melting point 23°C) and γ-form (melting point 19°C) are produced. These forms will eventually return to the stable form but this may take several days. The melting point is a problem in hot climates and can be reduced further by the addition of a soluble drug. The latter effect can be counteracted by adding beeswax (up to 10%), but care must be taken not to raise the melting point too high, as the suppository would not melt in the rectum. In addition, theobroma oil is prone to oxidation. Theobroma oil shrinks only slightly on cooling and therefore tends to stick to the suppository mould; thus requiring a mould lubricant.

Synthetic fats

These are hydrogenated vegetable oils. Synthetic fatty bases have many of the advantages but there are a few potential problems:

- The viscosity of the melted fats is lower than that of theobroma oil. As a result there is a greater risk of drug particles sedimenting during preparation leading to a lack of uniform drug distribution. This problem is partly compensated for in that these bases set very quickly
- These bases become brittle if cooled too rapidly, so should not be refrigerated during preparation
- These bases are produced in series of grades, each with different hardness and melting point ranges. These can be used to compensate for melting point reduction by soluble drugs. However, release and absorption of the drug in the body may vary depending on the base being used.

Further information on these bases can be found in the *Pharmaceutical Codex* (1994).

Water-soluble and water-miscible bases

Glycerol-gelatin bases

These bases are a mixture of glycerol and water stiffened with gelatin. The commonest is Glycerol Suppositories Base BP, which has 14% weight in weight (w/w) gelatin, and 70% w/w glycerol. In hot climates, the gelatin content can be increased to 18% w/w. Pharmaceutical grade gelatin is a pathogen-free, purified protein produced by the hydrolysis of the collagenous tissue, such as skins and bones, of animals. Some people may have ethical problems with the use of such a product.

Two types of gelatin are used for pharmaceutical purposes: Type A, which is prepared by acid hydrolysis and is cationic, and Type B, which is prepared by alkaline hydrolysis and is anionic. Type A is compatible with substances such as boric acid and lactic acid, while Type B is compatible with substances like ichthammol and zinc oxide. The 'jelly strength' or 'bloom strength' of gelatin is important, particularly when it is used in the preparation of suppositories or pessaries.

Glycerol-gelatin bases have a physiological effect which can cause rectal irritation because of the small amount of liquid present. As they dissolve in the mucous secretions of the rectum, osmosis occurs producing a laxative effect. The solution time depends on the content, quality of the gelatin and the age of the suppository. Because of the water content, microbial contamination is more likely than with the fatty bases. Preservatives may be added to the product, but can lead to problems of incompatibility. In addition, glycol-gelatin bases are hygroscopic and therefore require careful storage.

Macrogols

These polyethylene glycols can be blended together to produce suppository bases with varying melting points, dissolution rates and physical characteristics. Drug release depends on the base dissolving rather than melting (the melting point is often around 50°C). Higher proportions of high molecular weight polymers produce preparations which release the drug slowly and are also brittle. Less brittle products which release the drug more readily can be prepared by mixing high polymers with medium and low polymers. Details of combinations which are used are found in the *Pharmaceutical Codex* (1994). Macrogols have several properties which make them useful as suppository bases including the absence of a physiological effect, are not prone to microbial contamination and have a high water-absorbing capacity. As they dissolve, a viscous solution is produced which means there is less likelihood of leakage from the body.

The macrogol bases have a number of disadvantages. They are hygroscopic, which means they must be carefully stored, and this could lead to irritation of the rectal mucosa. This latter disadvantage can be alleviated by dipping the suppository in water prior to insertion. They become brittle if cooled too quickly and also may become brittle on storage. Incompatibility with several drugs

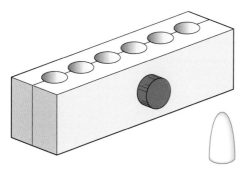

Figure 37.1 • Dispensing suppository mould.

Table 37.1 Lubricants for use with suppository bases	
Base	**Lubricant**
Theobroma oil	Soap spirit
Glycerol-gelatin base	Almond oil, liquid paraffin
Synthetic fats	No lubricant required
Macrogols	No lubricant required

and packaging materials, e.g. benzocaine and plastic, may limit their use. In addition, crystal growth occurs, with some drugs causing irritation to the rectal mucosa and may prolong dissolution times.

Preparation of suppositories

Suppositories are made using a metal or plastic suppository mould. Traditional metal moulds (Fig. 37.1) are in two halves which are clamped together with a screw. The internal surface is normally plated to ensure that the suppositories have a smooth surface.

Before use the mould should be completely cleaned by washing carefully in warm, soapy water and thoroughly dried, taking care not to scratch the internal surface. The exact shape can vary slightly from one mould to another.

Preparation of suppositories containing an active ingredient which is insoluble in the base

The bases used, most commonly, for extemporaneous preparation of suppositories and pessaries are the synthetic fats and glycerol-gelatin base.

1. When calculating the quantity of ingredients it is necessary to prepare excess due to unavoidable wastage. Usually, an excess of two should be calculated for, e.g. to prepare 12 suppositories, calculate for 14.
2. The mould should be carefully washed and dried.
3. Ensure that the two halves fit together correctly. This is necessary to ensure that there is no leakage of material. They usually have code letters and/or numbers which should match.
4. For some bases the mould will need to be lubricated. The lubricants are given in Table 37.1.
5. If a lubricant is necessary, apply it carefully to the two halves of the mould using gauze or other non-fibrous material. Do not use cotton wool as fibres may be left on the mould surface and become incorporated into the suppositories.
6. Invert the mould to allow any excess lubricant to drain off.
7. Accurately weigh the required amount of base. If large lumps are present the material should be grated.
8. Place in a porcelain basin and warm gently using a water bath or hot plate. Allow approximately two-thirds of the base to melt and remove from the heat. The residual heat will be sufficient to melt the rest of the base.
9. Reduce the particle size of the active ingredient, if necessary. Either grinding in a mortar and pestle or sieving (see Ch. 30).
10. Weigh the correct amount of medicament and place on a glass tile (ointment slab).
11. Add about half of the molten base to the powdered drug and rub together with a spatula.
12. Scrape the dispersion off the tile using the spatula and place it back in the basin.
13. If necessary, put the basin back over the water bath to remelt the ingredients.
14. Remove from the heat and stir constantly until almost on the point of setting. If the mixture is not stirred at this stage the active ingredient will sediment and uniform distribution of the drug will not be achieved.

15. Quickly pour into the mould, slightly overfilling each cavity to allow for contraction on cooling. Do not start pouring the suppositories while the mixture is still very molten. If this is done, a suspended drug will sediment to the bottom of the mould and the base shrinks excessively so that the tops become concave.

16. Leave the mould and its contents to cool for about 5 min and then, using a spatula, trim the tops of the suppositories. Do not leave the suppositories too long before trimming, as they will be too hard and trimming becomes very difficult.

17. Allow cooling for another 10–15 min until the suppositories are completely firm and set. Do not try to speed up the cooling process by putting the mould in a refrigerator. Synthetic fats in particular are inclined to become brittle and break if cooled too quickly.

18. Unscrew the mould and remove the suppositories.

19. Each perfect suppository should then be wrapped in greaseproof paper and packed in an appropriate container and labelled.

When preparing suppositories where the active ingredient is either a semi-solid, is soluble in the base or is a liquid which is miscible with the base, the melting point of the base will be lowered. In these situations, a base with a higher than normal melting point should be used if available. The base is melted as normal and the active ingredient is added directly to the base and incorporated by stirring.

Moulds are made in four sizes: 1 g, 2 g, 4 g and 8 g. Unless otherwise stated, the 1 g size is used for suppositories. The same moulds are used to prepare pessaries, when the two larger sizes are generally used. A suppository mould is filled by volume, but the suppository is formulated by weight. The capacity of a suppository mould is nominal and each mould will have minor variations. Therefore, the weight of material contained in different moulds may be different and will also depend on the base being used. It is therefore essential that each mould be calibrated for each different base.

Mould calibration

The capacity of the mould is confirmed by filling the mould with the chosen base. The total weight of the perfect suppositories is taken and a mean weight calculated. This value is the calibration value of the mould for that particular base (see Example 37.1).

> ### Example 37.1
>
> A 1 g suppository mould is to be used to prepare a batch of suppositories. The base to be used is a synthetic fat. Some base is melted in an evaporating basin over a water bath or hot plate. When about two-thirds of the base has melted the basin is removed from the heat. The contents of the basin are stirred and the remaining base melts with the residual heat. Continue stirring the base until it is almost on the point of setting (it starts to thicken, becomes slightly cloudy and small crystals can be seen on the surface). The base is then poured into the mould cavities, slightly overfilling to allow for shrinkage. They are trimmed after about 5 min and left to set for a further 10–15 min. The mould is then opened and the suppositories removed. Only the perfect products should be weighed. Any which are chipped or damaged should be discarded.
>
> From the above exercise, five perfect suppositories were obtained. The total weight was 5.05 g. The mould calibration figure is therefore 5.05/5 = 1.01 g. This is the value which should be used for that particular combination of mould and base.

Displacement values

The volume of a suppository from a particular mould is uniform but its weight can vary when a drug is present because the density of the drug may be different from that of the base. For example, a drug which has twice the density of the base will occupy half the volume which the same weight of base occupies, and a drug whose density is four times that of the base will occupy a quarter the volume which the same weight of base occupies. Allowance must be made for this by using displacement values (DV).

The displacement value of a drug is the number of parts by weight of drug which displaces 1 part by weight of the base.

Displacement values for a variety of medicaments are given in Table 37.2. Other reference sources such as the *Pharmaceutical Handbook* (Wade 1980) and the *Pharmaceutical Codex* also give information on displacement values. Minor variations may occur in the values quoted so it is always advisable to indicate the source of your information (see Example 37.2).

Displacement values in the literature normally refer to values for theobroma oil. These values can

Table 37.2 Displacement values with respect to fatty bases

Medicament	Displacement value
Aspirin	1.1
Bismuth subgallate	2.7
Chloral hydrate	1.4
Cinchocaine hydrochloride	1.0
Codeine phosphate	1.1
Hamamelis dry extract	1.5
Hydrocortisone	1.5
Ichthammol	1.0
Liquids	1.0
Metronidazole	1.7
Morphine hydrochloride	1.6
Paracetamol	1.5
Pethidine hydrochloride	1.6
Phenobarbital	1.1
Zinc oxide	4.7

also be used for other fatty bases. With glycerol-gelatin suppository base, approximately 1.2 g occupies the same volume as 1 g of theobroma oil. Using this information, the relevant displacement values can be calculated.

There may be occasions when information on the DV of a drug is not available. In these situations the DV must be determined (see Example 37.3).

Calculation of quantities when the active ingredient is stated as a percentage

A displacement value is not required when calculating quantities stated as percentages (see Example 37.4).

When there is more than one active ingredient present the quantity of each medicament is calculated and the amount of base is calculated using the displacement value for each ingredient (see Example 37.5).

Example 37.2

Prepare six suppositories each containing 250 mg bismuth subgallate.

Not all material can be removed from the evaporating basin, so quantities are calculated for an excess of two suppositories. Therefore calculate for eight suppositories.

DV of bismuth subgallate = 2.7 (*Pharmaceutical Codex*), i.e. 2.7 g of bismuth subgallate displaces 1 g of base.

A 1 g mould will be used with mould calibration = 0.94.

To calculate the amount of base required, a simple equation is used:

$$\text{Amount of base} = (N \times y) - (N \times D)/DV$$

where N is the number of suppositories to be made, y is the mould calibration, D is the dose in one suppository, DV is the displacement value.

Using the terms in the equation for this example:

$N = 8$

$Y = 0.94$

$D = 250\,\text{mg} = 0.25\,\text{g}$

$DV = 2.7$

Using the equation:

Amount of base required

$= 8 \times 0.94 - 8 \times 0.25/2.7 = 7.52 - 0.741$

$= 6.779\,\text{g} = 6.78\,\text{g}$

Example 37.3

To calculate the DV of a drug:

A batch of unmedicated suppositories is prepared and the products weighed.

A batch of suppositories containing a known concentration of the required drug is prepared and the products are weighed.

Weight of six unmedicated suppositories = 6 g

Weight of six suppositories containing 40% drug = 8.8 g

Weight of base is then = 60% = 60/100×8.8 = 5.28 g

Weight of drug in suppositories = 40% = 40/100 × 8.8 = 3.52

Weight of base displaced by drug = 6 × 5.28 = 0.72 g.

If 0.72 g of drug is displaced by 3.52 g of base, then 1 g of base will be displaced by 3.52/0.72 g = 4.88 g.

Therefore displacement value of drug = 4.9 (rounded to one decimal place).

Example 37.4

Prepare eight suppositories containing 18% zinc oxide.
Calculate for 10 suppositories (two excess).

Mould calibration = 1

Weight of base required to fill mould = 10 × 1 = 10

Zinc oxide is 18% of total = 1.8 g

Weight of base required = 10−1.8 = 8.2 g

Example 37.5

Calculate the quantities required to make 15 suppositories each containing 150 mg hamamelis dry extract and 560 mg of zinc oxide.

A 2 g mould, with mould calibration of 2.04, will be used.

Calculate for 17 suppositories (two excess).

DV of hamamelis dry extract = 1.5 (*Pharmaceutical Codex*)

DV of zinc oxide = 4.7 (*Pharmaceutical Codex*)

Weight of hamamelis dry extract = 17 × 0.15 = 2.55 g

Weight of zinc oxide = 17 × 0.56 = 9.52 g

Weight of base = 17 × 2.04−(2.55/1.5 + 9.52/4.7) = 34.68−(1.7 + 2.03) = 30.95 g.

Preparation of suppositories using a glycerol-gelatin base

The formula for Glycerol Suppository Base BP is:

Gelatin	14%
Glycerol	70%
Water	to 100%

1. The gelatin strip is cut into small pieces, approximately 1 cm square, trimming off any hard outer edges.
2. The required amount of gelatin is weighed and placed in a previously weighed porcelain evaporating basin.
3. Sufficient water to just cover the gelatin is added and the contents left for about 5 min.
4. When the gelatin has softened (hydrated), any excess water is drained off. This step is not necessary if powdered gelatin is being used.

5. The exact amount of glycerol is then weighed into the basin.
6. The basin is heated gently on a water bath or hot plate and the mixture gently stirred until the gelatin has dissolved. Do not stir vigorously as this will create air bubbles which are very difficult to remove. At this stage the base may need to be heat treated as noted below.
7. When the gelatin is dissolved, the basin is removed from the heat and weighed. If the weight is less than the required total (basin plus ingredients), water is added to give the correct weight. If the contents of the basin are too heavy, it must be heated further to evaporate the excess water.
8. When the correct weight is achieved, the active ingredient is added, with careful stirring.
9. The mixture is then poured into the prepared mould and lubricated with an oil such as almond oil or liquid paraffin. The mould must not be overfilled because glycerol-gelatin base cannot be trimmed.
10. The preparation is left to set. After removing from the mould, each suppository should be smeared with liquid paraffin before being wrapped in greaseproof paper.

Note: Pharmaceutical gelatin should not contain any pathogens, but as a precaution, the base may be heat treated. This is done by heating the base for 1 h at 100°C in an electric steamer. This should be done before the base is adjusted to weight (at Stage 7 above).

This base is commonly used for the preparation of pessaries, as described in Example 37.6.

Containers for suppositories

Glass or plastic screw-topped jars are the best choice of container for extemporaneously prepared suppositories and pessaries. Cardboard cartons may be used but these offer little protection from moisture or heat for hygroscopic materials.

Shelf-life

Suppositories and pessaries are relatively stable preparations, if well packaged and stored at a low temperature. Unless other information is available, an expiry date of 1 month is appropriate.

Example 37.6

Prepare 12 pessaries containing 10% ichthammol.
A 4 g mould (calibration value 4.0) is used.

Calculate for 14 pessaries to allow for wastage. Additional base is required because it is denser than the oily bases. The density factor is 1.2.

Mould calibration for glycerol-gelatin base is $4.0 \times 1.2 = 4.8$ g.

A displacement value is not required because the ichthammol is expressed as a percentage.

Formula for the base:

Gelatin	14 g
Glycerol	70 g
Water	to 100 g

Formula for the pessaries:

Ichthammol	10% w/w
Glycerol-gelatin base	90% w/w

The total weight required to prepare the pessaries is 14×4.8 g $= 67.2$ g. For ease of calculation prepare 70 g. Quantities are therefore:

Ichthammol	7 g
Base	63 g

It is advisable to make a small excess of base, taking care to choose quantities which give easily weighable amounts, i.e. do not try to weigh to several decimal points. In this case 65 g can be prepared.

Using the method described above, prepare 65 g of the base, taking care that the correct type of gelatin is chosen. Because the active ingredient is ichthammol, Type B should be used. When the 65 g of base has been prepared, 2 g should be removed from the basin, leaving the required 63 g. The base is removed from the heat, allowed to cool a little before 7 g of ichthammol is added with careful stirring. The mixture is then poured into the lubricated mould and left to set.

Labelling for suppositories

Adequate information should appear on the label so that the patient knows how to use the product. In addition, the following information should appear: 'Store in a cool place' and 'For rectal use only' or 'For vaginal use only', whichever is appropriate.

Patient advice

In addition to what appears on the label, patients should be told to unwrap the suppository or pessary (this may appear to be unnecessary advice but there is sufficient evidence to show that it is not always done) and insert it as high as possible into the rectum or vagina. It may be helpful to provide the patient with a diagram and instruction leaflet, such as that produced by the National Pharmaceutical Association. When suppositories are for children it is likely that an adult will have to carry out the insertion.

KEY POINTS

- Both rectal and vaginal administration can be used for local or systemic drug action
- Bases may be fatty or water miscible
- Synthetic fatty bases are easier to use than theobroma oil
- Glycerol-gelatin base produces a laxative effect
- Type A (anionic) or Type B (cationic) gelatin can be used to avoid incompatibilities
- Macrogol bases are blends of high and low molecular weight polymers which dissolve in rectal contents
- Suppository moulds have nominal capacities of 1, 2, 4 and 8 g and must be calibrated with the base to be used
- When using theobroma oil and glycerol-gelatin base, the mould has to be lubricated
- To allow for contraction on cooling, overfilling with oily bases is required
- Each mould should be calibrated for each base
- Because glycerol-gelatin base has a higher density than fatty bases, moulds hold approximately 1.2 times the nominal weight
- The displacement value is the number of parts by weight of drug which displaces one part by weight of base
- Unless the density of the drug and base are the same, a displacement value is required to calculate the amount of base displaced by the drug
- Labels should include either 'For rectal use only' or 'For vaginal use only', and 'Store in a cool place'

38

Powders and granules

Arthur J. Winfield

STUDY POINTS

- The pharmaceutical uses of powders
- Bulk and divided powders
- The mixing of powders
- Diluents used with powders
- Calculations required when preparing powders
- How to dispense powders
- The folding of powders

Introduction

A powder may be defined as a solid material in a finely divided state. Granules are powders agglomerated to produce larger free-flowing particles. Powders and granules can be used to prepare other formulations, such as solutions, suspensions and tablets. A powdered drug on its own can be a dosage form for taking orally (called a simple powder), when they are usually mixed with water first, or for external application as a dusting powder. Alternatively, the drug may be blended with other ingredients (called a compound powder).

Powders for internal use

Powders for oral administration will comprise the active ingredients with excipients such as diluents, sweeteners and dispersing agents. These may be presented as undivided powders (bulk powders) or divided powders (individually wrapped doses).

Individually wrapped powders tend not to be official formulae and are rarely prescribed these days (see Examples 38.1 and 38.2). Magnesium Trisilicate Powder Compound BP (see Example 38.4) and Compound Kaolin Powder BP are examples of bulk powders for internal use. Proprietary powders and granules include Dioralyte®, Electrolade® (both oral rehydration salts), Normacol® (sterculia) and Fybogel® (ispaghula husk).

Bulk powders

Supplying as an undivided powder is useful for non-potent, bulky drugs with a large dose, e.g. antacids, or when the dry powder is more stable than its liquid-containing counterpart. A bulk powder can be supplied to the patient although this is rarely seen nowadays because the dosage form is inconvenient to carry and there are possible inaccuracies in measuring the dose.

Individually wrapped powders

Individually wrapped powders are used to supply some potent drugs, where accuracy of dose is important. Extemporaneously produced powders are wrapped separately in paper. They are convenient dosage forms for children's doses of drugs which are not commercially available at the strength required, such as levothyroxine (thyroxine) or ibuprofen (see Example 38.2). Sealed sachets of powders are available commercially, e.g. Paramax® (paracetamol and metoclopramide) and oral rehydration salts. They are mixed with water prior to taking and are useful for patients who have difficulty swallowing or where rapid absorption of the drug is required.

Granules for internal use

Some preparations are supplied to the pharmacy as granules, for reconstitution immediately before dispensing, e.g. antibiotic suspensions. This protects drugs which are susceptible to hydrolysis or other degradation in the presence of water until the time of dispensing in order to give an adequate shelf-life.

Particle size

The particle size of a powder is described using standard descriptions given in the *British Pharmacopoeia* (BP). These refer to either the standardized sieve size that they are capable of passing through in a specified time under shaking, or to the microscopically determined particle size. Thus, powders for oral use would normally be a 'moderately fine' or a 'fine' powder. The former is able to pass through a sieve of nominal mesh aperture 355 μm and the latter one of 180 μm. Comminution is the process of particle size reduction. On a small scale, this can be achieved using a mortar and pestle when it is usually called trituration. This is a common first step in extemporaneous dispensing, after which the powder should be passed through the appropriate sieve before weighing.

Mixing the powder

Ingredients of powders should be mixed thoroughly, using the technique of 'doubling-up' (sometimes called geometric dilution) to ensure an even distribution. This process involves starting with the ingredient which has the smallest bulk. In Example 38.1, this is hyoscine hydrobromide. The other ingredient(s) are added progressively in approximately equal parts by volume. In this way the amount in the mortar is approximately doubled at each addition. Mixing in between additions continues until all the ingredients are incorporated. The powder can then be packed.

Preparing individually wrapped powders

The minimum weight of an individually wrapped powder is 120 mg. Dilution of a drug with a diluent, usually lactose, is often necessary to produce this weight.

Occasionally, manufactured tablets or capsules may be used to prepare oral powders (see Example 38.2). This involves either crushing the tablet in a mortar and

---

Example 38.1

Prepare 4 powders each containing 300 μg of hyoscine hydrobromide.

Calculation and method of preparation. Calculate for five powders. Use lactose as the diluent, each powder to weigh 120 mg.

Hyoscine hydrobromide (5×300)

$= 1500 \mu g = 1.5 mg$

Lactose ($5 \times 120 mg$) to 600 mg

The minimum weighable quantity (using a Class B balance) is 100 mg.

Step A

Make a 1 in 10 dilution of hyoscine hydrobromide with lactose:

Hyoscine hydrobromide 100 mg

Lactose 900 mg

Mix by doubling-up and remove 100 mg (triturate A).
100 mg of triturate A contains
$100/1000 \times 100 = 10 mg$ hyoscine hydrobromide.

Step B

Make a 1 in 10 dilution of triturate A with lactose:

Triturate A	100 mg
Lactose	900 mg

Mix by doubling-up and remove 150 mg (triturate B). 150 mg of triturate B contains $10/1000 \times 150 = 1.5 mg$ hyoscine hydrobromide.

Step C

Triturate B	150 mg

Lactose (($5 \times 120 mg$) $- 150 mg$) $= 450 mg$

Mix by doubling-up; 120 mg portions of this final powder will contain 300 μg of hyoscine hydrobromide. Weigh 120 mg aliquots and wrap in a powder paper.

---

pestle, or emptying the contents of the capsule and adding a suitable diluent. Lactose is the most commonly used diluent because it is colourless, odourless, soluble, and has good flow properties. Some patients may be unable to tolerate lactose and suitable inert alternative diluent include, light kaolin and starch.

Powder calculations

Quantities should be calculated to allow for loss of powder during manipulation. It is usual to allow for at least one extra powder. If the total amount of active ingredient required is less than the minimum weighable quantity, dilutions will be necessary. In this process, also called trituration, the minimum quantity of the active ingredient(s) is weighed and diluted, over several steps if necessary, in order to obtain the dose(s) required. Example 38.1 illustrates the process where two dilution steps are required (see also Ch. 19).

Folding papers

White glazed paper, called demy paper, is used for wrapping powders. A suitable size is 120 mm × 100 mm. The wrapping should be carried out on a clean tile or larger sheet of demy to protect the product. The papers should be folded with their long edges parallel to the front of the bench. Follow the steps illustrated in Figure 38.1 in order to fold the paper:

- The long edge, furthest away from the dispenser, should be turned over to about one-seventh of the paper width (step A)
- The powder should be weighed accurately and placed on the paper towards the folded edge of the centre of the paper (step B)
- The unfolded long edge (nearest the dispenser) should then be brought over the powder to meet the crease of the folded edge and the flap closed over it (step C)
- The folded edge should then be folded over (towards the dispenser) so that it covers about half the powder packet (step D)
- The short edges of the powder packet should be folded over, using a powder cradle if available, so that the flaps are of equal lengths and the folded powder fits neatly into a box or jar (steps E and F). Before making these folds, ensure that there is no powder in the ends to be folded, otherwise it may fall out and be lost.

The creases can be sharpened with a spatula, taking care not to tear the paper or use excessive pressure which would compress the powder inside the pack.

The powders can be packed in pairs, back to back, or in one bundle, with the final powder placed back to back. They should be held together with an elastic band. In a well-wrapped product, there will be no powder in the fold or flaps, so that all the powder is available for easy administration when unwrapped.

Manufactured powders are subject to a uniformity of weight test, or uniformity of content test if

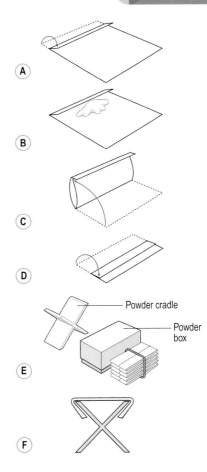

Figure 38.1 • Steps for the folding of individually wrapped powders.

each dose contains <2 mg of active ingredient or the content of active ingredient represents <2% of the total weight.

Shelf-life and storage of internal powders

Extemporaneously prepared powders should have an expiry of between 2 and 4 weeks. Proprietary powders often have a longer shelf-life because of the protective packaging. Some powders may be hygroscopic, deliquescent or volatile and will need to be protected from decomposition. Storage for these powders should be moisture proof and airtight.

Containers for internal powders

Extemporaneously prepared individually wrapped powders are often dispensed in a paperboard box. However, it is preferable to use a screw-top glass or plastic container which provides an airtight seal and protection against moisture. Proprietary powders in individual sachets which are moisture proof may be dispensed in a paperboard box. Bulk powders are packed in an airtight glass or plastic jar. A 5 mL spoon should also be supplied with bulk powders.

Special labels and advice for internal powders

Powders are usually mixed with water or another suitable liquid before taking, depending on their solubility. Powders for babies or young children can be placed directly into the mouth on the back of the tongue, followed by a drink to wash down the powder. Bulk powders should be shaken and measured carefully before dissolving or dispersing in a little water and taking.

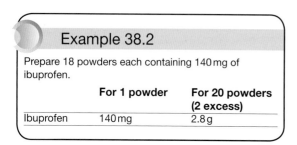

Example 38.2

Prepare 18 powders each containing 140 mg of ibuprofen.

	For 1 powder	For 20 powders (2 excess)
Ibuprofen	140 mg	2.8 g

Formulation notes. A diluent is not required, since the weight of each powder will be above the minimum 120 mg required. Pure ibuprofen powder can be used. However, if it is not available, manufactured 200 mg ibuprofen tablets (not modified release) can be used to prepare these powders.

Method of preparation. Take 14×200 mg ibuprofen tablets (contain 2.8 g ibuprofen) and weigh them. This is necessary to allow for the weight of the tablet excipients. Grind to a fine powder in a mortar and pestle. Pass the resulting powder through a 250 μm sieve and lightly remix. Divide the original weight of tablets by 20, and weigh aliquots of the resulting amount of powder. Pack into individual powder papers. Fasten the 18 powders together with an elastic band and pack in an amber glass jar or plastic container with a screw cap.

Shelf-life and storage. Store in a cool, dry place. A shelf-life of 2–3 weeks is appropriate.

Powders for external use

Powders, with or without medicament, are frequently applied to the skin. Dusting powders contain one or more substances in fine powder and may be dispensed as single-dose or multidose preparations (see Example 38.3). They are used to treat a variety of skin conditions or to soothe skin. Examples are antifungal powders for athlete's foot or talc dusting powder for the prevention of chafing and skin irritation. Zinc oxide and starch are added to formulations to absorb moisture and talc is used for lubricant properties. Talc, kaolin and other natural mineral materials are liable to contamination with bacteria such as *Clostridium tetani*, *C. perfringens* and *Bacillus anthracis*. These ingredients should be sterilized by dry heat or the final product should be sterilized. Dusting powders should be sterile if they are to be applied to large areas of open skin or wounds. They should not be used where there is a likelihood of large volumes of exudate, as hard crusts will form.

Preparing powders for external use

A sieve size of 180 μm should be used to obtain the finely divided powder. The constituents should be mixed using the doubling-up method, as described previously.

Shelf-life and storage for powders for external use

Dry powders should remain stable over a long period of time if packaged and protected from the atmosphere. For extemporaneously prepared products, an expiry of 4 weeks is appropriate.

Containers for powders for external use

Powders for external use may be packed in glass, metal or plastic containers with a sifter-type cap.

Some are also available commercially in pressurized containers, containing other excipients such as a propellant and lubricants.

Special labels and advice for powders for external use

'For external use only' and 'Store in a cool, dry place'.

Examples of official powders for external use include Zinc Oxide Dusting Powder Compound BPC, Chlorhexidine Dusting Powder BP and Talc Dusting Powder BP. There are now few proprietary examples of powders for external use one being Daktarin® (miconazole).

Example 38.3

Prepare 100 g of Zinc, Starch and Talc Dusting Powder BPC.

	Master formula	For 100 g
Zinc oxide	25%	25 g
Starch	25%	25 g
Sterilized purified talc	50%	50 g

Method of preparation. Sieve the powders, using a 180 μm sieve, weigh and mix them by doubling-up in a mortar and pestle. Pack in an amber glass jar or plastic container with a screw cap (with a perforated, reclosable lid if possible).

Shelf-life and storage. Store in a dry place. An expiry date of 4 weeks is advisable.

Example 38.4

Prepare 200 g of Compound Magnesium Trisilicate Oral Powder BP 1988.

	Master formula	For 200 g
Magnesium trisilicate	250 mg	50 g
Chalk	250 mg	50 g
Heavy magnesium carbonate	250 mg	50 g
Sodium bicarbonate	250 mg	50 g

Method of preparation. Sieve the powders, using a 250 μm sieve, weigh and mix them by doubling-up, using a mortar and pestle. Pack in an amber glass jar or plastic container with a screw cap.

Shelf-life and storage. Store in a dry place. A 4-week expiry date is reasonable if kept dry.

KEY POINTS

- Powders may be prepared as bulk powders, divided powders or granules
- Powders may be used internally or externally
- The particle size of a fine powder should be less than 180 μm
- The minimum weight of a divided powder is 120 mg
- Lactose is a good diluent for internal powders
- Trituration is the process used to obtain small doses which are below the minimum weighable quantity
- Ideally powders should be packed in a glass or plastic container
- A 5 mL spoon should be provided with bulk powders for oral use
- When dispensing divided powders, an excess of one or two should be prepared to allow for losses during processing

Oral unit dosage forms

Arthur J. Winfield

STUDY POINTS

- Different types of tablets
- Excipients used in tablets and capsules
- Dispensing commercially produced tablets and capsules
- Extemporaneous dispensing of capsules and cachets

Introduction

Tablets and capsules (oral unit dosage forms) are the most popular way of delivering a drug for oral use. They are convenient for the patient and are usually easy to handle and identify. They are produced by the pharmaceutical industry, where quality assurance ensures a high accuracy of dose within each individual dosage form. They are free from the problems of stability found in aqueous mixtures and suspensions. Packaging in blister packs can also enhance the stability of these dosage forms. The main disadvantages are that there is a slower onset of action relative to liquids and some people have difficulty swallowing solid oral dosage forms, e.g. the very young or very old.

Tablets

Tablets are solid preparations each containing a single dose of one or more active ingredient(s). They are normally prepared by compressing uniform volumes of particles, although some tablets are prepared by moulding.

Many different types of tablet are available, which may be in a variety of shapes and sizes. The types include dispersible, effervescent, chewable, sublingual and buccal tablets, lozenges, tablets for rectal or vaginal administration and solution tablets. Some tablets are designed to release the drug after a time lag, or slowly for a prolonged drug release or sustained drug action (see Ch. 29). The design of these modified-release tablets uses formulation techniques to control the biopharmaceutical behaviour of the drug. In addition to the drug(s), several excipients must be added. These will aid the process of tableting and ensure that the active ingredient will be released as intended. Excipients include:

- *Diluents*. These add bulk to make the tablet easier to handle. Examples include lactose, mannitol, sorbitol and calcium carbonate
- *Binders*. These enable granules to be prepared which improves the flow properties of the mixture during manufacture. Examples include polyvinylpyrrolidone and microcrystalline cellulose
- *Disintegrants*. These encourage the tablet to break into smaller particles after ingestion. Examples include modified cellulose and modified starch
- *Lubricants, glidants, antiadherents*. These are essential for the flow of the tablet material into the tablet dies and preventing sticking of the compressed tablet in the punch and die. Examples of lubricants are magnesium and calcium stearate, sodium lauryl sulphate and sodium stearyl fumarate. Colloidal silica is usually the glidant of choice. Talc and magnesium stearate are effective antiadherents
- *Miscellaneous agents* may be added, such as colours and flavours in chewable tablets.

Some tablets have coatings, such as sugar coating or film coating. Coatings can protect the tablet from environmental damage, mask an unpleasant taste, aid identification of the tablet and enhance its appearance. Enteric (gastro-resistant) coatings on tablets resist dissolution or disruption of the tablet in the stomach, but not in the intestine. This is useful when a drug is destroyed by gastric acid, is irritating to the gastric mucosa, or when bypassing the stomach, aids drug absorption.

Dispensing of tablets

Many tablets in the UK and other countries are packaged by the manufacturer into patient packs suitable for issue to the patient without repacking by the pharmacist. Patient information leaflets are also contained in these patient packs. When dispensing these packs to patients, the pharmacist must ensure that they are labelled correctly, according to the prescriber's instructions (see Ch. 31), and that the patient is counselled on the use of the medication (see Ch. 25).

For some controlled-release tablets, variations in bioavailability may occur with different brands. It is important that patients are given the brand that they are stabilized on in order to maintain therapeutic outcome. Examples where this is important include theophylline, lithium and phenytoin.

Tablets may also be supplied in a bulk container. The required number of tablets needs to be counted out (see Ch. 30) and placed in a suitable container for dispensing to the patient (see Ch. 32). It is important to minimize errors by ensuring that the correct bulk container has been selected and the correct drug dispensed. The pharmacist should verify this by checking the label of the bulk container and by examining the shape, size and markings on the dispensed tablets where appropriate, with the prescription. A copy of the patient information leaflet should be included.

Some tablets are supplied in a strip-packed form where each tablet has its own blister. A development of this is the calendar pack where the day or date on which the tablet is to be taken is indicated on the pack.

Shelf-life and storage of tablets

Most tablets should be stored in airtight packaging, protected from light and extremes of temperature.

When stored properly, they generally have a long shelf-life. The expiry date will be printed on the package or the individual strip packs. Some tablets need to be stored in a cool place, e.g. Ketovite® and Leukeran® (chlorambucil) (both stored between 2 and 8°C). Some tablets contain volatile drugs, e.g. glyceryl trinitrate, and must be packed in glass containers with tightly fitting metal screw caps (see Ch. 32).

Containers for tablets

Strip or blister packs are dispensed in a paperboard box and tablets counted from bulk containers are placed in amber glass or plastic containers with airtight, child-resistant closures.

Special labels and advice on tablets

Most tablets should be swallowed with a glass, or 'draught', of water. A draught of water refers to a volume of water of about 50 mL. This prevents the dosage from becoming lodged in the oesophagus, which can cause problems such as ulceration. Tablets may be coated and shaped to aid swallowing.

Some tablets should be dissolved or dispersed in water before taking, e.g. effervescent tablets. Other tablets, particularly those with coatings or modified-release properties, should be swallowed whole. There are also some tablets which should be chewed or sucked before swallowing. Appropriate labels should be placed on the container (see Ch. 31).

Coated tablets, e.g. enteric (gastro-resistant) coatings, require specific advice on avoiding indigestion remedies at the same time of day, as these will affect the pH of the stomach, and therefore cause premature breakdown of the enteric coating on the tablet.

Buccal and sublingual tablets are not swallowed whole because they will not have their intended therapeutic effect. Figure 39.1 illustrates the positioning for buccal tablets. Sublingual tablets are placed under the tongue.

Capsules

Capsules are solid preparations intended for oral administration made with a hard or soft gelatin shell. One (or more) medicament is enclosed within this gelatin container. Most capsules are swallowed

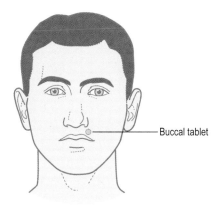

Figure 39.1 • Positioning of a buccal tablet.

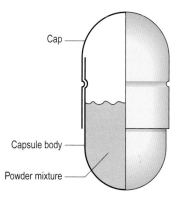

Figure 39.2 • Hard gelatin capsule shell: body and cap.

whole, but some contain granules which provide a useful premeasured dose for administering in a similar way to a powder, e.g. formulations of pancreatin. Some capsules enclose enteric-coated pellets, e.g. Erymax® (erythromycin). Capsules are elegant, easy to swallow and can be useful in masking unpleasant tastes. Capsules may also be used to hold oils for inhalation, e.g. Karvol® or for rectal and vaginal administration, e.g. Gyno-Daktarin® (miconazole nitrate) (see Ch. 37).

Soft shell capsules

A soft gelatin capsule consists of a flexible solid shell containing powders, non-aqueous liquids, solutions, emulsions, suspensions or pastes. Such capsules allow liquids to be given as solid dosage forms, e.g. cod-liver oil. They also offer accurate dosage, improved stability and overcome some of the problems of dealing with powders. They are formed, filled and sealed in one manufacturing process.

Hard shell capsules

Empty capsule shells are made from gelatin and are clear, colourless and essentially tasteless. Colourings and markings can be easily added for light protection and to ease identification. The shells are used in the preparation of most manufactured capsules and for the extemporaneous compounding of capsules. The shell comprises two sections, the body and the cap, both being cylindrical and sealed at one end. Powder or particulate solid, such as granules and pellets, can be placed in the body and the capsule closed by bringing the body and cap together (Fig. 39.2). Some capsules have small indentations on the body and cap which 'lock' together.

Compounding of capsules

Occasionally hand filling of capsules may be required, particularly in a hospital pharmacy or when preparing materials for clinical trials. A suitable size of capsule shell should be selected so that the finished capsule looks reasonably full. Hard shell capsules are available in eight sizes. These are listed in Table 39.1, with the corresponding approximate capacity (based on lactose). The bulk density of a powder mixture will also affect the choice of capsule size.

Calculations for compounding capsules

The recommended minimum weight for filling a capsule is 100 mg. If the required weight of the drug is smaller than this, a diluent should be added by trituration (see Ch. 38). If the quantity of the drug for a batch of capsules is smaller than the minimum weighable amount, 100 mg on a Class B balance, then trituration will also be required. Lactose and starch are commonly used diluents. To allow for small losses of powder, an excess should be calculated, e.g. two extra capsules (see Ch. 38).

Filling capsules

The number of capsules to be filled should be counted and set to one side. This avoids the danger of contaminating empty capsules. The powder to be encapsulated should be finely sifted (180 μm

Table 39.1 Sizes of hard gelatin capsules and their approximate capacities

Capsule no.	000	00	0	1	2	3	4	5
Content (mg)	950	650	450	300	250	200	150	100

sieve) and prepared. Magnesium stearate (up to 1% weight in weight (w/w)) and silica may be added as a lubricant and glidant respectively, to aid filling of the capsule. Various methods of filling capsules on a small scale are possible.

Filling from a powder mass

The prepared powder can be placed on a clean tile or piece of demy paper and powder pushed into the capsule body with the aid of a spatula until the required weight has been enclosed. The empty capsule body could also be 'punched' into a heap of powder until filled. Alternatively, create a small funnel from demy paper and fill the capsule body with the required weight. Gloves should be worn to protect the capsules from handling.

Filling with weighed aliquots

Weighed aliquots of powder may be placed on paper and channelled into the empty capsule shell. A sharp fold in the paper helps direct the powder. Alternatively, simple apparatus is available for small-scale manufacture of larger numbers of capsules. A plastic plate with rows of cavities to hold the empty capsule bodies is used, different rows holding different sizes of capsules. A plastic bridge containing a row of holes corresponding to the position of the capsule cavities can then be used to support a long-stemmed funnel. The end of the funnel passes into the mouth of the capsule below. The stem of the funnel should be as wide as possible for the size of the capsule to assist with powder flow. A weighed aliquot of powder can then be poured into the capsule via the funnel. A thin plastic rod or wire may be used to 'tamp' the powder to break blockages or to lightly compress the material inside the capsule. After filling the capsule, the cap can be fitted loosely and the weight checked before sealing.

Capsules are subject to tests for uniformity of weight and content of active ingredient, and uniformity of content where the content of active ingredient is <2 mg or <2% by weight of the total capsule fill.

Shelf-life and storage of capsules

If stability data are not available for extemporaneously filled capsules, then a short expiry date (up to 4 weeks) should be given. Manufactured capsules will be assigned expiry dates on the container and the packed strips or blister packs. Most capsules need to be stored in a cool, dry place.

Containers for capsules

The containers used for capsules are similar to those for tablets. Some capsules are susceptible to moisture absorption, and desiccants may be included in the packaging.

Special labels and advice on capsules

Capsules should be swallowed whole with a glass of water or other liquid. Advice may be sought from the pharmacist about whether it is acceptable to empty the contents of a capsule onto food or into water for ease of swallowing. In giving this advice, the release characteristics of the dosage form should be considered; for instance, whether it is an enteric-coated or prolonged-release formulation.

Other oral unit dosage forms

Pastilles

These contain a glycerol and gelatin base. They are sweetened, flavoured and medicated and are popular over-the-counter remedies for soothing coughs and sore throats.

Example 39.1

Prepare 8 capsules each containing haloperidol 10 mg and 1% w/w magnesium stearate.

	For 1 capsule	For 10 capsules
Haloperidol	10 mg	100 mg
Magnesium stearate	1 mg	10 mg
Lactose	89 mg	890 mg

Formulation notes. Magnesium stearate is added to act as a lubricant to aid flow of the powder into the capsule; 10 mg is not weighable, so a trituration must be carried out. Lactose acts as a diluent to bring the weight of each capsule fill to 100 mg.

Trituration for magnesium stearate:

Magnesium stearate   100 mg
Lactose   900 mg

Take a 100 mg portion of this mixture, which will contain 10 mg of magnesium stearate and 90 mg of lactose.

Method of preparation. Sieve the powders using a 180 µm sieve. Prepare the magnesium stearate triturate. Weigh 100 mg of haloperidol, and mix this with the magnesium stearate triturate in a mortar and pestle. Gradually add 800 mg of lactose to this mixture, by doubling-up. This gives a total powder quantity of 1000 mg (equivalent to 10 × 100 mg capsules). Fill the capsule shells (size 4 or 5) with 100 mg aliquots, checking the weight of each capsule before sealing. Pack eight capsules in an amber glass or plastic tablet container with a child-resistant closure.

Storage and shelf-life. Store in a cool, dry place and protect from light. Expiry date of 2 weeks, since stability in capsule form is unknown.

KEY POINTS

- Tablets and capsules are the most common dosage forms
- Excipients are added to improve manufacture, handling and release of the drug
- Tablets and capsules should be swallowed normally with about 50 mL of water
- Some tablets are designed to be chewed, dissolved, swallowed whole or delivered by the buccal or sublingual route
- Tablets cannot be made extemporaneously, but capsules are filled when preparing for clinical trials
- Capsule size is selected so that they look reasonably full
- The minimum weight of contents in an extemporaneous capsule is 100 mg
- Medicated glycerol-gelatin-based pastilles are popular for coughs and sore throats

Section 6

Specialized pharmacy products and services

Production of sterile products

Derek G. Chapman

STUDY POINTS

- The requirements for sterile production
- Grades of clean areas
- Design and operation of clean areas
- Isolators
- Environmental monitoring
- Preparation of aseptic products

Introduction

The production of sterile medicinal products has special requirements. These products must be produced in conditions that ensure that they are pure. They must also be free from viable organisms and pyrogens with limited, or ideally no, particulate contamination. It is thus important that only carefully regulated and tested procedures are used to manufacture sterile products.

Owing to their special manufacturing requirements, sterile medicines are prepared in special facilities known as clean rooms. These rooms are designed to reduce the risk of microbial and particulate contamination at all stages of the manufacturing process.

The clean area used to produce sterile products is commonly designed as a suite of clean rooms. With this system, the operators enter the clean rooms by way of a changing room. Within this area, the operators put on clean room clothing before entering into the clean rooms. The changing room has a lower standard of environmental quality. A clean room with a lower environmental standard is also used to prepare solutions. These solutions are then sterilized by filtration before being transferred into the filling room. The clean room used to fill and seal the product containers is the highest quality of clean room. This will reduce the risk of product contamination.

Sterile products that are marketed in the European Union must be produced in conditions which conform with the conditions given in the revised Annex 1 of Good Manufacturing Practices (Volume IV) of *The Rules Governing Medicinal Products in the European Union*. This guidance on the procedures for manufacturing sterile products describes the cleanliness of the clean room environment and recommends how pharmaceutical clean rooms should be built and used.

Sterile product production

Production of sterile products should be carried out in a clean environment with a limit for the environmental quality of particulate and microbial contamination. This limit for contamination is necessary to reduce the risk of product contamination. In addition, however, the temperature, humidity and air pressure of the environment should be regulated to suit the clean room processes and the comfort of the operators.

Clean areas for the production of sterile products are classified into grades A, B, C and D. These grades are categorized by the particulate quality of the environmental air when the clean area is operating in both a 'manned' and 'unmanned' state. In

Table 40.1 Air-borne particle contamination for manned and unmanned clean rooms

Grade	Maximum number of particles per cubic metre equal to or above the size indicated			
	Clean room at rest		Clean room operating	
	0.5 μm	5 μm	0.5 μm	5 μm
A	3500	1	3500	1
B	3500	1	350 000	2000
C	350 000	2000	3 500 000	20 000
D	3 500 000	20 000	Varies with procedure	Varies with procedure

Table 40.2 Limits for microbial contamination of an operating clean room

Grade	Viable organisms per cubic metre of air	90 mm settle plate per 4 h	55 mm contact plate	Glove print (5 fingers)
A	<1	<1	<1	<1
B	10	5	5	5
C	100	50	25	N/A
D	200	100	50	N/A

addition, these areas are graded by the microbial monitoring of the environmental air, surfaces and operators when the area is functioning. The standards are shown in Tables 40.1 and 40.2.

There are two common procedures used to manufacture sterile products. The first method involves the preparation of products that will be terminally sterilized. The second method involves the aseptic filling of containers that are not exposed to terminal sterilization. Aseptic filling requires a higher environmental quality for the preparation of solutions and the filling of containers. The qualities of the clean rooms used for these production procedures are detailed in Tables 40.3 and 40.4.

Table 40.3 Conditions for preparing terminally sterilized products

Procedure	Required standard before terminal sterilization
Preparation of solutions for filtration and sterilization	Grade C is used for products which support microbial growth
	Grade D acceptable if solutions subsequently filtered
Filling small and large volume parenterals	Grade C. For products with a high risk of contamination such as wide-necked containers, a Grade A laminar airflow workstation with Grade C background
Preparation and filling of ointments, creams, suspensions and emulsions	Grade C

Table 40.4 Conditions for the production of aseptically prepared products

Procedure	Required standard
Handling of sterile starting materials	Grade A with Grade B background or Grade C if solution filtered later in production process
Preparation of production solutions	Grade A with Grade B background or Grade C if sterile during filtered production
Filling of aseptically prepared products such as small and large volume parenterals	Grade A with Grade B background
Preparation and filling of ointments, creams, suspensions and emulsions	Grade A with Grade B background

Premises

The sterile production unit must be separated from the general manufacturing area within the hospital pharmacy or factory. This sterile production unit must not be accessible to unauthorized personnel.

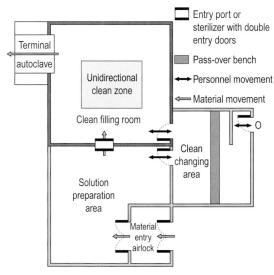

Figure 40.1 • Rooms for the production of terminally sterilized medicines.

The unit is designed to allow each stage of production to be segregated. It should also ensure a safe and organized workflow and reduce the need for personnel to move around the clean rooms. The unit is built and the equipment positioned to protect the product from contamination. The layout must allow efficient cleaning of the area and avoid the build up of dust. Premises are also arranged to decrease the risk of mix up or contamination of one product or material by another.

The filling room is typically serviced from an adjacent preparation room. This allows supporting personnel to assemble and prepare materials. Staff within the filling room area then use these materials. Figure 40.1 shows the layout of rooms for the production of terminally sterilized medicines such as small or large volume injections.

Design and construction

Access to clean and aseptic filling areas is limited to authorized personnel. Operators enter clean rooms by way of changing rooms. Within the changing room the operators can don and remove their clean room garments.

A low physical barrier, commonly known as a pass-over (or cross-over) bench, extends across the changing room. It forms a physical barrier that separates the different areas for changing by the operators.

Special precautions are needed to avoid contamination of clean and aseptic filling areas when materials are passed through airlocks or hatchways. Thus, sterilizers and entry ports are fitted with double-sided doors. The doors are interlocked to prevent both doors being opened simultaneously.

Surfacing materials

All clean room surfaces, including the floors, walls and ceilings, should be smooth, impervious and unbroken. This will decrease the release and build-up of contaminating particles and organisms. The surfaces are made of materials that allow the use of cleaning agents and disinfectants. The ceilings are sealed to prevent the entry of contaminants from the space above them. Uncleanable recesses within the clean room should be avoided. This will reduce the collection of contaminating particles. Thus, the junction between the wall and the floor is commonly coved. The presence of shelves, ledges, cupboards and equipment is minimized. Windows should be non-opening and sealed. This will prevent the ingress of contaminants.

Services

Piped liquids and gases should be filtered before entering the clean room. This will ensure that the liquid or gas at the work position will be as clean as the clean room air. The pipes and ducts must be positioned for easy cleaning. All other fittings such as fuse boxes and switch panels should be positioned outside the clean rooms.

Sinks and drains must be excluded from areas where aseptic procedures are performed in clean room areas. They should be avoided in the whole unit wherever possible. In areas where sinks and drains are installed they must be designed, positioned and maintained to decrease the risk of microbial contamination. They are thus often fitted with easily cleanable traps. The traps may contain electrically heated devices for disinfection.

There should be a limited number of entry doors for personnel and ports for materials. Entry doors should be self-closing and allow the easy movement of personnel.

Airlock doors, wall ports, through-the-wall autoclaves and dry heat sterilizers should be fitted with interlocked doors. This will prevent both doors being opened simultaneously. An alarm system should be fitted to all the doors to prevent the opening of more than one door.

Lights in clean rooms are fitted flush with the ceiling to reduce the collection of dust and avoid disturbing the airflow pattern within the room. Similarly, equipment should be positioned in clean rooms to avoid the distribution and the collection of particles and microbial contaminants.

Environmental control

Potential sources of particles and microbial contaminants occurring within the clean room are:

- The air supply of the room
- Inflow of external air
- Production of contaminants within the room.

Each of these possible sources can be minimized as described below.

Air supply

The air supply to a Grade A, B or C clean room must be filtered to ensure the removal of particulate and microbial contamination. This is carried out by filtering the air with high-efficiency particulate air (HEPA) filters. The HEPA filter should be positioned at the inlet to the clean room or close to it. A prefilter may be fitted upstream of the HEPA filter. This will prolong the life of the final filter. A fan is required to pump the air through the filter.

The HEPA filters use pleated fibreglass paper as the filter medium. Parallel pleats of this filter material increase the surface area of the filter and increase the airflow through the filter. This structure allows the filter to retain a compact volume. Aluminium foil is used to form spacers in the traditional type of HEPA filter. Spacers are not used in the more modern 'mini-pleat' type of filter design. These mini-pleat filters are now widely used. They have a shallower depth in construction than the traditional HEPA filter. Within the structure of the filter, the filter material is sealed to an aluminium frame (Fig. 40.2). At least one side of the filter is protected with a coated mild steel mesh. HEPA filters exhibit:

- A high flow rate
- High particulate holding capacity
- Low-pressure drop across the filter.

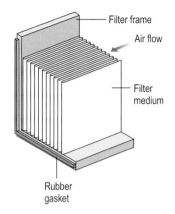

Figure 40.2 • Section through a mini-pleat high-efficiency filter, showing its construction.

HEPA filters remove larger particles from the air by inertial impaction, the medium-sized particles by direct interception and the small particles by Brownian diffusion. The HEPA filters are least efficient at removing particles of about 0.3 μm. However, the efficiency of removing particles is affected by the air velocity and the filter packing. Larger and smaller particles will be removed more efficiently.

With a new HEPA filter fitted in a clean room, the air exits from the filter face at a rate of about 0.45 m/s and has a 99.997% efficiency at removing 0.3 μm particles. The pressure difference across the depth of a new filter is about 130 Pascal (Pa). At the end of the effective life of the filter the pressure drop across the filter will increase to about 490 Pa. To retain the operating efficiency of the filter, the fan forcing air through the filter must be able to maintain this pressure difference. Sensors are fitted upstream and downstream of the filters to indicate the pressure differential across the filter. An automatic alarm system should be fitted to indicate failure in the air supply or filter blockage.

The HEPA filters for clean room use must conform with the British Standard 5295 (1989) aerosol test. The filters may have faulty seals and can be damaged during delivery or installation. It is thus important that they are tested in situ before use.

The filter material possesses a uniform resistance and is constructed with a large number of parallel pleats. This results in the air downstream of the filter face flowing uniformly with a unidirectional configuration.

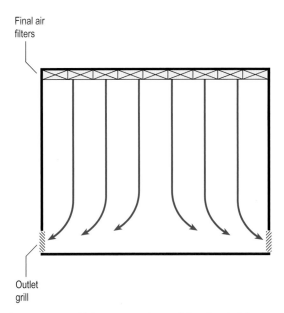

Figure 40.3 • Airflow pattern in a unidirectional airflow clean room.

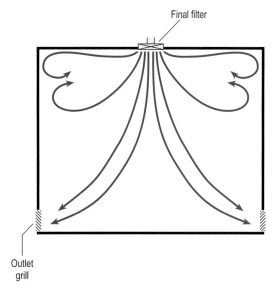

Figure 40.4 • Airflow pattern in a non-unidirectional airflow clean room.

The number of air changes in clean rooms is affected by:

- The room size
- The equipment in use
- The number of operators in the area.

In practice 25–35 air changes per hour are common. The airflow pattern within the clean room must be carefully regulated to avoid generating particles from the clean room floor and from the operators. Various options for ventilating clean rooms may be categorized by the airflow pattern within the room. These are:

- Unidirectional airflow systems
- Non-unidirectional airflow systems
- Combination airflow systems.

Unidirectional airflow systems

Air enters the room through a complete wall or ceiling of high-efficiency filters. This air will sweep contamination in a single direction to the exhaust system on the opposing wall or floor (Fig. 40.3). In the interests of economy, the exhaust grill may be fitted low down on the wall. The velocity of the air is about 0.3 m/s in downflow air from ceiling filters and 0.45 m/s in crossflow air. These are highly efficient airflow systems. However, one major

disadvantage of these rooms for pharmaceutical use is that they are expensive to construct. They also use much more conditioned air than rooms with non-unidirectional airflow. This greatly increases their operating costs. Owing to these factors, unidirectional airflow clean rooms are seldom used for pharmaceutical purposes.

Non-unidirectional airflow systems

Air enters the clean rooms through filters and diffusers that are usually located in the ceiling. It exits through outlet ducts positioned low down on the wall or in the floor at sites remote from the air inlet (Fig. 40.4). With the use of this system, the filtered inlet air mixes with and dilutes the contaminated air within the room. As the clean room air has been previously heated and cleaned, it can be recirculated to save energy, a little fresh air being introduced with each air change cycle.

Various designs of diffuser are used with this ventilation system. These affect the air movement and the cleanliness of the rooms. The perforated plate diffuser produces a jet flow of air directly beneath it. This jet of air will carry contamination at its edges. However, it does produce high-quality air directly under the diffuser. It is thus important that production procedures are located directly below the diffuser. By contrast, the air released from the bladed diffuser will mix with the clean

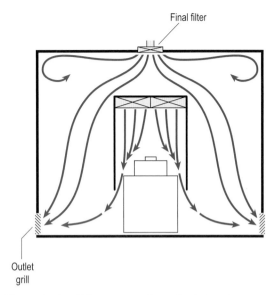

Figure 40.5 • Airflow patterns in a mixed-flow clean room with non-unidirectional airflow background environment and unidirectional airflow protection for a critical area.

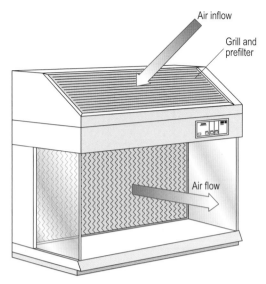

Figure 40.6 • Horizontal laminar airflow unit. (Courtesy of John Bass Ltd.)

room air. This diffuser thus produces a reasonably constant quality of air throughout the room.

Combination systems

In many pharmaceutical clean rooms, it is common to find that the background area is ventilated by a non-unidirectional airflow system. Meanwhile, the critical areas are supplied with high-quality air from unidirectional airflow units.

The combination airflow system is often selected for pharmaceutical clean room applications as it:

• Produces controlled room pressure
• Separates the manufacturing process from the general clean room
• Is cheaper to use.

Several types of unidirectional flow workstations or benches are used in this combination-type room. Various vertical unidirectional airflow systems are used in combination clean rooms. With one system, the critical area is surrounded by a plastic curtain with vertical unidirectional downflow air 'washing' over the manufacturing process and exiting under the plastic curtains into the general clean room area (Fig. 40.5). An alternative system is often used with the small-scale combination-type clean room in hospital pharmacies. With this system,

a horizontal airflow cabinet (Fig. 40.6) is used as the workstation. With these cabinets, a fan forces air through a HEPA filter located at the rear wall of the workstation. The air that exits from the filter first washes over the critical work area before washing over the arms and upper body areas of the operator. Contamination arising from the operator is thus kept downstream of the critical procedures. Grade A environmental conditions are achieved at the critical work area. A similar workstation known as a vertical laminar airflow cabinet (Fig. 40.7) could also be used in the combination room. This cabinet passes air vertically downwards from the ceiling of the cabinet over the critical working area. It produces a Grade A environmental quality. The air exits from the front of the workstation.

In recent times, there has been a trend towards protecting the critical procedures within combination clean rooms by using isolator cabinets. The isolator cabinet gives a localized high-quality environment. Isolators give protection from potential contamination in clean rooms as they are positively pressurized with air supplied through HEPA filters. The operator works outside the confines of the isolator using glove ports to perform procedures within the enclosed chamber. The gloved hands of clean room operators can transfer microbial contamination into critical working areas within the clean room. To indicate that the required clean room standards have been achieved (Table 40.2),

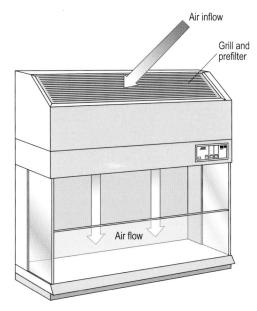

Figure 40.7 • Vertical laminar airflow unit. (Courtesy of John Bass Ltd.)

the fingertips of a gloved hand are depressed onto the surface of a suitable solid growth medium. This medium is incubated to show any contamination.

There is also a need to avoid contaminated external air passing into the clean room environment. Thus, the clean room air pressure must exceed that of the surrounding areas. The pressure differential between different standards of clean room should be 10–15 Pa. This level should be comparatively easy to monitor and will decrease the unregulated outflow of air. Adjusting grills known as pressure stabilizers located in the walls of rooms regulate the outflow of clean room air and the room pressure. The air moves from an area of high pressure to an area of lower pressure. To maintain the room pressure, it is important that the rooms are airtight. However, a small quantity of air will exit from the rooms by way of door spaces.

Temperature and humidity control

The temperature and the humidity are adjusted to suit the procedures being carried out within the clean room and maintain the comfort of the operators. A target temperature of about 20°C with a relative humidity of about 35–45% is usually preferred.

Personnel

The clean room environment is supplied with high-quality air at positive pressure. The main source of contamination in these areas arises from skin scales that are released by the clean room operators.

To limit clean room contamination by personnel, there is a need to:

- Restrict the number of operators working in the clean room
- Restrict operator conversations
- Instruct operators to move slowly
- Minimize general movement throughout the room
- Avoid operators interrupting the airflow between the inlet filter and the work area.

The clean room operator is constantly shedding dead skin scales from the body surface. Not all of these skin particles are contaminated with bacteria. Males shed more particles that are contaminated with bacteria than females. In addition, individual males and females show variable rates of bacterial dispersal. This dispersal from the individual is affected by:

- Personal characteristics
- General health and skin condition.

Body movements of personnel will increase the number of contaminated particles released from the skin surface. Each individual releases more than 10^6 skin scales/min during normal walking movements. There is a need to contain the dispersion of skin particles from the operators in clean rooms and protect both the environment and the product. Containment of particles is achieved by the operators wearing clean room clothing. This clothing is made from synthetic fabrics that filter out particulate and microbial contamination from the operators without the fabrics releasing contamination. However, this clothing is not absolute and particles can pass through the garments. Operators wearing clean room undergarments reduce this effect. The outer garments are close fitting at the neck, wrists and ankles, but these sites still provide an exit route for particulate matter.

Clean garments should be used for each work session and must provide operator comfort. Disposable single-use garments are available, although most production units employ reusable garments. The clothing is specially laundered in an area with similar standards to those used in the clean room. Garments are laundered by a wet-wash process using particle-free solutions. This is followed by an antibacterial rinse and hot air drying and then the garments are packaged in sealed bags to avoid particulate contamination. This cleaning process fulfils the needs of most pharmaceutical clean room applications, which are a balance between cost and acceptability. For a higher level of sterility assurance the garments are gamma irradiated using ^{60}Co, each garment receiving an approved dose of 25 kGy. This treatment is expensive and decreases the life of the garments. The donning of clean room clothing without contaminating the outer surface of the garments is a rather difficult procedure that is performed in the changing room.

Table 40.5 Clothing for clean room use

Clean room grade	Description of clothing
A/B	Head cover and face mask
	Single- or two-piece trouser suit
	Overboots and sterile powder-free rubber or plastic gloves
C	Hair (and beard) cover
	Single- or two-piece trouser suit
	Clean room shoes or overshoes
D	Hair (and beard) cover
	Protective suit
	Appropriate shoes or overshoes

Changing room

Entry of personnel into clean rooms should be through a changing room fitted with interlocking doors. These doors act as an airlock to prevent the influx of external air. This access route is intended for the entry of personnel only. The changing room is subdivided into three areas. Movement through these areas must comply with a strict protocol. They are often colour coded as black, grey and white, black representing the dirtiest area while white represents the cleanest area.

The black area is where jewellery, cosmetics, factory or hospital protective garments and shoes are removed. Long hair may be contained and a mobcap donned to contain the hair completely. The pass-over bench forms a physical separation between the black and the grey areas in the changing room. The operator sits on the pass-over bench, swings his/her legs over the bench and fits clean room covers over the feet before they are placed on the floor of the grey area.

The operator then stands up in the grey area. Wrappings on the various garments are opened to avoid contacting the outer surface of the packaging following the hand-washing procedure. Then the operator washes hands and forearms using an antiseptic solution. Special attention is paid to cleaning the fingernails. The hands are then dried using an automatic air-blow drier as towels shed particles when used for drying hands.

Clothing garments are donned in sequence from head to foot. Throughout this procedure, care must be taken to avoid the hands contacting the outer surface of the clean room clothing. First, the head and shoulder hood is fitted, ensuring that all the hair is contained within the head cover. A face mask is fitted to prevent the shedding of droplets. The one-piece coverall (or alternatively two-piece trouser suit) is put on. Care must be taken to avoid these garments contacting the floor surface. The shoulder cover of the head and shoulder hood is tucked into the coverall. Then the zip is closed and the studs fastened. Overboots are then fitted over the clean room shoes. The overboots are kept in position with ties that are suitably fastened for operator comfort. For entry into aseptic filling rooms an antiseptic cream is applied to the hands. The clean room powder-free gloves are then donned. Care is needed to avoid contacting the outer surface of the gloves. The cuffs of the coverall are secured within the gloves and the gloved hands disinfected. The operator now enters into the white clean room area and begins work. During the work procedures, the gloved hands of the operators are regularly disinfected. Key features of the clothing are given in Table 40.5.

Cleaning

A strict cleaning and disinfection policy is essential to minimize particulate and microbial contamination in the clean room. Operators release microbial and particulate contamination within the clean room. These contaminants are mostly deposited onto horizontal surfaces. However, other areas of the clean room can become contaminated due to direct contact with the operators' clothing. It is thus essential that a strict cleaning and disinfection policy is implemented within the clean room to minimize both the particulate and the microbial contamination.

There are two main methods of cleaning. Vacuuming is effective at removing gross particulate contamination of particles greater than 100 μm. However, vacuuming is not very effective at removing smaller particles. Small particles are removed by wet wiping. It is important that the wet wipe is sterile and must not generate particulate contamination. The use of wet wipes involves the use of cleaning agents that will remove particulate contamination and have an antibacterial effect.

The ideal cleaning agent should be:

- Effective in removing undesirable contamination
- Harmless to surfaces
- Fast drying
- Non-flammable
- Non-toxic
- Cost-effective.

Anionic or cationic surfactants are used as cleaning agents within the clean room. The disinfectants of choice for clean room use are generally quaternary ammonium compounds, phenols, alcohols and polymeric biguanides. The disinfectant solutions should be freshly prepared before use. Different types of disinfectants should be used in rotation to prevent the development of resistant microbial strains. Most surfactants or detergents will dissipate surface static electricity but the most effective and widely used antistatic agents used in clean rooms are cationic surfactants.

Trained personnel regularly clean critical production areas of clean rooms. A less stringent cleaning protocol is required in the general clean room areas. This applies to the walls and floors where contamination cannot directly contaminate the product. As part of the cleaning protocol, regular microbiological monitoring should be carried out to determine the effectiveness of the disinfection procedures.

Isolators

Commercial manufacturers are using isolators increasingly for the aseptic filling of products, with combination isolators being used. Isolators are also used for sterility testing of products. Robots have

Table 40.6 Microbial contamination of batch-produced sterile products

Place of production	Microbial contamination
Industrial production	
Terminal sterilization by dry or moist heat or irradiation	1 in at least 10^6 containers
Aseptic preparation in sealed gassed isolator using sophisticated transfer system	1 in 10^6
Aseptic preparation in conventional clean room using sophisticated laminar airflow system	1 in 10^5
Aseptic preparation in conventional clean room	1 in 10^4
Aseptic complex preparation of large-volume total parenteral nutrition fluids	1 in 10^3
Production in hospital pharmacy	
Terminal sterilization by dry or moist heat containers	1 in at least 10^6
Aseptic preparation in an isolator with surfaces cleaned and wiped with sterile alcohol. Extensively used in many pharmacies	1 in 10^3
Aseptic preparation in a well-managed clean room	1 in 10^3 (or less)

been used in isolators for repetitive processes such as sterility testing but they are expensive. Isolators are used in hospital pharmacy departments as an alternative to clean rooms for the small-scale aseptic processing of sterile products. Aseptic procedures performed in the best isolators cannot reach the same levels of sterility assurance achieved by terminal heat sterilization (see Table 40.6). However, when suitably operated they can produce a sterility assurance level better than the conventional clean room. Isolators are often selected for aseptic manipulations of sterile products as they are:

- Relatively inexpensive
- Easily designed for a specific purpose
- Capable of providing operator protection from the product.

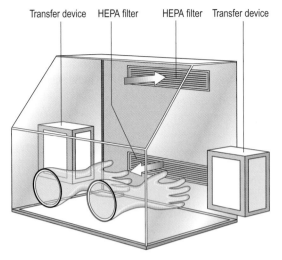

Transfer device   HEPA filter   HEPA filter   Transfer device

Figure 40.8 • Isolator cabinet.

Isolators are composed of a chamber that controls the environment surrounding the work procedure (Fig. 40.8). The inlet and exhaust air passes through HEPA filters. The airflow pattern within the isolator chamber may be either unidirectional, non-unidirectional or a combination of both. Vertical unidirectional airflow has the advantage of rapidly purging particles from the isolator chamber. This is an advantage for aseptic processes. The air within the isolator chamber should be frequently changed to maintain the aseptic chamber environment. Particle and microbial contamination of the environment within the isolator chamber must conform with the Grade A standard as detailed in Tables 40.1 and 40.2.

The operator remains outside the isolator chamber environment. To perform manual manipulations within the chamber, the operator inserts his hands and arms into the chamber. Entry occurs by way of a glove port using either a one-piece full-arm-length glove or a glove and sleeve system. With the glove and sleeve system, the easily changeable glove is attached to a sleeve that is attached to the wall of the chamber through an airtight seal. Using either of these glove systems, the operator is able to perform aseptic manipulations in comfort up to a distance of about 0.5 m within the chamber. The glove system avoids contamination arising from the operator and maintains the integrity of the isolator chamber environment. As cytotoxic materials can diffuse through the gloves it is important that they are changed regularly. To

perform the work procedure within the chamber, materials must be introduced and prepared products removed without compromising the chamber environment. This transfer procedure is a critical factor in the operation of the isolator and is carried out using a transfer system. The transfer system separates the external environment from the controlled isolator environment. It restricts airflow between these areas while allowing the transfer of materials between them. The transfer system is fitted with an interlocked double door entry system. This will provide an airlock that avoids both doors being opened to the external environment simultaneously. A filtered air inlet and exhaust is fitted to the transfer system. However, a risk of microbial contamination during the transfer does exist. The isolator must be positioned in a suitable background environment of at least a Grade D classification. This is typically achieved by positioning the isolator in a dedicated room that is only used for the isolator and its related activities.

Isolators are divided into positive and negative pressure isolators.

Positive pressure isolator

This isolator operates under positive pressure and protects the product from contamination arising from an external source and from the aseptic process itself. It is used for the aseptic preparation of pharmaceutical products and can be used as a sterility test chamber.

Negative pressure isolator

This isolator will protect the product from contamination arising from an external source and from the aseptic manipulation. In addition, however, this isolator should protect the operator from hazardous materials such as cytotoxic preparations or radiopharmaceuticals in the isolator chamber. This type of isolator operates under negative pressure. The exhaust air is ducted to the outside through at least one HEPA filter and through an adsorption material such as activated carbon. Rigid negative pressure isolators should be used for radiopharmaceutical manipulations. In this situation, the isolator is frequently used with a lead-free vision panel and a lead glass protector around the product. Alternatively, isolators are available with lead acrylic glass windows.

The chambers of isolators are gas sterilized. The ideal sterilant for use in the isolator chamber should have the following properties:

- Non-corrosive to metals and plastics
- Rapidly lethal to all microorganisms
- Good penetration
- Harmless.

The sterilants in most general use for pharmaceutical applications in isolators do not comply with all of these ideal properties. Those used are peracetic acid vapour and hydrogen peroxide vapour. To reduce the risk of chemical contamination of the sterile product, the sterilant contact time should be carefully regulated. The sterilant must be flushed from the isolator before beginning the aseptic manipulations.

Currently marketed isolators are constructed with either a flexible canopy or a rigid containment medium. The rigid type of isolator is often preferred, owing to the reduced risk of the chamber being punctured. This occurs more readily with the flexible canopy design. Rigid isolators are often constructed from a stainless steel frame with a moulded acrylic window. A further isolator known as a half-suit isolator is currently in use. This is a flexible canopy isolator that is made from material such as nylon-lined polyvinyl chloride. It is designed using a half-suit sealed to a wall of the chamber. This system allows the torso of the operator to be introduced into the suit that is located within the chamber of the isolator. To improve visibility, a transparent helmet is sealed to the neck of the suit that is ventilated by a pressurized air supply. This provides operator comfort over prolonged work sessions. The advantage of the half-suit isolator is that the operator can easily access a large area of the chamber and manoeuvre heavier and larger materials. The half-suit isolator is used as dedicated production equipment for the aseptic compounding of products such as total parenteral nutrition (TPN) fluids.

During a 2-week period in September 1992, eight children died from infection after receiving contaminated TPN fluids at four different hospitals in South Africa. These fluids had been prepared in flexible film isolators. The investigation of this incident revealed that the production equipment was suitable for its purpose but inadequate procedures had allowed contamination and subsequent growth of pathogenic bacteria in the TPN fluids. It should therefore be carefully noted that the use of isolators requires trained staff and good manufacturing practices to maintain product quality.

Isolator tests

Isolators must be frequently tested to ensure that they operate as a sealed chamber and conform with the required level of air quality and surface contamination. They are thus subjected to both physical and microbial tests.

Physical tests include:

- *Integrity tests*. These tests will detect leaks that compromise the integrity of the isolator chamber. The procedure is routinely carried out by sealing the chamber and recording changes in the chamber pressure over time
- *Glove inspection*. The glove and sleeve are visually inspected and leak tested for pin holes
- *HEPA filter test*. The integrity of the HEPA filter should be tested with an aerosol generator and a detector
- *Air-borne particle count*. This is carried out in the isolator chamber and the transfer device using a particle counter.

Microbial tests use microbial growth media suitable for the growth of potential contaminants. The tests include:

- *Active air sampling*. This test determines the number of organisms in the air of the isolator chamber. The procedure uses impact and agar impingement samplers
- *Settle plates*. Settle plates containing growth media are exposed in the chamber for 2–4 h. Particles and organisms settle by gravity onto the agar surface. The plates are then incubated
- *Surface tests*. Surfaces are sampled using direct contact plates that are then incubated. Following sampling, it is important to remove materials deposited onto the sampled surfaces during the test. Alternatively, surfaces are sampled using sterile moistened swabs. The swabs are then streaked onto solid growth media and incubated. Soluble swabs may be dissolved in sterile diluent and the viable count determined
- *Finger dabs*. The fingertips of the gloved hand are pressed onto the surface of solid growth medium. The medium is then incubated

- *Broth fill test*. This test challenges both the manipulative procedure of the operator and the facilities. The test simulates routine aseptic procedures by using nutrient medium in place of a product to produce broth-filled units. These units are incubated to indicate microbial contamination.

Environmental monitoring

Following construction of a clean room, it must be tested to ensure that it is providing the required quality of environment. These verification tests are rigorously performed and are similar to the tests that are used to monitor the clean room. The monitoring tests ensure that the clean room continues to provide satisfactory operation.

To ensure that the pharmaceutical clean room is providing the required environmental standards, the following are determined.

Air quality

The air supplied to the clean room must not contribute to particulate or microbial contamination within the room. The HEPA filters for the inlet air must be tested to ensure that neither the filter fabric nor the filter seals are leaking. This is done by introducing a smoke with a known particle size upstream of the filter. The clean room surface of the filter is then scanned for smoke penetration using a photometer or a particle counter.

Air movement

Adequate ventilation throughout the clean room can be determined by air movement tests. These are carried out at the time of clean room validation. Air movement within the clean room is determined by measuring the decay profile of smoke particles released into the clean room. Smoke particle release is also used to ensure that a clean area within a unidirectional workstation is not being contaminated with air from the clean room environment.

The outflow of air from a clean room with a higher standard of cleanliness to an area with a lower standard is indicated by the pressure differential between the rooms. This is determined using a manometer or magnehelic gauge.

Air velocity

The velocity of the air at several points in a clean room area of critical importance should be determined. This is done both at validation of the clean room and at timed intervals. The procedure involves the use of an anemometer.

Air-borne particulate and microbial contamination

The particle count and the microbial bioburden of the clean room provide the basis for the air classification system for grading a clean room, as detailed in Table 40.1. The points for sampling and the number of samples taken at each position are determined by the size and the grade of the clean room. Air-borne particles are normally sized and counted by optical particle counters.

Microbial monitoring

There should be very few viable organisms present in the clean room air. However, operators within the clean room disperse large numbers of skin particles. Many of these particles are contaminated with bacteria. The dispersal of contaminated particles by the clean room operator is greatly decreased by the wearing of occlusive clothing together with appropriate air ventilation. Sampling for microbial contamination is necessary when people are present in the clean room during production. Monitoring of the microbial contamination during production will ensure that both the use of clean room clothing by the operators and the air ventilation system are producing the required environmental standards. Air sampling is carried out by volumetric sampling or by the use of settle plates. With volumetric sampling, a measured volume of air is drawn from the environment and contaminants are impinged onto a suitable microbial growth medium. The medium is then incubated and the colonies of microbial growth counted. Settle plates rely on bacteria-carrying particles being deposited onto the exposed solid surface of sterile microbial growth media contained in a 90 or 140 mm diameter Petri dish. When positioning the plates, care is needed to avoid accidental contamination. Owing to the small number of microbial contaminants in the clean room, the settle plates are preferably exposed for about 4 h.

The surfaces of the clean room should also be tested for microbial contamination, notably in areas that may be contacted by the clothing of the operators. This is achieved by using contact plates or by using sterile moistened swabs. The contact plates allow a sterile agar surface to be pressed onto the clean room surface. These plates are then incubated to reveal microbial growth. Swabbing procedures are carried out as previously detailed in isolator tests.

Aseptic preparation

Parenteral products such as injections, infusions and eye products must be sterile for administration to the patient (see Chs 41 and 42). The preferred method of manufacturing parenteral medicines is to place the product in its final container and then seal this package. The product is then protected from further contamination and is terminally sterilized. At worst, this achieves the risk of one product in a million being contaminated following terminal sterilization by dry or moist heat or by irradiation. Some products cannot withstand this sterilization process. An alternative approach known as aseptic preparation must then be used to prepare these medicines. This procedure is carried out in industry with selected products but is extensively used in hospital pharmacy where products are specially compounded to meet the specific needs of patients (see Chs 44 and 46).

As shown in Table 40.6, aseptic preparation of parenteral products provides the lowest level of assurance of sterility of all the methods currently used to produce these formulations. In the pharmaceutical industry, pre-sterilized medicines are aseptically filled into sterile containers. The filling process must avoid recontamination of the sterile medicine and its container during this process. A sterility assurance level of 10^{-6} is achieved, but to achieve this requires highly sophisticated industrial production procedures. In hospital pharmacy, pre-sterilized product components are aseptically compounded using sterile apparatus and then aseptically added to appropriate packaging for subsequent patient administration. It is critical that the sterile product components and the packaging are not recontaminated with organisms or particulate matter during these aseptic procedures. In order to achieve this, the sterile product components and the sterile package must be manipulated in a high-quality environment.

The aseptic preparation and filling of products is performed in a localized Grade A zone that is achieved by a laminar airflow cabinet with a Grade B background. The Grade A environment within an isolator cabinet is also suitable for the compounding of aseptic preparations. It is important that this quality environment is continuous throughout the aseptic preparation process. Great reliance is not only placed on the facility and equipment used to produce the product, but also on the ability of the trained operators to avoid product contamination. It achieves a sterility assurance level of about one in a thousand. The manufacture of aseptic products also needs a stringent quality assurance system to ensure production of a quality product that is fit for its intended purpose. The quality assurance system should have documented, validated and audited procedures with in-process monitoring and standard operating procedures defining each step of the production process.

There is a need for awareness of the potential risk of infection that can occur during the aseptic preparation of pharmacy products. This has been shown by the tragic outcome of the supply of contaminated parenteral nutrition fluids to children at the Royal Manchester Children's Hospital in 1994. These fluids were aseptically compounded in an isolator. Microorganisms were unknowingly transferred from a sink into the isolator chamber on components used to prepare the feeds. The contaminating organisms grew in fluid remaining in assembled tubing used to prepare the feeds in the isolator. Reuse of this tubing resulted in contamination of the feeds that infected the patients. During these events, it was shown that the equipment was not faulty, only the manner in which it had been used. This demonstrates the importance of adequately disinfecting the components being transferred into the isolator and for a total quality system for the manufacture of aseptic products.

In order to aseptically prepare a parenteral medicine, it is critical that validated procedures are stringently followed. This must go hand in hand with the other components of the quality assurance system for the preparation of aseptically prepared products of quality that are right first time and every time.

Testing for sterility

Sterility testing is the final method of assuring sterility of the manufactured product. The test is required in most countries for assuring the sterility of aseptically prepared sterile products. Aseptic manufacturing units in hospital pharmacy often perform the test retrospectively following patient administration. A few commercial manufacturers are exempt from performing the sterility test on products that have been terminally sterilized and prepared using highly developed quality assurance procedures incorporating validated and controlled sterilization procedures. This has been referred to as parametric release.

Sterility testing attempts to indicate the presence or absence of viable microorganisms in containers selected from a batch of product. A decision is made as to the sterility of the entire batch from the results obtained by testing the sample. The test has both technical and numerical limitations and thus only provides a partial indication to the state of sterility of each product within a manufactured batch. The numerical limitation arises as only 10% of a batch of parenteral product is sampled, but the probability of accidental contamination in an aseptically manufactured batch can be as high as one in a thousand (10^{-3}), while the probability of contamination of a terminally sterilized batch is at worst only one in a million (10^{-6}).

The details of the test for sterility are provided in the *British Pharmacopoeia* (BP 2012) and this test conforms with the standards of the *European Pharmacopoeia* (EP 2013). These are also very similar to the test in the *Japanese Pharmacopoeia* (2012) and *United States Pharmacopoeia* 36 (USP 2013).

KEY POINTS

- Particulate and microbial contamination of sterile products is minimized by preparation in a clean environment
- Quality of clean areas is graded A, B, C, D in decreasing stringency for particulate and microbial content
- Premises must allow segregation of stages of production and protect products from contamination by all possible means of design and operation
- Access to clean areas is restricted and special clothing must be worn

- Environmental control, particularly of the air supply to the room, is required to ensure a minimal contamination hazard
- HEPA filters have a 99.997% efficiency at removing 0.3 μm particles, the size at which their efficiency is lowest
- Airflow may be designed as unidirectional, non-unidirectional or as a combination system
- In addition to general air quality, localized areas of higher quality can be produced either by airflow design in enclosed areas or by isolator cabinets
- The main source of contamination in clean rooms is the skin scales from operators
- Clean room clothing, made from synthetic fabrics, is designed to minimize release of operator contaminants
- Changing areas are designed and used to minimize the entry of contamination on personnel
- During cleaning, vacuuming and wet wiping are used to remove large and small particles, respectively
- Isolators give protection to both the product and the operator at relatively low cost
- Type II isolators protect the operator from hazardous materials in addition to providing the Type I facilities of protection of the product from contamination
- Isolator interiors are sterilized using a gas sterilant
- Isolator integrity is tested using physical and microbial tests
- A range of environmental tests is used in clean rooms to monitor air quality, movement and velocity, air-borne particles and microbial contamination
- Aseptic preparation is involved with repackaging sterile products for patient use without terminal sterilization
- Aseptic preparation is performed in laminar airflow cabinets in clean rooms or in isolator cabinets to avoid product contamination
- A stringent quality assurance system is required for aseptic production to ensure a quality product is prepared
- The test for sterility has numerical limitations due to the sample size – cannot guarantee to detect small levels of product contamination

Parenteral products

41

Derek G. Chapman

STUDY POINTS

- Reasons for parenteral administration
- Routes available for parenteral administration
- Forms and types of parenteral product
- Design of containers for the administration of parenteral products
- Formulation and uses of parenteral products

Introduction

In practice, parenteral products are often regarded as dosage forms that are implanted, injected or infused directly into vessels, tissues, tissue spaces or body compartments. Parenteral products are often used for drugs that cannot be given orally. This may be because of patient intolerance, the instability of the drug, or poor absorption of the drug if given by the oral route. From the site of administration the drug is transported to the site of action. With developing technology, parenteral therapy is being used outside the hospital or clinic environment: at a patient's home or their workplace, allowing self-administration.

Parenteral therapy is used to:

- Produce a localized effect
- Administer drugs if the oral route cannot be used
- Deliver drugs to the unconscious patient
- Rapidly correct fluid and electrolyte imbalances
- Ensure delivery of the drug to the target tissues.

Parenteral injections are either administered directly into blood for a fast and controlled effect or into tissues outside the blood vessels for a local or systemic effect. An intravenously administered (IV) injection will rapidly increase the concentration of drug in the blood plasma, but this concentration falls due to the reversible transfer of the drug from blood plasma into body tissues, a process known as distribution. An IV infusion administers a large volume of fluid at a slow rate and ensures that the drug enters the general circulation at a constant rate. A steady state is reached when the rate of drug addition equals the rate of drug loss in the blood plasma. When infusion is stopped, elimination of the drug from the body generally follows first-order kinetics.

Following subcutaneous (SC) and intramuscular (IM) injection, there is a delay in the systemic effects of the drug due to the time taken for the drug to first pass through the walls of the capillaries before entering into the blood. This occurs by passive diffusion that is promoted by the concentration gradient across the capillary wall. The drug concentration in the blood plasma rises to a peak level and then falls due to distribution to the tissues followed by metabolism and excretion.

Administration procedures

IV injections and infusions

The vein that is selected for administering the formulation depends on the size of the delivery needle or catheter, the type and volume of fluid to be administered and the rate at which the fluid is to be administered. The fluids are administered into a

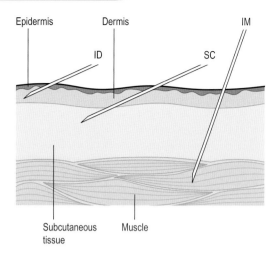

Figure 41.1 • Injection routes. ID, intradermal; SC, subcutaneous; IM, intramuscular.

superficial vein, commonly on the back of the hand or in the internal flexure of the elbow. The intravenous route is widely used to administer parenteral products, but it must not be used to administer water-in-oil emulsions or suspensions.

SC injections

These are injected into the loose connective and adipose tissue immediately beneath the skin in the abdomen, the upper back, the upper arms and the lateral upper hips (Fig. 41.1). Typically, the volume injected does not exceed 1 mL. Following administration, the site of the injection, the body temperature, age of the patient and the degree of massaging of the injection site will all affect the drug distribution.

IM injections

Small-volume aqueous solutions, solutions in oil and suspensions are administered directly into the body of a relaxed muscle, such as the gluteal muscle in the buttock, the deltoid muscle in the shoulder and the vastus lateralis of the thigh (Fig. 41.1).

Other routes of parenteral administration include intradermal, intra-arterial, intracardiac, intraspinal and intra-articular.

Products for parenteral use

Parenteral products include injection, infusion and implantation.

Injections

These are subdivided into small- and large-volume parenteral fluids. Small-volume parenteral fluids are sterile, pyrogen-free injectable products. They are packaged in volumes up to 100 mL. Small-volume parenteral fluids are packed as:

- Single-dose ampoules
- Multiple-dose vials
- Prefilled syringes.

Single-dose ampoules

Most small-volume parenteral fluids are currently packaged as either ampoules or vials. Glass ampoules are thin-walled containers made of Type I borosilicate glass (see Fig. 32.2). Injections packaged in glass ampoules are manufactured by filling the product into the ampoules, which are then heat sealed. To achieve the quality required of these products, the packaged solution must be sterile and practically free of particles. These products are prepared in clean room conditions (see Ch. 40). Opening glass ampoules may contaminate the product with glass particles; this is a hazard to the patient. Modern glass ampoules have weakened necks to reduce the number of particles.

Plastic ampoules are prepared, filled and sealed by a procedure known as blow-fill-seal in which the semi solid plastic is blow moulded and formed into ampoules. These containers are filled with the product and immediately sealed. This system is only used to package simple solutions due to absorption of the drug by the plastic. When the ampoule is opened only a few particles are released into the solution.

Ampoules should have a reliable seal that can be readily leak tested and will not deteriorate during the lifetime of the product. Ampoules do not contain added antimicrobial preservatives. The ampoule must contain a slight excess volume of product. This is necessary to allow the nominal injection volume to be drawn into a syringe.

Multiple-dose vials

These are composed of a thick-walled glass container that is sealed with a rubber closure. The closure is kept in position by an aluminium seal (see Fig. 32.4), then covered with a plastic cap. The cap is removed before a needle, attached to a syringe, is inserted through the rubber closure to withdraw a dose of product. The contents of the vial may be removed in several portions.

There are disadvantages with the use of glass vials. Fragments of the closure may be released into the product when the needle is inserted through the closure. There is also the risk of interaction between the product and the closure. Repeated withdrawal of injection solution from these containers increases the risk of microbial contamination of the product. These products must, therefore, contain an antimicrobial preservative unless the medicine itself has antimicrobial activity. An example of such a multidose product is insulin.

Prefilled syringes

With these devices, the injection solution is aseptically filled into sterile syringes. The packed solution has a high level of sterility assurance and does not contain an antimicrobial preservative. The final product is available for immediate use. Prefilled syringes are becoming increasingly common.

Administration of small-volume parenteral products

Hypodermic syringes and needles are extensively used for administering small volumes of parenteral formulations to the patient. These syringes have been sterilized by ethylene oxide gas or by gamma irradiation following packaging. Various sizes of hypodermic syringes are available. They are composed of a barrel, having a graduated scale, together with a plunger and a headpiece, known as a piston (Fig. 41.2). These components are often made of polypropylene.

Formulation of parenteral products

Vehicles for injections

The vehicle provides the highest proportion of the formulation and should not be toxic nor have any therapeutic activity.

Water for Injections

Water for Injections is the most extensively used vehicle in parenteral formulations, Water for Injections

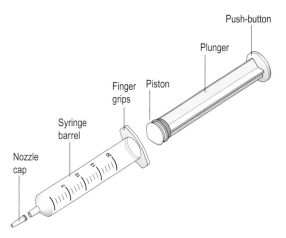

Figure 41.2 • Hypodermic syringe for single use.

must be free of pyrogens and have a high level of chemical purity. The BP considers that Water for Injections can only be prepared by distillation.

Sterilized water for injections

This is prepared by packing a volume of Water for Injections in sealed containers. These containers are then moist-heat sterilized which yields a sterile product that remains free of pyrogens.

Pyrogens

Pyrogens are fever-producing substances. Water is the greatest source of pyrogens in parenteral products. Pyrogens can be removed in the preparation of water for injections by distillation. Water that is free from pyrogens is termed apyrogenic.

Microbial pyrogens arise from components of Gram-negative and Gram-positive bacteria, fungi and viruses. Non-microbial pyrogens are for example some steroids and plasma components.

Parenteral products must be prepared in conditions that reduce microbial contamination because bacteria contaminating aqueous solutions can release pyrogens. Contaminated solutions will become more pyrogenic with the passage of time. Therefore, these products must be sterilized shortly after preparation.

Dry heat at 250°C for 30 min is the most common method of inactivating pyrogens.

Non-aqueous solvents

Water-miscible co-solvents, such as glycerin and propylene glycol, are used as vehicles in small-volume parenteral fluids. They are used to increase the solubility of drugs and to stabilize drugs degraded by hydrolysis.

Metabolizable oils are used to dissolve drugs that are insoluble in water. For example, steroids, hormones and vitamins are dissolved in vegetable oils. These formulations are administered by intramuscular injection.

Additives

Various additives, such as antimicrobial agents, antioxidants, buffers, chelating agents and tonicity-adjusting agents, are included in injection formulations. Their purpose is to produce a safe and elegant product. Both the types and amounts of additives to be included in formulations are given in the appropriate monograph in the BP.

Antimicrobial agents

Antimicrobial agents are added to inhibit the growth of microbial organisms that may accidentally contaminate the product during use, for example, multiple-dose vials. The antimicrobial agents must be stable and effective in the parenteral formulation. Rubber closures have been shown to take up antimicrobial preservatives from the injection solution. Preservative uptake is more significant with natural and neoprene rubber and much less significant with butyl rubber closures.

Antioxidants

Many drugs in aqueous solutions are easily degraded by oxidation. Small-volume parenteral products of these drugs often contain an antioxidant. Bisulfites and metabisulfites are commonly used antioxidants in aqueous injections. Antioxidants must be carefully selected for use in injections to avoid interaction with the drug. Injections may, in addition to antioxidants, also contain chelating agents such as EDTA or citric acid, which remove trace elements.

Buffers

The ideal pH of parenteral products is pH7.4. If the pH is above pH9, tissue necrosis may result, while below pH3, pain and phlebitis can occur.

Buffers are included in injections to maintain the pH of the packaged product. Changes in pH can arise through interaction between the product and the container. Acetate, citrate and phosphate buffers are commonly used in parenteral products.

Tonicity-adjusting agents

Isotonic solutions have the same osmotic pressure as blood plasma and do not damage the membrane of red blood cells. Hypotonic solutions have a lower osmotic pressure than blood plasma and cause blood cells to swell and burst because of fluids passing into the cells by osmosis. Hypertonic solutions have a higher osmotic pressure than plasma and as a result the red blood cells lose fluids and shrink. Thus, the BP states that aqueous solutions for large-volume infusion fluids, together with aqueous fluids for subcutaneous, intradermal and intramuscular administration, should be made isotonic. Intrathecal injections must also be isotonic to avoid serious changes in the osmotic pressure of the cerebrospinal fluid. Aqueous hypotonic solutions are made isotonic by adding either sodium chloride, glucose or, occasionally, mannitol. The latter two agents are incompatible with some drugs. If the solution is hypertonic, it is made isotonic by dilution.

Injection solutions are often made isotonic with 0.9% sodium chloride solution. The amount of solute, or the required dilution necessary to make a solution isotonic, can be determined from the freezing point depression. The freezing point depression of blood plasma and tears is −0.52°C. Thus, solutions that freeze at −0.52°C have the same osmotic pressure as body fluids. Hypotonic solutions have a smaller freezing point depression and require the addition of a solute to depress the freezing point to −0.52°C.

The amount of adjusting substance added to these solutions may be calculated from the equation:

$$W = (0.5 - 2a)/b$$

where W=percentage concentration of adjusting substance in the final solution, a=freezing point depression of the unadjusted hypotonic solution, b=freezing point depression of a 1% weight in volume (w/v) concentration of the adjusting substance.

An extensive list of freezing point depression values is detailed in the *Pharmaceutical Codex* (1994: 53–64) (Example 41.1).

Other methods that are used to estimate the amount of adjusting substances required to make a solution isotonic include:

- Sodium chloride equivalents
- Molar concentrations
- Serum osmolarity.

Example 41.1

A 100 mL volume of a 2% w/v solution of glucose for intravenous injection is to be made isotonic by the addition of sodium chloride.

A 1% w/v solution of glucose depresses the freezing point of water by 0.1°C and a 1% solution of sodium chloride depresses the freezing point of water by 0.576°C.

The depression of freezing point of the unadjusted solution of glucose (a) will therefore be:

$$(a) = 2 \times 0.1 = 0.2$$

A 1% w/v solution of sodium chloride depresses the freezing point of water by 0.576°C (b).

Substituting these values for a and b in the above equation:

$$W = (0.52 - 0.2)/0.576 = 0.32/0.576 = 0.555$$

The intravenous solution thus requires the addition of 0.555 g of sodium chloride per 100 mL volume to make it isotonic with blood plasma.

Example 41.2

Sodium chloride has one sodium and one chloride ion. Thus, 1 mole of sodium chloride provides 1 mole of both sodium and chloride ions. The weight of sodium chloride, which provides a 1 mmol quantity is 58.5 mg. This weight corresponds to its relative molecular mass and provides 1 mmol of both sodium and chloride ions.

Magnesium chloride has one magnesium and two chloride ions. The weight in milligrams that provides 1 mmol of magnesium and 2 mmol of chloride ions is 203 mg. This weight corresponds to the relative molecular mass of this salt. The quantity of salt in milligrams containing 1 mmol of a particular ion can be determined by dividing the relative molecular mass of the salt by the number of the particular ions that it contains. Weights of common salts that provide 1 mmol are given in the 12th edition of the *Pharmaceutical Codex* (1994: 49–50).

in grams. The number of moles of each of the ions of a salt in solution depends on the number of each ion in the molecule of the salt (Example 41.2).

Details of these methods are given in the *Pharmaceutical Codex* (1994: 64–67).

Units of concentration

The concentration of the components in parenteral products may be expressed in various ways (see also Ch. 19):

- *Percentage weight/volume*. Examples include: magnesium sulfate injection 50%, sodium chloride intravenous infusion 0.9%
- *Weight per unit volume*. Examples include: atropine sulfate 600 μg/mL or ephedrine hydrochloride injection 30 mg/mL
- *Millimoles per unit volume*. Examples include: potassium chloride solution, strong (sterile) contains 2 mmol each of K^+ and Cl^- per mL; Calcium Chloride Injection BP contains 2.5 mmol of Ca^{2+} and 5 mmol of Cl^- in 5 mL.

During the formulation of injections and infusions, the units of interest are the ions of electrolytes and the molecules of non-electrolytes. For molecules, 1 millimole (mmol) is the weight in milligrams corresponding to its relative molecular mass. A mole of an ion is its relative atomic mass weighed

Special injections

These are more complex formulations than solutions for injection.

Suspensions

Suspensions for injection contain <5% of drug solids with a mean particle diameter within the range 5–10 μm. Owing to the presence of particles in these formulations, these injections are more difficult to process and sterilize than solutions for injection. During the manufacture of suspensions for injection, the components are prepared and sterilized separately. They are then aseptically combined (see Ch. 29). The final product cannot be filter sterilized, owing to the presence of particles in the formulation. Powders for use in sterile suspensions can be sterilized by gas, but gas residues must be avoided.

Dried injections

With these products the dry sterile powder is aseptically added to a sterile vial. Alternatively, a sterile filtered solution can be freeze dried in a vial. The dry drug powder is reconstituted with a sterile vehicle before use.

Non-aqueous injections

Drugs that are insoluble in an aqueous vehicle can be formulated in solution using an oil as the vehicle. Several oils are used in these formulations, including arachis oil and sesame oil, which are easily metabolized. These viscous injections give a depot effect with slow release of the drug and are administered by intramuscular injection.

Large-volume parenteral products

These are formulated as single-dose injections that are administered by intravenous infusion. They are sterile aqueous solutions or emulsions with water for injections as the main component. It is important that they are free of particles. During the administration of these fluids, additional drugs are often added to the fluids (see Ch. 40). This may be carried out by the injection of small-volume parenteral products to the administration set of the fluid, or by the 'piggyback' method. In this procedure, a second, but smaller, volume infusion of an additional drug is added to the intravenous delivery system.

Large-volume parenteral products include:

- Infusion fluids to deliver drugs or restore fluid or electrolyte imbalance
- Total parenteral nutrition (TPN) solutions
- Intravenous antibiotics
- Patient-controlled analgesia
- Dialysis fluids
- Irrigation solutions.

All of these products have direct contact with blood or are introduced into a body cavity.

Large-volume parenteral fluids must be terminally heat sterilized. While water for injections is the main component of these products, they also incorporate other ingredients including:

- Carbohydrates, e.g. dextrose, sucrose and dextran
- Amino acids
- Lipid emulsions which contain vegetable or semisynthetic oil
- Electrolytes such as sodium chloride
- Polyols, including glycerol, sorbitol and mannitol.

Most large-volume parenteral fluids are clear aqueous solutions, except for the oil-in-water emulsions. The production of emulsions for infusion is highly specialized as they are destabilized by heat.

Production of large-volume parenteral products

The fluids are produced and filled into containers in a high-standard clean room environment (see Ch. 46). The use of stringent quality assurance procedures is essential to ensure the quality of the products.

In commercial manufacturing facilities, the fluids are packaged from a bulk container into the product container using high-speed filling machines. Just before the fluid enters the container, particulate matter is removed from the fluid by passing it through an in-line membrane filter. Immediately after filling, the neck of each glass bottle is sealed with a tight-fitting rubber closure that is kept in place with a crimped aluminium cap. The outer cap is also aluminium and an outer tamper-evident closure is used.

When using plastic bags, the preformed plastic bag is aseptically filled and immediately heat sealed. As an alternative, a blow-fill-seal system can be used. Blow-fill-seal production decreases the problems with product handling, cleaning and particulate contamination. Following filling of the product into containers, the fluids are examined for particulate matter and the integrity of container closures established.

Moist heat is used to sterilize parenteral products, irrigation solutions and dialysis fluids as soon as possible after the containers have been filled. Plastic containers must be sterilized with an over-pressure during the sterilization cycle to avoid the containers bursting.

Containers and closures

Large-volume parenteral fluids are packaged into:

- Glass bottles
- Polyvinyl chloride (PVC) collapsible bags
- Semi-rigid polythene containers.

The containers and closures that are used for packaging parenteral products must:

- Maintain the sterility of the packed fluids
- Withstand sterilization
- Be compatible with the packed fluid
- Allow withdrawal of the contents.

Glass bottles are rarely used these days, but may be used for products that are incompatible with plastic containers. If used they require the use of an air inlet filter device for pressure equilibration within the container. Particles of glass can be released into the injection fluids. Damage to the neck of the bottles may result in contamination of the container contents from the external environment. Owing to these difficulties with glass containers, plastic containers have become widely used.

PVC collapsible bags are used to package most infusion fluids. They are designed with a port for the attachment of the administration set and an additive port for the addition of small-volume parenteral fluids.

PVC collapsible bags are:

- Resistant to impact
- Flexible and collapse during fluid administration and do not require an air inlet system.

The disadvantages of plastic bags are that:

- They permit a high moisture penetration
- They adsorb some drugs
- They require an extended sterilization time due to the heat resistance of the PVC
- Moist heat sterilization requires air ballasting to avoid pouch explosion.

Semi-rigid plastic containers are used for volumes of 100 mL for electrolyte solutions, 3 L for TPN solutions and up to 5 L for dialysis solutions.

Semi-rigid containers:

- Are more drug compatible than PVC containers
- Are difficult to break
- Do not fully collapse
- Need extended heat sterilization times
- Need air equilibration.

Semi-rigid bags are designed with two ports. One port allows the attachment of the administration set. The other port permits the addition of small-volume parenteral products or small-volume infusion fluids. They have a graduated scale that can be read either in an inverted or upright position (Fig. 41.3). To enable containers of large-volume parenteral fluids to be suspended from a drip stand for administration, bags are made with an eyelet opening that suspends the bag.

Administration of large-volume parenteral fluids

Most large-volume parenteral fluids are administered to the patient by a parenteral route using the

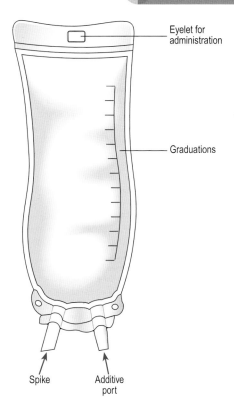

Figure 41.3 • Semi-rigid infusion bag.

standard infusion set specified in British Standard 2463 (Part 2, 1989). These sets are packaged as sterile units intended for single use (Fig. 41.4). Fluid moves through them by gravity.

Labelling

Batch-produced products have identical labels attached to both the product and the outer packaging carton that is used for transport. With flexible plastic containers, the labelling requirements are commonly printed directly on to the container prior to filling. With bags containing TPN fluids, a label is placed on the bag itself and an identical label is attached to the outer plastic cover on the bag. Labels are attached to infusion fluid containers. The labels on parenteral fluids should include the following details:

- Product identity and details of the contained volume
- Solution strength in terms of the amount of active ingredient in a suitable dose-volume
- Batch number and product expiry date

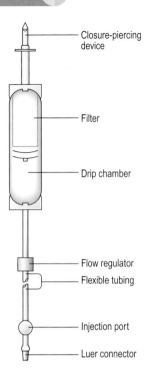

Closure-piercing device

Filter

Drip chamber

Flow regulator

Flexible tubing

Injection port

Luer connector

Figure 41.4 • Diagram of a typical administration set.

- Storage requirements
- For TPN solutions, the name of the patient, the unit number, ward and infusion rate.

Containers often carry a warning label to discard the remaining product when treatment is completed.

Aseptic dispensing

Most parenteral fluids are terminally moist heat sterilized. However, some products are aseptically compounded from sterile ingredients in the hospital pharmacy. These products are prepared and dispensed for individual patients. Examples of aseptically prepared products are TPN fluids (see Ch. 44) and the aseptic reconstitution of freeze-dried formulations. These freeze-dried products are often reconstituted using either water for injections or 0.9% sodium chloride injection. Aseptic dispensing is performed in a Grade A clean room environment or a Grade A isolator chamber (see Ch. 40). The dispensing of these products relies on good aseptic procedures to ensure the sterility of the product. Owing to the absence of terminal sterilization, it is important that manufacture is performed using rigorous quality

assurance procedures. Aseptically dispensed products are given a very limited expiry time.

Admixtures

These are prepared by adding at least one sterile injection to an intravenous infusion fluid for administration. The injections to be added are packed in an ampoule or vial, or may be reconstituted from a solid. These additions should be carried out using aseptic procedures in a Grade A environment within an isolator cabinet or clean room facility. This environment is required to maintain the sterility of the product and avoid contamination of the product with particulate matter, microorganisms and pyrogens. Following the additions, a sealing cap may be placed over the additive port of the infusion bag to prevent further, potentially incompatible, additions at ward level. Hospital pharmacies often have a centralized intravenous additive service (CIVAS), as detailed in Chapter 46. These facilities ensure that additions to infusion fluids are carried out in a suitable environment.

Infusion devices

There are situations that require strict control of the volume of fluids that are infused into a patient. Accurate flow control with infusion devices is vital for patient safety and for optimum efficacy of the infusion. A range of delivery systems are available that regulate the volume of fluid administered and are used both in the hospital and for the self-administration of fluids by patients at home.

The selection of an infusion device for the self-administration of medicines by patients requires careful consideration of several factors including:

- Delivery volume and control of flow rate
- Complexity of the administration procedure
- Type of therapy being administered
- Frequency of dosing
- Reservoir volume available in the infusion device.

Irrigation solutions

These solutions are applied topically to bathe open wounds and body cavities. They are sterile solutions for single use only. Examples of irrigation fluids are 0.9% w/v sodium chloride solution or sterile water for irrigation. Most irrigation fluids are now available in rigid plastic bottles. Urological irrigation solutions are used for surgical procedures. They are usually sterile water or sterile glycine solutions and are used to remove blood and maintain tissue integrity during an operation.

Water for irrigation is sterilized distilled water that is free of pyrogens. The water is packed in containers and is intended for use on one occasion only. The containers are sealed and sterilized by moist heat.

Peritoneal dialysis fluids

Peritoneal dialysis involves the administration of dialysis solutions directly into the peritoneum by way of an indwelling catheter. The fluid is then drained after a 'dwell-time' to remove toxic waste products from the body. Peritoneal dialysis solutions are sterile solutions manufactured to the same standards as parenteral fluids. The composition of peritoneal dialysis fluid simulates potassium-free extracellular fluid. These fluids are packaged in volumes of 3–5 L in plastic containers that are similar to the bags used for TPN (see Ch. 44).

Haemodialysis

In this dialysis procedure, blood is removed and returned to the patient by way of a catheter, or a double needle arrangement, using a fistula where an artery and vein are joined together. The dialysis procedure involves the use of an artificial disposable membrane within a 'dialyser' machine that acts as an artificial kidney. An electrolyte fluid, simulating body fluid, bathes one side of the membrane, with blood from the patient on the other side. There is no direct contact between the blood and the dialyser fluid. Thus fluids for haemodialysis are not required to be sterile or free of pyrogens or particulate matter.

Blood products

These products are not usually identified as sterile products although they are commonly packaged as sterile large-volume parenteral fluids. These biological products include albumin, human plasma and blood protein fractions. All these products must be treated to inactivate virus contamination prior to packaging. This is usually achieved by specialized heat treatment or filtration. These products are unstable to heat sterilization. Therefore, they are filter sterilized and then aseptically filled into containers in large-scale production facilities. Most of these products are packed as liquids, although a few blood protein fractions such as factor VIII and factor IX are freeze dried. The collection, management and distribution of these products are carried out by the blood transfusion service.

KEY POINTS

- Convention uses the term 'parenteral' for dosage forms which are placed directly into the body
- The three main routes are IV, IM and SC
- Parenteral products are sterile forms used for injection, infusion or implantation
- Small volumes are packed in glass or plastic ampoules
- Multiple-dose injections must have an antimicrobial preservative
- Water for injections must be used as the aqueous ingredient in all injections
- Water for irrigations is used in large volumes to irrigate body cavities and other areas
- Pyrogens cause fever and must be eliminated from water for injections and water for irrigations
- Additives to injections include antimicrobial preservatives, antioxidants, buffers, tonicity adjusters and co-solvents
- Injection solutions for SC, intradermal, IM, intrathecal and large-volume IV use should be made isotonic
- Large-volume parenteral products, include infusion fluids, TPN, dialysis fluids and irrigation solutions
- All large-volume parenteral products must be sterilized after filling into their final containers
- Large-volume parenteral products may be packaged in glass bottles, semi-rigid or collapsible plastic containers
- When aseptic dispensing is required, rigorous quality assurance is essential and a short expiry date is given to the product

Ophthalmic products

R. Michael E. Richards

R. Michael E. Richards

STUDY POINTS

- The formulation, preparation and uses of ophthalmic preparations
- The packaging and labelling requirements for ophthalmic preparations
- Advising patients on the use of eye medication and on any adverse effects
- The anatomy and physiology of the eye in relation to the administration of medication and the wearing of contact lenses
- The properties of contact lenses in relation to their physicochemical composition
- The wearing of and caring for contact lenses and the various products available to facilitate comfort, effectiveness, convenience and safety
- The role of antimicrobial preservatives in ophthalmic products
- Advising patients on the possible adverse effects of concurrent medication and the sensible use of cosmetics when wearing contact lenses

Introduction

The human eye is a remarkable organ and the ability to see is one of our most treasured possessions. Thus, the highest standards are necessary in the compounding of ophthalmic preparations and the greatest care is required in their use. It is necessary that all ophthalmic preparations are sterile and essentially free from foreign particles.

These preparations may be categorized as follows:

- Eye drops including solutions, emulsions and suspensions of active medicaments for instillation into the conjunctival sac
- Eye lotions for irrigating and cleansing the eye surface, or for impregnating eye dressings
- Eye ointments, creams and gels containing active ingredient(s) for application to the lid margins and/or conjunctival sac
- Contact lens solutions to facilitate the wearing and care of contact lenses
- Parenteral products for intracorneal, intravitreous or retrobulbar injection
- Ophthalmic inserts placed in the conjunctival sac and designed to release active ingredient over a prolonged period
- Powders for the preparation of eye drops and eye lotions.

Medicaments contained in ophthalmic products include:

- Anaesthetics used topically in surgical procedures
- Anti-infectives such as antibacterials, antifungals and antivirals
- Anti-inflammatories such as corticosteroids and antihistamines
- Antiglaucoma agents to reduce intraocular pressure, such as beta-blockers
- Astringents such as zinc sulphate
- Diagnostic agents such as fluorescein which highlight damage to the epithelial tissue
- Miotics such as pilocarpine which constrict the pupil and contract the ciliary muscle, increasing drainage from the anterior chamber
- Mydriatics and cycloplegics such as atropine, which dilate the pupil and paralyse the ciliary muscle and thus facilitate the examination of the interior of the eye.

Anatomy and physiology of the eye

Figure 42.1 gives an indication of the relevance of the external structures of the eye and the structure of the eyelids to the application of medication and the wearing of contact lenses (see p.406 also).

Formulation of eye drops

The components of an eye drop formulation are given below:

- Active ingredient(s) to produce desired therapeutic effect
- Vehicle, usually aqueous but occasionally may be oil
- Antimicrobial preservative to eliminate any microbial contamination during use and thus maintain sterility; it should not interact adversely with the active ingredient(s)

- Adjuvants to adjust tonicity, viscosity or pH in order to increase the 'comfort' in use and to increase the stability of the active ingredient(s); they should not interact adversely with other components of the formulation
- Suitable container for administration of eye drops which maintains the preparation in a stable form and protects from contamination during preparation, storage and use.

The single most important requirement of eye drops is that they are sterile. Historically, instances of microbially contaminated eye drops have been reported; the contaminating organism, *Pseudomonas aeruginosa*, is difficult to treat successfully and can cause loss of the eye.

Antimicrobial preservatives

Multiple-dose eye drops contain an effective antimicrobial preservative system, which is capable of withstanding the test for efficacy of antimicrobial

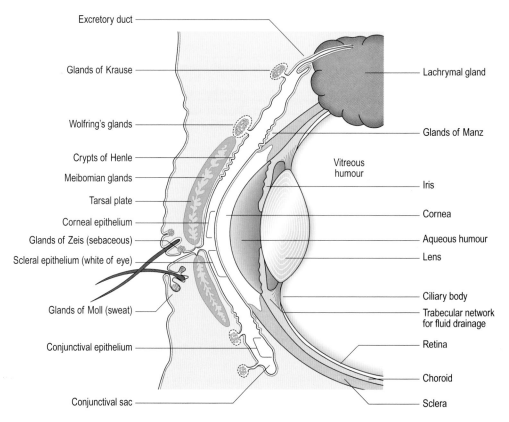

Figure 42.1 • Section of the eye showing the glands which produce the fluids that form the precorneal film and the tears, the epithelial sites of drug action and absorption and the internal sites of pharmacological action.

preservatives of the *British Pharmacopoeia* (BP 2007). This ensures that the eye drops are maintained sterile during use and will not introduce contamination into the eyes being treated. Normal healthy eyes are quite efficient at preventing penetration by microorganisms. Eyes that have damaged epithelia are compromised and may be colonized by microorganisms. This has to be guarded against. The lack of vascularity of the cornea and certain internal structures of the eye make it very susceptible and difficult to treat once infection has been established.

No single substance is entirely satisfactory for use as a preservative for ophthalmic solutions. The systems that have been used, based on work of the author and others in the 1960s, have formed the basis of effective preservation over the subsequent years.

Eye drops specifically formulated for use during intraocular surgery should not contain a preservative because of the risk of damage to the internal surfaces of the eye. Diagnostic dyes should preferably be supplied as single-dose preparations. Preservatives which are suitable for a selection of eye drops are given in Box 42.1.

Box 42.1

Preservatives suitable for specific eye drops

Benzalkonium chloride 0.01% w/v	Chlorhexidine acetate 0.01% w/v	Phenylmercuric nitrate[a] 0.002% w/v
Atropine sulphate	Cocaine	Tetracaine
Carbachol	Cocaine and homatropine	Chloramphenicol
Cyclopentolate		Fluorescein[b]
Homatropine		Hydrocortisone and neomycin
Hyoscine		Lachesine
Hypromellose		Neomycin
Phenylephrine		Sulfacetamide
Physostigmine		Zinc sulphate
Pilocarpine		Zinc sulphate and adrenaline
Prednisolone		

[a]The acetate may also be used.
[b]This is preferably used as single dose preparations.

Benzalkonium chloride

This quaternary ammonium compound is the preservative of choice. It is in over 70% of commercially produced eye drops and over a third of these also contain disodium edetate, usually at 0.1% w/v.

Benzalkonium chloride is not a pure material, but is a mixture of alkylbenzyldimethyl ammonium compounds. This permits a mixture of alkyl chain lengths containing even numbers of carbon atoms between 8 and 18 and results in products of different activities. The longer the carbon chain length, the greater the antibacterial activity but the less the solubility. Therefore the manufacturer should seek to maximize the activity within the constraints of solubility. This means maximizing the proportions of C_{12}, C_{14} and C_{16}. It should be noted that Benzalkonium Chloride BP contains 50% w/v benzalkonium chloride.

Benzalkonium chloride is well tolerated on the eye up to concentrations of 0.02% w/v but is usually used at 0.01% w/v. It is stable to sterilization by autoclaving. The compound has a rapid bactericidal action in clean conditions against a wide range of Gram-positive and Gram-negative organisms. It destroys the external structures of the cell (cell envelope). It is active in the controlled aqueous environment and pH values of ophthalmic solutions. Activity is reduced in the presence of multivalent cations (Mg^{2+}, Ca^{2+}). These compete with the antibacterial for negatively charged sites on the bacterial cell surface. It also has its activity reduced if heated with methylcellulose or formulated with anionic and certain concentrations of non-ionic surfactants. Benzalkonium chloride is incompatible with fluorescein (large anion) and nitrates and is sorbed from solutions through contact with rubber.

The antibacterial activity of benzalkonium is enhanced by aromatic alcohols (benzyl alcohol, 2-phenylethanol and 3-phenylpropanol) and its activity against Gram-negative organisms is greatly enhanced by chelating agents such as disodium edetate. These agents chelate the divalent cations, principally Mg^{2+}, of Gram-negative cells. These ions form bridges and bind the polysaccharide chains which protrude from the outer membrane of these cells. Thus, the integrity of the membrane is compromised and the benzalkonium chloride activity enhanced. This is particularly valuable in preserving against contamination with *Pseudomonas aeruginosa*.

The surface activity of benzalkonium chloride may be used to enhance the transcorneal passage of non-lipid-soluble drugs such as carbachol. Care must be taken since the preservative can solubilize the outer oily protective layer of the precorneal film. This film has an internal mucin layer in contact with the corneal and scleral epithelia, a middle aqueous layer and an outer oily layer. The oil prevents excessive aqueous evaporation and protects the inner surface of the lids from constant contact with water. The blink reflex helps maintain the integrity of the precorneal film. For these reasons, it is important not to use benzalkonium chloride to preserve local anaesthetic eye drops which abolish the blink reflex. The combined effect of the two agents causes drying of the eye surface and irritation of the cornea.

Chlorhexidine acetate or gluconate

Chlorhexidine is a cationic biguanide bactericide with antibacterial properties in aqueous solution similar to benzalkonium chloride. Its activity is often reduced in the presence of other formulation ingredients. It is used at 0.01% w/v. Its antibacterial activity against Gram-negative bacteria is enhanced by aromatic alcohols and by disodium edetate. Activity is antagonized by multivalent cations. Stability is greatest at pH 5–6 but it is less stable to autoclaving than benzalkonium chloride. Chlorhexidine salts are generally well tolerated by the eye although allergic reactions may occur.

Chlorobutanol

This chlorinated alcohol is used at 0.5% w/v and is effective against bacteria and fungi. Chlorobutanol is compatible with most ophthalmic products. The main disadvantages are its volatility, absorption by plastic containers and lack of stability at autoclave temperatures.

Organic mercurials

Phenylmercuric acetate and nitrate and thiomersal are organic mercurials. They are slowly active, at concentrations of 0.001–0.004% w/v, over a wide pH range against bacteria and fungi. Absorption by rubber is marked.

The organic mercurials should not be used in eye drops which require prolonged usage because this can lead to intraocular deposition of mercury (mercurialentis). Allergy to thiomersal is also possible.

Tonicity

Where possible, eye drops are made isotonic with lachrymal fluid (approximately equivalent to 0.9% w/v sodium chloride solution). In practice, the eye will tolerate small volumes of eye drops having tonicities in the range equivalent to 0.7–1.5% w/v sodium chloride. Nevertheless it is good practice to adjust the tonicity of hypotonic eye drops by the addition of sodium chloride to bring the solution to the tonicity of the lachrymal fluid. (See Ch. 19 for methods for calculating the amount of sodium chloride required.) Some preparations are themselves hypertonic and so no adjustment should be made.

Viscosity enhancers

There is a general assumption that increasing the viscosity of an eye drop increases the residence time of the drop in the eye and results in increased penetration and therapeutic action of the drug. Most commercial preparations have their viscosities adjusted to be within the range 15–25 millipascal seconds (mPas). However, gently pressing downwards on the inside corner of the closed eye restricts the drainage channel into the nasal cavity and prolongs contact time. This has been recommended to increase the therapeutic index of antiglaucoma medications. Under normal conditions, a large proportion of a typical 50 μL drop will have drained from the conjunctival sac (capacity 25 μL) within 30 s. There will be no trace of the drop after 20 min.

Hypromellose

The hydroxypropyl derivative of methylcellulose is the most popular cellulose derivative employed for enhancing viscosity. It has good solubility characteristics (soluble in cold but insoluble in hot water) and good optical clarity. Typical concentrations in eye drop formulations are 0.5–2.0% w/v.

Polyvinyl alcohol

This is used at 1.4% w/v as a viscosity enhancer. It has a good contact time on the eye surface and good optical qualities. It withstands autoclaving and it can be filtered through a 0.22 μm filter.

Polyvinylpyrrolidone, polyethylene glycol and dextrin have also been used as viscolizing agents.

Box 42.2

Buffers suitable for some specific eye drops

Borate buffer (boric acid/borax): pH range 6.8–9.1

- Chloramphenicol eye drops: BP 1993 – pH 7.5
- Hypromellose eye drops: BPC 1973 – pH 8.4

Phosphate buffer (sodium acid phosphate/sodium phosphate): pH range 4.5–8.5

- Neomycin eye drops: BPC 1973 – pH 6.5
- Prednisolone sodium phosphate eye drops: BPC 1973 – pH 6.6

Citrate buffer (citric acid/sodium citrate): pH range 2.5–6.5

- Benzylpenicillin eye drops – pH 6.0
- Idoxuridine eye drops – pH 6.0

pH adjustment

The best compromise is required after considering the following factors:

- The pH offering best stability during preparation and storage
- The pH offering the best therapeutic activity
- The comfort of the patient.

Most active ingredients are salts of weak bases and are most stable at an acid pH but most active at a slightly alkaline pH.

The lachrymal fluid has a pH of 7.2–7.4 and also possesses considerable buffering capacity. Thus a 50 µL eye drop which is weakly buffered will be rapidly neutralized by lachrymal fluid. Where it is possible, very acidic solutions, such as adrenaline acid tartrate or pilocarpine hydrochloride, are buffered to reduce a stinging effect on instillation. Suitable buffers are shown in Box 42.2.

Antioxidants

Reducing agents are preferentially oxidized and are added to eye drops in order to protect the active ingredient from oxidation. Active ingredients requiring protection include adrenaline (epinephrine), proxymetacaine, sulfacetamide, tetracaine, phenylephrine and physostigmine.

Sodium metabisulphite and sodium sulphite

Both may be used as antioxidants at 0.1% w/v. The former is preferred at acid pH and the latter at alkaline pH. Both are stable in solution when protected from light. Sodium metabisulphite possesses marked antimicrobial properties at acid pH and enhances the activity of phenylmercuric nitrate at acid pH. It is incompatible with prednisolone phosphate, adrenaline (epinephrine), chloramphenicol and phenylephrine.

Chelating agents

Traces of heavy metals can catalyse breakdown of the active ingredient by oxidation and other mechanisms. Therefore, chelating agents such as disodium edetate may be included to chelate the metal ions and thus enhance stability. Disodium edetate is a very useful adjuvant to ophthalmic preparations at concentrations of up to 0.1% w/v to enhance antibacterial activity and chemical stability. It has also been used at higher concentrations as an eye drop for the treatment of lime burns in cattle.

Bioavailability

The effect of pH on the therapeutic activity of weak bases such as atropine sulphate has already been indicated under the section on pH adjustment. At acid pH, these bases exist in the ionized hydrophilic form. In order to penetrate the cornea, the bases need to be at alkaline pH so that they are in the unionized lipophilic form. Thus at tear pH (7.4) they are able to penetrate the outer lipid layer of the lipid–water–lipid sandwich, which constitutes the physicochemical structure of the cornea. Once inside the epithelium the undissociated free base will partially dissociate. The water-soluble dissociated moiety will then traverse the middle aqueous stromal layer of the cornea. When the dissociated drug reaches the junction of the stroma and the endothelium it will again partially associate, forming the lipid-soluble moiety and thus cross the endothelium. Finally, the drug will dissociate into its water-soluble form and enter the aqueous humour. From here it can diffuse to the iris and the ciliary body which are the sites of its pharmacological action (see Fig. 42.1). Thus, the most effective penetration of the lipophilic–hydrophilic–lipophilic corneal membrane is by active ingredients having both hydrophilic and lipophilic forms. For example, highly water-soluble steroid phosphate esters have poor corneal penetration but the less water-soluble, more lipophilic steroid acetate has much better corneal penetration.

Storage conditions

To minimize degradation of eye drop ingredients, storage temperature and conditions must be considered at the time of formulation. The stability of several drugs used in eye drops is improved by refrigerated storage (2–8°C), e.g. chloramphenicol.

Containers for eye drops

Containers should protect the eye drops from microbial contamination, moisture and air. Container materials should not be shed or leached into solution, neither should any of the eye drop formulation be adsorbed or absorbed by the container. If the product is to be sterilized in the final container, all parts of the container must withstand the sterilization process.

Containers may be made of glass or plastic and may be single- or multiple-dose containers. The latter should not contain more than 10 mL. Both single-dose and multiple-dose packs must have tamper-evident closures and packaging.

Single-dose containers

The 'Minims'® range is the most widely used type of single-dose eye drop container in the UK. It consists of an injection-moulded polypropylene container which is sealed at its base and has a nozzle sealed with a screw cap. This container is sterilized by autoclaving in an outer heat-sealed pouch with peel-off paper backing.

Plastic bottles

Most commercially prepared eye drops are supplied in plastic dropper bottles similar to the illustration in Figure 42.2. Bottles are made of polyethylene or polypropylene and are sterilized by ionizing radiation prior to filling under aseptic conditions with the previously sterilized preparation.

Glass bottles

Most extemporaneously prepared eye drops are supplied in 10 mL amber partially ribbed glass bottles.

The components of the eye dropper bottle are illustrated in Figure 42.3.

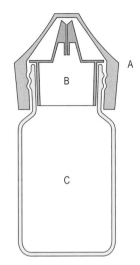

Figure 42.2 • Plastic eye drop bottle. (A) Rigid plastic cap. (B) Polythene friction plug containing baffle that produces uniform drops. (C) Polythene bottle.

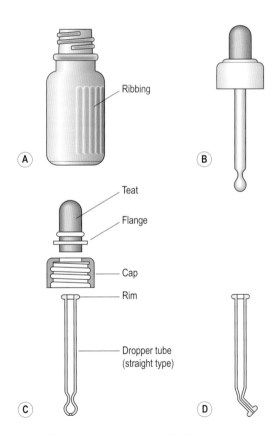

Figure 42.3 • Eye dropper bottle. (A) Bottle. (B) Assembled closure. (C) Components of closure. (D) Dropper tube (angled type).

Bottles can be made of neutral glass and can be autoclaved more than once, or soda glass which has had the internal surfaces treated during manufacture to reduce the release of alkali when in contact with aqueous solutions, but can only be autoclaved once. The teat can be made of good-quality natural or synthetic rubber. The former will withstand autoclaving at 115°C for 30 min but will not withstand the high temperatures of dry-heat sterilization. The latter teats, made from silicone rubber, will withstand dry-heat sterilization and are suitable for use with oily eye drops. Silicone rubber is permeable to water vapour and for this reason aqueous eye drops in bottles having silicone rubber teats are given a limited shelf-life of 3 months. This can be lengthened by supplying the sterile eye drops in an eye drop bottle sealed with an ordinary screw cap together with a separately wrapped and sterilized silicone rubber dropper unit. The dropper is carefully substituted for the cap when the eye drops are about to be used.

Teats and caps are used once only. All components are thoroughly washed with filtered distilled or deionized water, dried and stored in a clean area until required.

Rubber teats sorb preservatives and antioxidants during autoclaving and storage. It is necessary that individual studies are undertaken during formulation to help counteract preservative and antioxidant loss.

Preparation of eye drops

Extemporaneous preparation of eye drops involves the following:
- Preparation of the solution
- Clarification
- Filling and sterilization.

Preparation of the solution

The aqueous eye drop vehicle containing any necessary preservative, antioxidant, stabilizer, tonicity modifier, viscolizer or buffer should be prepared first. Then the active ingredient is added and the vehicle made up to volume.

Clarification

The BP has stringent requirements for the absence of particulate matter in eye drop solutions. Sintered glass filters or membrane filters of 0.45–1.2 μm pore sizes are suitable. The clarified solution is either filled directly into the final containers which are sealed prior to heat sterilization or temporarily filled into a suitable container prior to filtration sterilization. Clarified vehicle is used to prepare eye drop suspensions which are filled into final containers and sealed prior to sterilization.

Sterilization

This can take the form of:
- Autoclaving at 115°C for 30 min or 121°C for 15 min
- Filtration through a membrane filter having a 0.22 μm pore size into sterile containers using strict aseptic technique. Filling should take place under Grade A laminar airflow conditions (see Ch. 46)
- Dry-heat sterilization at 160°C for 2 h is employed for non-aqueous preparations such as liquid paraffin eye drops. Silicone rubber teats must be used.

Immediately following sterilization, the eye drop containers must be covered with a readily breakable seal, such as a viskring, to distinguish between opened and unopened containers.

Labelling of containers

Labelling requirements are summarized in Table 42.1 and Box 42.3.

Instillation of eye drops

Patients who have not used eye drops before need an explanation of how to instil the drops satisfactorily.
- Wash hands
- Tilt head back and with one hand gently pull down lower eyelid to form a pouch between the eye and the eyelid
- Hold dropper bottle (or separate eye dropper containing eye drops) above the eye and drop a single drop into the preformed pouch. Do not touch the dropper on the eye or eyelid. (Using a well illuminated mirror will help.) Administration aids are available to assist the

Table 42.1 Labelling requirements for eye drop and eye ointment containers at the time of dispensing

Requirement	Include on label
State route of administration	'For use in the eye only'
Fully identify the product	The name and concentration of the active ingredient(s)
Statement on preservation	Confirm presence or absence of preservative
Directions for use	e.g. 'Add one drop to each eye morning and evening'
State an 'in use' expiry date	Day, month, year
Storage requirements	'Store in a cool place' or 'Protect from light'
Identify patient	Patient's name
Date of dispensing	Day, month, year

Note: When the stability of the final preparation requires it, eye drops may be provided in two containers as a dry powder and an aqueous vehicle. The labels should state 'Powder for eye drops' on one container and the directions for the preparation of the eye drops on the other package or container.
Based on the Department of Health guidance HSC(IS)122 1975, revised by the Royal Pharmaceutical Society of Great Britain 2001.

Box 42.3

Additional labelling requirements for use in specific locations

All locations

- Name and concentration of any anti microbial present

Hospital: wards

- Patient's name. The eye to be treated. Date of opening bottle and/or date to discard (7 days later)

Hospital: operating theatres

- Single dose for once only use. Marked with indication of active ingredient and concentration. No preservative. Outer package fully labelled

Hospital: clinics

- Single dose or multidose used once only

Domiciliary

- 'Avoid contamination of contents during use'. 'Discard 28 days after opening'. 'Keep out of the reach of children'.

Note: If both eyes are to be treated and the patient has an open infection and/or medical opinion dictates, a separate bottle is supplied for each eye and labelled accordingly.

---

self-administration of eye drops contained in plastic eye dropper bottles

- Release lower lid. Try not to blink more than usual as this removes the medicine from the eye
- Replace the dropper in the bottle or the cap on the bottle.

Formulation of eye lotions

The purpose of eye lotions is to assist in the cleaning of the external surfaces of the eye. This might be to help remove a non-impacted foreign body or to clean away conjunctival discharge. Eye lotions may also be used to impregnate eye dressings. Eye lotions intended for use in surgical or first-aid procedures should not contain antimicrobial preservatives and should be supplied in single-use containers. In keeping with their simple requirements these preparations should have simple formulations and the most common eye lotion consists of sterile normal saline. This preparation typifies the requirements of an eye lotion which are:

- Sterile and usually containing no preservative
- Isotonic with lachrymal fluid
- Neutral pH
- Large volume but not greater than 200 mL
- Non-irritant to ocular tissue.

Labels

These should include:

- Title identifying the product and concentration of contents
- 'Sterile until opened'
- 'Not to be taken'
- 'Use once and discard the remaining solution'
- Expiry date.

Preserved eye lotion would need the additional labelling:

- 'Avoid contamination of contents during use'
- 'Discard remaining solutions not more than 4 weeks after first opening'.

The lotions should be supplied in coloured bottles and sealed to exclude microorganisms.

Powders for the preparation of eye drops and powders for the preparation of eye lotions

These powders are supplied in a dry, sterile form for dissolving or suspending in an appropriate vehicle at the time of use to provide a solution or suspension which complies with the requirements for eye drops or eye lotions as appropriate. The powders may contain suitable excipients to aid dissolution or dispersion, to adjust the tonicity and to improve stability. Unless an exception has been authorized, eye drops in the form of a suspension must pass the same particle size limit test as that applied to the size of particles in eye ointments (see below). In addition, single-dose powders for eye drops and eye lotions should either comply with the test for the uniformity of dosage of the *European Pharmacopoeia* (EP), or where appropriate, with the tests for uniformity of content and/or uniformity of mass.

Formulation of eye ointments

Eye ointments are popular and duplicate many of the therapeutic options offered by eye drops. Ointments have the disadvantage of temporarily interfering with vision, but have the advantage over liquids of providing greater total drug bioavailability. However, ointments take a longer time to reach peak absorption.

Eye ointments must be sterile and may contain suitable antimicrobial preservatives, antioxidants and stabilizers. The *United States Pharmacopoeia* (USP 25) requires these ointments to contain one of the following antimicrobials: chlorobutanol, the parabens or the organic mercurials. In addition such ointments should be free from particulate matter that could be harmful to the tissues of the eye. The EP and BP (2007) have limits for the particle size of incorporated solids. Each $10\,\mu g$ of active solid should have no particles $>90\,\mu m$, not more than 2 particles $>50\,\mu m$ and not more than 20 particles $>25\,\mu m$.

The basic components of an eye ointment are:

Liquid paraffin	1 part
Wool fat	1 part (to facilitate incorporation of water)
Yellow soft paraffin	8 parts

Hard paraffin may be substituted as necessary to maintain an appropriate consistency in hot climates.

Containers for eye ointments

Eye ointments should be supplied in small sterilized collapsible tubes made of metal or a suitable plastic. The tube should not contain more than $10\,g$ of preparation and must be fitted or provided with a nozzle of a suitable shape to facilitate application to the eye and surrounds without allowing contamination of the contents. The tubes must be suitably sealed to prevent microbial contamination.

Preparation of eye ointments

Eye ointments are normally prepared using aseptic techniques to incorporate the previously sterilized finely powdered active ingredient or a sterilized concentrated solution of the medicament into the sterile eye ointment basis. Immediately after preparation, the eye ointment is filled into the sterile containers which are then sealed so as to exclude microorganisms. The screw cap should be covered with a readily breakable seal.

All apparatus used in the preparation of eye ointments must be scrupulously clean and sterile. Certain commercial eye ointments may be sterilized in their final containers using ionizing radiation.

Preparation of eye ointment basis

The paraffins and the wool fat are heated together and filtered, while molten, through a coarse filter paper in a heated funnel into a container which can withstand dry-heat sterilization temperatures. The container is closed to exclude microorganisms and together with contents, is maintained at 160°C for 2 h.

Ophthalmic inserts

These are sterile solid or semi-solid preparations for insertion in the conjunctival sac. They contain a reservoir of active material which is slowly released from a matrix or through a rate-controlling membrane over a known time period. Ophthalmic inserts each have their own sterile container which is labelled to state the total quantity of active substance per insert and, where applicable, its rate of release. The EP requires that in the manufacturing of ophthalmic inserts appropriate product dissolution behaviour is demonstrated.

Monitoring of eye preparations for adverse effects

Pharmacists should be available to counsel patients on the use of their eye medication and advise them about any adverse effects they may experience while using their medicines. Failing to use eye medication appropriately may also have serious consequences. It is important that the pharmacist is able to support the patient in using their medicine correctly. The pharmacist should also be alert to notice any signs/symptoms of adverse effects, that the patient may be experiencing resulting from medication, in order to give appropriate and timely advice. Table 42.2 indicates the signs/symptoms of adverse effects which may occur with eye preparations used in the treatment of primary open angle glaucoma. In addition to adverse effects associated with the eye it should be noted that undesirable

Table 42.2 Signs/symptoms of adverse effects which may occur with treatment for primary open angle glaucoma

Drugs used	General signs/symptoms of adverse effects	
Dose frequency as solutions/suspensions	Objective signs	Subjective signs
Beta-blockers	Blood pressure – hypotension	Difficulties in breathing, dry eyes
Timolol 2 × daily	Heart rate – slowed	Itchy and watery eyes
Timolol gel 1 × daily		Pain after instillation
Betaxolol 2 × daily		Blurring of vision
Carteolol 2 × daily		Palpitations
Levobunolol 1 or 2 × daily		Headaches, dizziness, anxiety
Metipranolol 2 × daily		
Parasympathomimetics (Miotics)	Heart rate – rarely affected	Variable blurring of vision
Pilocarpine 4 × daily		Reduction in night vision
Ocusert-Pilo[a] weekly		Transient headache
A slow-release gel formulation[a] 24-hourly		Ocular and periorbital pain
		Twitching eyelids
		Sweating, gastrointestinal upsets – rare
Sympathomimetics	Heart rate – quickened	Smarting and redness of eye
	Blood pressure – hypertension	Itchy, watery eyes
Adrenaline (epinephrine) 2 × daily	Conjunctival deposits of oxidized adrenaline[b]	Nasal obstruction
Guanethidine 2 × daily	Conjunctival fibrosis on prolonged guanethidine use[b]	Dilated pupil, could precipitate acute glaucoma – dangerous
Dipivefrine[a] 2 × daily		Headache, blurring vision

[a]These formulations can reduce adverse effects.
[b]These are specific effects.

systemic effects can also occur with eye medication. Such systemic effects have been reported for certain potent ophthalmic medicines. This is due to excess solution draining from the eye surface through two small channels, the lachrymal canaliculi, into the lachrymal sac and on via the nasolachrymal duct and the gastrointestinal tract. Consequently, it is necessary to seek to avoid the instilling of excess eye drops.

Patients who are using an eye drop preparation for a chronic condition may become sensitive to the preservative in the formulation. This may happen with contact lens products also. Changing to a formulation having the same active ingredient but having a different or no preservative should solve the problem.

Contact lenses and their solutions

The ready accessibility of the eye and its external structures facilitates the fitting and wearing of lenses on the precorneal film and on the surface of the eye. Optometrists prescribe and fit contact lenses and monitor their use. Pharmacists should refer patients having persistent problems with wearing their lenses to their optometrist.

Popularity, problems, risks

The popularity of contact lenses results from their cosmetic appeal, optical advantages and their usefulness in sporting activities. Many prefer extended-wear soft lenses to daily-wear soft and hard lenses because of their relative convenience.

The problems that occur with the wearing of contact lenses result from inadequate education of the wearer about lens care. Extended-wear lenses in particular have been marketed in a manner which maximizes the volume of sales at the expense of adequate consumer education. That is, the marketing of lenses has overemphasized the convenient and carefree aspects of overnight lenses to the extent of trivializing the wearing of contact lenses. This has often resulted in poor patient compliance with suggested regimes of lens wear and care. It is estimated that more than 50% of those who wear contact lenses care for them unhygienically.

The risks associated with the wearing of contact lenses include recurrent corneal abrasions, corneal scarring and corneal vascularization. However, the most serious complication is microbial ulcerative keratitis or corneal ulcer, caused by microbial invasion of the cornea. Left untreated this can lead to loss of vision. Fortunately, the natural defences of the cornea are very effective and the normal cornea resists microbial infection as long as the surface epithelium is intact.

It has been shown that the risk of corneal ulcers is 9–15 times greater for extended-wear lenses worn overnight than for daily-wear soft lenses worn only during the day. The risk increases with the number of consecutive days that lenses are worn without removal.

A serious, but fairly rare, complication that can arise from using non-sterile water in the care of lenses is infection with the free-living opportunistic pathogen *Acanthamoeba*. This is found in most soil and water habitats. *Acanthamoeba* keratitis is hard to diagnose and to treat and can lead to serious loss of vision. *Acanthamoeba* infection has also resulted from wearing soft lenses while bathing in a Jacuzzi; consequently this practice is contraindicated.

The aim of formulators and providers of contact lens systems must be to supply the safest possible system with known and acceptable risks; that is, both convenience and safety must be the aim.

Relevant properties of the eye

Anatomy and physiology

Figure 42.1 indicates the structures of the eye which are particularly relevant to the use of topical medications, contact lenses and contact lens products. First, it is important to note that the cornea, the lens and the humour compartments are avascular and that this property facilitates the transmission of light and vision. Second, exchange of nutrients and waste products in these situations takes place almost entirely by diffusion processes through the aqueous humour, through the lens and cornea and through the lachrymal fluid. Contact lenses reduce the diffusion of oxygen to the cornea and thus can affect corneal metabolism.

Secretions

The secretions of the eye have an important role and influence on the wearing of contact lenses. Lachrymal fluid, commonly known as tears, performs the important functions of lubricating, hydrating, cleaning and disinfecting the anterior surface of the eye. The latter function is performed by the enzyme lysozyme (1,4-*N*-acetylglycosaminidase) which catalyses the hydrolysis of 1,4-glycosidic linkages between *N*-acetyl muramic acid and *N*-acetyl-glucosamine in the peptidoglycan layer of the bacterial cell wall. The peptidoglycan layer of Gram-positive cells is accessible to the action of lysozyme.

The fluid forming the precorneal film is produced by differing groups of glands. It contains mucus (Henle and Manz), water (Krause and Wolfring) and oil (Meibomian, Moll and Zeis). These fluids are stratified in three distinct layers. The surface-active mucoid layer spreads on the corneal surface and associates with the intermediate aqueous layer externally. The aqueous layer is surfaced with an oily layer which lubricates and protects the mucous membranes of the internal lid surfaces.

Tear electrolyte content

This is broadly similar to that of serum except that the potassium ion is approximately four to six times greater (24 mEq/L compared with 4–6 mEq/L in serum). The protein content of tears is mainly albumin and globulin and is approximately a tenth of that in serum (0.7% compared with 7%).

Tear production

Tears are produced by the lachrymal glands in response to four distinct types of stimuli: emotional via psychological factors, sensory via external irritants, continuous via automatic nervous control and systemic via chemicals in the bloodstream affecting the nerves innervating the lachrymal glands.

Tear pH

This is slightly alkaline at 7.2. Tears have sufficient buffering capacity to adjust rapidly the pH of small volumes of weakly buffered solutions to pH 7.2.

Eyelids

These perform a protecting and a cleaning function. The outer margins of the eyelids close slightly before the inner margins and sweep the fluids across the eye towards the lachrymal canaliculi at the inner angle of the eye from where it can pass via the lachrymal sac into the nasal cavity and gastrointestinal tract. Systemic absorption of excess eye medicament may take place through this mechanism.

Bacterial flora

There is a common misconception that lachrymal fluid is sterile. It has been known since 1908 that staphylococci and diphtheroids can be found regularly in normal conjunctiva. Gram-negative enteric bacilli have also been isolated from the conjunctivas and lids of about 5% of people. This shows that care is necessary when wearing contact lenses to avoid abrading the corneal epithelium.

Contact lenses

Sir John Herschel used a refractive glass shell in 1823 to protect the cornea from a diseased lid. Dr Eugen Fickfirst used the term 'contact lens' in 1887. Fick's blown glass lenses were intended to correct defective vision. In 1948, Tuohy introduced the hydrophobic hard plastic corneal lens and in 1962, soft pliable lenses were introduced as the result of work in Prague University. These lenses have been very popular. Gas-permeable hard lenses have also been introduced which allow oxygen perfusion to the cornea. These lenses are more comfortable than the original hard lenses. The first extended-wear lenses were introduced in 1981.

The aim in making contact lenses is to produce lenses which will:

- Correct the patient's vision
- Maintain their position on the eye
- Allow respiration of the cornea
- Permit free flow of tears round or through the lens
- Not release toxic substances
- Not introduce microbial contamination
- Be wearable throughout the day
- Be easy to handle and economical to use.

Hard lenses

Polymethylmethacrylate (PMMA) or 'Perspex' has optical properties similar to spectacle crown glass. PMMA has hydrophobic properties conferred by the large proportion of methyl groups compared with hydrophilic carboxy ester groups. This means that lachrymal fluid does not readily wet lenses made of this material. Therefore, the lenses need to be wetted before mounting on the precorneal film to reduce or eliminate patient discomfort. Hence the need for a wetting solution to facilitate wear and the need for a storage, hydrating, decontaminating solution to facilitate care of the lenses when not being worn. The original hard lens composition had some major disadvantages for the wearer. Free passage of oxygen and carbon dioxide to and from the corneal epithelium could not take place. Corneal oedema and distortion were a common result. Thus, modern lenses have been designed to be gas permeable. These lenses are physiologically more user-friendly and have greater wearer acceptance.

The original gas-permeable lenses consisted of cellulose acetate butyrate (CAB), which was readily wettable and proved quite acceptable. More recently, lenses based on silicone and fluorine have been produced which have greater gas permeability. Silicone methacrylate copolymers are very popular. The silicone composition controls the permeability properties and the PMMA composition controls the degree of rigidity. Similarly, fluorosilicone methacrylate copolymers, which have very high oxygen permeability properties and good wetting properties, are proving to be popular. These gas-permeable lenses are cared for using hard lens solutions. These lenses are less subject than soft lenses to deposits of lipids, protein and other substances from the lachrymal fluid. They also have better optical qualities and are generally easier to care for.

Soft lenses

Soft lenses are made from the hydroxyethyl ester of polymethacrylic acid (poly-HEMA). The large number of polar hydroxyl groups confers hydrophilic properties to the polymer. Poly-HEMA is flexible and can absorb about 47% of its own weight of water. Thus, lenses of this material are comfortable and easy to wear but more difficult to care for than hard lenses. A particular problem is uptake of antibacterial preservatives and subsequent release and irritancy during wear. Although a wetting solution is not needed, cleaning, storing, hydrating and decontaminating functions are required of solutions.

Copolymers of poly-HEMA with vinylpyrrolidine (VP) are also produced which can absorb up to 80% by weight of water depending on the

HEMA/VP ratio. The higher water content lenses have the advantage of greater gas permeability and comfort than the poly-HEMA lenses which may occasionally cause corneal oedema. However, they are more fragile and difficult to care for than poly-HEMA, have a greater tendency to attract deposits, more solution problems and less precise optical properties.

Disposable lenses

Disposable lenses may be discarded after 1 month, 1 week or even 1 day. The latter would obviate the need for the use of solutions and theoretically increase the safety and acceptability of lens wear. However, the original intention of these lenses was for extended wear without removal. It has already been pointed out that the additional risks that are associated with extended wear makes this unattractive and even a dangerous practice. These lenses would seem to offer the greatest advantage to those people who wear lenses on an irregular basis for social and sporting activities and for those children who may need soft lenses.

Hard lens solutions

A 'wetting solution' and a 'soaking/storing/decontaminating solution' are required for the wear and routine care of hard lenses. The first is suitable for placing in the eye but the second must not have contact with the eye.

Wetting solution

Purpose

- Achieves rapid wetting by the lachrymal fluid and thus promotes comfort
- Facilitates insertion of lens
- Provides cushioning and lubrication
- Enables cleaning after removal
- Must be non-irritant during daily use.

Formulation

- Wetting and viscolizing agents – polyvinyl alcohol and hypromellose
- Viscosity 15–20 mPas for comfort

- pH 6.8
- Tonicity 0.9–1.1% sodium chloride
- Antimicrobials – benzalkonium chloride 0.004% plus disodium edetate 0.1%.

Storing solutions

Purpose

- Achieves cleaning and microbial inactivation
- Hydrating.

Formulation

- Surface-active agent not inactivating antimicrobials
- pH 7.4
- Antimicrobials – benzalkonium chloride 0.01% plus disodium edetate 0.1%.

Soft lens solutions

Cleaning solutions

Purpose

- To remove deposits such as lipoprotein adhering to the lens after wear.

Formulation

- Viscolizing surface-active agent such as hypromellose to enable suitable gentle friction with fingertips
- Antibacterial – fast-acting benzalkonium chloride 0.004% may be used if contact time is only 20–30 s.

Storing solutions

Purpose

- Hydrating
- Cleaning
- Inactivation of microbial contamination.

Formulation

- Isotonic≡0.9% w/v sodium chloride
- Antibacterial.

Hydrogen peroxide – was introduced into commercially available care systems in 1984. Hydrogen peroxide is a powerful oxidizer and this is the source of its antimicrobial activity. It has good activity against *Acanthamoeba*.

$$2H_2O_2 > 2H_2O + O_2 + Energy$$

Decomposition is more rapid at alkaline than acid pH and many substances catalyse the reaction. These properties are utilized in the formulation of storage, disinfecting and cleaning solutions. For example, a solution containing 3% hydrogen peroxide at acid pH is used to disinfect lenses over a period of 6 h. This is then followed by suitable inactivation with sodium pyruvate, platinum or the enzyme catalase, to facilitate subsequent safe wearing of the lenses. The procedure is referred to as the two-step system because a separate neutralization step follows the disinfecting step. One-step systems have also been developed for greater patient convenience. The inactivating substance is incorporated with the 3% hydrogen peroxide and the lenses in the disinfecting solution. This system needs to be calibrated to slowly neutralize hydrogen peroxide, but to allow it to have antimicrobial activity over a 6 h period to ensure effectiveness against *Acanthamoeba* cysts. Some commercial systems may neutralize the effect of the hydrogen peroxide over a period of 30 min or so, which is too rapid to guarantee effectiveness.

Polyquad – a polyquaternium compound is used as an antimicrobial in soft lens solutions because it is not sorbed by lenses and it has low toxicity to corneal and ocular tissues.

(Thermal disinfection is an alternative disinfection process and the American FDA stipulates heating the lenses in a suitable solution in a lens case at a minimum of 80°C for 10 min. Heating reduces the life of the lens and it is also inconvenient.)

Enzyme protein digest

Purpose

- Occasional cleaning procedure followed by suitable washing and cleansing before wear. Frequency will vary with the individual and his/her state of health. Influenza or hay fever, for example, will increase the need.

Formulation

- Proteolytic enzyme, such as papain, as a solution tablet to produce a suitable solution when dissolved in a stated volume of sterile aqueous vehicle.

Lipid digest or combined protein and lipid digest systems are also available.

All-purpose solutions

The all-purpose solutions initially represented a compromise for hard lens wearers finding it difficult to comply with a two-solution regimen. Single-solution lens care systems are now widely available for use with soft lenses, which incorporate an enzyme cleaner combined with a disinfection solution. For example, the serine protease subtilisin A, obtained from the bacterium *Bacillus subtilis*, is used in the presence of hydrogen peroxide to remove protein contamination from contact lenses. Certain all-purpose lens solutions incorporate polyhexamide (polyhexamethylene biguanide) 0.00006–0.0004% as the antimicrobial agent. It is reported to be active against a wide range of bacteria and against *Acanthamoeba*.

All-purpose solutions for soft lenses have become very popular.

Containers

Contact lens solutions are usually packed in plastic containers. It is imperative that the low concentrations of antimicrobials present in these products are not reduced to ineffective levels due to sorption effects with the plastic.

Contact lens storage cases are also of importance to the contact lens wearer. It is important that these containers are kept in a hygienic condition by keeping them scrupulously clean and using the disinfecting/storage solutions strictly in accordance with the manufacturers' instructions. Storage cases should be changed periodically.

Advice to patients

General considerations

Contact lens wearers presenting at the pharmacy with a persistent red eye indicating an infection should not be recommended antibacterial eye drops. They should be referred to an ophthalmologist. This is to guard against the possibility that the person has an infection with *Acanthamoeba*. Such an infection would be more difficult to diagnose after partial treatment.

Disease states leading to a dry eye syndrome such as Sjögren syndrome, which is mostly confined to menopausal women having osteoarthritis, will also adversely affect the ability of a person to wear contact lenses.

Hard lenses and to a lesser extent soft lenses interrupt the oxygen supply to the cornea and with prolonged wear produce increasing hypoxia. After approximately 16 h of wear, this corneal hypoxia results in a dip in the corneal glycogen level with resultant oedema. Irritation, itchiness, photophobia and blurred vision can result. The patient should be advised not to over-wear the lenses and they may also be recommended to instil sterile sodium chloride 2% w/v every 3–4 h, after the lenses have been removed, until the oedema has resolved. They should be warned that the hypertonic drops may cause temporary stinging on instillation.

Adverse effects of medicines

Pharmacists should be aware that many medicines taken systemically can also cause problems for wearers of contact lenses and be prepared to offer appropriate counselling.

Certain medicines can affect the eye surface and lachrymal fluid production and thereby influence the comfort of contact lens wear. Medication having anticholinergic properties such as sedative antihistamines, chlorphenamine, antispasmodics, hyoscine, tricyclic antidepressants and neuroleptics can all reduce lachrymal fluid production. Diuretics will also reduce tear volume and topical timolol can cause transitory dry eyes. The consequent lack of lubrication may cause lens discomfort and increased lens deposits.

Oral contraceptives may cause corneal oedema, decreased aqueous and increased mucus and protein production and thus lead to lens intolerance. Pregnancy may also be associated with increased lens awareness and discomfort possibly associated with reduced tear flow and changes in corneal thickness and the curvature of the eye. Clomifene and primidone have also been reported to cause lid and corneal oedema.

Cholinergic drugs and also ephedrine and reserpine will increase tear volume. Aspirin produces low concentrations of salicylic acid in the lachrymal fluid. This can be absorbed by soft lenses and subsequently cause irritation. Isotretinoin may cause conjunctival inflammation and consequently cause discomfort to contact lens wearers.

Discolouration, via the lachrymal fluid, particularly with soft lenses, may occur with the administration of certain medicines such as labetalol, nitrofurantoin, phenothiazines, phenolphthalein, rifampicin, sulfasalazine and tetracyclines. Rifampicin for example will stain the lenses and tears orange.

Lenses must be removed before diagnostic dyes such as fluorescein are instilled. In fact it is a general rule that patients should be counselled not to place any ophthalmic preparation on to the eyelids or surface of the eye, while contact lenses are in place. Certain eye drops may be instilled while hard lenses are being worn. Sterile 'Comfort drops' may be instilled while lenses are being worn to help maintain the hydration and lubrication of the eye surfaces and lenses when required. Numerous commercial solutions are available. The basic requirements are that the drops should be isotonic, have good wetting properties and be slightly viscous.

Concurrent use of cosmetics

Soft lenses should always be inserted before applying eye makeup but rigid gas-permeable lenses may be put on after. All lenses should be put on before applying nail polish, hand creams, perfumes or using nail polish remover. Aerosol products should be used with caution so that spray does not get between the lens and the eye. All eye makeup should be water based and powders should be avoided. Mascara (not waterproof) should only be applied to the tips of the eyelashes.

The pharmacist should be aware of the various situations mentioned above when offering advice and discussing customers'/patients' questions.

KEY POINTS

- Ophthalmic preparations must be sterile
- Eye drops may be solutions, suspensions or emulsions and contain:
  - Active ingredient
  - Liquid vehicle free from particulate matter; particle size limits for suspensions

- Antimicrobial preservative
- Adjuvants: tonicity, viscosity, buffering, antioxidants, chelating, dispersing, emulsifying
- Eye drops are contained in a glass or plastic bottle
- Eye lotions are:
  - Isotonic
  - Neutral pH
  - Large volume but not greater than 200 mL
  - Non-irritant
  - Contained in a fluted, coloured bottle
- Eye ointments contain:
  - Semi-solid base
  - Active ingredient
  - Antimicrobial preservative
  - Adjuvants: antioxidants, stabilizers
- Eye ointments are:
  - Free from harmful particulate matter; particle size limits
  - Contained in a metal or plastic tube
- Ophthalmic inserts:
  - Contain a reservoir of active material
  - Incorporate a slow-release mechanism
- Properties of the eye affecting formulation of products include:
  - Anatomy and physiology
  - Secretions
  - Lids
  - Bacterial flora
- Contact lenses may be:
  - Hard lenses including gas permeable
  - Soft lenses including disposable
- Contact lens solutions may be:
  - Hard lenses – (i) wetting and cleaning; (ii) storing and disinfecting or (iii) all purpose
  - Soft lenses – (i) cleaning; (ii) storing and disinfecting or (iii) all purpose
- Enzyme cleaning agents are required for all lenses
- Pharmacists should be able to counsel patients on:
  - Possible adverse effects of eye medication
  - Common problems encountered by lens wearers
  - Adverse effects of concurrent medications
  - Concurrent use of cosmetics

Inhaled route

Peter M. Richards

STUDY POINTS

- The rationale for using the inhaled route
- The appropriate use of the most widely prescribed inhaled medicines
- The role of the peak flow meter
- The different types of inhaler, and inhaler technique
- Nebulized therapy

The role of the pharmacist

Inhaled products are specialized dosage forms, which are designed to deliver medicines directly to the lung. A variety of inhaler devices are in use, all of which require the user of the inhaler to adopt an appropriate inhaler technique. Failure to use the correct inhaler technique will result in treatment failure. The pharmacist, who is usually the person who gives (dispenses) the inhaler to the patient, is ideally placed to demonstrate the appropriate inhalation technique for that inhaler. Using an inhaler is a skill, subject to the development of 'bad habits', which can lead to poor technique. Inhaler technique should therefore be regularly checked to ensure that the technique is optimal; again the pharmacist is ideally placed to perform this function.

Pharmacists can also provide education to patients beyond a discussion of a patient's inhalers and other medicines, to include education about the patient's disease (e.g. asthma) and its management. Pharmacists also run asthma clinics and may do so as supplementary or independent prescribers. A few pharmacists have specialist respiratory consultant posts in secondary care. A pharmacist wishing to undertake a specialist role in respiratory medicine will need to gain appropriate experience and undertake further training.

This chapter describes the most frequently prescribed inhaled therapies in the context of asthma and chronic obstructive pulmonary disease (COPD). The most widely prescribed inhaler devices are outlined along with instructions in their use.

Introduction

Many patients on inhaled therapy will be using more than one inhaler and may also have been prescribed a peak flow meter (PFM) to aid in monitoring their condition. In order for pharmacists to be able to provide useful education and advice to these patients, pharmacists will need to understand the condition being treated and the role of the medicines and devices prescribed. This chapter will provide that understanding in the context of the two most common airways diseases treated with inhaled medicines, namely asthma and COPD. It is beyond the scope of the chapter to discuss the diseases themselves, or the role of oral therapy and non-drug management of these conditions. It should be remembered that the most important interventions in COPD are smoking cessation and pulmonary rehabilitation.

There are significant differences in the way that inhalers are prescribed for asthma and COPD. In COPD, the emphasis of treatment is on the use of bronchodilators, and it may be appropriate for a COPD patient to have a long-acting inhaled beta-agonist without an inhaled steroid. This is different from asthma treatment where a long-acting beta-agonist should always be prescribed with an inhaled steroid. The scope of this chapter is limited to commonly used inhaled treatments and devices used for these inhaled treatments. By being familiar with national treatment guidelines for asthma and COPD, pharmacists can be assured that the advice that they give patients is likely to be consistent with that given by other healthcare professionals. These guidelines are: BTS/SIGN Asthma Guideline, 2011 (January 2012 revision): http://www.brit-thoracic.org.uk/guidelines/asthma-guidelines.aspx and NICE CG101 Chronic Obstructive Pulmonary Disease: http://guidance.nice.org.uk/CG101/NICEGuidance/pdf/English.

Asthma is a very common condition in the UK, affecting at least 5% of adults and up to 10% of children; therefore many people will experience symptoms attributable to asthma at some time in their life.

COPD has been an under-publicized condition. Prevalence of COPD in the UK is thought to be 2–4% of the total population with 1.5% of the population with diagnosed COPD. The decline in lung function leading to COPD is age-related but this decline can be rapidly accelerated in some smokers. COPD is thus an increasing problem in an ageing population.

Asthma and COPD are not mutually exclusive and some patients will have features of both diseases; this is often referred to as 'mixed disease'. The prevalence of asthma, COPD and related conditions means that pharmacists will not only frequently encounter patients on inhaled therapy during dispensing, but will also encounter patients on inhaled therapy when giving advice on the sale of over-the-counter medicines.

The inhaled route

The inhaled route delivers medicines to the lungs. Inhaled medicines may have a local effect on the lungs or may be absorbed to give a systemic effect. The inhaled route is generally used when the lung is the target organ, e.g.:

- The antibiotic colistimethate sodium is nebulized to treat lung infections associated with cystic fibrosis
- The antiviral zanamivir is presented as a dry-powder inhaler for treating influenza.

Using the inhaled route when the lung is the target organ has a number of advantages:

- A smaller dose can be used. The normal adult oral dose of salbutamol is 4 mg, but the normal inhaled dose of salbutamol is 200 µg
- The risk of unwanted systemic effects is reduced
- A faster onset of action may be achieved with some drugs, e.g. salbutamol
- Topically active drugs with poor oral bioavailability can be used.

The main disadvantage of the inhaled route is that inhaling a drug is more difficult than swallowing a tablet. Some drugs are ineffective by the inhaled route, e.g. theophylline.

Using the inhaled route does not result in the entire quantity of drug in the inhaler device reaching the lung. Even if an inhaler device is used perfectly, it is unlikely that any more than 20% of the drug reaches the lung. The majority of the rest of the drug remains in the oropharynx and is normally swallowed.

The lungs are designed to prevent the inhalation of anything other than gas. However, particles with a diameter of approximately 5 µm can be inhaled and have sufficient mass to settle in the lung. Particles larger than 10 µm remain in the oropharynx. Particles smaller than 1 µm are inhaled, but are then exhaled. Decreasing particle size increases the chance of penetration further down the tracheobronchial tree. It may be that a particle needs to be less than 3 µm to reach the 8th to 23rd branch generation. These particle sizes apply to the adult lung, and a smaller particle size of the order of 2.5 µm may be optimal in infant lungs.

The specific target in the lung for medicines used in asthma and COPD is the bronchiole. Branching from bronchi, bronchioles are the first airways in the lung not to contain cartilage and are less than 1 mm in diameter. The absence of cartilage means that smooth muscle contraction reduces the size of the airway. Inflammation also results in reduction in size of the airway (Fig. 43.1).

Inhaled medicines used for asthma and COPD

Short-acting beta$_2$ agonists (SABAs)

Salbutamol and terbutaline are widely used SABAs. They act on beta$_2$ receptors in the smooth muscle

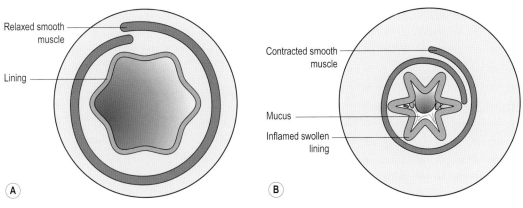

Figure 43.1 • Airways obstruction in asthma. (A) Unobstructed airway. (B) Obstructed airway.

of bronchioles to reverse bronchospasm. Symptoms caused by bronchospasm include wheeze, coughing, breathlessness and a feeling of tightness of the chest. For this reason, SABAs are often referred to as 'relievers' and should be used 'as required' to relieve symptoms. If a reliever inhaler is required for asthma more than twice a week most weeks, the addition of a 'preventer' (usually a steroid) inhaler should be considered.

Points to note

- The inhaler itself is not dangerous – but asthma is potentially life-threatening
- Appropriate, 'as required' use of a reliever inhaler provides a useful marker of the severity of the condition
- Frequent usage of a reliever inhaler may indicate severe uncontrolled asthma
- There is no risk that using the reliever inhaler whenever needed will result in a diminishing response, but worsening asthma will not respond to a reliever inhaler alone – additional treatment is required
- If the reliever inhaler is not relieving symptoms, urgent medical attention is required
- If reliever inhaler usage has increased, or is being used more than twice a week most weeks, review of treatment is required
- The reliever inhaler can be used immediately before sport/exercise to prevent exercise-induced asthma in susceptible individuals
- A reliever inhaler is normally blue.

Unwanted effects of inhaled beta$_2$ agonists are rare but tremor can occur.

SABAs are also prescribed for symptom relief in COPD.

Short-acting muscarinic antagonists (SAMAs)

The most commonly prescribed SAMA is ipratropium. Smooth muscle relaxation is achieved by opposing the parasympathetic nervous system. Ipratropium's role in COPD is now limited to being an alternative to salbutamol for as required relief of symptoms.

Long-acting beta$_2$ agonists (LABAs)

Salmeterol, formoterol and indacaterol are inhaled LABAs. Salmeterol and formoterol are licensed for use in both asthma and COPD and are used twice daily. Indacaterol is licensed for COPD only and is used once daily. These inhalers are sometimes referred to as 'protectors'.

Points to note

- LABAs should be used regularly and not on an 'as required' basis
- A reliever inhaler (SABA in asthma) should be used to relieve breakthrough symptoms
- For asthma, inhaled steroids (preventer inhalers) should be continued
- For COPD it is appropriate to use a LABA without concomitant inhaled steroids

For COPD, a long-acting bronchodilator is the next step to a short-acting bronchodilator. A SABA (or SAMA) will also be required to relieve breakthrough symptoms.

Long-acting muscarinic antagonists (LAMAs)

Tiotropium bromide, glycopyrronium bromide and aclidinium bromide are inhaled LAMAs indicated for maintenance bronchodilator therapy in COPD. They are not licensed for asthma.

Inhaled corticosteroids (ICS)

The anti-inflammatory actions of steroids are able to control the inflammatory processes in asthma. No steroid inhaler is licensed for use in COPD. Two combination inhalers (LABA + ICS) at specific doses are licensed for COPD.

The inhaled route allows small doses of steroid to be used, minimizing the risk of systemic effects. The ideal inhaled steroid's properties would include:

- Poor absorption from the gastrointestinal tract to minimize systemic effects due to the swallowed portion
- Complete metabolism in the 'first pass' through the liver
- High topical activity
- Metabolism in the lung to inactive metabolites (absorption from the lung circumvents the 'first pass' through the liver).

Using a spacer device with the steroid inhaler, and/or rinsing the mouth with water and spitting immediately after using the inhaled steroid may reduce systemic effects and unwanted local effects in the mouth and throat.

Beclomethasone, budesonide, fluticasone ciclesonide and mometasone are examples of inhaled steroids. They are used once or twice daily depending on their license. Inhaled steroids are often referred to as 'preventers'.

Inhaled steroids should normally be introduced:

- After a severe exacerbation of asthma
- If an asthmatic is using his short-acting beta$_2$ agonist more than twice a week
- If asthma is causing waking one night a week or more.

The above measures form the basis for assessing control of asthma; in addition, limitation of exercise due to asthmatic symptoms and measures of lung function can be considered.

Points to note

- Inhaled steroids should be used regularly, not on an 'as required' basis
- Inhaled steroids have no immediate effect
- Improved asthma control will take a minimum of 1–3 days, and it may be 14–28 days before maximum improvement is seen after starting or increasing the dose of inhaled steroid
- Steroid inhalers are normally brown, orange or maroon.

Unwanted systemic effects of inhaled steroids are extremely rare provided that the total daily dose is less than the equivalent of 800–1000 µg beclomethasone dipropionate.

Unwanted local effects of inhaled steroids include:

- Oral candidiasis (thrush)
- Dysphonia.

Combination LABA/ICS inhalers

There are a number of different combinations presented in a variety of inhaler devices, these include:

- Salmeterol + fluticasone, three strength combinations as a metered dose inhaler (MDI) and three strength combinations as a dry powder inhaler (DPI)
- Formoterol + budesonide, three strength combinations as a DPI
- Formoterol + beclomethasone, one strength combination as a MDI
- Formoterol + fluticasone, three strength combinations as a MDI

In general, these combination inhalers are used as regular preventative therapy with the dose adjusted to achieve long-term control of asthma; a short-acting beta agonist inhaler being used for control of breakthrough symptoms. However, a budesonide 200 µg/formoterol 6 µg dry powder inhaler has been granted a licence for preventer (maintenance) and reliever use for asthma. Thus, some asthmatics who are using a budesonide 200 µg/formoterol 6 µg inhaler may only need to have one inhaler. A budesonide 200 µg/formoterol 6 µg inhaler can only be used for relief of symptoms if also being used as a regular preventer.

It is not licensed for use before exercise to prevent exercise-induced asthma; an additional short-acting beta$_2$ agonist should be used for this purpose.

Fluticasone 500 µg/salmeterol 50 µg dry powder inhaler and budesonide 400 µg/formoterol 12 µg dry powder inhaler, twice daily, are licensed for patients with COPD whose forced expiratory volume in 1 s (FEV$_1$) is less than 50–60% predicted and who are frequent exacerbators (two or more exacerbations per year).

The peak flow meter

The peak flow meter (PFM) is a simple inexpensive device, prescribable on the NHS, which gives a useful objective measure of airways obstruction. A peak flow meter and its correct use is illustrated in Figure 43.2. The PFM measures peak expiratory flow rate (PEFR). PEFR is expressed in litres per minute (L/min). Flow rate of gas through a tube is proportional to the diameter of the tube when the pressure exerted on the gas is constant. Thus, the maximum rate at which individuals can expel air from their lungs is proportional to the patency of the tubes in their lungs. A reduced PEFR indicates that there is obstruction to airflow in the lungs.

Asthmatics will obtain useful information about their condition by using the PFM twice daily and charting their results for 2–4 weeks in the following situations:

- To confirm a diagnosis of asthma (a diurnal variation of PEFR of more than 20% is characteristic of asthma)
- To establish the level of control of asthma on current therapy
- To track improvement of control of asthma following the introduction of a new treatment
- To ensure asthma control is maintained when treatment is stepped down
- As an aid to self-management of asthma.

Normal values are available for PEFR in graph or chart form or on 'wheels'. In adults, normal values for PEFR vary by age, sex and height; for children, PEFR varies just by height. Normal or average values of PEFR are just that and values of 50–100 L/min above or below a predicted value fall within the normal range. An increase of at least 20% in PEFR following the use of an inhaled short-acting beta$_2$ agonist such as salbutamol is diagnostic of asthma. This is known as a reversibility test.

1 Set marker to zero
2 Stand up, hold PFM horizontally, avoiding touching or blocking the movement of the marker
3 Breathe in deeply then blow into the PFM as fast and hard as possible
4 Note reading, reset marker and repeat twice
5 The peak flow is the highest of the three readings

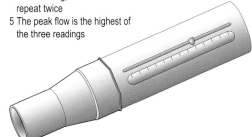

Figure 43.2 • The correct use of a peak flow meter (PFM).

The PFM is of less value in COPD as the airways obstruction tends to be fixed rather than variable, and lung volumes may be more important. Spirometry, which measures FEV$_1$ and forced vital capacity (FVC), is a more useful test of lung function in COPD.

Types of inhaler device

Aerosol inhalers

Metered dose inhaler (MDI)

An MDI (Fig. 43.3) delivers an aerosol of drug dissolved or suspended in a propellant. Immediately an MDI is actuated, some of the propellant rapidly evaporates to produce droplets of appropriate size to be inhaled into the lung. Further evaporation of propellant may occur in the mouth and the so-called 'cold-freon effect' occurs if there is further evaporation of propellant (freon) when the aerosol impacts on the back of the throat. The sensation produced by the cold-freon effect can be sufficient in a minority of individuals to stop the inhalation and means that these individuals cannot use MDIs. The propellants currently used are generally hydrofluoroalkanes (HFAs). Chlorofluoroalkanes, also known as chlorofluorocarbons (CFCs), were formerly used as propellants, but are now banned by international treaty because of their ozone-depleting properties. It should perhaps be noted that while HFAs do not have the ozone-depleting

Physical components

Formulation

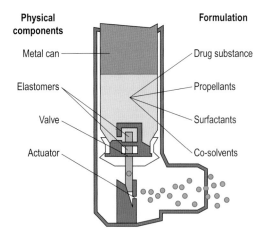

- Metal can — Drug substance
- Elastomers — Propellants
- Valve — Surfactants
- Actuator — Co-solvents

Figure 43.3 • The main elements of a metered dose inhaler.

effects of CFCs, both CFCs and HFAs are 'greenhouse' gases.

Surfactants such as oleic acid and co-solvents such as ethanol may be used to facilitate the production of an appropriate suspension or solution of drug in propellant.

The propellants, which are gases at room temperature, are maintained as liquids by filling under pressure into the metal aerosol canister.

A metered dose is achieved by having an appropriate size reservoir in the valve, which fills by gravity as the valve re-seats after each actuation.

The correct method of using an MDI is shown in Figure 43.4.

Common errors in using an MDI include:

- Inability to coordinate actuation of the inhaler with inspiration
- Taking a short, sharp inspiration, instead of a long, steady inspiration (this is often at least in part due to not exhaling before using the inhaler)
- Actuating the inhaler twice (or more) on one inspiration.

Breath-actuated MDI

Inhaling through a breath-actuated MDI triggers a mechanism that 'fires' (actuates) the aerosol. These inhalers are particularly useful for those patients who have difficulty coordinating inspiration with actuation of the MDI.

Easi-Breathe® is a type of breath-actuated MDI; its correct use is shown in Figure 43.5.

Autohaler® is another breath-actuated MDI. Using an Autohaler® is essentially the same as using

HOW TO USE A METERED DOSE INHALER

1 Shake the inhaler then remove cap
2 Breathe out slowly and gently
3 Place the mouthpiece in your mouth
4 When you start to breathe in, press down on the canister and continue to breathe in deeply and slowly
5 Hold your breath for 10–15 seconds
6 Remove the mouthpiece from your mouth, then breathe out
7 For a further dose, repeat steps 1 to 6 after a 30 second wait
8 Replace the cap and store in a cool place

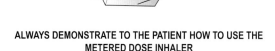

A Metered Dose Inhaler

ALWAYS DEMONSTRATE TO THE PATIENT HOW TO USE THE METERED DOSE INHALER

Figure 43.4 • How to use a metered dose inhaler.
(*Source*: Education for Health).

an Easi-Breathe® except that the Autohaler® is primed by raising a lever on the top of the inhaler, whereas the Easi-Breathe® is primed by opening the mouthpiece cover.

Common errors when using a breath-actuated MDI include:

- Not achieving a sufficiently high inspiratory flow rate to actuate the device
- Stopping inhaling immediately the inhaler actuates.

MDI + spacer

A chamber device (spacer) may be attached to an MDI (Fig. 43.6).

A spacer consists of a plastic chamber with a port at one end for the MDI and in most cases a one-way valve and mouthpiece at the other end.

An MDI + spacer is best used by firing a single dose from the MDI; inhalation should then start as soon as possible.

A spacer may be used with an MDI for the following reasons:

- To overcome difficulty in coordinating inspiration with actuation of the MDI, as

HOW TO USE THE EASI-BREATHE®

1 Shake the inhaler then open the cap
2 Breathe out slowly and gently
3 Place the mouthpiece in your mouth and close your mouth tightly around it
4 Keeping the inhaler upright, breathe in slowly and deeply. Don't stop breathing in when the inhaler 'puffs'.
5 Hold your breathe for 10–15 seconds, then remove mouthpiece
6 For a further dose, repeat steps 1–5 after a 30 second wait
7 Replace cap and store in a cool place

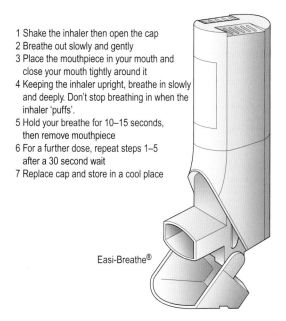

Easi-Breathe®

ALWAYS DEMONSTRATE TO THE PATIENT HOW TO USE THE EASI-BREATHE®

Figure 43.5 • How to use the Easi-Breathe®.
(*Source*: Education for Health.)

HOW TO USE A SPACER DEVICE e.g. VOLUMATIC®

Single breath technique

1 Shake the inhaler and remove the cap
2 Insert the inhaler into the device
3 Place the mouthpiece of the device into your mouth
4 To release a dose of the drug, press down once on the canister
5 Breathe in slowly and deeply
6 Hold your breath for about 10 seconds, then breathe out into the mouthpiece of the device
7 Breathe in again, then remove the mouthpiece from your mouth
8 For a further dose, repeat steps 1–7, after a 30 second wait

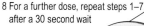
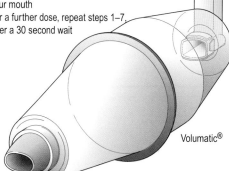

Volumatic®

ALWAYS DEMONSTRATE TO THE PATIENT HOW TO USE THE SPACER DEVICE

Figure 43.6 • How to use a spacer device, e.g. Volumatic®. Method for patients who can use the device without help.
(*Source*: Education for Health).

the inspirable particles remain available for inhalation for some seconds after actuation
- To decrease deposition of non-respirable particles in the oropharynx. The larger particles are deposited in the spacer, rather than the oropharynx. This may be particularly important for high-dose inhaled steroids
- To allow those unable to distinguish between inspiration and expiration (e.g. young children) to benefit from inhaled therapy by simply inhaling and exhaling across the one-way valve
- To deliver a large dose of bronchodilator in an acute attack. Current guidelines advocate inhaling single doses serially. There has also been a practice of actuating a number of doses into the larger volume spacers (e.g. Volumatic®) and then breathing tidally across the one-way valve.

A mask may be attached or be integral to a spacer. The mask can then be placed over the mouth and nose of babies or infants to enable them to benefit from inhaled therapy. The correct use of a spacer and face mask is shown in Figure 43.7.

Examples of spacers are Volumatic®, Nebuhaler® and AeroChamber®.

Dry powder inhaler (DPI)

Medicines for inhalation can be presented as a micronized powder. The powder may be pure drug as in some Turbohalers®, or be drug and a carrier powder such as lactose, as in Diskhaler® and Accuhaler®.

When a carrier powder is used, the drug particles are adhered by weak electrostatic forces to the much larger carrier particles. As the drug/carrier powder is inhaled from the inhaler, the small respirable drug particles fly off the larger non-respirable carrier particles. The lactose carrier thus remains in the mouth. Patients using DPIs that employ a carrier powder should be reassured that even when using the inhaler correctly they will have carrier powder left in the mouth.

**HOW TO USE A LARGE VOLUME
SPACER AND MASK**

1 Remove the mouthpiece cover from the inhaler
2 Attach the mask to the spacer mouthpiece
3 Shake the inhaler and insert into the spacer device
4 Tip the spacer to an angle of 45° or more to enable the
  valve to remain open
5 Apply the mask to the child's face covering nose and mouth
  with as tight a seal as possible
6 Press the inhaler canister once to release a dose of the medication,
  keep the mask on the child's face to allow 5 or 6 breaths
7 Wait for 30 seconds before repeating
8 When using this method to administer inhaled
  steroids, remember to wash the child's
  face after each treatment

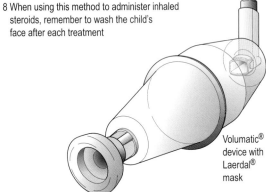

Volumatic®
device with
Laerdal®
mask

**ALWAYS DEMONSTRATE TO THE PATIENT HOW TO USE THE
LARGE VOLUME SPACER AND MASK**

Figure 43.7 • How to use a large-volume spacer and
face mask.
(*Source*: Education for Health.)

HOW TO USE THE TURBOHALER®

1 Remove the cap by unscrewing
2 Whilst holding the Turbohaler® upright, twist the base clockwise
  then back again until a click is heard
3 Breathe out slowly and gently, then place mouthpiece between teeth
  and lips and breathe in deeply and slowly
4 Hold breathe for about 10 seconds, remove
  Turbohaler® from mouth and then
  breathe out
5 Repeat steps 2 and 4, if another dose
  is required
6 Replace cap
7 Twenty doses are left when a red line
  shows in the window at the side of the
  Turbohaler®. The Turbohaler® is empty
  when the red line completely fills the
  window.

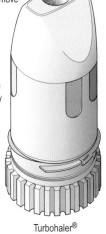

Turbohaler®

**ALWAYS DEMONSTRATE TO THE PATIENT HOW TO USE THE
TURBOHALER®**

Figure 43.8 • How to use the Turbohaler®.
(*Source*: Education for Health).

HOW TO USE THE ACCUHALER®

1 Open the outer case of the Accuhaler®. Ask your
  pharmacist if unsure how to do this.
2 With the mouthpiece facing you, slide the lever away from
  you until you hear a click. This procedure moves the dose
  counter on and makes the dose available
3 Breathe out slowly and gently, then place the mouthpiece
  between teeth and lips
4 Breathe in deeply and slowly
5 Remove the mouthpiece and
  hold breath for about
  10 seconds
6 Repeat steps 2–5 for a
  second dose
7 Close the Accuhaler®
8 The dose counter is red when
  5 doses are left

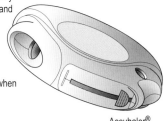

Accuhaler®

Patients inhaling pure drug from a Turbohaler®
providing only drug may experience little or no taste.

The correct method of using the Turbohaler®
is shown in Figure 43.8 and the Accuhaler® in
Figure 43.9.

All inhalers are boxed with instruction leaflets.
However, the best way to learn how to use an
inhaler is to have the technique demonstrated, then
to attempt to use the inhaler under supervision so
that any errors can be corrected. Many patients
will benefit from pharmacists providing this service. Similarly, for pharmacists to best learn how
to provide this service, they too should be shown
how to use the inhaler and how to spot common
errors. Medical representatives from companies
that market inhalers are usually more than happy
to train pharmacists how to use, demonstrate and
check inhaler technique. As part of this service, the
medical representative will provide placebo inhalers, to allow the pharmacist to demonstrate the
correct inhaler technique, instruction leaflets and

**ALWAYS DEMONSTRATE TO THE PATIENT HOW TO USE THE
ACCUHALER®**

Figure 43.9 • How to use the Accuhaler®.
(*Source*: Education for Health.)

other patient education material. Pharmacists can also signpost patients to demonstration videos on websites such as www.asthma.org.uk.

The use and care of a DPI differs from that of an MDI, as shown in Table 43.1.

Nebulizers

Medicines for inhalation can be presented as solutions or suspensions for nebulization. A nebulizing system (Fig. 43.10) usually consists of a compressor supplying compressed air to a nebulizing chamber, which delivers the nebulized drug to the patient via a mouthpiece or face mask. The face mask is most commonly used but when deposition of the nebulized drug on the face is undesirable (e.g. a steroid),

then a mouthpiece is preferable, or the face under the mask should be protected with petroleum jelly. A mouthpiece is also needed with inhaled ipratropium to prevent the potential precipitation of closed angle glaucoma.

The principle of jet nebulization is shown in Figure 43.11. The gas used to drive the nebulization process may be oxygen or air, but in either case a minimum flow rate of 8 L/min at a pressure of at least 69 kPa (10 psi) is required.

Patients using more than one nebulized medicine may have two different solutions mixed in the nebulizing chamber to be nebulized together. The summary of product characteristics (SPC) may give advice on other solutions and diluents that may be appropriately mixed with a given medicine for nebulization. It is possible that one

Table 43.1 Differences in the use and care of metered dose inhalers and dry powder inhalers	
MDI	**DPI**
Coordination of actuation and inhalation required	No coordination required as the release of powder and inhalation is a two-step process
Long, slow inhalation is the ideal to allow vaporization of propellants	Inhalation should be vigorous to disperse drug particles
The outer plastic housing of the inhaler (aerosol canister removed) can be washed to prevent blockage of actuator	Inhalers containing drug, e.g. Turbohaler®, must never be washed
Exhalation prior to inhalation can be into the inhaler	Exhalation must never be into the inhaler

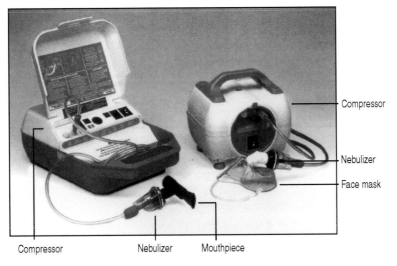

Figure 43.10 • Nebulization equipment.

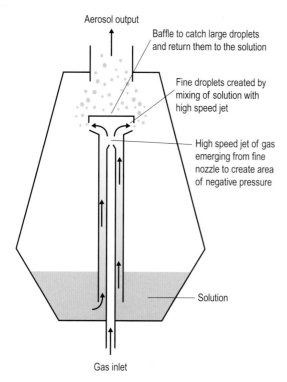

Aerosol output

Baffle to catch large droplets
and return them to the solution

Fine droplets created by
mixing of solution with
high speed jet

High speed jet of gas
emerging from fine
nozzle to create area
of negative pressure

Solution

Gas inlet

Figure 43.11 • The principle of jet nebulization.

solution will precipitate the other; this can normally be detected by the mixed solutions in the nebulizer chamber changing from clear to cloudy. Such a change means that the mixed solutions are not compatible and should not be nebulized together. Consideration should also be given to the total volume of the mixed solutions, as the larger the volume, the longer it will take to be nebulized.

Nebulizers are used when high doses of drug are required and/or when the patient is unable to use any form of inhaler. Nebulizers do not require the patient to learn any technique and are effective on normal or shallow breathing.

Nebulizers are used in the treatment of severe acute asthma and this is best done under medical supervision:

- To ensure that an adequate objective and maintained response to treatment is achieved (e.g. by measuring PEFR before and after nebulization)
- To assess if other treatment is indicated, e.g. oral or parenteral steroids
- To plan follow-up and possible review of chronic medication.

Nebulized treatment may also be used in the latter stages of COPD often in conjunction with domiciliary oxygen therapy. Domiciliary oxygen cylinders do not provide sufficient flow rates to produce adequate nebulization, so a compressor unit should be used.

Drugs for nebulization are normally presented as unit dose vials; examples of these are Nebules® and Respules®.

KEY POINTS

- Asthma and COPD are common conditions, treatment of which is largely dependent on the inhaled route
- The vast majority of inhaled treatments for asthma and COPD can be divided into two pharmacological classes of drugs: inhaled bronchodilators and inhaled steroids
- Inhaled bronchodilators can be further subdivided into $beta_2$ agonists and muscarinic agonists. Each of these classes can be further subdivided into short acting and long acting
- National and international management guidelines are available for asthma and COPD and treatment is based on a step-wise approach
- A range of inhalation devices is available to deliver drugs directly to the lungs. This has clear advantages including using much lower doses compared with oral therapy
- The use of inhalers is technique dependent and patients require training in their use
- Medicines to be inhaled are presented as aerosol inhalers, dry powder inhalers or liquids to be nebulized
- The most widely prescribed inhaler device is the aerosol metered dose inhaler (MDI). The MDI may be used in conjunction with a spacing device (a 'spacer'). A modified form of the MDI, triggered to actuate by inhalation, is a breath-actuated MDI. Both the 'spacer' and the breath-actuated MDI overcome the main difficulty of using an MDI, the need to coordinate inhalation with actuation of the MDI, and allow a wider range of individuals to successfully use an MDI
- Dry powder inhalers (DPIs) were originally developed to overcome the difficulty some patients have coordinating inhalation with actuation of an MDI
- DPIs vary widely in appearance and the method by which the powder is made available for inhalation, but all rely on inhalation to mobilize the powder from the inhaler and through the mouthpiece
- Liquids for nebulization are either solutions or permanent suspensions. It may be that solutions

are more reliably nebulized and inhaled than permanent suspensions

- Caution should be exercised when mixing two liquids for nebulization in the nebulizer, as one liquid can cause precipitation in the other
- The peak flow meter is a simple prescribable device which gives an objective measurement of lung function, and can be useful from time to time for asthmatics, e.g. when commencing a new treatment. It may also be used to aid self-management of asthma

- Many asthmatic and COPD patients will have at least two or three different inhalers. They will obtain greatest benefit from their inhalers if they understand something about their condition, the rationale for the different inhalers and how and when to use them
- Pharmacists with an understanding of asthma and COPD treatment and the correct use of inhalers can provide advice, education and training for patients on inhaled therapy which can markedly improve patients' quality of life.

Parenteral nutrition and dialysis

44

Lindsay Harper and Liz Lamerton

STUDY POINTS

- Provision of nutritional support for patients
- Indications for total parenteral nutrition (TPN)
- Components and compounding of a TPN/home parenteral nutrition (HPN) formulation
- Addition of medicines to a TPN or HPN bag
- HPN training and potential problems
- Administration of a TPN/HPN formulation
- British Parenteral Nutrition Group and British Association of Parenteral and Enteral Nutrition
- Introduction to home-care for patients on dialysis
- Haemodialysis (HD), peritoneal dialysis (PD), including continuous ambulatory peritoneal dialysis (CAPD), intermittent peritoneal dialysis (IPD) and automated peritoneal dialysis (APD)
- Dialysis solutions
- Provision of services from a hospital renal unit, including home dialysis

Introduction

Today, an increasing number of patients are requesting and being provided with healthcare services at home. Such services include the provision of home parenteral nutrition and home dialysis. This chapter will explore the provision of parenteral nutrition and dialysis for patients in hospital and will explain how these services can be transferred to the home-care setting.

Provision of nutritional support

Studies have shown that up to 50% of medical and surgical patients can suffer from nutritional deficiencies. If nutritional support is indicated, enteral feeding should be considered as the first option. Patients can receive nutrients orally or via a tube feed, e.g. by nasogastric feeding. This is only possible if the gastrointestinal tract is functional. If this is not the case, parenteral nutrition may be considered. Short-term (e.g. postoperative) intravenous (IV) administration of fluids, such as 5% dextrose or saline may be sufficient. This could provide the patient with around 500 calories per day but does not provide any protein, vitamins, minerals or trace elements.

Patients who need longer-term nutrition support may require total parenteral nutrition (TPN) which is a method of administering adequate nutrients via the parenteral route. The components of a TPN formulation are added to a sterile infusion bag and administered to the patient via a catheter. Administration can be via a peripheral Venflon, a peripherally inserted central catheter (PICC) or a central line. However, TPN fluids are normally highly concentrated mixtures, which on a long-term basis could cause damage to peripheral veins. For this reason, peripheral veins are only used for TPN administration lasting up to 4 weeks.

If parenteral nutrition is supplied to patients at home, it is known as home parenteral nutrition (HPN) and is more likely to be provided by a commercial company than a hospital TPN unit. Patients on HPN administer their nutrition via a central line into a central vein.

Parenteral nutrition formulations are prepared under strict aseptic conditions (see Ch. 40) following guidelines published by the MHRA in *Rules and Guidance for Pharmaceutical Manufacturers*

(2002) and by the DH in *Aseptic Dispensing for NHS Patients* (Farwell 1995).

HPN is becoming increasingly prevalent. Guidelines have been published by the British Association of Parenteral and Enteral Nutrition (BAPEN) and the National Institute for Health and Care Excellence (NICE) to ensure that adequate provision is made for patients receiving HPN. Patients who are suitable candidates for HPN will be, initially, stabilized on TPN bags while in hospital. They can then undergo appropriate training to enable them to administer their TPN bags at home. If the patient is unable to care for their line, then a carer or nurse would be trained to administer the TPN at home. However, HPN patients will still need to return to the hospital for regular check-ups. This means that pharmacists involved in the care of HPN patients will require a working knowledge of the procedures adopted to provide care for patients in hospital and at home. They may also have to liaise with the patient's GP and the community nurse.

This chapter concentrates on the provision of adult TPN, although neonatal TPN is available.

Indications for TPN

TPN can be required for finite periods of time or for life. Some of the main indications for TPN are:

- Gastrointestinal disease, including Crohn's disease, ulcerative colitis, pancreatitis and malabsorption syndrome
- Major trauma including severe burns, severe septicaemia
- Major abdominal surgery; severely malnourished patients may benefit from early peri and postoperative parenteral nutrition if surgery has resulted in a non-functioning gastrointestinal tract
- Malignancy of the small bowel
- Radiation enteritis, when TPN is considered if enteritis is severe after treatment of a primary malignancy
- High-dose chemotherapy, radiotherapy and bone marrow transplantation. Patients are often ill for a limited time (3–6 weeks) and are unable to eat. TPN can be administered during this period to ensure that the patient's nutritional requirements are adequately met.

Several other conditions may require the nutritional support of TPN, e.g. patients in a prolonged coma or AIDS patients.

Assessment of the patient in hospital

TPN aims to provide patients with all their nutritional requirements in one formulation which can then be infused directly into the body via the veins, either central or peripheral. In order to determine exactly what the patient's nutritional requirements are, clinical and biochemical assessments must take place. The Malnutrition Universal Screening Tool (MUST) is used to identify patients who may benefit from TPN. The patient's body weight, height and body mass index (BMI) can be recorded and comparison made with their ideal body weight which would be available from standard charts. In most hospitals a dietitian would review the patient and calculate their nutritional requirements.

Factors investigated will include urea and electrolytes, full blood counts, liver function tests, triglycerides, blood glucose and fluid balance. Trace elements are only monitored if the patient receives TPN for longer than 28 days. The NICE guidelines for nutrition support contain a section on the monitoring required for TPN patients.

Each hospital has its own particular way of designing a TPN regimen. Most hospitals use a range of standard formulations which are routinely used to treat TPN patients. Standard bags can be altered if the need arises. In general, additions to the finished TPN bags outside of the pharmacy aseptic unit are not recommended in order to minimize microbial contamination.

More recently, pharmaceutical companies have introduced a range of three-in-one ready-to-use multichambered TPN bags. These bags have three chambers, which contain amino acid, dextrose and lipid. When a bag of TPN is required, the seal separating the chambers can easily be broken and the three solutions are mixed together in one chamber. Before mixing, these bags have a long expiry date of around 2 years and do not need to be stored in the fridge. Many hospitals have swapped to using these bags as they are cost-effective and reduce the time for manufacture. Trace elements and vitamins need to be added to these bags before use.

Some hospitals tailor regimens to individual patients and carry out a number of calculations to determine baseline requirements for each component. In this way they can build up a formulation by matching up the patient's requirements to commercially available solutions which contain the required components in the correct proportions. Individualized bags tend to be used in patients on long-term TPN. Patients on HPN will always have bags tailored exactly to their nutritional needs.

The nutrition team

In most hospitals where TPN is supplied, there will be a nutrition team to coordinate the delivery of the parenteral nutrition service. This team can include the following:

- Consultant
- Senior registrar/registrar
- Pharmacist
- Clinical psychologist
- Nutrition nurse(s)
- Dietitian(s)
- Biochemist(s).

The role of these individuals in provision of patient care can vary from one hospital to another. In general, the consultant is responsible for prescribing the TPN formulation and liaising with the patient's GP to provide care for HPN patients, although with the introduction of non-medical prescribing, this role is increasingly taken over by nurses and pharmacists.

The pharmacist can provide information on aseptic techniques for handling and setting up TPN bags, formulation requirements, potential complications or stability problems, and storage conditions required. In some hospitals, the pharmacist's role can be extended to include the following:

- Training nursing staff in the techniques required for IV administration of TPN fluids
- Helping with patient training for HPN
- Monitoring of patients in HPN clinics
- Liaising with the staff from the home-care company
- Advising on the patient's drug therapy
- Liaising with the patient's community pharmacist.

The nutrition nurse and dietitian will together give advice on a day-to-day basis regarding the nutritional status of the patients and will advise on necessary dietary requirements.

Commercial companies supplying home-care services have a nutrition nurse who provides medical care, support and advice (on a 24-hour basis if required), a patient coordinator who deals with the ordering of HPN bags and ancillaries, and a designated delivery person who will supply the necessary equipment and HPN bags to the patient's home.

In the rare circumstances that the HPN is supplied by the hospital pharmacy, patients can be provided with the support from the hospital and their GP.

Components of a TPN formulation

TPN formulations can contain the following components:

- Water
- Protein source – measured in grams of nitrogen
- Energy source – carbohydrate and fat
- Electrolytes
- Trace elements
- Vitamins and minerals.

Baseline water requirements

Water accounts for over 50% of body weight. To prevent patients becoming dehydrated, daily water losses and gains must be carefully considered. Water can be lost through urine and faeces and through 'insensible losses', i.e. through the skin and lungs. Patients with burns and gastrointestinal losses will require increased volume. Patients with renal and cardiac failure should be given reduced volumes.

Several methods are available for estimating daily fluid requirements, but most take into consideration body weight and measured urine output, and an allowance is made for insensible losses. The average adult requires between 1500 and 4000 mL of fluid per day. A TPN regimen will need to provide this volume of fluid on a daily basis.

Protein source

Protein requirements vary from one patient to another and are highly dependent on the metabolic status of the patient. Undernourished patients requiring parenteral nutrition are, generally, said to have a negative nitrogen balance. This means that the amount of nitrogen excreted in urine and faeces is greater than the amount of nitrogen administered.

Lack of nitrogen in the body can result in poor wound healing and interference with the body's defence mechanisms. To overcome this problem, a

A postoperative surgical patient requires 0.2 g/kg/24 h of nitrogen. The patient weighs 47 kg.

Nitrogen requirements per day $= 0.2 \times 47$ kg
$= 9.4$ g nitrogen

This requirement can then be matched up to commercially available solutions. Each gram of amino acid nitrogen is equivalent to 6.25 g of protein, e.g. Vamin 9 contains 9.4 g of nitrogen per litre. This is equivalent to 60 g of protein and will provide the patient with the required daily nitrogen intake. However, care must also be taken when selecting an amino acid solution for inclusion in a TPN formulation, as most commercially available solutions are hypertonic in nature and have a pH between 5 and 7.4. The pH of the amino acid solution may have an effect on the overall stability of the formulation and must be considered carefully.

utilizable source of nitrogen must be administered to the patient. This is achieved by administering amino acid solutions in a TPN formulation. Nitrogen requirements can be estimated from a 24-hour urine collection. This is done by analysing the total amount of urea excreted and by considering the individual patient's body weight and clinical 'type'.

Energy sources

Carbohydrates and fats are chosen to provide optimal energy sources for TPN patients. The relative proportions of each will be dependent on the clinical requirements of the patient and formulation considerations. The carbohydrate of choice is normally dextrose and is available in solution with concentrations ranging from 5% to 70% weight in volume (w/v). Like amino acid solutions, dextrose solutions are hypertonic and have a low pH (3–5). If high concentrations of dextrose are added to the TPN bags, they must only be given centrally.

The fat component in a TPN formulation is administered in the form of an oil-in-water emulsion. Fat emulsions are isotonic with plasma, have neutral pH and provide a high calorie source in a low volume. As a result, they are often used in combination with dextrose to provide the necessary calorie content, thereby avoiding the potential problems encountered with excessive dextrose administration.

Fat emulsions provide the patient with essential fatty acids and also act as a vehicle for fat-soluble vitamins which are required in the TPN formulation. Fat is not required in every TPN formulation, but fat deficiency can occur in patients who do not receive fat components for periods longer than 1 month.

Commercially available preparations are based on soya bean oils and are composed of varying combinations of long and medium chain triglycerides. Newer fat solutions have been developed, incorporating olive oil and fish oils, which are claimed to protect patients on long-term parenteral nutrition from complications. Larger and longer trials are required to prove these claims. The energy content of commercially available solutions for both carbohydrates and fats is expressed in kcal/L, e.g. Intralipid 10% provides 550 kcal/500 mL; dextrose 5% provides 210 kcal/500 mL.

Electrolytes

The main electrolytes of clinical significance in a TPN formulation include sodium, potassium, magnesium, calcium, phosphate and chloride. The requirement for electrolytes can be met in the form of injectable solutions of varying percentage content. Electrolyte content of each is expressed in terms of mmol/L. The individual role of each electrolyte in a TPN formulation is given in Table 44.1.

Trace elements

Trace elements act as metabolic cofactors and are said to be essential for the proper functioning of several enzyme systems in the body. Despite being termed essential, they are only required in very small quantities, expressed in micromoles. The main trace elements required in a TPN formulation are zinc, copper, manganese and chromium.

Vitamins and minerals

Vitamin requirements fall into two categories: fat soluble and water soluble. Four fat-soluble vitamins (vitamins A, D, E and K) and nine water-soluble vitamins (vitamins B_1, B_2, B_3, B_5, B_6, B_{12}, C, folic acid and biotin) are said to be essential.

Vitamins and minerals are normally included in foods taken in orally and must therefore be included in TPN formulations for patients on long-term parenteral

Table 44.1 Role of electrolytes used in TPN formulations

Electrolyte	Principal function	Daily intravenous requirement	Symptoms of deficiency	Symptoms of excess	Common sources
Sodium	Main extracellular cation Regulation of water balance Neuromuscular contractility	1–2 mmol/kg	Weakness, lethargy, confusion, convulsions, appetite, nausea and vomiting	Lethargy, coma, convulsions, muscle rigidity, thirst	Sodium chloride Sodium acetate Sodium phosphate
Potassium	Main intracellular cation Regulation of acid–base balance Neuromuscular contractility	1–2 mmol/kg	Muscle weakness, ileus, arrhythmias, alkalosis	Muscle weakness, paraesthesia, bradycardia, nausea and vomiting	Potassium chloride Potassium phosphate
Magnesium	Cofactor for enzyme systems Neuromuscular contractility	0.1–0.2 mmol/kg	Lethargy, cramps, tetany, paraesthesia, arrhythmias, excitability, hypokalaemia, hypocalcaemia	Decreased muscular activity, lethargy, depression	Magnesium sulfate Magnesium chloride
Calcium	Mineralization: bones + teeth Neuromuscular contractility	0.1–0.15 mmol/kg	Paraesthesia, tetany, fitting, confusion, arrhythmias	Nausea, anorexia, lethargy, muscle weakness, confusion	Calcium gluconate Calcium chloride
Phosphate	Main intracellular anion Acid–base balance Energy	0.5–0.7 mmol/kg	Weakness, tingling	Non-specific effects on calcium balance	Phosphate salts of sodium and potassium, hydrogen
Chloride	Main extracellular anion Acid–base balance	1–2 mmol/kg	Alkalosis	Acidosis	Chloride salts of above cations

From Walker and Edwards 2003, reproduced by permission.

nutrition. The NICE guidelines published in 2006 recommend that patients must receive vitamins and trace elements daily in their TPN bags.

Compounding of TPN and HPN formulations

Compounding can take place within a hospital pharmacy using aseptic dispensing facilities within a clean room or within a designated compounding unit in a commercial pharmaceutical company.

Preparation and training

For patients in hospital, a suitable TPN regimen will be prescribed. On receipt of the prescription, the pharmacist checks the suitability and compatibility of the formulation, the required volume of each component is calculated and details are transferred to a worksheet. Patient details are entered into a computer and labels generated for the worksheet and the final product. In the preparation area, items required for the compounding process are collected together in an appropriate tray ready for transfer to the clean room facility. Batch numbers and expiry dates for each product used are recorded on the worksheet. The pharmacist checks all details, including calculations, before the compounding procedure begins.

Compounding of a TPN formulation is carried out under strict aseptic conditions (in a Grade A environment) using a laminar airflow (LAF) cabinet within a clean room facility. Chapter 40 gives details regarding clean room facilities, gowning-up procedures for entry to clean rooms and working procedures for using LAF cabinets. SOPs should be available for all staff carrying out aseptic dispensing procedures.

TPN/HPN bags

The components of a TPN formulation are sterile and are prepared under sterile conditions as the formulation is eventually infused directly into the bloodstream of the patient. It is therefore essential that the bags used to hold the TPN formulation are also sterile. In the past, only polyvinyl chloride (PVC) bags were used for TPN formulations. However, because of the problems of leaching of plasticisers from PVC bags containing a fat component, ethylvinyl acetate (EVA) bags (which contain no plasticizers) are now recommended. However, EVA bags have been shown to be permeable to oxygen; hence multilayer EVA bags are now available for formulations requiring prolonged storage.

Bags are usually supplied with a pre-mounted sterile filling set attached. The filling set consists of a number of hollow plastic tubes (up to six) with a plastic spike attached to the end of each. The spikes are used to pierce the rubber septum of the bottles and bags of amino acids, glucose and fat emulsion to enable filling of the components into the TPN bag. Clamps fitted with air vents are attached to each filling tube to clamp off the source bottles and bags when they are empty. Filling sets are used for compounding purposes only and are disconnected and replaced with a sterile hub before being sent out to the patient. Every HPN bag is supplied with a sterile giving set which allows the bag to be infused into the patient.

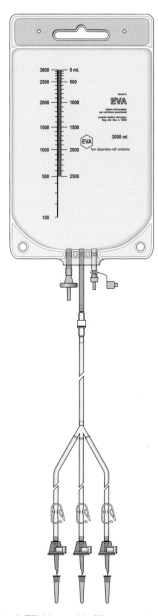

Figure 44.1 • A TPN bag with filling set attached.

TPN bags vary in size, ranging from small 250 mL bags used for neonatal TPN up to 4 L bags for adult TPN. Figure 44.1 shows a TPN bag with filling set attached.

Addition of components to a TPN bag

Components are added into the TPN bag in a strictly defined procedure. Small-volume additives can be added directly into large-volume fluids (but not directly into the fat component) or directly into the additive port on the bag (depending on manufacturers' recommendations). Amino acid solutions and glucose are added into the bag first, followed by any fat emulsion if required. To prevent precipitation of vitamins, they are, generally, only added immediately before administration.

Filling of the TPN bags can be achieved under gravity. The bag is placed on the floor of the LAF cabinet and the solution components suspended from a retort stand, enabling the solution to flow freely into the bag. If several bags require to be compounded in a limited time period, the bag can be placed in a vacuum chamber to speed up the filling process. Electronic devices, known as compounders, are also available. They are usually under microprocessor control and can be pre-programmed to fill TPN bags with set volumes of individual components.

When all the components are added, the bag can be clamped off and the filling set removed. The bag is gently shaken to ensure adequate mixing of all components. The TPN bag and compounding materials are transferred back to the preparation area. A visual inspection of the bag is made, including checking of the additive port, for integrity. All necessary documentation is completed and the TPN bag is labelled. Details to be included on the label are shown in Box 44.1.

The TPN bag is then sealed into a dark-coloured outer plastic bag (to protect the formulation from light) and an outer label that is identical to the label on the bag itself is attached.

To maintain stability of the formulated product, it is refrigerated until required. All TPN and HPN formulations must be stored in a designated pharmaceutical grade refrigerator. Coolboxes packed with ice packs can be used for transportation of formulations to the ward or the patient's home.

Compounding of HPN formulations by commercial companies

A designated compounding unit is used for preparing HPN formulations. Conditions used will be the same as those used in the hospital sector and the same government regulations apply. The compounding unit must hold a manufacturing licence prior to supplying TPN bags (see Ch. 4).

The commercial company providing the home-care service must be in receipt of a prescription for the HPN formulation prior to compounding.

However, when the health care is transferred to the home-care setting in Scotland, the patient's GP will take on the responsibility for supplying the HPN prescription. In England and Wales, the primary care commissioner is responsible for providing the HPN prescription, although with the current changes to the NHS in England and Wales the responsibilities may change. Subsequent prescriptions will then be forwarded to the commercial company in advance of the patient's requirements. The hospital nutrition team will issue the prescriptions for the patients at home. The patient coordinator will deal with orders for sundries and ancillaries such as pumps, dressings, needles, etc.

Potential complications arising during compounding and administration of TPN formulations

The components of a TPN formulation will individually and collectively contribute to the overall stability of the resulting formulation. However, with several hospitals now using standard TPN formulations, many of these problems can be overcome. For hospital pharmacies which have a manufacturing licence, standard bags can be made up in advance of requirements and stored in a refrigerator for periods of 30 days or more. The shelf-life given to individual formulations must be based on validated stability studies previously carried out on the formulation. The stability of any regimen will be confirmed before manufacture.

Box 44.1

Details to be placed on a label of a TPN bag

- Patient name (ward and unit number if hospital patient)
- Components of the bag (expressed in mmol)
- Total volume (mL)
- Energy content (kcal)
- Nitrogen content (g)
- Infusion rate (mL/h)
- Route of administration
- Expiry date and storage conditions

Individual components of the formulation such as vitamins, electrolytes and fat can cause formulation complications. Vitamin stability is very poor, particularly in the presence of light and with extended storage time. Stability is also affected by solution pH, hence the need for careful consideration of the overall formulation.

The requirement for administration of calcium and phosphate in a formulation can lead to precipitation of calcium phosphate. This reaction is said to be affected by factors such as the relative amounts of each component present, solution pH, concentration of amino acid solutions present and the mixing process used. To overcome this type of problem, manufacturers of parenteral nutrition fluids can supply tables which give details of the amount of each component that can be safely combined to ensure stability of the formulation is maintained. These tables are specific to an individual formulation and details cannot be interchanged between formulations.

The presence of fat in a TPN formulation can cause stability problems. As storage time increases, the fat component of the formulation becomes less stable, resulting in a process of 'cracking' where the oil and water phases of the emulsion separate out. If the formulation is administered to the patient in this unstable condition, this can lead to potentially dangerous fat deposits arising in the lungs and other body tissues.

The factors a pharmacist must consider when formulating a TPN bag with a fat component are:

- The order in which components are added to the bag
- The types and amount of electrolytes present and their relative proportions – divalent and trivalent cations reduce stability
- The pH of the resultant mixture – higher pH improves stability
- Conditions arising during storage and administration
- The type of plastic bag used – EVA bags preferred.

Addition of medicines to a TPN or HPN bag

Stability studies have been carried out on a number of medicines to determine their compatibility and stability in a TPN bag. So far, studies have confirmed the suitability of only a limited range of medicines which includes: heparin, insulin, aminophylline, cimetidine, famotidine, ranitidine and certain antibiotics. Reference to manufacturers' literature and compatibility studies will provide current recommendations. Although stability is available on the drugs listed above, the addition of drugs to TPN is not recommended. This is because the drugs may affect the long-term stability of the TPN bag and it will affect the pharmacokinetics of the drugs added to the TPN. Most hospitals in the UK allow no additions to the TPN bags.

Administration of TPN/HPN formulations

For patients requiring TPN for longer than 4 weeks, central venous access is required. During their stay in hospital, patients have a catheter inserted into the subclavian vein under anaesthesia. It has an exit site on the lower chest wall, allowing patients easy access for care of the catheter site.

Catheters can be made of materials such as polyvinyl chloride or silicone. For long-term feeding, a permanent catheter (a Hickman catheter or a Portacath) is used. It is held in place by a Dacron cuff (an internal woven plastic used to connect arteries and veins under the skin). Good aseptic techniques are essential to ensure that the catheter site does not become contaminated. Infection around the catheter site can be difficult to treat successfully and may eventually result in removal of the catheter and replacement at another site.

Catheter sites should only be used for administration of TPN fluids and not for blood sampling or administration of other medicines. In some instances, a triple lumen catheter can be used with one line being kept for administration of the TPN bag only. To infuse the TPN formulation into the patient, the catheter is connected via an extension set to a volumetric infusion pump. These devices use positive pressure as the driving force to allow accurate infusion at pre-set rates (see Ch. 41).

The infusion period varies from 24h in hospital to around 12–14h for home patients (as HPN can often be administered overnight). Most pumps now have the ability to be programmed to give an infusion rate which 'steps up' at the beginning and 'steps down' at the end of the infusion period, avoiding potential problems with high concentrations of dextrose in the formulation. They are also fitted with an alarm which will alert the patient if a technical fault arises.

Potential problems for HPN patients

Mechanical problems

Problems of pneumothorax, or air embolism, are more likely to occur in the hospital environment in the early stages of catheter placement and are dealt with before the patient commences on HPN. However, daily connection and disconnection of the catheter hub may result in cracking and possible leakage of the HPN fluid. Repair kits are available, and if used promptly when the problem first arises, catheter replacement may not be necessary.

Internal line blockage of the catheter can arise. Patients are taught to flush out the catheter port with heparinized saline to prevent thrombus formation. Blockage of the line arising during administration of the HPN fluid can cause changes in flow rate which are recognized by the pump, and the alarm is activated.

Metabolic problems

Metabolic complications include:

- Problems with electrolyte levels leading to conditions such as hypernatraemia or hyponatraemia
- Problems with glucose levels leading to hyperglycaemia or hypoglycaemia
- Balancing of fluid intake (to ensure adequate hydration is achieved)
- Altered liver enzymes which can be resolved by amending the TPN prescription
- Metabolic bone disease, monitored by regular bone scans.

The majority of the metabolic complications which can affect HPN patients can be overcome by careful monitoring of the patient initially in hospital and with regular check-ups and home visits by the nutrition nurse.

Catheter-related complications

Catheter-related infections can arise as a result of poor management of the catheter exit site. Infection is distinguished by pain, redness and tenderness around the site and rigors when feeding through the line. To minimize such infections, staff are trained to use strict aseptic procedures when changing TPN bags and use of the catheter port is restricted to administration of the TPN bag only. HPN patients are taught the same aseptic techniques and are required to carry out these procedures at all times when changing bags at home. Home-care patients are also taught to be aware of their own physical condition and to be alert to any deterioration in their medical condition at the earliest possible time. Patients are asked to contact their nutrition nurse if they experience any signs or symptoms of infection around the catheter site.

Psychological and social problems

Patients receiving TPN in hospital or at home must learn to adapt to the changes occurring in their lifestyle. Some patients have, over a prolonged period of time, suffered from a general deterioration in their health and as a result adapt well to the initiation of parenteral nutrition as it improves their quality of life. Other patients require TPN as a result of major trauma and these patients find the dramatic changes in their lifestyle very difficult to cope with.

While in the hospital receiving treatment, patients have the constant support of medical and nursing staff to help them to cope with any practical difficulties encountered. The clinical psychologist will review many patients before discharge and coping strategies will be discussed. The ability of patients to adapt to HPN is highly dependent on a number of factors:

- Patient's underlying medical condition
- Physical ability and capability of the patient
- Training and counselling prior to leaving hospital
- Home circumstances, particularly support from family members and the patient's GP
- Ability to deal with physical and emotional changes in lifestyle, e.g. dependence on others.
- Disruption to normal sleeping pattern during administration of the HPN bag overnight and loss of 'social' eating can be difficult for many patients, particularly in the initial stages of HPN.

To enable a smooth transition from hospital to home to be achieved, patients require the services of the nutrition nurse and other healthcare workers to teach them the necessary skills required for handling, setting up their HPN bags and disconnecting them once the procedure is complete.

Training for HPN patients

Health care which can be provided at home has a number of advantages. Patients have a better quality of life and can become more independent as their confidence in providing self-care increases. However, motivation and confidence to carry out the required manipulations at home are essential. Thus, training in the hospital environment is required to build up the necessary skills and techniques.

A discharge plan is required for each patient working towards home-care. The British Association for Parenteral and Enteral Nutrition (BAPEN), a registered charity formed in 1992, has laid down guidelines for the provision of nutritional care at home. Individual hospitals will develop their own guidelines based on the advice given by BAPEN. The scope of BAPEN includes guidelines on the following matters:

- Details which should be included in a patient discharge plan
- Knowledge and practical skills which must be achieved by patients prior to discharge
- Guidelines for GPs on the provision of HPN
- Advice on how to liaise with the patient's GP to ensure that everyone is aware of their responsibilities
- Information regarding the supplier of the HPN bags and equipment and how this service will be provided
- Details of appropriate people who patients can contact for advice and help with any problems they have.

The length of time required for training can vary depending on the patient's underlying medical condition and personal approach to training. Patients must be taught aseptic techniques and the importance of ensuring that they are carried out correctly. They must demonstrate their skills and competence on several occasions prior to leaving the hospital. Areas covered during the training period include:

- Aseptic techniques for setting up and disconnecting the HPN bag
- Care of the catheter site

- How to deal with problems of the catheter blocking
- Setting the pump for infusion of the HPN bag
- Dealing with simple mechanical problems with the pump.

Information booklets on HPN and educational videos can be used with patients to reinforce the training received in hospital.

Services provided by home-care companies

Patients receiving home-care will require certain practical arrangements to be put in place before HPN can be initiated. Home-care companies who provide services to HPN patients normally provide the following items for patient use: a refrigerator for storing HPN bags; a trolley for patients to set up their HPN bags aseptically; a drip stand and an infusion pump. Patients are required to have adequate storage space to keep any extra components which may be required for HPN administration and easy access to hand washing facilities for use prior to setting up their HPN bag. A home assessment will be completed by the home-care company and a nutrition nurse from the hospital before discharge to ensure the patient's home circumstances are suitable for HPN.

Support services provided for HPN patients

Patients will be metabolically stable prior to transfer to the home-care setting, hence frequency of monitoring will be reduced to a minimum. Patients can have monthly check-ups at the hospital initially, reducing to 3-monthly as they adapt to life on HPN. During visits, patients may be seen by the multidisciplinary nutrition team and reviewed by each member of the team. The pharmacist on the team will arrange any changes in the patient's TPN prescription. Routine monitoring can be carried out during these visits, including the following:

- Checking the patient's underlying medical condition
- Reviewing the patient's nutritional status, particularly in relation to their weight
- Routine haematological and biochemical tests

- Checking for any complications
- Reviewing the patient's psychological state.

The nutrition nurse will make home visits if required to check on aseptic techniques and any practical difficulties being encountered by patients and/or their partner or carer.

Patients on HPN can benefit from the support of others undergoing nutrition therapy at home. This is made possible by an organization called 'PINNT' (Patients on Intravenous and Nasogastric Nutrition Therapy). This charitable organization aims to support and bring together people who have similar medical conditions and could benefit from the moral support of others who understand the problems they face. PINNT provides practical help in areas such as provision of portable equipment for people on HPN who wish to go on holiday, help with holiday arrangements, including appropriate travel insurance and general advice on benefits available to HPN patients. A newsletter is produced on a regular basis and close links are kept between PINNT and BAPEN to ensure that patient needs are adequately met.

The British Parenteral Nutrition Group

Pharmacists in the UK can keep up-to-date with the working of organizations like PINNT and BAPEN by joining the British Parenteral Nutrition Group (BPNG). Currently, BPNG has a large membership, most of whom are hospital pharmacists working in the NHS. However, membership also includes dietitians, nutrition nurses, research workers and members of commercial companies who work in the field of TPN and HPN. The BPNG exists to further the practice of TPN through a number of activities including research, contributing to the work of BAPEN and arranging symposia on practical and scientific developments in the field. This group is also one of five constituent groups which make up BAPEN.

Introduction to kidney disease and dialysis therapy

In December 2010, there were over 50 000 adult patients receiving renal replacement therapy in the UK. Patients requiring renal replacement therapy (RRT) have end-stage renal disease/failure (ESRF) which may have occurred acutely or may be the result of chronic kidney disease. Transplantation is the most common treatment modality (48%) with haemodialysis accounting for 44% and peritoneal dialysis 8% of RRT. Home therapies make up 9% of RRT. Home therapy was used by 17.6% of prevalent dialysis patients in 2010, with 2.9% on home haemodialysis and the remaining patients having either continuous ambulatory peritoneal dialysis or automated peritoneal dialysis. While still small in number, more patients are now receiving home haemodialysis, with numbers increasing by 23% since 2009, from 636 patients to 780 patients.

Chronic kidney disease

Chronic kidney disease (CKD) is relatively common, affecting approximately 1 in 10 people in the general population. The most common cause is diabetes. Glomerulonephritis and hypertension are also responsible and less common causes include pyelonephritis. CKD may also be inherited, e.g. polycystic kidney disease. Some common drug therapies may also lead to kidney disease.

ESRF is the result of progressive kidney disease, which leads to an irreversible and life-threatening loss of function. Patients with ESRF may be suitable for RRT or may choose conservative treatment. There are a number of types of RRT, e.g. kidney transplantation, haemodialysis or peritoneal dialysis. Unfortunately, over 30% of patients are unsuitable for transplantation and for a number of patients, a suitable donor may not be found. For these patients, transplantation may not therefore be an option and chronic RRT is required. For most patients with ESRF who wish to have RRT, there are two choices, either long-term haemodialysis (HD) or peritoneal dialysis (PD) therapy, although patients may not be suitable for both modalities and may change from one to the other at various times according to need.

RRT with dialysis replaces only some of the functions of the kidneys and is an artificial method of filtering toxins and breakdown products from the blood. It does not replicate normal renal function and does not provide any of the metabolic functions of the kidney such as insulin metabolism or the hormonal functions such as erythropoietin production. RRT with HD or PD uses a combination of dialysis therapy to remove unwanted solutes by the process of diffusion and haemofiltration and ultrafiltration to remove water.

Epidemiology

In 2010, the incidence rate in the UK was 107 per million population. The median age of all incident patients was 64.9 years and for non-whites 57.1 years. Diabetic renal disease is identified as the single most common cause in 24% of patients. There is no identified relationship between social deprivation and presentation pattern according to the renal registry data.

Dialysis

Dialysis is commenced to treat, or to prevent, life-threatening hyperkalaemia, acidosis or hypervolaemic pulmonary oedema or to treat complications of CKD, e.g. pericarditis, uraemic neuropathy or seizures.

Haemodialysis

HD is a process where blood is filtered to remove waste products. The patient is connected to a dialysis machine where blood is removed from the patient's body and filtered by passing it over an artificial semi-permeable membrane into dialysis fluid. The waste products are retained within the dialysis fluid and the blood returned into the body.

To facilitate HD, access to the patient's blood-stream must be established, either using a surgically created arteriovenous fistula, where an artery is joined to a vein during a minor surgical operation, a graft, and the join between the artery and vein is made using a synthetic tube, or by inserting a permanent or temporary central vascular catheter into a large vein, such as the subclavian, jugular or femoral vein.

HD usually takes 3–4 hours each time and will be required, on average, three times a week for most patients. The blood is removed and passed over a membrane with a large surface area to allow solutes to be exchanged between the blood and dialysis fluid. Dialysis membranes are sterile, disposable membranes made of cellulose or polycarbonate materials. Pressure is applied to the blood in the machine to induce an ultrafiltration process and allow removal of excess water in addition to the removal of toxins.

Dialysis fluid is composed of similar constituents to plasma:

- Sodium
- Potassium
- Chloride
- Calcium
- Magnesium
- Glucose
- Bicarbonate, citrate or lactate is added to buffer the solution.

To promote potassium removal from the blood, the dialysate potassium concentration is variable and is usually lower than that in the plasma. To prevent the blood clotting in the dialysis circuit, unfractionated heparin, low molecular weight heparin or prostacyclin may be used.

During the HD process, there are a number of potential complications such as low blood pressure, air embolus and blood loss.

HD may be carried out in a variety of settings providing the appropriate equipment and water supply is available. Locations include specialist hospital units or in the patient's own home. The dialysis process follows the same principles in all settings.

Hospital-based haemodialysis

Patients occasionally have direct responsibility for their treatment; however, it is more common for the dialysis to be managed by a team of doctors, nurses and other healthcare professionals. Patients travel to the unit for HD according to an arranged schedule.

In a satellite unit, patients sometimes play a more active role in their treatment. They are supervised by trained staff but may prepare the dialysis machine or carry out the dialysis process themselves.

Home haemodialysis

Home HD may be suitable for a limited number of patients. NICE (TAC 48) recommends that all suitable patients should be offered home HD.

There are a number of advantages to home HD:

- Greater independence for the patient
- Excellent long-term outcome
- Improved blood pressure control
- Lower hospital admission rates
- Fewer limitations on timing of dialysis
- Greater flexibility

- No transport difficulties
- Optimal use of resources.

There are a number of factors that determine a patient's suitability for home HD. For example, patients must be able and motivated to learn and perform dialysis at home and be capable of maintaining and monitoring their own treatment observations. They must be medically stable and be free of complications that make dialysis difficult. Patients also require good functioning vascular access, support from family or carers and suitable space and facilities must be available. Any patients considered suitable for home HD will be assessed, including their home circumstances. They will undergo a comprehensive training programme to develop skills and techniques in addition to developing confidence and self-reliance.

Peritoneal dialysis

In PD, the dialysis fluid is passed directly into the patient's body and, in contrast to HD, no blood removal occurs. The peritoneal membrane which lines the abdominal cavity has a large surface area and a good capillary blood supply. It is this semi-permeable membrane that is used to perform PD and allows excess water and waste products to be removed from the blood.

Dialysis fluid is instilled into the peritoneal cavity through a surgically inserted indwelling catheter, which goes through the abdominal wall. The distal end of the catheter has tiny holes in it to allow the dialysis fluid to flow freely into the peritoneal cavity. Fluid is removed from the blood by ultrafiltration down an osmotic pressure gradient. Solutes and toxins cross the peritoneal membrane through diffusion and solvent drag with water.

There are two main methods of PD: continuous ambulatory peritoneal dialysis (CAPD) and automated peritoneal dialysis (APD).

In CAPD, patients generally carry out three or four PD exchanges every 24 h and this is the most common form of home dialysis. In APD, patients are connected to a machine for 8–12 h, often overnight. The machine utilizes a pump delivery system which warms the dialysis fluid prior to administration and delivers a carefully programmed volume of dialysis fluid which exchanges throughout the infusion period. The home patient or a carer will set the machine every night by connecting it to the catheter. This method of dialysis has advantages for the patient as it allows freedom from dialysis during the day.

A variety of dialysis fluids are available and each patient will be prescribed a specific tailored regimen of dialysis fluids. The volume will be determined in part by the available abdominal space. For adults, the range is 1–7 L.

The composition of the dialysate consists of sodium, calcium, glucose or dextran to increase or decrease osmolality.

The dialysis exchange requires strict aseptic technique and a number of different systems may be employed. The most popular is a disconnect system. Dialysis fluid is warmed to body temperature and both this and a drainage bag are attached to the abdominal catheter. Fluid is drained out from the abdominal catheter into the empty bag and new dialysate is instilled from the warmed bag. The bags are then disconnected and the fluid left in place for 4–8 h. The dialysate in the abdominal cavity drains in and out under gravity and by capillary blood flow.

The advantages of PD include the following:

- Independence – as the dialysis does not require hospital attendance or complex plumbing or machinery
- Continuous dialysis process is preferable, as the haemodynamic fluctuations are minimized
- Blood loss is avoided compared with HD, resulting in less anaemia
- Cost savings compared with HD
- Less fluid and dietary restriction.

Disadvantages include:

- Infections of the peritoneum
- Glucose absorption from the dialysate
- Protein loss
- Treatment failure if the peritoneum is damaged.

Community dialysis teams

Community dialysis teams provide support to patients undertaking dialysis at home – both HD and PD. Most teams are multidisciplinary with highly trained medical and nursing staff making decisions regarding the treatment and providing the care and support through regular home visits to monitor patients. The team will usually have strong links with the wider multidisciplinary team, which includes dietitians, pharmacists, renal technicians and social workers.

Each member of the renal team will have specific responsibilities:

- The medical and nursing team will be involved with prescribing of dialysis programmes and clinical monitoring
- The dietitian advises on nutritional intake and any dietary restrictions required
- The pharmacist provides medicines advice and may have a role in the ordering and supply of dialysis fluids and ancillary products
- The social worker provides advice and practical help for patients
- The renal technician is responsible for the programming, servicing and functioning of dialysis machines.

UK Renal Pharmacy Group

The UK Renal Pharmacy Group (UKRPG) is affiliated to the British Renal Society and is a specialist interest group for pharmacists and pharmacy technicians working in the field of renal medicine or with an interest in renal pharmacy. The UKRPG uses its clinical pharmacy experience to compile *The Renal Drug Handbook* and *Introduction to Renal Therapeutics*; both publications are excellent reference sources for further reading.

KEY POINTS

- Up to half of medical and surgical patients may have nutritional deficiencies
- TPN/HPN formulations are prepared under strict aseptic conditions
- Before starting TPN, a full assessment of the patient's nutritional needs must be made
- The nutrition team contribute their expertise to provide good patient care by meeting regularly to monitor patient needs
- A TPN formulation may contain water, protein, carbohydrate, fat, electrolytes, trace elements, vitamins and minerals

- Most TPN patients have a negative nitrogen balance and so require amino acids
- Care must be taken when administering dextrose in a TPN/HPN formulation to prevent problems of hyper or hypoglycaemia
- Strictly defined procedures are followed when adding ingredients to TPN bags during preparation
- Stability of TPN formulations is one of the major issues which must be carefully considered
- Controlling quantities can minimize incompatibilities such as that between calcium and phosphate
- TPN bags containing a fat component become less stable on prolonged storage and could result in fat deposits arising in lungs and capillaries if administered in this unstable condition
- For TPN lasting longer than 4 weeks, a central vein should be used
- A number of problems can arise during TPN/HPN administration. For HPN patients, adequate training to deal with problems arising at home is essential
- HPN patients are required to make psychological and social adjustments, but can also have an improvement in quality of life
- BAPEN has laid down standards for home nutritional care which are used as the basis for patient training prior to discharge
- Dialysis is used to remove toxic metabolites, correct acid–base balance and avoid fluid overload
- In haemodialysis, the patient's blood is passed over a semi-permeable membrane to allow exchange of small solutes with dialysis fluid
- Peritoneal dialysis uses the peritoneal membrane as the semi-permeable membrane, the dialysis fluid staying in the peritoneal cavity during the exchange
- CAPD has a number of advantages and disadvantages for patients
- HD solutions do not need to be sterile, but PD solutions must be sterile and aseptic technique used in handling
- Home dialysis patients will require training and support

Radiopharmacy

45

David Graham

STUDY POINTS

- Types of radionuclides and the principles of their medical use
- Examples of alpha-emitters, beta⁻- and beta⁺-emitters, electron capture and isomeric transitions
- Radionuclide production of beta⁺-emitters
- Principles of using a molybdenum-technetium generator
- Preparation of ^{99m}Tc radiopharmaceuticals
- Safety in radiopharmacy

Introduction

Elements that emit radiation are known as radio-nuclides and have a number of applications in medicine. Radiopharmacy in hospital practice is concerned with the manufacture or preparation of radioactive medicines known as radiopharmaceuticals. These have two main applications in medicine:

- As an aid to the diagnosis of disease (diagnostic radiopharmaceuticals)
- In the treatment of disease (therapeutic radiopharmaceuticals).

Diagnostic radiopharmaceuticals may be classified into two types:

- Radiopharmaceuticals used in tracer techniques for measuring physiological parameters (e.g. ^{51}Cr-EDTA for measuring glomerular filtration rate)
- Radiopharmaceuticals for diagnostic imaging (e.g. ^{99m}Tc-methylene diphosphonate (MDP) used in bone scanning).

In diagnostic imaging, gamma-emitting radionuclides are used, since their interaction with tissue is much less than that of particulate emitters and will cause significantly less damage to tissue. Radiopharmaceuticals are administered to the patient, usually by the intravenous (IV) route, and distribute into a particular organ. The radiation is then detected externally using a special scintillation detector known as a gamma-camera. These are used by nuclear medicine departments to image the distribution of the radiopharmaceutical within the patient's body. Using the gamma-camera in conjunction with a computer system it is not only possible to produce static images of an organ, but also to examine how the radiopharmaceutical moves through an organ. These dynamic images describe how the organ is functioning. It is also possible to create images in three dimensions, a process known as single photon emission computerized tomography (SPECT) when used in combination with gamma-emitting radionuclides such as ^{99m}Tc and positron emission tomography (PET) when used in combination with positron-emitting radionuclides such as ^{18}F.

It is important to note that for the safe production of radiopharmaceuticals, the radiopharmacy must be designed to comply with, and procedures must follow, good manufacturing practice and good radiation protection practice. Radiopharmacists working in this field are part of a multidisciplinary team which includes physicians, physicists, radiochemists and technicians from the field of pharmacy as well as nuclear medicine. As part of this team, they not only ensure that the radiopharmaceuticals will give high-quality clinical information, but also that they are safe for both patient and user alike.

Radionuclides used in nuclear medicine

Alpha-emitters

Alpha-decay is the process whereby a nucleus emits a helium nucleus, or alpha-particle. This commonly occurs with heavy nuclei (e.g. ^{226}Ra: $^{226}_{88}$Ra → $^{222}_{86}$Rn + alpha).

Because they are heavy and positively charged, alpha-particles travel only short distances in air (~5 mm) and only micrometre distances in tissues. Their ionizing nature would result in a highly localized radiation dose if taken internally and hence they tend not to be used as diagnostic radiopharmaceuticals but may have a place as therapeutic agents.

Some alpha-emitters (e.g. ^{137}Cs) when encapsulated are used as sealed sources, emitting X-rays or gamma-rays for radiotherapy applications. Here the body is exposed to radiation externally in an attempt to treat malignant tumours.

Beta-emitters

Beta-decay occurs in two ways, one that involves the emission of a negatively charged beta$^-$-particle, or electron, and the other that involves the emission of a positively charged beta$^+$-particle, or positron.

Beta$^-$-emitters

Radionuclides which decay by beta$^-$-decay tend to have nuclei that are neutron rich. They attempt to reach a more stable state by the transformation of a neutron into a proton with the emission of a beta$^-$-particle (e.g. ^{32}P: $^{32}_{15}$P → $^{32}_{16}$S + beta$^-$). Despite beta$^-$-particles having a range in air of up to several metres, their range in tissues is only a few millimetres. Because of this and their highly ionizing nature, beta$^-$-emitters tend to be used in therapeutic radiopharmaceuticals (Table 45.1).

The principle of therapeutic treatment with radionuclides is to target the radionuclide to a specific tissue within the body in an attempt to selectively damage or destroy that tissue. Ideally, therapeutic beta$^-$-emitting radionuclides should have energies of 0.5–1.5 MeV and a half-life of several days to provide a prolonged radiobiological effect.

The most widely used example of this is ^{131}I-sodium iodide, which is used in the treatment of hyperactive thyroid disease and in certain thyroid tumours. Here the physiological property of thyroid tissue is exploited to target the radionuclide to the site of action. Since thyroid tissue avidly takes up iodine in the normal synthesis of the hormone levothyroxine, radioactive iodine is also taken up and held in the thyroid tissue. Hence, the radiation damage is targeted to the thyroid tissue specifically and the normal excretion of any excess iodine results in no significant damage to other organs and tissues.

Table 45.1 Examples of radionuclides used in nuclear medicine

Mode of decay	Radionuclide	Radiopharmaceutical	Half-life	Clinical use
Beta$^-$-emitters	^{131}I	Sodium iodide capsules	8 days	Thyrotoxicosis, thyroid carcinomas
	^{89}Sr	Strontium chloride injection	50 days	Palliation of pain from bone metastases
Beta$^+$-emitters	^{15}O	^{15}O$_2$ gas	2.04 min	Brain blood flow imaging
	^{11}C	^{11}C-methionine	20.4 min	Prostate cancer
	^{13}N	^{13}N ammonia	9.97 min	Cardiac perfusion
	^{18}F	Fluorodeoxy-glucose injection	109.8 min	Tumour detection
Electron capture	^{111}In	Indium chloride solution	67 h	Antibody labelling
	^{123}I	Sodium iodide injection	13 h	Thyroid imaging
Isomeric transition	^{99m}Tc	Sodium pertechnetate injection	6 h	See Table 45.2
	^{81m}Kr	Krypton gas	13 s	Lung ventilation imaging

Beta$^+$-emitters (positrons)

Radionuclides that emit positrons are becoming more widely used in nuclear medicine. In this transformation, a proton-rich nuclide attempts to achieve stability by converting a proton to a neutron with the emission of a positron (e.g. $^{11}C:^{11}_{6}C \rightarrow ^{11}_{5}S + beta^+ + gamma$). The positron is very short-lived, since it interacts with an electron resulting in an annihilation reaction and the conversion of both particles into electromagnetic (EM) radiation. This EM radiation is in the form of two gamma-rays, each having energy of 0.511 MeV, which are emitted at an angle of 180° to each other.

When used in conjunction with a specialized gamma-camera with detectors placed 180° apart, it is possible to create images in all three dimensions with the position of the radiopharmaceutical being very precisely known. This type of imaging technique is known as positron emission tomography (PET). There are a number of positron emitting radionuclides which are becoming important tools in diagnostic imaging. Currently ^{18}F-labelled glucose, known as ^{18}F-fluoro deoxy-glucose (^{18}F-FDG), is the most commonly used PET radiopharmaceutical in hospital practice and as a result the production processes for it will be described in simplified form and used as an example (see below). However, it should be noted there are four main positron emitters used to prepare radiopharmaceuticals (see Table 45.1). PET imaging with ^{18}F-FDG, in combination with X-ray computerized tomography (CT) is rapidly becoming an important imaging technique in the diagnosis of cancer.

Electron capture

Nuclei that are proton rich may, as an alternative to positron emission, capture electrons from the atom's electron orbital. This process results in the transformation of a proton to a neutron within the nucleus. The subsequent rearrangement of the electrons orbiting the nucleus results in a characteristic emission of X-rays or gamma-rays (e.g. $^{123}I:^{123}_{53}I +$ electron$\rightarrow ^{123}_{53}Te$ + gamma).

Radionuclides which decay by electron capture are useful in diagnostic imaging since they emit gamma-rays; examples are given in Table 45.1.

Isomeric transition

Some radionuclides exist for measurable periods in excited, or isomeric, states prior to reaching ground

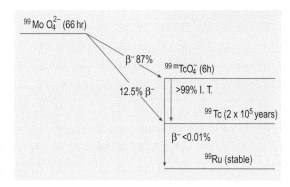

Figure 45.1 • Diagrammatic representation of ^{99}Mo decay.

state. This form of decay involves the emission of a gamma-ray and is known as isomeric transition. When radionuclides exist in this transitional state, they are known as metastable, which is denoted by the letter 'm' and written thus: ^{99m}Tc.

A simplified decay scheme for ^{99m}Tc-technetium is shown in Figure 45.1 where ^{99m}Tc's parent radionuclide, molybdenum (^{99}Mo), decays by beta$^-$-emission to the ground state ^{99}Tc either directly or indirectly.

The indirect route, which is the most common, involves the isomer ^{99m}Tc, which in turn decays from its metastable state to ^{99}Tc by isomeric transition.

Radionuclides which decay by this process are used in diagnostic imaging since they emit gamma-rays (see Table 45.1). It should be noted that ^{99m}Tc is the most widely used radionuclide in hospital radiopharmacy today, making up the radionuclide component of around 90% of the radiopharmaceuticals produced. For these reasons the production processes for ^{99m}Tc-radiopharmaceuticals will be especially emphasized (see below).

Principles of ^{99m}Tc-radiopharmaceutical production

The physical and chemical properties of ^{99m}Tc make it nearly ideal for imaging purposes as outlined below:

- It has a 6-h half-life ($T_{1/2}$); long enough to allow imaging to take place in the working day, while also being short enough that patients are not radioactive for long periods (in 24 h, or 4 half-lives, the radioactivity will have decayed by 94%)

- ^{99m}Tc emits gamma-rays of 140 keV energy: ideal for use with the modern gamma-camera
- There are no particulate emissions that, if present, would add to the patient's radiation dose
- By purchasing a device known as a ^{99}Mo/^{99m}Tc -generator, ^{99m}Tc can be made readily available to the hospital site in a sterile and pyrogen-free form
- ^{99m}Tc has versatile coordination chemistry and will allow a large number of ligands to complex with it. By using different ligands in the radiopharmaceutical's formulation, a wide range of radiopharmaceuticals can be prepared in the radiopharmacy, providing for the many different investigations carried out in nuclear medicine departments (Table 45.2).

The production of ^{99m}Tc – the molybdenum/technetium generator

Radionuclides with long half-lives (e.g. ^{131}I, $T_{1/2}$=8 days) can be easily transported from production site to the user hospital. With shorter half-life radionuclides, e.g. ^{99m}Tc, this supply system would be extremely difficult. As a result, a device known as the radionuclide generator is used to provide ^{99m}Tc to the hospital site.

Radionuclide generators work on the principle that they contain a relatively long-lived 'parent' radionuclide that decays to produce a 'daughter' radionuclide. The chemical nature of parent and daughter are different, allowing separation of the daughter from the parent.

The molybdenum/technetium generator consists of ^{99}Mo (long-lived 'parent') absorbed onto an alumina-filled column, the ^{99}Mo being present in the form of molybdate (^{99}MoO$_4$$^{2-}$). ^{99}Mo decays to its 'daughter' radionuclide ^{99m}Tc, as pertechnetate, ^{99m}TcO$_4$$^-$ (see Fig. 45.1). The amount of ^{99m}TcO$_4$$^-$ grows as a result of the decay of ^{99}Mo, until a transient equilibrium is reached. At this point the amount of ^{99m}Tc in the column appears to decay with the half-life of ^{99}Mo (Fig. 45.2).

By drawing a solution of sodium chloride 0.9% weight in volume (w/v) through the column, ^{99m}Tc is removed from the column in the form of sodium pertechnetate, Na^{99m}TcO$_4$. This process is known as eluting the generator and the resulting solution as the eluate. This process results in the production of a sterile solution of sodium pertechnetate that may now be used to make ^{99m}Tc -radiopharmaceuticals.

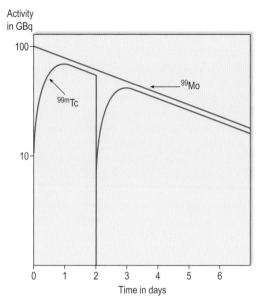

Figure 45.2 • Radioactivity changes with time in a molybdenum/technetium generator column.

^{99}Mo remains on the column where it decays to produce further ^{99m}Tc, the equilibrium being re-established about 23 h after elution. Elution of the generator is repeated daily to provide the radiopharmacy with a supply of ^{99m}Tc for 7–14 days, beyond which the yield of ^{99m}Tc becomes too small to be useful. Hospital radiopharmacies tend to buy generators on a weekly basis to provide a continuous supply of ^{99m}Tc.

Design of a ^{99m}Tc-generator

The design of a typical generator will be described by reference to the GE Healthcare generator, Drytec® (Fig. 45.3). The main components of this generator are:

- A needle connected to the top end of the alumina column by tubing (it is this needle upon which a vial of IV Sodium Chloride Intravenous Infusion BP 0.9% w/v will be placed)
- A sterile alumina column to which is bound ^{99}Mo
- An elution needle which is connected to the bottom end of the alumina column
- Two 0.22 µm filters.

These components are housed within a compact plastic casing. The alumina column is encased in lead to give protection from the radiation.

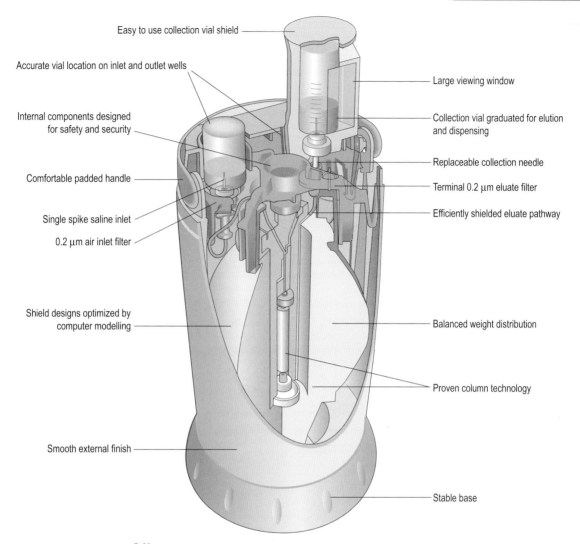

Easy to use collection vial shield

Accurate vial location on inlet and outlet wells

Internal components designed for safety and security

Comfortable padded handle

Single spike saline inlet

0.2 µm air inlet filter

Shield designs optimized by computer modelling

Smooth external finish

Large viewing window

Collection vial graduated for elution and dispensing

Replaceable collection needle

Terminal 0.2 µm eluate filter

Efficiently shielded eluate pathway

Balanced weight distribution

Proven column technology

Stable base

Figure 45.3 • The Drytec® 99mTc-generator. (Courtesy of GE Healthcare plc.)

Operating the generator is fairly straightforward. A vial of Sodium Chloride Intravenous Infusion BP 0.9% w/v, supplied with the generator, is first placed on the left hand needle (see Fig. 45.3). A sterile evacuated vial, also supplied with the generator, is placed in a lead pot designed for the elution process. Then, by placing this on the elution needle, the vacuum draws sterile Sodium Chloride Intravenous Infusion BP 0.9% w/v from the vial through the column and into the evacuated vial. When eluate has been collected, air enters the elution vial after first passing through the column. This dries the column as well as removing excess vacuum in the elution vial. The elution process is

now complete and the vial may be removed from the generator.

The sterility of the eluates is maintained throughout the useful life of the generator by the following means:

- The eluting solution is terminally sterilized Sodium Chloride Intravenous Infusion BP 0.9% w/v
- Air entering the system passes through a 0.22 µm filter
- A terminal eluate 0.22 µm filter is placed between the column and the elution needle
- Between elutions, the needle is protected by a single-use, disposable, sterile needle guard.

The elution of the generator should be carried out in a Grade A environment (see Ch. 40).

Preparation of ^{99m}Tc-radiopharmaceuticals

The daily supply of ^{99m}Tc is provided by the elution of the generator, resulting in a sterile solution of sodium pertechnetate that is subdivided to provide the radioactive component of the radiopharmaceutical. Some nuclear medicine investigations use sodium pertechnetate alone as the radiopharmaceutical (see Table 45.2). In this case, preparation of sodium pertechnetate injection requires only the subdivision from the generator eluate with perhaps some further dilution with Sodium Chloride Intravenous Infusion BP 0.9% w/v.

Other investigations, and these are in the majority, use radiopharmaceuticals that involve the chemical transformation of the sodium pertechnetate into another radiochemical form.

In order to make the preparation of ^{99m}Tc-radiopharmaceuticals as simple as possible, commercially available 'kits' are used to manufacture these radiopharmaceuticals. These kits allow the radiopharmacist, in the hospital environment, to transform the pertechnetate, via complex chemical reactions performed within the vial, into the desired radiopharmaceutical. This is achieved by the simple addition of pertechnetate into the vial followed by shaking to dissolve the contents.

A kit consists of a pre-packed set of sterile ingredients designed for the preparation of a specific radiopharmaceutical. Most commonly, the ingredients are freeze dried, enclosed within a rubber-capped nitrogen-filled vial. Normally, the kit contains sufficient materials to prepare a number of patient doses. In a typical formulation, the following may be found:

- The compound to be complexed to the ^{99m}Tc. These are known as ligands (e.g. methylene diphosphonate)
- Stannous ions (e.g. stannous chloride or fluoride) which are present as a reducing agent.

Table 45.2 Examples of ^{99m}Tc-radiopharmaceuticals

Radiopharmaceutical	Organ or tissue of distribution	Main clinical application
^{99m}Tc-sodium pertechnetate	Thyroid	Imaging the thyroid gland and ectopic tissue
	Salivary gland	Dynamic images of accumulation and drainage to show gland function
	Gastric mucosa	Presence of Meckel's diverticulum containing gastric mucosa
^{99m}Tc-methylene diphosphonate (MDP)	Skeleton	Bone metastases from carcinoma of lung, breast and prostate
^{99m}Tc-macro-aggregates of albumin (MAA)	Lung blood flow	Lung perfusion studies most commonly for the diagnosis of pulmonary embolism
^{99m}Tc-exametazime (HMPAO)	Brain blood flow	Regional cerebral imaging in stroke and tumours
		Diagnosis of Alzheimer's dementia
^{99m}Tc-exametazime (HMPAO) labelled leucocytes	Infection or inflammation	Identification of abscesses associated with pyrexia of unknown origin. Extent of inflammatory bowel disease
^{99m}Tc-tetrofosmin	Heart	Cardiac perfusion imaging
^{99m}Tc-sestamibi (MIBI)	Heart	Cardiac perfusion imaging
^{99m}Tc-tin colloid	Liver	Location of hepatic tumours, abscesses and cysts. Detection of cirrhosis
^{99m}Tc-mercapto triglycine (MAG 3)	Kidney	Dynamic studies to study kidney function
^{99m}Tc-dimercapto-succinic acid (DMSA)	Kidney	Static imaging showing the kidney structure

The reduction of $^{99m}TcO_4^-$ to a lower valance state is required to allow the ligands to form a complex with the ^{99m}Tc

- Other compounds that act as stabilizers, buffers or antioxidants.

Given below is an example of how ^{99m}Tc-radiopharmaceutical production may be performed. The compounding procedures must be carried out within the facilities described in Chapter 40 using aseptic technique and carried out as 'closed' procedures (GMP).

The production method (Fig. 45.4) involves two simple steps:

Step 1. The freeze-dried kit is reconstituted by aseptically transferring the necessary activity of sodium pertechnetate using a sterile syringe and needle. This step may also include a further dilution of the eluate with a suitable diluent. The amount of activity withdrawn for the reconstitution of the kit vial depends on two factors:

- The number of patient doses to be manufactured
- The amount of activity required at injection time for each of the patient doses. The calculation would take into account the decay of ^{99m}Tc.

Manufacturers normally specify a maximum activity that may be added to the vial.

Step 2. The reconstituted kit is aseptically subdivided to provide each patient dose with sufficient activity to allow proper imaging after administration.

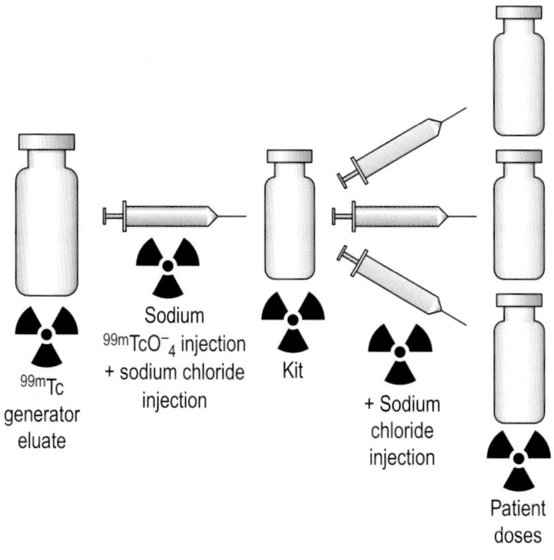

As in Step 1, a diluent may be added to the final dose to give the desired radioactive concentration.

^{99m}Tc-radiopharmaceuticals must be administered on the day of production, for the following reasons:

- *Sterility.* Aseptically prepared pharmaceuticals should ideally be administered within a few hours of production, in accordance with GMP
- *Radioactivity.* ^{99m}Tc has a half-life of only 6 h

Radiochemical stability. ^{99m}Tc-complexes are generally stable for a period between 4 and 8 h after production.

Principles of ^{18}F-fluoro deoxyglucose (^{18}F-FDG) production

In the manufacture of ^{18}F-FDG there are two main processes. First there is the production of the radionuclide itself, which is produced in a cyclotron facility. This is followed by the radiosynthesis of the ^{18}F-FDG, which is carried out in an automated apparatus, known as a synthesis module. The resulting solution of ^{18}F-FDG has then to be sterilized and may have to be sub-dispensed in some way so as to provide the injection in a ready to administer form. Since the ^{18}F-FDG has been synthesized, it will require analysis and other quality control checks prior to administration to the patient.

Radionuclide production

A cyclotron is a device used to produce radionuclides. It accelerates atomic or subatomic particles in a circular orbit, increasing the energy of the particles until a high-energy beam of particles is created. Once the particles have reached their maximum energy they are extracted using high voltage and allowed to bombard target materials. The composition of the target material and the nuclear reactions that take place determine the radionuclides that are produced.

For ^{18}F production, the most common nuclear reaction used is the ^{18}O (p,n) ^{18}F reaction, where protons are produced from hydrogen gas and are accelerated until, at a required energy, a 'beam' of the protons are allowed to bombard a target of ^{18}O-enriched water ($H_2^{18}O$). ^{18}O is a naturally occurring isotope of oxygen, but much less

Figure 45.4 • Schematic representation of the preparation of patient doses of radiopharmaceuticals.

Labels in figure: ^{99m}Tc generator eluate — Sodium $^{99m}TcO_4^-$ injection + sodium chloride injection — Kit — + Sodium chloride injection — Patient doses abundant than the normal ^{16}O. By forcing a proton into the ^{18}O nucleus the now unstable nucleus ejects a neutron and the result is the production of ^{18}F – a positron-emitting radionuclide.

Radio-synthesis

2-[^{18}F] fluoro-2-deoxy-D glucose (^{18}F-FDG) may be prepared by various chemical pathways, but whatever radio-synthetic route is used it must be rapid to minimize the radiation risk and be of high yield. An automated apparatus, the synthesis module, is used to synthesize the ^{18}F-FDG to assure production efficiency and keep radiation exposure to a minimum. There are now commercially available synthesis modules such as the TRACERlabFx Synthesizer® as shown in Figure 45.5, which are supplied with good manufacturing practice (GMP) standard raw materials and reagents for use in the module. Using this equipment, the following synthetic pathway is performed:

1. The ^{18}F-fluoride is adsorbed by an anion-exchange resin.
2. The retained ^{18}F-fluoride is eluted using an aqueous potassium carbonate solution.

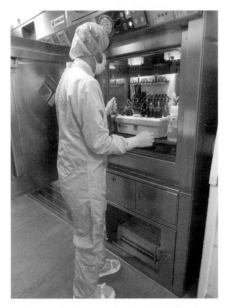

Figure 45.5 • Synthesis module for ^{18}F-FDG production (TRACERlabFx Synthesizer®). (Courtesy of GE Healthcare plc.) Module located in lead-shielded (5.5 cm) specialized fume cupboard known as 'hot cell'.

3. A phase transfer catalyst (Kriptofix 222) dissolved in acetonitrile is then added, to bind the potassium ion and to enhance the nucleophilic reactivity of the ^{18}F-fluoride.
4. After evaporation of the solvents, the ^{18}F-fluoride is allowed to react with the reagent mannose triflate at elevated temperature (1,3,4,6-O-Acetyl-2-O-trifluoromethanesulfonyl-beta-D-mannopyranose). The structure of mannose triflate is similar to that of glucose with a leaving group (triflate) and four acetyl protecting groups to ensure the mannose ring undergoes nucleophilic substitution at the second carbon atom.
5. Hydrolysis under acidic or alkaline conditions also at elevated temperature yields 2-[^{18}F] fluoro-2-deoxy-D glucose (^{18}F-FDG).

Sterilization and sub-dispensing

Sterilization of the ^{18}F-FDG is achieved either by filtration through a 0.2 μm filter, although there are automated systems that use high temperature short sterilization cycles (e.g. 10 min cycle consisting of 4 min heat up; 135°C for 3.5 min; 2.5 min cool down). Sub-dispensing or fractionation of the bulk solution into patient doses is then carried out using robotic dispensing systems that perform the aseptic transfers since the radiation hazard is too great for regular manual aseptic transfer. This aseptic manipulation is carried out within a specialized isolator specifically designed for handling PET radiopharmaceuticals.

Quality control

Since the ^{18}F-FDG has been synthesized, it must undergo stringent testing as outlined in the monograph given in the *European Pharmacopoeia*. A detailed description is beyond the scope of this chapter, but in summary the tests will include:

- Identification test
- Determination of pH
- Sterility test
- Determination of bacterial endotoxins
- Determination of chemical purity
- Determination of radionuclide purity
- Determination of radiochemical purity
- Determination of the radioactivity.

Facilities required for the production of radiopharmaceuticals

The majority of radiopharmaceuticals are intended for IV administration; therefore it is of paramount importance that these preparations are sterile. They also contain radionuclides with short half-lives that require their preparation and administration on the same day. Because of the thermal lability of some of these products, it is not possible to use terminal sterilization by autoclaving and hence these injections must be prepared using aseptic techniques. Here, highly skilled operators work with sterile ingredients within clean room facilities containing either laminar flow safety cabinets or isolators. The facilities for carrying out such manipulations are more fully described in Chapter 40, but there is specialized equipment as well as design criteria specifically for handling radiopharmaceuticals. More information can be found in Further Reading (see Appendix 4).

Radiation protection in the radiopharmacy

There are three basic principles to radiation protection:

- *Shielding*. By placing shielding around the radioactive source, the radiation dose rate may be reduced. Materials used as shielding must be appropriate to the type of radiation being emitted by the radionuclide. Plastic, Perspex and metals of low molecular weight such as aluminium are appropriate materials for shielding beta -emitters. For gamma-emitters, high molecular weight metals such as lead and tungsten should be used. The thickness of shielding material necessary for gamma-emitters is dependent on the gamma-ray energy – the greater the energy, the thicker the shield required
- *Distance*. The radiation dose from a radioactive source is inversely proportional to the square of the distance (i.e. by doubling the distance the radiation dose is quartered)
- *Time*. Minimizing the time spent handling a radioactive source will reduce the radiation dose. It is important for new operators to practice

the handling operation prior to working with radioactive materials.

In working practice, all three of these principles may be used in isolation or together, to reduce the radiation dose to the operator. For example, in the dispensing operation outlined in Figure 45.4, all vials containing radioactive material would be contained in a 3mm lead pot. This will attenuate ^{99m}Tc's gamma-rays by a factor of approximately 1000. The syringes used to carry out the transfers would be only half full (i.e. 1 mL of radioactive solution would be transferred with a 2 mL syringe) in order to maximize the distance between the operator's fingers and the source, without compromising the accuracy of the dispensing operation.

The syringes, during the operation, should also be contained within a syringe shield. These are made of materials such as lead, tungsten, lead glass or lead acrylic, the latter two being transparent. Lead and tungsten syringe shields have lead glass/acrylic windows incorporated to allow the operator to see the graduations on the syringe. Alternatively, the whole syringe shield may be made of lead glass/acrylic which would have the advantage of giving greater visibility.

Handling the vials outside their lead pots should be carried out using long forceps and not with the fingers. The dispensing process should be carried out over a 'drip tray' that allows easy containment of any accidental spillage. It also should be carried out within a laminar flow safety cabinet or negative pressure isolator that provides operator protection as well as product protection (see Ch. 40).

The staff working in the radiopharmacy will be constantly monitored to assess their radiation exposure and to ensure compliance with safety legislation. Whole-body dose may be monitored with film badges and the radiation dose to the finger pulp with thermo luminescent dosimeters.

KEY POINTS

- Radiopharmaceuticals may be used in therapy or diagnosis, the latter either as tracers or in imaging
- PET-CT imaging with ^{18}F-FDG is becoming an important imaging technique in the diagnosis of cancer
- ^{18}F-FDG may be prepared by first producing ^{18}F in a cyclotron, followed by the radio-synthesis of the ^{18}F-FDG, which is carried out in an automated apparatus, known as a synthesis module

- ^{99m}Tc is the most widely used radionuclide
- A molybdenum/technetium generator will provide a daily supply of ^{99m}Tc for 7–14 days, as sodium pertechnetate
- Reacting with a suitable ligand can chemically modify sodium pertechnetate. Different ligands give different bio-distributions, resulting in the wide range of scans that may be performed with ^{99m}Tc
- Radiation protection should be provided for operators using a combination of shielding, distance and time

Specialized services

Geoff Saunders

STUDY POINTS

- Pharmacy aseptic compounding services and the range of medicines prepared in them
- Equipment and procedures used in centralized cytotoxic reconstitution services
- Occupational health risks of cytotoxic drugs and the effective management of these risks
- Benefits of centralized, pharmacy-operated aseptic compounding services
- Scope and operation of a centralized intravenous additive service (CIVAS)

Introduction

This chapter describes the specialized services provided by hospital pharmacy departments in the provision of various aseptic dosage forms. These services may include: chemotherapy reconstitution services, centralized intravenous additive services (CIVAS), radiopharmacy services (see Ch. 45) and home-care services. In each case, the service involves the provision of aseptically-prepared medicines which are often tailored to the specific needs of individual patients. This chapter introduces the scope, practice and pharmaceutical challenges of aseptic compounding services.

Cancer chemotherapy

The majority of chemotherapy doses are administered as injections or infusions. This offers the advantages of assured bioavailability, control over the rate and sequence of drug administration and also the ability to stop administration immediately in the event of adverse effects. However, the parenteral route may be associated with complications such as infection, extravasation and thromboembolism. The majority of these drugs are given in the hospital setting.

Cytotoxic drugs are available as sealed vials containing freeze-dried powders or sterile, concentrated solutions and are designed to provide an adequate shelf-life (usually >2 years). The freeze-dried powders require reconstitution with an appropriate diluent. Either may then require further dilution before being filled into syringes, infusion bags or infusion devices for administration.

Ambulatory infusion devices can be filled for use in the community by patients receiving home chemotherapy.

Occupational exposure risks

Cytotoxic drug exposure has been associated with various acute toxicities including headache, rash, nausea and dizziness. However, the more serious risks are related to the potential mutagenic, carcinogenic and teratogenic effects. Routes of exposure include ingestion, inhalation, needle-stick injury and skin contact – the most significant risk for occupational exposure.

In the UK, the requirements for safe handling of cytotoxic drugs are set out and enforced by the Health and Safety Executive. Pharmacy staff preparing cytotoxic agents must be fully trained in the necessary aseptic and safe handling techniques and must be fully aware of the potential health risks and the precautions that are required. Current opinion suggests that resources should be invested in appropriate equipment, staff training and competency assessment.

Published guidelines include the following areas of safe practice:

- Personnel training and competency
- Facilities and containment systems
- Techniques and precautions
- Dealing with spillage
- Disposal
- Labelling, packaging and distribution

Useful guidelines on cytotoxic handling include *The Cytotoxics Handbook* and further references are available in Appendix 4.

Provision of a pharmacy-based chemotherapy preparation service

Protection of both the product and the staff involved in its preparation is technically demanding and requires carefully developed systems and procedures together with extensive validation, which must be integrated with the principles of good pharmaceutical manufacturing practice (GMP). Capacity plans should ensure that the service is capable of meeting current and future demand; for example, the rising demand for targeted therapies.

Despite the challenges outlined above, it is important that pharmacy staff 'own' chemotherapy preparation services and take a clear lead. In the UK, from NPSA Alert 20 on injectable medicines, it is clear that application of the risk assessment guidelines places all cytotoxic drugs in the high-risk category. It is therefore essential that these medicines are prepared by specialized hospital pharmacy aseptic units or by appropriate commercial providers. Pharmacy staff offer a unique combination of skills and expertise, including the practice of aseptic technique, a wide clinical knowledge of cancer chemotherapy, familiarity with formulation and drug stability issues, the application of GMP, quality assurance (QA) and quality control (QC) to aseptic preparation and considerable experience in working with SOPs, batch documentation and checking procedures. These are key attributes that help to ensure the provision of safe, effective chemotherapy and contribute towards minimizing the risks of occupational exposure to drugs used in the treatment of cancer.

Training required for staff preparing cytotoxics

All personnel involved in preparing and handling cytotoxics require training and competency assessment in the appropriate techniques. On a practical level, all staff must be aware of the following, over and above standard aseptic technique and the application of GMP to aseptic preparation:

- Procedures required on receipt of a prescription for chemotherapy
- Completion of worksheets or batch documents
- Techniques for the safe handling and manipulation of cytotoxic drugs
- Safe storage and transportation of chemotherapy
- Background information on commonly used chemotherapy drugs and protocols
- Local and national policies and procedures.

Validation of operator techniques

Prior to commencing work on reconstitution of cytotoxics, an operator's competence in this field must be assessed.

- The operator is asked to carry out broth transfer simulations where solutions are transferred from one vial or container to another
- The broth-filled vials can then be incubated and examined for microbiological growth
- Operators must achieve negative results (no growth after incubation) on each occasion before they are deemed capable of preparing cytotoxic agents
- Typically, each operator and each process would be re-validated at least every 3 months and training procedures should be reviewed on a regular basis
- Operators routinely incorporate environmental monitoring tests such as settle plates and finger-dab plates into the production schedule as part of the QA process
- Expert guidance on the validation and monitoring of aseptic compounding has been published by the NHS
- Operator technique in the safe handling of cytotoxic drugs can be assessed by simulating

aseptic transfer processes using a sterile solution containing a fluorescent dye as splashes or spillage can be visualized using a portable ultraviolet lamp
- As with assessment of aseptic technique, safe handling should be evaluated using a combination of simulation and expert observation.

Documentation required for cytotoxics

On receipt of a prescription for a cytotoxic agent, a number of procedures must be undertaken. Figure 46.1 shows the areas of work in which a pharmacist may have involvement.

When the prescription is received, it is clinically checked by an experienced oncology pharmacist. The prescription must be validated against an approved chemotherapy protocol. It is essential that patients receive the correct number of cycles of treatment at the correct intervals. The British Oncology Pharmacy Association Standards for Prescription Verification for Systemic Anti Cancer Therapy provides detailed guidance.

Information from the prescription is transferred to a worksheet or batch document and details of medicine(s) required, diluent and volume for reconstitution are recorded together with the number of drug vials required. Details of batch numbers and expiry date for each component used, all dose and dilution calculations, preparation methods, container(s) to be used, time and date of preparation, and expiry of the final product are also required. Additionally, a sample label is attached to the worksheet. Most chemotherapy preparation units use preprinted worksheets for each chemotherapy protocol, with a pharmacist-approved master document from which copies are made. Alternatively, some units use computer-based systems which contain a database of all approved chemotherapy protocols and produce batch documents and labels.

Labels should include the following information:
- Patient's name, hospital number and ward or clinic name
- Drug name, total quantity and final volume of infusion
- Vehicle in which the drug is prepared (e.g. 0.9% sodium chloride)
- Batch number, expiry date and storage conditions required
- Hospital pharmacy name and address
- Route of administration and infusion rate
- Inclusion of the term 'cytotoxic'.

When the worksheet is complete, the materials required are collected together and then subjected to an initial check before transfer to the designated clean room. After preparation has been completed, the finished product(s) and used or part-used vials are returned in the tray, together with batch documents, for labelling, inspection and release. Some cytotoxic agents require protection from light and are sealed in opaque plastic overwraps which will also require labelling. The pharmacist responsible for the release of the prepared medicines will check all details on the worksheets and will reconcile the number of drug vials used in the preparation. If correct, the pharmacist will sign the worksheet or batch

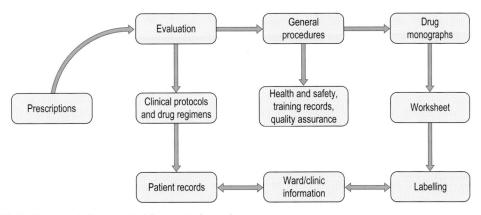

Figure 46.1 • Documentation required for cytotoxic services. (From Allwood et al. 2002, reproduced with permission.)

documents to signify approval, and the medicines are dispatched. All documents must be retained for up to 13 years after the date of preparation.

Cytotoxic preparation areas

In the UK, and in many parts of Europe, pharmaceutical isolators are used for cytotoxic preparation. In addition to providing aseptic conditions for preparation of the product, isolators are designed to protect the operator and the clean room environment from cytotoxic contamination. To achieve this, many isolators operate under negative pressure with respect to the clean room, and the exhaust air is externally ducted via a high-efficiency particulate air (HEPA) filter. All isolators should be located in a classified clean room.

It is generally accepted that isolators offer greater operator protection than open-fronted Class II safety cabinets. The main disadvantages of isolators include limited access for equipment and difficulties in cleaning and removing cytotoxic residues. Gas sterilizable isolators enable sterilization of the outer surface of vials and components used in the preparation process. Gases such as vapourized hydrogen peroxide are pumped into the isolator to sterilize the inside of the isolator and the outer surface of components in situ, prior to manipulation.

Techniques and precautions

When handling cytotoxics, it is vital that the appropriate protective clothing is worn. Operators using clean room facilities must wear appropriate clean room clothing, with the addition of chemotherapy gowns or armlets. These garments are non-shedding and have an absorbent surface and impermeable backing. Full clean room suits are worn beneath the chemotherapy gown so it is important to ensure that the clean room temperature is carefully controlled. Gloves designed specifically for cytotoxic handling are available and these are normally fabricated from a nitrile material. Gloves should be worn for handling cytotoxic drug vials outside the clean rooms as these can be contaminated with cytotoxic residues on the outer surface.

Product segregation is crucial in all aseptic work to avoid any risk of product mix up and only one product or one batch of product, is prepared at any one time.

Reconstitution procedures

When carrying out reconstitution procedures, certain precautions must be taken:

- Vials and outer packs of consumables should be sprayed with sterile 70% alcohol and wiped with a sterile swab before being introduced into the clean room and the process repeated before introducing these materials into the isolator or Class II cabinet workstation. Rubber stoppers on vials should be swabbed with a sterile swab prior to removal of liquid
- Transfer of liquids to and from vials requires the insertion of a venting needle with hydrophobic filter into the vial or the use of a vented reconstitution device. These devices ensure pressure equalization and reduce the risk of aerosol generation
- Luer lock syringes with wide-bore needles should be used for all procedures to allow free flow in the fluid pathway and to avoid the risk of syringes and needles becoming disconnected during fluid transfer
- To ensure that no further additions are made outside the pharmacy preparation area, all completed products in syringe form should be sealed with a blind hub before removal from the cytotoxic cabinet (Fig. 46.2). An additive plug or cap must be placed on each minibag once additions are complete.

The vials that contain cytotoxic agents are effectively a closed system which contains either a powder requiring reconstitution or a drug concentrate requiring withdrawal from the vial into a syringe. In each case, equalization of pressure within the vial is required to allow withdrawal from it and is achieved by inserting a sterile 0.2 mm hydrophobic filter venting needle into the vial to facilitate liquid transfer. Ordinary needles with no hydrophobic filter must not be used for venting due to the risk of leakage of cytotoxic solution from the needle. Alternatively, reconstitution devices are available to help with the reconstitution process. Some of these devices consist of a small plastic spike with an integral hydrophobic filter. These devices are useful for rapid transfer of solutions, but the large needle bore can produce large holes in the rubber bung of cytotoxic vials, thus increasing the risk of leakage. The CytoSafe needle is a commonly used example of this type of product. This device consists of a needle which is vented to allow equilibrium of

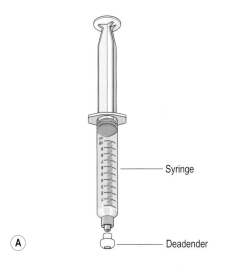

Syringe

Deadender

(A)

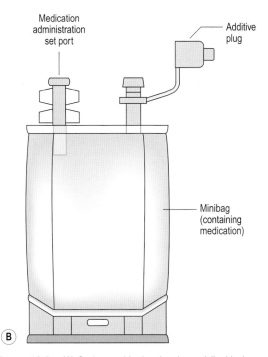

Medication
administration
set port

Additive
plug

Minibag
(containing
medication)

(B)

Figure 46.2 • (A) Syringe with deadender or blind hub
in position. (B) Minibag with additive plug.

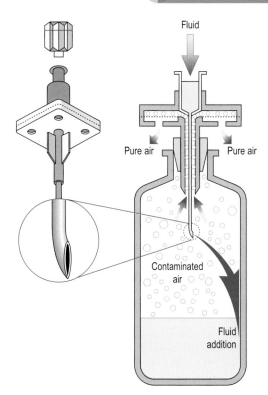

Fluid

Pure air   Pure air

Contaminated
air

Fluid
addition

Figure 46.3 • (A) CytoSafe needle and (B) reconstitution
set-up.

These devices virtually eliminate the risks of cytotoxic aerosol formation and operator needle-stick
injuries. An example of this type of device is the
Tevadaptor (Fig. 46.4). This system comprises a vial
adaptor to access the drug vial, and a syringe adaptor which fits securely onto a Luer lock syringe and
enables needle-free docking with the vial adaptor.
The closed reconstitution systems have been shown
in studies to be effective in reducing cytotoxic
contamination.

Dealing with cytotoxic spillage

In the event of a cytotoxic spillage, the problem
should be dealt with immediately to prevent the
spread of contamination. A written policy on dealing with spillages should be prepared. Most policies
are based on a spillage kit which contains all the
required materials to deal with a spill. Spillage kits
should be available in pharmacy preparation units,
in wards/clinics and in transport vehicles.

pressure between the vial and the syringe. It is useful for reconstitution of large vials or when more
than one vial is required for a dose (Fig. 46.3).
However, care must be taken when withdrawing
or adding liquid to a vial as the filter may become
blocked.

'Closed systems' using needle-free technologies have been designed for cytotoxic handling.

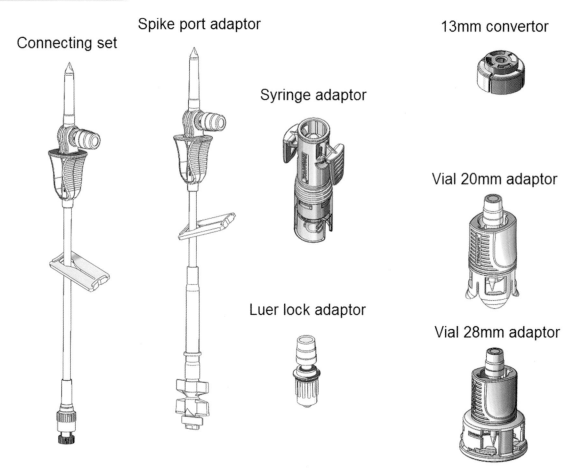

Figure 46.4 • Tevadaptor closed cytotoxic reconstitution and fluid transfer system. (All rights reserved to Teva Medical Ltd © 2013).

If the spillage has come in contact with the skin, the contaminated area should be washed thoroughly with soap and water. Contact with eyes should be dealt with by irrigation with a sodium chloride eyewash and medical help sought. In the event of a needle-stick injury, the puncture wound should be encouraged to bleed and the area should again be thoroughly washed. All incidents should be reported.

Disposal of cytotoxic waste

Cytotoxic waste materials are regarded as 'hazardous waste' and should be placed in a purple coloured plastic bag, sealed and labelled with a cytotoxic warning label ready for disposal by incineration. Sharp objects including needles, syringes, ampoules and vials should be placed in a sharps bin which is made of rigid plastic and does not allow leakage of cytotoxic waste. When the sharps bin is full, it should be sealed with 'cytotoxic' warning tape and disposed of by incineration.

Packaging of cytotoxic infusions

Cytotoxic infusions should be packaged in a labelled, hermetically sealed overwrap. This has two functions: containment of any leak from the infusion and protection of staff from any cytotoxic residues. Ideally, the infusions should be transported in a rigid, closed plastic box to protect from any mechanical trauma.

Management of the chemotherapy workload

It is evident from the above text that chemotherapy preparation is very labour-intensive. There is a clear tendency to move from in-patient treatment of cancer patients on hospital wards to chemotherapy outpatient clinics. This can place significant workload pressures on pharmacy chemotherapy units, partly because several patients often arrive for treatment at the same time, and also because blood test results and other patient-specific data are required before the oncologist is able to confirm the chemotherapy dose and allow treatment to proceed.

Various strategies have been employed to manage these problems. In many centres, it is possible to organize patients' blood samples 2 days before the patient is due to visit the outpatient clinic for treatment. This enables prescriptions to be 'pre-written' so that pharmacy can prepare batch documents and tray-up consumables on the day before treatment.

Many oncology centres have adopted the approach of 'dose-banding'. Individual patient doses are calculated in the normal way, but the dose is then fitted to predefined dose ranges or 'bands'. These standard doses are provided from a limited range of standard pre-filled syringes or infusion bags, either singly or in combination. In practice, five or six standard pre-fills are needed to provide the required range of standard doses.

There is no doubt that managing chemotherapy services is a very challenging task. Operating a patient-focused service that meets clinical needs within the confines of limited resources requires innovation, organization and regular communication with medical and nursing colleagues. The service should be carefully monitored and key outcomes such as errors and patient waiting times should be audited on a regular basis.

Centralized intravenous additive service (CIVAS)

The Breckenridge Report (1976) made recommendations that IV infusions should be prepared, where possible, by hospital pharmacies. The provision of an IV additive service did not commence until the 1980s and then only in a limited number of hospitals.

Currently, a large proportion of hospital pharmacists in the UK and many European countries provide a CIVAS, and this is augmented by a growing number of commercial compounding units. Despite these developments, it is estimated that of all infusions prepared in UK hospitals, less than 40% are prepared in pharmacy CIVAS units.

Scope of a CIVAS

A CIVAS is set up to provide a range of parenteral dosage forms suitable for administration to patients. A CIVA service can provide the following:

- IV antibiotics, antivirals, antifungals and steroids
- Patient-controlled analgesia, and other opioid infusions for postoperative analgesia and palliative care
- Epidural analgesics infusions
- Ambulatory infusion devices for various IV therapies at home
- Electrolyte infusions (that are not commercially available).

Given that CIVAS are resourced to provide only a proportion of the IV additive/compounding needs of a hospital, they normally prioritize the services offered according to clinical risk. Accordingly, CIVAS-produced infusions often include antibiotics for neonates and paediatric patients which require extensive dilution to the required doses. Economic factors can also influence which infusions are prepared in CIVAS units. Many IV medicines contain no preservative and are designed for single use only. However, subject to validated infusion stability, it is possible for a CIVAS unit to prepare a batch of infusions for several days' use, or even longer, so reducing or eliminating drug wastage.

Provision of a CIVAS

The main goals of providing a CIVAS should include:

- Improved patient safety
- Improved use of hospital resources
- Improved services to patients, particularly with home infusions
- Improved pharmacy control and reduced risk of medication errors.

Although there are compelling reasons for the provision of pharmacy CIVAS in all major hospitals, it is important in presenting a balanced argument to be aware of potential disadvantages to the hospital and healthcare system:

- Increased pharmacy expenditure diverting funds from other healthcare services
- Pharmacy CIVAS, once established, should be available 24 hours a day, including weekends and public holidays
- There is a potential risk of de-skilling ward staff in the preparation of drug infusions
- Some wards and departments may be difficult to service, e.g. accident and emergency, because doses of some drugs may be required urgently
- The capacity of the CIVAS is not infinite but there will always be pressures to add new drugs to the service as soon as these enter clinical use.

Many of these problems can be overcome through good communication, both within the pharmacy department and with medical and nursing staff. A service level agreement is a useful device for ensuring that all stakeholders know their responsibilities and that the service operates within the confines of the available resources.

Quality assurance

All procedures used during preparation of CIVAS doses must be fully validated and documented. Procedures must also be audited and be subject to in-process monitoring. Staff preparing IV products should complete appropriate batch documents and adhere to authorized SOPs and published guidelines. As with the chemotherapy preparation service described previously, there are various elements to be considered as part of the decision-making process for the release of CIVAS medicines for administration to patients. Clean room overpressures should be recorded at least daily, and HEPA filter integrity checks should be carried out at least on an annual basis or in the event of any deviation from defined operating conditions.

Records will be kept for all IV medicines prepared and will include the batch numbers of products used during reconstitution procedures. This ensures that in the event of a product recall or any problems with an IV medicine, a full audit trail documenting all aspects of the process can be reviewed.

Validation of procedures

Validation of processes and operator technique for CIVAS is almost identical to the validations necessary for chemotherapy preparation.

Infusion stability and shelf-life assignment

The assignment of a shelf-life or expiry date to any aseptically prepared medicine is a rigorous, evidence-based process which requires expert interpretation of physical and chemical stability data and a clear understanding of the level of protection afforded to prevent microbiological contamination during the aseptic preparation process.

In the UK, aseptic medicines prepared requiring pharmacist supervision of the process, are restricted to a maximum shelf-life of 7 days, and then only if there is evidence to support this. On the other hand, aseptic medicines made under a manufacturer's 'specials' licence issued by the MHRA can be assigned any reasonable shelf-life providing this is supported by rigorous evidence.

Stability data for CIVAS infusions, including cytotoxic drugs, can be sourced from a number of reference books. In many cases, it will be necessary to search the scientific and professional literature for original stability study reports and, on some occasions, the drug manufacturer may be willing to share extended stability data. Whatever the source of information, stability data should always be subjected to critical appraisal before it is used in the assignment of infusion shelf-lives.

Assessment of infusion stability is a key responsibility of any pharmacist managing a CIVAS. In the case of infusions which are outsourced from commercial compounding units, it is essential that clear and robust evidence is available to support the assigned shelf-life. Care must be exercised when attempting to extrapolate published stability data to infusions with variations in the concentration, diluents or container used. Expert review and a written justification are required to validate a shelf-life where there is any variation to the conditions under which the stability data were obtained.

Consideration must also be given to the transportation and storage of aseptically prepared medicines. Cold chain transport systems must be fully validated to ensure that the stability of infusions is not compromised and the storage temperatures should be monitored at least daily, but preferably by continuous monitoring and data logging.

KEY POINTS

- Cancer chemotherapy can include treatment with cytotoxic drugs and biological 'targeted' therapies
- There are significant occupational exposure risks to healthcare workers who handle cytotoxic drugs
- Compliance with safe handling guidelines, combined with use of protective equipment, containment facilities and validated technique can minimize unplanned cytotoxic exposure
- Use of strict aseptic conditions minimizes the risk of microbiological contamination during preparation
- Detailed SOPs for preparation and administration of chemotherapy must be prepared and implemented

- All personnel involved in provision of a centralized cytotoxic reconstitutions service must be trained and validated in all relevant procedures and techniques
- Transfer of solutions between cytotoxic drug vials and syringes must be carried out using a hydrophobic venting pin or a purpose designed transfer device to avoid the generation of aerosols
- Drug stability is a key issue in assigning infusion shelf-lives, particularly those used for home infusion
- Increased use of chemotherapy outpatient or day-case clinics can place significant pressures on the workload of the pharmacy chemotherapy unit
- New strategies such as 'dose-banding' are useful to manage chemotherapy workload
- A CIVAS can provide a wide range of aseptically prepared medicines for hospital and domiciliary use
- Potential benefits of CIVAS include reduced risk of medication errors, improved use of resources, better services to patients and pharmacy control
- Most doses are provided from CIVAS as either pre-filled syringes or minibags

Appliances

47

Ian Smith

STUDY POINTS

- What appliances do pharmacists dispense?
- What makes an ideal wound dressing?
- What can be supplied for dressing a wound?
- What appliances are available for urinary incontinence?
- The appliances available for a patient with a stoma
- How to supply graduated compression hosiery
- How to supply a truss

Introduction

In addition to dispensing medicines, pharmacists have traditionally had a role in dispensing and supplying appliances. Appliances are sometimes termed as medical devices. In the European Union, there is a requirement that all appliances have a CE marking on them. This indicates that the product conforms to the relevant medical device directives laid down by the EU. There are some medical devices, which are exempt from the CE marking requirement an example of which would be made to measure hosiery.

In the UK, only the appliances which are listed in the *Drug Tariff* can be supplied on an NHS prescription.

The main types of appliance which pharmacists supply are wound dressings, incontinence and stoma products. Pharmacists are also required to supply and to measure and fit hosiery and trusses. Other appliances which pharmacists can supply include needles and syringes, bandages, ear syringes and peak flow meters.

Wound dressings

When the skin becomes damaged, it will undergo a process of wound healing. The speed and mechanism of the healing of the wound will depend on the degree of tissue loss and the depth and site of the wound. One major concern is that the wound may become infected.

The wound healing process consists of four overlapping phases:

1. *Haemostasis*. This is not always considered a phase in all publications. Bleeding is stopped by a combination of vasoconstriction and coagulation. It happens immediately the wound has occurred and can last from a few seconds to a few days, depending on the wound.
2. *Inflammation*. This is cleansing and removal of debris. This phase starts a few hours after haemostasis and can last a few days. The inflammatory response leads to redness, heat and swelling. Macrophages and polymorphs in the blood begin to clean the wound of debris, damaged tissues and bacteria. This leads to the production of exudate and the wound can become macerated.
3. *Proliferation*. This is characterized by granulation and vascularization. This starts after a few days and continues for a few weeks. It is the stage when the wound is rebuilt.
4. *Maturation or epithelialization*. At this final stage of wound healing, the collagen is remodelled.

From the phases required for healing, it can be seen that for effective wound healing the wound needs an adequate blood supply and nutrients, particularly vitamin C. Therefore some conditions which affect the flow of blood to the wound might affect the speed of the healing process, such as diabetes or vascular disease. Certain drugs can also affect the wound healing process, such as cytotoxics.

In the past, wound dressings were used mainly to protect the wound and keep the area clean and warm. A greater understanding of the wound healing process has led to more advanced dressings. Understanding the different types of dressings and the wounds which they treat requires a degree of specialism.

An ideal wound dressing should:

- provide a moist, warm environment
- remove excess exudate
- be oxygen permeable but not permeable to bacteria
- protect the wound from further damage
- be easily removed and not required to be changed too frequently
- not cause harm through being toxic, causing an allergic response or leaving particles
- be cost-effective with a good shelf-life.

Wound dressings can be categorized in the following ways.

Basic wound contact dressings

- *Low adhesive dressings*: these are tulle (open weave fabric with yellow or white soft paraffin, e.g. Paratulle®) or knitted viscous primary dressing (e.g. N-A Dressing®)
- *Absorbent dressings*: these are further categorized into those for lightly, moderate to heavy and heavy exudating wounds
- *Lightly exudating wound dressings* are absorbent perforated dressings with an adhesive border (e.g. Mepore®) and absorbent perforated plastic film faced dressings (e.g. Melolin®)
- *Moderate to heavy absorbent dressings* include absorbent cellulose dressings with a fluid repellent backing (e.g. Mesorb®)
- *Heavy exudating wound dressings* include a number of polymer dressings, some of which also contain cellulose (e.g. DryMax Extra®).

Advanced wound dressings

- *Hydrogel dressings*: these are used to give the wound moisture as they are a polymer matrix which contains 96% water

- *Vapour permeable film and membrane*: these are impermeable to fluids and bacteria but permeable to air and water vapour. They are available with or without an absorbent pad
- *Soft polymer dressings*: these are available with or without an absorbent pad or biocellulose
- *Hydrocolloid dressings*. A number of hydrocolloids are available, e.g. pectin and gelatin. These form a gel when exposed to the exudate and promote moist wound healing. These dressings are combined with a semi-permeable film and come with or without adhesive
- *Foam dressings*: these contain polyurethane foam which absorbs the exudate. They can be adhesive or non-adhesive and can come with or without a plastic film backing. They are categorized further in the BNF into those for lightly, lightly to moderate and moderate to heavy exudating wounds
- *Alginate dressings*: these are made from the alginic acid derived from brown seaweed. These dressings are highly absorbent which makes them useful in exuding wounds. They are available as dressings or sheets and can be adhesive or non-adhesive
- *Capillary action dressing*. Hydrophilic fibres in the dressing draw up the exudate. Low adhesive wound contact layers on either side of the fibres prevent any the fibres contaminating the wound
- *Odour absorbent dressings*: these dressings contain activated charcoal to reduce the odour coming from the wound
- *Antimicrobial dressings*: these dressings contain honey, silver, iodine or other antimicrobials to lower the number of bacteria in an infected wound.

Urinary incontinence

There are two main types of urinary incontinence:

1. Stress incontinence is caused by an action which raises intra-abdominal pressure such as sneezing, coughing or laughing.
2. Urge incontinence, of which enuresis is one type, is when the patient gets the urge to urinate but does not reach the toilet in time.

Stress and urge incontinence account for 90% of cases. Urinary incontinence is more common in females than males and the incidence increases in both sexes with age.

There are a number of appliances available for the management of urinary incontinence in men and women. In the UK, some of these devices are available on the NHS and these are listed in the *Drug Tariff*. Incontinence pads and garments are not available on the NHS in the UK.

Urinary catheters

These are tubes which are passed into the bladder to allow the drainage of urine from the bladder.

The main types of urinary catheters are Nélaton and Foley. Nélaton catheters are long tubes. Foley catheters have a balloon that is inflated by filling it with a liquid which is normally sterile water. This balloon acts as a self-retaining device and holds the catheter in place in the bladder. The balloons come in different sizes, which are expressed in millilitres: 3 mL and 5 mL balloons are used in children and 10 mL and 30 mL in adults.

Catheters come in different lengths and diameters and are also made from different materials.

Materials

The material the catheter is made from will affect how long it can remain in place. Latex is suitable only short term. The latex can be coated with Teflon® or silicone and this will increase the time it can be left in the bladder and not removed. Catheters made of silicone can be kept in place the longest.

Diameter

The Charrière (Ch) system is used to describe the different diameters. Only even numbers are used in this system and the bigger the number the larger the external diameter of the tube, ranging from 6 Ch (2 mm) to 30 Ch (10 mm). Sizes between 14 Ch and 18 Ch are the most common diameters used in adults. Paediatric catheters are usually between 6 Ch and 10 Ch.

Length

Differences in anatomy will mean that males require longer tubes than females. In males, the tubes are about 40 cm long and in females about 20 cm, hence the catheters are described as male, female or paediatric.

In males, an alternative to using a catheter is to use a latex sheath which fits over the penis. Some sheaths require another device to keep them in place.

Catheters or sheaths can then be connected to a drainage bag which will collect the urine. The volume of urine the bag holds varies. Some are intended to be worn on the leg so the patient can be mobile and some are intended for use when the patient is in bed. The drainage bag can be emptied of urine via a tap at times convenient to the patient or carer.

Stoma

Stomas or ostomies can be made surgically from the bowel, either the colon (colostomy) or ileum (ileostomy) or can be made from the ureters (urostomy – a piece of bowel is also used) or ureterostomy. An opening on the surface of the body is made through which the bowel or ureters drain the waste materials from the body. The stoma can be either permanent or temporary.

The colostomy is the most common type of stoma for which a pharmacist will supply appliances.

Colostomy and ileostomy appliances

The main type of appliance a pharmacist or appliance contractor supplies is used to collect the waste material which is being discharged from the stoma. The stoma, unlike the rectum, does not have sphincter muscles so the drainage of waste cannot be controlled. The appliance consists of a bag for collection with some system for attaching the bag to the body. In addition to these collection devices, stoma caps, bag covers, deodorants and skin protectors are available.

Stoma bags

For a collection system to be effective it should have the following features:

- Comfortable to wear
- Does not leak and protects the skin from irritation
- Does not smell
- Not visible or noticeable (does not emit a noise)
- Easy to empty and change
- Able to hold the required amount of waste.

Stomas vary in size. This means that it is important to get a bag with the right diameter hole to fit the stoma and to prevent leaking and damage to the surrounding skin. The size of the stoma may change with time so it is important that patients get reassessed.

The bags used for stomas can be drainable or non-drainable. The choice of appliance will depend on the nature of the waste being discharged. This can range from liquid to solid depending where along the bowel the stoma is, i.e. the nearer the stoma is to the rectum, the more solid will be the discharge.

If the appliance consists of the bag and is the means of attaching it to the body, it is called a one piece appliance. If the method of attaching the bag to the body is separate from the bag, it is a two piece appliance. With a two piece system you do not need to change the attachment on the body every time you change the bag.

The appliance can be adhesive so it sticks to the body or non-adhesive, which normally means it is held in place by a belt.

Some bags come with filters which are useful to prevent the bag from expanding if the patient is passing flatus.

Stoma caps or plugs can be used instead of a bag when the patient is able to predict when the bowel movement will happen. They may also be useful for short-term use when a patient is doing exercise or swimming.

Bag covers are used to cover the bag to make it less visible or to make the bag more comfortable to wear.

Unless the skin around the stoma is smooth and flat and the appliance fits precisely, it is possible that the waste from the stoma will come into contact with the skin. This can then lead to irritation and pain. Skin fillers and protectors are available to prevent this from happening.

Graduated compression hosiery

Graduated compression hosiery available on the NHS comes in three classes which are based on the degree (amount of pressure) of compression they give at the ankle, measured in millimetres of mercury (mmHg). They are mainly indicated for varicose veins but can also be used in the treatment and prevention of leg ulcers and oedema.

The three classes are:

- Class 1 – light support (14–17 mmHg)
- Class 2 – medium support (18–24 mmHg)
- Class 3 – strong support (25–30 mmHg).

Hosiery comes in different lengths (thigh length or below knee), different knits (circular, flat bed, net), different sizes (e.g. small, medium and large) and different colours.

One of the roles of a pharmacist is to ensure that the hosiery is the right size for the patient and that they know how to put it on. The NHS pays an additional professional fee for the measuring and fitting of hosiery.

Sometimes a patient may not be a standard or stock size and in this situation, the pharmacist will be required to measure the patient and will then order a made to measure stocking from the manufacturer.

There are also a number of accessories available for supply with hosiery to either help in putting them on or keeping them in place when they are on.

Trusses

Trusses are appliances used for abdominal hernias. A hernia occurs when an organ of the body protrudes through a cavity that is normally meant to keep it contained. If the abdominal muscle weakens, there is a chance that a hernia or rupture can occur. This is where the bowel protrudes through the abdominal wall. This is usually due to the fact that the abdominal wall has a number of weak points and with age, these weaken further. Hernias can also arise from an event, which increases the pressure on the abdomen, such as coughing, lifting and straining on defecation. Hernias can be repaired by surgery. If a patient cannot undergo surgery or is waiting to have surgery, a truss can be fitted.

The purpose of the truss is to plug the hole in the abdominal wall and therefore prevent the bowel from coming through it. This helps prevent the hernia from becoming larger and reduces the chance the hernia will become strangulated. Strangulation is when the blood flow is restricted, due to the fact the bowel is trapped by the abdominal wall and can lead to complications where the bowel swells and may burst and peritonitis could ensue.

Other types of hernia

There are a number of hernias for which trusses are available:

- *Umbilical hernia*: happening around the umbilicus. Very rare and can be fitted with an elastic band umbilical truss

- *Femoral hernia*: more common in women and happens where the femoral blood vessel leaves the abdomen at the top of the leg. A spring truss with a femoral pad can be fitted to this hernia
- *Incisional hernia*: happens where the abdomen has been cut during surgery.

Inguinal and scrotal hernias

The commonest abdominal hernia happens at the point where the inguinal canal, which in men carries the spermal cord (vas deferens) to the testes, leaves the abdomen. This is called an 'inguinal hernia'. The bowel can follow the canal downward and can end up in the scrotal sac. If the lump caused by the bowel is below the pubic arch the hernia is called a 'scrotal hernia'.

When a pharmacist receives a prescription for a truss it should contain the following information:

- The position of the hernia – inguinal, scrotal, and which side it is on
- The type of belt – elastic band or spring
- The number of pads – single or double. The patient may have a hernia on both sides of the abdomen
- The type of pad used – inguinal or scrotal.

It is part of the service agreement with the NHS that pharmacists measure and fit trusses and an endorsement on a prescription of 'measured and fitted' attracts an additional professional fee.

Hiatus hernia

This is common and is a result of the stomach going into the chest cavity through the hiatus, which is the point where the oesophagus goes through the diaphragm. As this is internal, it would not warrant treatment with a truss.

KEY POINTS

- Pharmacists are required to supply appliances as well as medicines
- There are four stages involved in wound healing
- There are large numbers of wound dressings available to dress different types of wound
- Catheters vary in material, length and diameter
- There are different types of stoma
- Graduated compression hosiery comes in three classes
- Pharmacists may be required to measure and fit hosiery and trusses

Section 7

Pharmacy services

Public health and pharmacy interventions

Jennie Watson

48

STUDY POINTS

- Pharmacy and its role in public health
- Accessibility of pharmacy
- Services that can be delivered by pharmacists to support the public health agenda

Introduction

Public health and its role in society has been described in Chapter 13. This chapter describes the part pharmacy plays in providing public health services to the public.

Traditionally, pharmacy has tended to work closely with health service commissioners to provide dispensing services. As the profession develops with time, it will need to work outside its traditional areas and increase its involvement in other areas, such as the provision of public health advice and services.

In many countries, the responsibility for public health sits between local government and health services. Pharmacists will, therefore, need to look towards local government in the future both as a commissioner of services and as the organization which will determine public health strategy.

Access

Community pharmacy has, traditionally, had the reputation as the only healthcare profession which is readily accessible to the general public without an appointment.

Over the past few years, as more pharmacies have opened in the UK, particularly pharmacies which open at least 100 hours each week, this accessibility has increased. For example, in England it is estimated that 1.8 million people visit a pharmacy every day, which means that in England, an average person will visit a pharmacy 14 times a year. Many of these will be people using the pharmacy for non-traditional purposes, i.e. not to have a prescription dispensed or to purchase an OTC medicine. These people will use the pharmacy to seek advice about general health care and to access other services. Because many of the people accessing pharmacies are not ill, pharmacists are ideally placed to offer advice to help people stay healthy. The profession's unrivalled access to this portion of the population makes it extremely valuable in supporting general well-being and reducing the incidence of long-term health problems in the general population.

Thus, pharmacy is ideally located to be at the heart of the patient-centred health service.

Healthy living pharmacies

This is a concept developed in the UK in 2010. The aim is to increase the public's awareness of community pharmacy as a centre within a neighbourhood, where anyone could go and access information to improve or maintain their health. These pharmacies do not necessarily offer more services than other local pharmacies but they do have 'health trainers'. These people are usually identified from the medicines counter assistants and are people who are passionate about well-being. Their role is to proactively approach people in the pharmacy to help them with either current health issues or to help them make positive changes to their lifestyle. Health trainers are a recognized role in the NHS but this is the first time they have played a significant role in pharmacy.

Healthy Living Pharmacies are accredited by local commissioners. In the future, it may be that for a pharmacy to be commissioned for new enhanced services, it will have to meet the standards required to be a Healthy Living Pharmacy.

Services

Pharmacy is beginning to move away from dispensing as its sole purpose, and to offer other services, many of which are covered elsewhere in this book. This chapter looks at some of the services and interventions pharmacists and their teams can offer to support the public health agenda.

Smoking cessation

For many years, pharmacists and medicines counter assistants have been selling nicotine replacement therapies (NRT) as an aid to stop smoking. As perceptions of smoking have changed, it has become routine for many healthcare professionals to ask patients whether or not they smoke and this has also become routine for pharmacists. Encouraging a smoker to quit is probably the biggest positive intervention that can be made to their health. Since many smokers will use a pharmacy to buy products to treat minor illnesses (particularly coughs and colds), the pharmacy team is ideally placed to encourage a smoker to quit.

For some pharmacy teams, the intervention will be solely based around motivational conversations and the sale of an appropriate NRT product from the wide range available. In other pharmacies, the patient will be able to access a commissioned smoking cessation service. This may involve an in-depth consultation with a smoking cessation advisor (usually drawn from the medicines counter assistant population), during which there will be agreements about why the patient wants to stop, when they intend to stop, the support available (in some pharmacies this can involve groups of quitters meeting weekly to discuss progress) and decisions about the right NRT product for the patient. The patient will then be supplied with the product free of charge, if they are exempt from prescription charges.

In other pharmacies, the pharmacist may be involved in offering a smoking cessation service if they have been authorized to supply Champix® (a selective nicotine-receptor partial agonist) under a PGD (see Ch. 4).

Another group of pharmacies will process the vouchers issued to patients to obtain a free supply of NRT by smoking cessation advisors, who work elsewhere in the community, e.g. nurses in clinics.

Cardiovascular checks

In the UK, cardiovascular disease (CVD) is one of the main causes of premature morbidity and mortality. It is recognized that when cardiovascular disease has been diagnosed as a result of a cardiovascular event (such a minor stroke or myocardial infarction), effective treatments are available to reduce the risk of a second event. However, we do not have an effective national screening programme to reduce the risk of the first cardiovascular event happening.

Screening would be most effective if carried out for both male and females who are aged between 40 and 74 years of age. Often, this is a group of people who do not routinely access care from their GP, but who will access treatment for minor ailments from a pharmacy.

Some pharmacies have been commissioned to carry out CVD risk assessments, particularly in those areas where the target numbers for patients being screened has not been met by GP surgeries.

The CVD risk screening covers the following:

* Body mass index (BMI) and waist/hip ratio
* Random blood glucose
* Total cholesterol and LDH/HDH lipid ratio
* Blood pressure
* Smoking status
* Alcohol consumption
* Activity levels.

Using the information obtained from the screening tests, the pharmacist calculates the risk of a cardiovascular event occurring in the next 10 years, for the patient. Depending on the level of risk the pharmacist and patient agree either lifestyle changes to reduce risk or referral to the GP for other preventative measures (e.g. medication).

Alcohol intake screening

It is believed that at least one in three adults in the UK drinks more alcohol each week than is regarded as safe. It is also believed that a large number of these people do not realize that their alcohol consumption is at a level that is anticipated to cause health problems in the future.

Pharmacists are being encouraged to include discussions about alcohol intake as a normal part of the conversation with a patient. Currently, this seems very alien and intrusive to many pharmacists. This matches the feelings experienced in the 1990s when pharmacists were first asked to start including discussions about smoking status as part of most conversations. It would be unusual now not to be questioned about smoking status when asking for medication for a cough or cold in a pharmacy and so pharmacists can now plan to increase their patients' awareness of the problems caused by drinking alcohol to excess.

In some places, pharmacists have been commissioned to provide services to increase awareness of safe drinking levels. Pharmacists can target 'at risk' patients, who may include:

- Patients accessing emergency hormonal contraception through the pharmacy
- Pregnant women
- Men over 45
- Customers who buy hangover cures or products for indigestion
- Customers who need treatment for falls.

Customers are asked to complete a questionnaire or use a scratch card to identify their drinking patterns. Depending on what the questionnaire/scratch card highlights, the outcome may be:

- brief counselling provided at the pharmacy together with supporting leaflets
- referring the patient in a specialist alcohol service for more in-depth guidance.

Services for drug-user clients

Pharmacists play an important public health role with the services they provide for drug-user clients. They can include:

- Observed, supervised consumption of prescription medicines
- Needle and syringe supply and exchange
- Supply of other injecting equipment
- Safe injecting technique training
- Blood-borne virus testing.

(These are covered in more detail in Chapter 50.)

Screening for chronic disease

Pharmacists can also be involved in screening for long-term (chronic) disease/conditions, e.g. screening to identify patients with, or at risk of, developing Type 2 diabetes.

It is estimated that one in four people with Type 2 diabetes are, at any one time, undiagnosed. The consequences of this delay in diagnosis are:

- Patients may have symptoms without being aware they have diabetes so do not know why they are feeling unwell
- Patients are often diagnosed late as a result of a preventable complication of the disease being found. These complications would include retinopathy identified during a routine sight test or peripheral neuropathy being identified after a series of falls
- Early diagnosis means that patients are less likely to develop complications resulting in a better quality of life and less support required from the NHS.

Pharmacists have been commissioned to provide a service in certain parts of the UK with a high rate of undiagnosed diabetics. The service targets patients through:

- opportunistic screening of 'at risk' patients
- referrals from other agencies such as social services.

After identification of the 'at risk' patient, the patient is asked to complete a lifestyle questionnaire. The pharmacist or a trained colleague then carries out the following tests:

- Blood glucose (either fasting or random)
- BMI and waist/hip measurements
- Blood pressure.

Depending on the results obtained, the pharmacist will either:

- Recommend lifestyle improvements to reduce risk factors for Type 2 diabetes (e.g. weight management programme, smoking cessation programme)
- Refer to a GP for confirmation of a diagnosis and treatment.

Treatment and prevention of infectious disease

A key public health requirement is to monitor and reduce infection from what are termed 'communicable diseases'. While all infections have the potential to be passed on, public health priorities focus on the infections or diseases that tend to spread easily and have serious health consequences. Both the common cold and influenza are such types of infections. In particular, the health consequences of influenza can be serious, may require hospital admission and can cause death.

Pharmacy has a role to play here, in four areas:

- Provision of vaccination to prevent infection
- Screening to identify specific infections
- Provision of treatment of specific communicable diseases
- Increasing patient compliance with medication for a communicable disease with a long treatment period.

None of these are part of key or essential services, but like many of the other services given in this chapter, they are commissioned in response to a local need.

Provision of vaccination

Vaccination is only effective as a widespread infection control if a large percentage of the population is vaccinated. For some infections, vaccination is designed to ensure that patients with other conditions/diseases, that make them susceptible to complications from the infection, are vaccinated. This is the case for the influenza vaccine, where the NHS vaccinates groups of people with underlying medical conditions such as asthma or heart disease.

Pharmacies provide vaccination as a way of increasing access. Patients will access vaccination services through pharmacy, rather than from a GP surgery, for one of two main reasons:

- The opening hours of pharmacies tend to be over more days and more hours per day than those of a GP surgery. This is particularly relevant for patients who work and would have to take time off to be vaccinated. Pharmacy plays a substantial role in both identifying patients who should be vaccinated and also vaccinating those patients who are unwilling to be vaccinated at their GP surgery

- Pharmacy is seen by some patients as more anonymous than attending the GP surgery. Some pharmacies provide human papillomavirus (HPV) vaccination for older female teenagers, whose age means that they missed the national vaccination programme at school. Some of these patients will not wish to be vaccinated at their GPs, as they perceive information about their sexual activity will be recorded in their patient record.

Screening to identify specific infections

Some pharmacies are commissioned to screen for sexually transmitted diseases and blood-borne viruses which are transmitted when drug-users share needles.

Since pharmacies are accessed by sexual health services and by drug-user clients, they are ideally placed to discuss infection risk and then test (usually using dry blood spot testing) for infections such as HIV, syphilis, hepatitis B and C. For these infections, the pharmacy is then unlikely to provide treatment but will help the patient identify how they would like to access treatment elsewhere in the health service.

For infections such as *Chlamydia*, pharmacists can be commissioned to provide testing kits and then if infection is confirmed, can be trained to provide antibiotic treatment under a PGD.

Provision of treatment of specific communicable diseases

Pharmacists have been trained, in some parts of the UK, to supply drugs to patients who have tested positive for MRSA as a result of hospital pre-admission tests. Since the test results are not available on the day of the pre-admission tests, a patient who tested positive for MRSA would normally have to return to the hospital for treatment. To ensure that patients are completing their treatment before they return to the hospital, some areas have increased access by transferring the treatment to the patient's local pharmacy.

Increasing patient compliance with medication for a communicable disease with a long treatment period

Tuberculosis (TB) is a disease that has increased in incidence due to changes in migration. The treatment involves a medication regime that lasts many months. If the patient fails to complete the regime, there is an increased risk of drug-resistant TB developing.

In areas with higher than average levels of TB infection in the population, pharmacies have been commissioned to provide increased support for patients to improve compliance with their drug regime. This can include:

- Daily or weekly dispensing with contact being made with the assigned TB nurse if the patient misses doses
- Observed supervised administration of doses, again with contact being made with the assigned TB nurse if the patient misses doses.

Public emergency support

In a public emergency, such as a pandemic, some legislation is temporarily suspended to allow the emergency to be dealt with quickly and effectively. The legislation affected can include that which governs the supply of medicines. This may mean that:

- some medicines can be withdrawn from the supply chain so that the best use is made of limited supplies
- some medicines can be supplied against an order rather than a prescription. This can reduce the time to supply some drugs and also ensures that some drugs are only issued under specific guidance (e.g. antiviral drugs in an influenza pandemic will be available in limited quantities and cannot be given to every infected person)
- some medicine supply functions can be carried out by people other than pharmacists (in the case of an epidemic, there may be too many pharmacists ill to continue with providing the population with drugs so registered technicians may be authorized to undertake some supply functions).

Although there was little need to put these options into operation, during the H1N1 influenza pandemic of 2009/2010, some pharmacies were commissioned to provide antiviral drugs against an authorization form rather than a prescription.

Sexual health services

Sexual health services available through pharmacies can be grouped into three main areas:

- Contraception
- Prevention and treatment of sexually transmitted diseases
- Pregnancy testing.

Most pharmacies will play some role in providing sexual health services from selling condoms and pregnancy testing kits to commissioned services to supply regular hormonal contraceptives. Many emergency hormonal contraception (EHC) services are commissioned to try to reduce the incidence of teenage pregnancy and so will be available to girls under 16 years of age. In the UK, girls under 16 who access contraceptive services have to be assessed under the Fraser Guidelines, and their competency recorded.

Contraception

Pharmacies will provide a variety of contraception services:

- The sale of condoms and kits to predict ovulation to help couple using natural methods of contraception
- Distribution of condoms to young people under the c-card scheme
- Provision of free of charge emergency hormonal contraception (EHC) under a PGD, or if the patient is not suitable for EHC, referral to another provider to discuss other emergency contraception options
- In some areas, pharmacists have been trained to provide a full family planning service for hormonal contraception (combined pill or progesterone only pill) – this includes assessment, supply and follow-up.

Prevention and treatment of sexually transmitted diseases

As well as the information covered earlier in this chapter, pharmacists will also supply condoms to women being supplied with EHC and in many cases, it is a requirement of the service to discuss whether the women needs to consider screening for sexually transmitted infections and in particularly *Chlamydia*.

Pregnancy testing

Pharmacists have traditionally carried out pregnancy testing or sold pregnancy testing kits. With more effective and accurate testing kits available to purchase, more women are purchasing testing kits to use at home.

However, in some areas, pregnancy testing in the pharmacy has become a commissioned service as a way of increasing the number of women who access midwifery services early in pregnancy. This is particularly important in areas where a lower than average proportion of the population is registered with a GP.

Conclusion

Pharmacy has the potential to be involved in many areas to support the public health agenda. To be successful at this, pharmacists need to be prepared to engage with commissioners and to explain what services they can deliver to support the public health agenda.

KEY POINTS

- Pharmacists are the most readily accessible healthcare professionals
- The public health agenda is one that has been supported by pharmacists in the past but the services provided have rarely been thought of as public health services
- Public health service provision must be decided by local need
- Key areas are prevention of long-term conditions, drug-user services, sexual health services, disease prevention and treatment
- Healthy Living Pharmacies are a concept that helps pharmacists and their teams to provide a wide range of public health interventions

Pharmacy services for vulnerable patients

Victoria Crabtree

STUDY POINTS

- Definition of vulnerable patients
- UK policies relating to vulnerable patients
- Pharmacy services for disabled patients, children and young people, the elderly and those unable to care for themselves
- How pharmacists can help protect children and vulnerable adults

Introduction

Vulnerable patients can be described as those: 'who are or may be in need of care services by reason of mental or other disability, age, or illness; and who is or may be unable to take care of him or herself, or unable to protect him or herself against significant harm or exploitation' (Taken from the 1997 consultation paper 'Who decides', issued by the Lord Chancellors Department). Pharmacists are often in a position to help and support vulnerable patients via the services that they provide, and they have a duty to help ensure the safety of children and vulnerable adults.

To identify how pharmacists can support vulnerable patients, the reasons why they may be vulnerable should be considered. Some patients with mental disabilities may have problems understanding disease and its treatment, or they may find it difficult to describe their symptoms or problems to healthcare professionals. These patients may require support to make decisions regarding their health. When dealing with patients with mental disabilities, there can sometimes be complications around consent to treatment. Usually patients should be fully informed

about disease and treatment options, and be able to consent to any treatments provided; however in certain cases, if a patient has a reduced mental capacity, then parents, carers and healthcare professionals are involved in the treatment decisions of that patient. In most cases where decisions are made without the involvement of the patient, the actions are in their best interests; however on the very rare occasions that patients do not receive the care that they require, they may not be in a position to recognize a lack or care, raise their concerns or object, leaving them vulnerable to harm.

Some people with physical disabilities may be considered vulnerable as they may be relying on others for their basic daily needs such as bathing, dressing and eating. Some physical disabilities may lead to communication problems which can render a patient vulnerable if they are unable to communicate their needs or raise concerns about harm or exploitation.

Babies and children are considered vulnerable for a number of reasons. Primarily children rely on adults to feed, clothe, wash, care for them and protect them from harm. When adults fail to do this, children are often unable to verbalize their needs or recognize the lack of care. When considering health care, younger children have reduced mental capacity to understand disease and treatment, and rely on parents and guardians to make decisions based on their best interests. When considering UK law, parents and guardians usually consent to the treatments given to children; however as children develop into young adults they acquire more legal rights with regard to consent, and decisions around treatment can become complex. They tend to involve the young person, parents, guardians, local heath authorities and occasionally courts of law.

As people age, some issues around vulnerability can start to emerge, particularly the frail elderly who may find that they are no longer able to take care of themselves. When a person is no longer able to care for themselves either due to frailty or serious illness, they can be considered vulnerable, as they may rely on others for their basic needs and support with undertaking treatments for illness. These patients may require the services of carers or may live in a residential care home. Due to frailty or illness they may not be in a position to report lack of care or abuse from their care providers.

Pharmacists may find themselves providing services to patients who are unable to protect themselves from harm or exploitation; these patients could include children, drug misusers or those in abusive and exploitative relationships. These groups may feel afraid or unable to discuss concerns with health professionals or care agencies.

UK policies relating to vulnerable patients

In recent years, there have been a number of documents published that health professionals should be aware of relating to vulnerable patients. Some of these documents have sadly been published in response to high profile cases such as the Victoria Climbié Enquiry Report (2003), The Bristol Royal Infirmary Enquiry (1998) and the Peter Connelly Serious Case Review ('Baby P') (2010), where vulnerable people have been let down by social and healthcare services. These documents aim to prevent harm from occurring with other vulnerable patients. Pharmacists need to be aware of the content and implications for their practice.

No Secrets: Guidance on developing and implementing multi-agency policies and procedures to protect vulnerable adults from abuse was published in 2000 for local authorities, social services, the police, health services, service users and carers. It gives guidance on how to work together and develop local protocols to deal with suspected abuse in vulnerable adults.

Subsequent to the Safeguarding Vulnerable Groups Act in 2006, the 'vetting and barring scheme' was developed to help prevent unsuitable people from working with children and vulnerable adults. The scheme is currently under review by the government. The scheme is run by the Independent Safeguarding Authority and is essentially a list to prevent individuals who pose a risk to vulnerable people, from working with them. This list is checked when pharmacy staff are required to undertake enhanced Disclosure and Barring Service (DBS) checks. Currently, pharmacists delivering some enhanced services such as emergency hormonal contraception are required to undertake a DBS check prior to accreditation for the service; however, it is likely in the future that pharmacists will have to undertake DBS checks when joining a new employer.

In 2011, *Safeguarding adults: the role of health service practitioners* was published. This is particularly relevant to pharmacists as it provides specific principles for all health practitioners to adhere to. The guidance reminds practitioners of their duties to safeguard adults, whilst providing assistance in how to prevent and respond to harm and abuse in patients.

Working Together to Safeguard Children: A guide to inter-agency working to safeguard and promote the welfare of children was updated in 2010. This document sets out how organizations and individuals should work together to safeguard and promote the welfare of children and young people. The guidance directs that the Local Safeguarding Children Boards should be working with pharmacists as they are involved in the delivery of services to children.

In addition to these documents that state a pharmacist's duties in relation to the protection of vulnerable patients, there are also a number of guidance documents that identify where pharmacists can contribute to and enhance the lives of vulnerable patients. These include the National Service Frameworks for children and young people, older people and mental health. National Service Frameworks aim to increase the quality of care that these groups receive and within them many pharmacist roles are identified.

Pharmacy services for disabled patients

Pharmacists have a duty to comply with the Disability Discrimination Act 1995. The Act requires pharmacy premises to accommodate those with physical disabilities, e.g. ensuring wheelchair access. The Disability Discrimination Act also requires pharmacies to make 'reasonable adjustments' to support those with disabilities. What amendments are made to ensure that pharmacies comply with the Disability Discrimination Act affects the services that are provided. It can be difficult for a pharmacist to establish exactly what adjustments are needed; therefore decisions are usually best made in partnership with the patient or carer and dependent on their needs. Many services that pharmacies already offer comply with the Disability Discriminations Act. For example, those with dexterity issues could benefit from the use of oversize packaging or the supply of screw caps or wing caps for tablet bottles. Some physically disabled patients may benefit from collection and delivery services. Patients with vision impairments may benefit from the provision of large font labels or talking labels. The medicine use review service is an ideal opportunity to support those with disabilities. For example, if a patient is having difficulty swallowing, then medication could be rationalized to aid adherence or alternative dosage forms could be suggested. If a patient has a mental disability that results in decreased adherence due to cognitive issues, then provision of a multi-dosage system or a simple tick chart can be provided to support medicine taking. Pharmacists should ensure that their services are available to those with mental disabilities; this most often requires pharmacists to take time to ensure that their explanations are appropriate, and pharmacists may need to provide additional support such as providing leaflets or carrying out demonstrations. Involving carers and family members in decision-making and explanations can be helpful when appropriate.

Pharmacy services for children and young people

Pharmacists are often involved in the provision of prescribed medication for babies, children and young people. Particular care is often required when clinically checking prescriptions or carrying out full medication reviews for this group of patients due to the differences in drug handling from adults. As children mature, their total body water decreases, therefore neonates and infants may need larger doses of water-soluble drugs. Neonates, infants and children have a higher metabolic rate than adults, sometimes resulting in the need for more frequent dosing or higher doses of drugs on a mg/kg basis.

Ideally, the drugs used in children will have undergone clinical trials in young age groups for the condition that is being treated. However, most drugs are only tested on adults for safety and efficacy, and are therefore unlicensed for use in children. When prescribing decisions are made, pharmacists can provide their expertise by evaluating current clinical evidence. Pharmacists should recommend using a licensed product where possible, or evaluate the safest and most effective unlicensed products available. Parents and carers may be alarmed at the use of unlicensed products, especially if they read an inappropriate patient information leaflet. Explaining the use of the unlicensed medicines to the parent or carer and involving the whole family in any treatment decisions can help overcome this. If a drug has not been tested in children, then calculating the dosage can be difficult and the age and weight of the child should be considered. If a high-risk medicine is being used, such as those with a narrow therapeutic range, then the weight of the child and the dose in mg/kg should be stated on all prescriptions to ensure safety.

Pharmacists are often the first health professionals that a parent or guardian will encounter if a child is suffering from a minor ailment. When providing over-the-counter (OTC) treatments for children, only OTC products designed and licensed for use in children should be supplied, as they will have been tested for safety and efficacy in this age group. These products are often pleasant tasting, colourful liquids, or melt in the mouth sweets, and are more palatable to children. Parents sometimes have concerns about sugar content, and artificial flavourings and colours; information can be given to help them make informed choices when treating their children. When advising on OTC treatments, this is an ideal opportunity to advise parents about the safe storage of medicines in the home, as these medicines may appear appealing to children.

Pharmacists are able to carry out medicine use reviews and medication reviews with children; this will usually be with the consent of the parent or guardian. These are ideal opportunities to involve the child or young person in decisions around their medication with the intention of increasing adherence. It has been recognized that some teenagers may be embarrassed to take medicines to school, or they may decide that they do not need to follow advice as they assert their own independence. To overcome these problems, pharmacists can support by communicating disease and treatment options to the young person in a way that they will understand, and providing practical support such as suggesting modified-release preparations to avoid school-time dosing or supplying discrete appliances such as insulin pens.

Pharmacies have a role in informing parents and children of local health promotion initiatives. This can include advice on healthy eating, immunization programmes and sexual health. Pharmacists are in an ideal position to promote breast-feeding, give advice on the use of formula milk and help parents to wean their babies correctly and at an appropriate time. Children have different dietary needs to adults; although children do not require the same volume of food as adults, they may need more energy-releasing foods to support their higher metabolic rate. As children develop into young adults, pharmacists can advise on what constitutes a healthy diet, promoting the intake of at least five portions of fruit and vegetables a day, with the hope that good eating habits are taken forward into adulthood.

Babies and children receive a number of different immunizations and parents often have concerns about their use. Pharmacists have a role in educating parents about the safety and importance of immunizations, and they can ensure that they are received at the correct age. It can be difficult for pharmacists to keep up-to-date with what the current recommendations are. The best resource to use in the UK is *The Green Book*, which is regularly published and updated by the department of health.

Pharmacists are often the first healthcare professionals that a young person may encounter for advice on contraception and sexual health. Pharmacists sell condoms, provide emergency contraception, sign-post to family planning clinics, provide *Chlamydia* screening and treatment programmes, and provide health promotion about sexually transmitted infections. Emergency hormonal contraception (EHC) can be sold to young people over the age of 16 where appropriate, and some pharmacists supply EHC to under-16-year-olds using a patient group direction (see Ch. 48 for further details).

When pharmacists are delivering sexual health services to young people, it is prudent to be aware of child protection and the local safeguarding children procedures. Pharmacists should be aware of repeated requests for EHC, and signs of sexual abuse. Pharmacists need to know what to do if it is suspected that a young person needs help. Usually this involves contacting the local child protection officer and sharing your concerns. The Sexual Health Act 2003 states that children under the age of 13 are unable to consent to sexual activity,

therefore if a young person under this age requests advice on sexual matters particularly EHC, then this should be taken seriously, and reported to social services, unless there are exceptional circumstances backed by documented reasons for not sharing the information.

Pharmacy services for the elderly

By 2025, one-quarter of the British population will be over the age of 60. Many older people lead active and independent lives late into old age; however some older people will become frail and increasingly rely on the NHS and social services.

As people age, their bodies undergo a number of changes. This increases the number and range of diseases that older people suffer from and changes their response to certain drugs. Older people may find that as family and friends move or pass away, they become more socially isolated and therefore vulnerable, as they may rely on others for their basic needs.

Older people are one of the main users of pharmacy services. Pharmacists may find themselves carrying a large proportion of medicine use reviews and New Medicine Services for older people, as it has been estimated that four out of five people over 75 take at least one prescribed medicine. In addition to these services, pharmacists can be involved in influenza immunization programmes, fall prevention programmes and full medication review services.

Pharmacists can be involved in ensuring that the elderly receive the influenza vaccination via a local enhanced service. It is recommended that all people over 65, those living in long-term residential care homes and those that care for elderly or disabled people receive an influenza vaccination.

Falls in older people have serious consequences and often result in a healthy active older person becoming vulnerable. Falling has been shown to be a major cause of accidental death in older people and many patients who suffer a fracture never live independently again. The fear of falling can limit what older people do in their day-to-day lives.

Older people are at an increased risk of falling, as their muscle mass is decreased, which results in a loss of physical strength and a reduction in mobility. Medicines have been implicated in causing older patients to fall. Hypnotic drugs such as benzodiazepines can cause drowsiness, and antihypertensives may cause hypotension and dizziness. Particular care should be taken when an older person suffers from osteoporosis, as these patients are much more likely to suffer fractures and consequent deterioration in quality of life. The National Service Framework (NSF) for older people states that if older people can be prevented from falling, they may live longer, healthier lives, not become vulnerable and therefore ease pressures on the NHS. Many pharmacists have undertaken specialist training to become fall prevention pharmacists. The fall prevention pharmacist reviews a patient's medication, and suggests strategies to withdraw drugs that can predispose a person to falls, and they may suggest the introduction of medicines to prevent osteoporosis. They also advise on how to avoid OTC medicines that increase the risk, such as sedating antihistamines.

When undertaking full medication reviews in older people, there are some factors with regard to drug handling that should be considered. Older people experience slower intestinal motility, reduced total surface area for absorption and decreased gastric emptying. Although these factors do not usually have a large effect on total drug absorption, they can slow the rate of drug absorption, resulting in a delayed response. Older people experience a decrease in muscle mass and a gain in adipose tissue. This can sometimes cause problems as lipid-soluble drugs are stored in the adipose tissue, increasing the chances of side-effects and toxicity; therefore lower doses of lipid-soluble drugs should be prescribed. The elderly experience reduced blood perfusion of the liver, resulting in the slower metabolism of some drugs; lower doses of these would therefore be required. The elderly may also require reduced dosages of some drugs as renal filtration becomes slower with age, increasing the chances of drug toxicity occurring.

For some older people, community pharmacies are not only places where prescriptions are collected, they are a source of advice, OTC medicines and social contact. When considering OTC medications, care should be taken to check for interactions with prescribed medications; it is good practice to record OTC sales in the patient medication record where appropriate, and it is important to remember that not all OTC products are suitable for the elderly. For example palatable thrush treatments should not be provided to those over 60 as the incidence of vaginal thrush in this group is low and symptoms would require investigation.

Pharmacy services for those unable to care of themselves

This group of patients relies on carers to support them living at home or they live in a residential care home and pharmacists deliver a number of services to support the patients, carers and the homes.

Some patients who need support to care for themselves are still able to live in their own homes with the help of carers or family. Pharmacists can often support this group of patients by providing multi-dosage systems, and pharmacists can carry out medicine use reviews in a patient's home with appropriate permission. Many patients and carers find pharmacy collection and delivery services helpful; however it is important that pharmacists maintain regular contact with the patient, especially if they are not visiting the pharmacy premises.

Some patients need to live in a care home to ensure that they are adequately looked after. There are a number of different types of care home in the UK which provide different levels of service. Residential care homes provide meals, accommodation, help with personal care such as dressing and bathing and support through short illnesses. This type of home often accommodates the frail elderly or those convalescing after illness. Nursing care homes have a qualified nurse on the premises 24 hours a day and therefore they are often used by those with more severe illness or a disability that requires frequent nursing care. Specialist care homes are available for those who have specific disabilities or needs such as dementia, where specially trained staff or adapted facilities are required. Pharmacists can provide different levels of service to care homes to help them look after their residents.

Pharmacists are involved in the provision of medicines, dressings and appliances to care homes. In some homes, residents have complete control of their medication, which includes ordering their medicines, choosing a pharmacy to dispense them and taking responsibility for taking them. If residents are able to do this they should be encouraged to and be provided with a lockable cupboard to store their medicines in. However, in many homes the staff take some responsibility for medication use. If a home takes responsibility for the residents' medication, then a suitably trained person orders the prescriptions from the residents' prescriber. The home usually has a local agreement with a pharmacy to supply all the medicines, dressings and appliances for the residents in that home. Although this reduces the residents' choice, it is much more convenient for the care home staff, and has benefits for patient safety.

When pharmacists supply homes, they can provide medicines in the manufacturer's original containers or they can put medicines into monitored dosage systems (MDS). MDS is a method of repackaging solid dosage forms into individualized blister packs and this is done to help residents or carers in the taking of the medicines. MDS is time-consuming to prepare; however, they may reduce administration errors as carers and residents can clearly see when to take the medication. Not all solid dosage forms can be repackaged into MDS. Drugs may deteriorate quickly if not in their original container, and before putting medication into an MDS, the manufacturers should be consulted.

It is important that adequate records of drug administration are kept, especially in homes with large numbers of staff, frequent shift changes and large numbers of residents. Medication administration record (MAR) charts are official records of the medicines that a resident is taking and should be completed every time a drug is administered. MAR charts are provided with the MDS and are kept up-to-date to reflect any medication changes.

In addition to providing medication to care homes, pharmacists can also provide care home advisory services to help homes reach the standards set by their regulator. The UK regulators include the Care Quality Commission (England), the Care and Social Services Inspectorate for Wales, the Scottish Commission for the Regulation of Care and the Regulation, Quality and Improvement Authority (Northern Ireland). Pharmacists may receive payment for these services via a local enhanced service.

When providing advisory services, the pharmacist usually makes an initial visit to the home, and then further annual visits to give advice. These visits entail checking that good practices are followed regarding the supply, administration, storage and destruction of medicines. The pharmacist should be aware of the regulatory body requirements and any advice given to the care home should be recorded. Pharmacists should use these opportunities to talk to the residents; advice can be given about medicines and recommendations added to each individual's care plan. Pharmacists can also use these visits to help the home develop safe policies and procedures for drug handling and help train the staff to adopt safe practices, e.g. helping homes develop protocols for dealing with medication errors. Some pharmacists provide training courses for care workers up to NVQ level, for which extra payment can be claimed.

While visiting a care home, the pharmacist may encounter a scenario where they suspect the residents are at risk of abuse from the care home workers. If a pharmacist becomes concerned that a vulnerable adult may be being harmed, they have a duty to act upon their concerns.

How pharmacists can help protect children

Children and young people are considered vulnerable, as they may not be able to protect themselves from people who harm or exploit them. Pharmacists may become involved in child protection if they have concerns about the welfare of a child and wish to report those concerns. Pharmacists could be asked to provide information on a child or young person to the police or social services, or pharmacists may be involved in a child protection plan.

All healthcare professionals have a duty to safeguard and support the welfare of children. If a pharmacist suspects that a child or young person is being abused, they have a legal duty to act upon their suspicions. Abuse can be physical, emotional, sexual or due to neglect. A pharmacist may suspect physical abuse if a child's injuries could not be accounted for by an explanation provided by the parent or carer, or a pharmacist may notice that a child or young person often presents in the pharmacy with injuries. Emotional abuse is more difficult to identify; however, pharmacists may have concerns if a child or young person becomes withdrawn, shows signs of self-harm or appears fearful of an adult. Pharmacists may encounter children or young people who are suffering from sexual abuse when they are supplying EHC, or the young person may describe sexual activities that are inappropriate for their age. Signs of neglect include failure to provide adequate shelter, food or clothing, which may become apparent to a pharmacist.

A pharmacist may notice behaviours in a parent or carer that are of concern. These may include a parent or carer delaying treatment, appearing detached from a child or not showing concern for injuries. Parents may appear reluctant to provide information or a pharmacist may witness aggression or violence towards a child.

If a pharmacist suspects any form of abuse, then they must follow the local child protection procedures. To find out your local child protection procedures, it is best to contact the local safeguarding children board within the local authority. If you believe that there is an immediate risk to a child, then it is appropriate to contact the police. It is not recommended that pharmacists investigate any suspicions of abuse themselves, but they should record their concerns and any actions taken.

Pharmacists may be asked to give information to social services if a child protection investigation occurs. It is important for pharmacists to cooperate with the police and social services, as all agencies involved in child protection should work together if abuse is suspected.

Pharmacists may be directly involved in a child protection plan. These are plans written by social services to help protect a child from harm. An example of how pharmacists can play a key role, is within the protection of children who are cared for by drug or alcohol-dependent parents. Pharmacists may be asked by social services for feedback on whether a parent is complying with a drug recovery programme, as this would have a positive impact on the safety of the child.

In situations such as these, conflicts of confidentiality may arise. However, if disclosure is necessary for the protection of children or to prevent serious injury to a person's health, then information should be shared.

emotional abuse may come to light or pharmacists may notice evidence of self-harm or self-mutilation; signs can also include inappropriate verbal abuse or patients displaying a fear of certain people. During sexual health consultations, sexual abuse and rape may be identified or disclosed; signs can include repeated requests for emergency hormonal contraception or signs of sexually transmitted diseases.

Pharmacists may find themselves in a situation where they suspect a carer of abusing vulnerable adults. Signs could involve a carer delaying access to treatment for a vulnerable adult, showing detachment from them or a lack of concern for their injury or illness. Carers may appear reluctant to give information or a pharmacist may witness aggressive behaviour towards a vulnerable adult.

If a pharmacist suspects abuse, then knowing what to do can be difficult. The adult's wishes should be taken into account at all times, and consent to share information should be sought. Pharmacists should not attempt to undertake investigations or discuss their concerns with the alleged perpetrator. If a pharmacist's employer has a safeguarding procedure in place this can be helpful when making decisions around disclosure. If a vulnerable adult is in immediate danger, then disclosure of information without consent may be necessary to ensure the safety of the patient and/or others. When sharing information around the safety of vulnerable adults this is usually with the local social services authority, NHS trust, police or GP.

How pharmacists can help protect vulnerable adults

It has been identified that the frail, some elderly and some adults with disabilities can be considered vulnerable, in addition to those in abusive relationships and some substance misusers, who can also be considered vulnerable.

As pharmacists may be a point of contact for these groups it is imperative that pharmacists can recognize any signs that would prompt intervention. Signs of physical abuse could include unusual injuries that are not easily explained, bite marks, scalds, fingertip bruising, fractures or repeated injuries. Vulnerable people who rely on others for their basic needs could show signs of neglect such as malnourishment, poor hygiene or appearing dirty and unkempt. When pharmacists are involved in conversations with patients,

KEY POINTS

- Vulnerable patients can include some people with disabilities, children and young people, some elderly, those who rely on carers for their basic needs, some substance misusers and some people in abusive relationships
- In recent years the UK government has produced clear advice for health professionals regarding their duty to protect vulnerable patients
- Pharmacy services should be accessible to those with disabilities
- Pharmacists can provide prescribing advice to ensure appropriate medicines and doses are used for children. Pharmacies are often the first place where parents receive advice about minor ailments and health promotion for their children, and pharmacists are often the first health professionals a young person may consult for sexual health advice

- Pharmacies are often used by older people for services and influenza immunization, fall prevention, medicine use reviews and new medicine services can be particularly helpful for this group
- Pharmacists can support those who need help to take care for themselves by providing compliance aids, collection and delivery services and services to residential care homes
- Pharmacists must be alert to the signs of abuse in children and vulnerable adults and be aware of local safeguarding procedures

Substance use and misuse

Jenny Scott

STUDY POINTS

- The main psychoactive substances taken for non-medicinal purposes
- The range of professional interventions used in the field of substance misuse
- The aim of pharmaceutical interventions and their operation
- The role of the pharmacist
- Key factors to consider when providing pharmaceutical care to people with drug misuse problems

Introduction

This chapter begins with some background information before it summarizes current thinking on drug misuse and drug dependence. It then looks at treatment provision in the UK and the range of interventions used, focussing on the practical provision of the two main pharmaceutical interventions: needle exchange and substitute pharmacotherapy provision.

Terminology

Terminology used in the field of drug misuse can be confusing, even for those who work in the area. There are political and philosophical differences behind the use of various terms, a discussion of which is outside the scope of this work. However, it is important to be aware that a variety of terms essentially refer to the same things.

'Drug use' in the context of this chapter, is the term commonly used to refer to the consumption of psychoactive substances without medical or healthcare instruction. The term 'drug misuse' refers to drug use that is problematical and incurs significant risk of harm. These two terms are often used interchangeably. 'Drug abuse' essentially refers to the same thing but its use is less common in recent publications. 'Substance' is sometimes used in place of 'drug' to include non-medicinal chemicals such as solvents, alcohol and nicotine.

'Dependence' or 'addiction' refers to the compulsion to continue administration of psychoactive substance(s) in order to avoid physical and/or psychological withdrawal effects. Dependence syndrome is defined by the World Health Organization (WHO) as:

> A cluster of behavioural, cognitive, and physiological phenomena that develop after repeated substance use and that typically include a strong desire to take the drug, difficulties in controlling its use, persisting in its use despite harmful consequences, a higher priority given to drug use than to other activities and obligations, increased tolerance, and sometimes a physical withdrawal state. The dependence syndrome may be present for a specific psychoactive substance (e.g. tobacco, alcohol, or diazepam), for a class of substances (e.g. opioid drugs), or for a wider range of pharmacologically different psychoactive substances.

Dependence can be classified in more detail, as found in the *Shorter Oxford Textbook of Psychiatry*.

'Drug user' is commonly used to refer to someone who participates in drug/substance use. The term 'drug misuser' refers to someone undertaking drug use in such a way that it is problematical and presents significant risk of harm. The two terms tend to be used interchangeably. Terms such as 'drug addict' and 'drug abuser' are less used in recent literature.

Historical note

Historical works on psychoactive drug consumption make interesting reading and help us to understand how current drug policy came to be formulated. They indicate that psychoactive drug use is not a new phenomenon in society – psychoactive drug use has been recorded as part of some societies more than 7000 years ago.

Substances that are used and their effects

Table 50.1 lists some commonly used psychoactive substances in western societies and summarizes their effects. (Nicotine is included for completeness: the role of the pharmacist in smoking cessation is covered in Ch. 48). The unwanted and harmful effects of some drugs relate to prolonged and excessive use, whereas others occur with single doses of smaller amounts. The method of administration also influences the extent of the risks, e.g. injecting opiates presents greater health risks than taking them by vaporization ('chasing the dragon'). Table 50.1 is presented as a guide, but it is not comprehensive.

Why do people use psychoactive drugs?

Benefits

Why people use psychoactive drugs is a multifaceted question to which there is no simple answer. As a crude summary, people do so because they expect to experience a benefit in some way. Any awareness of risks is weighed up against the perceived benefits and the decision to take the drug prevails.

The expected or perceived benefits may include: the attainment of pleasurable feelings (e.g. relaxation); increased social interaction (e.g. reduced inhibitions); alteration of the person's psychological condition to a more desirable state (e.g. escapism); physical change (e.g. anabolic steroids taken by bodybuilders) or avoidance of withdrawal symptoms in someone who is dependent on a drug. The reasons

for use may change over time with the same user, e.g. opiate use may be commenced to escape from reality but then continued to avoid the withdrawal effects.

Choice of drug used

The decision to use a drug may be influenced by many things, including:

- Availability and opportunity to try
- Legal status of the drug
- Perceived desired effects
- Perceived risks
- Specifically desired effects versus the risks as weighed up and assessed by the individual concerned
- Acceptability of the drug and/or method of administration to the individual, the individual's peer group and their wider society.

Risks

The incidence and nature of risks vary with the drug and how it is used, the individual concerned and the circumstances. Examples of such variables include the drug substance, the presence of impurities, the dose, the frequency of use, the route of administration, the legal status of the drug, related social and financial circumstances, the personality of the individual drug user and the interaction between drug use and lifestyle.

Weighing up benefits vs risks

If the benefits from drug use are experienced before the harm, or to a greater perceived extent than the harm, positive endorsement of drug taking occurs. Following positive endorsement, drug use may, but does not necessarily, continue.

Control and dependence

A lack of specific types of neurological control is sometimes given as the reason why some people develop addictions to specific psychoactive drug(s) whereas others do not. Published studies can be criticized as the models of behaviour are largely shown in animals not humans. Nevertheless, neurological processes manifest positive and negative reinforcement

Table 50.1 Some common psychoactive drugs used/misused and selected information on their effects

Common name	Active/main psychoactive component	Most common method(s) of administration	Effect on central nervous system	Examples of desired effects (e.g. reasons for taking)	Examples of unwanted effects/harm from use
Acid/LSD	Lysergic acid diethylamine	Orally dissolved on the tongue	Hallucinogenic	Altered sensory perceptions, e.g. visual hallucinations, time distortion, detachment from reality	Panic attacks, frightening altered perceptions, dysphoria, delusions, psychosis, tachycardia. After-effects include 'flashbacks'
Alcohol	Ethanol	Orally in drinks, e.g. wines, spirits, beers, etc.	CNS depressant	Relaxation, disinhibition, promotes social interaction	Aggressive mood, diuresis, dehydration, hypoglycaemia, sedation, vomiting, depression, anxiety, liver cirrhosis, acute hepatitis, gastric cancer
Caffeine	Caffeine	Orally often in drinks, e.g. tea, coffee, and some soft drinks. Tablets.	CNS stimulation	Increased alertness, combats fatigue, promotes stamina	Diuresis, insomnia, restlessness, anxiety, poor concentration, tremor, headaches
Cannabis	Delta-9-tetrahydrocannabinol (THC) plus other cannabinoids	Hashish (resin) or marijuana (dried flower heads and leaves), both of which are smoked often with tobacco in hand-rolled cigarettes	CNS depressant	Relaxation, enhances mood, disinhibition, sociability	Anxiety, panic reactions, sedation, tachycardia, coughing, lung disorders, loss of motivation
Ecstasy	3,4-methylenedioxy-methamphetamine (MDMA) (other similar amphetamine derivatives also used)	Oral ingestion in tablet form often in association with attendance at dance music event	CNS stimulation, hallucinogenic	Physical and mental stimulation, confidence, sociability, happy, elevated mood, increased energy	Sweating, tachycardia, headache, dry mouth, rhabdomyolysis, hyperpyrexia, hyponatremia, renal failure. After-effects include depression, insomnia, anxiety, lethargy
Heroin	Diamorphine	Inhalation of vapour produced when heated on tin foil, intravenous injection	CNS depressant	Intense pleasure including euphoria, warmth, relaxation, detachment from emotional distress	Initially nausea and vomiting, constipation, drowsiness, confusion, dry mouth, sweating, in overdose – respiratory depression, pulmonary oedema, hypoxia, arrhythmias

(Continued)

Table 50.1 (Continued)

Common name	Active/main psychoactive component	Most common method(s) of administration	Effect on central nervous system	Examples of desired effects (e.g. reasons for taking)	Examples of unwanted effects/ harm from use
Tobacco	Nicotine	Cigarette smoking, chewing tobacco	CNS stimulation	Social activity, mood elevation, increases concentration, promotes relaxation	Various cancers, cardiac disease, chronic obstructive airways disease, cough, halitosis
Cocaine	Cocaine hydrochloride (cocaine powder), cocaine base ('crack')	Nasal administration though snorting, injecting, smoking (free base)	CNS stimulation	Euphoria, alertness, increased confidence, excitement, physical stimulation. Intense exhilaration (injection and crack)	Cardiac toxicity, tachycardia, palpitations, hypertension, chest pain, sweating, tremor, mental and anxiety, psychosis. After-effects include dysphoria, depression, fatigue, intense craving
Speed	Amphetamine	Nasal administration through snorting, orally, intravenous injecting	CNS stimulation	Physical and mental stimulation, confidence, increased energy	Sweating, tachycardia, hypertension, anxiety, paranoia and psychosis. After-effects include fatigue and depression

of drug seeking and taking behaviours, with genetic variations influencing these.

The level of control a drug user has over his use will influence the balance between the benefits and harms experienced. With controlled use, harms can be prevented or contained, e.g. the quantity of alcohol consumed may be controlled to avoid unwanted effects. In uncontrolled use, harms can escalate. Uncontrolled use is a characteristic of drug dependence.

When a person loses control over his drug consumption, or rather drug consumption controls the person, this may be described as dependence. Drug dependence can present a significant amount of harm to the individual and to society. There is a clear association between drug dependence and social deprivation. Socially deprived areas tend to have a greater incidence of drug problems. However, drug problems are also found in non-deprived areas.

Withdrawal

When a person stops using a substance they are dependent on, they often experience withdrawal. Withdrawal can be described in two forms.

Physical withdrawal effects

These are physical signs and symptoms experienced when the drug is removed. Examples include seizures in alcohol withdrawal, stomach cramps and severe influenza-type symptoms experienced in opiate withdrawal, palpitations and anxiety in cocaine withdrawal, insomnia in nicotine withdrawal. Physical withdrawal effects can be severe and tend to be of shorter duration than psychological withdrawal effects. For example the acute physical withdrawal stage from heroin lasts usually no more than 7 days.

Psychological withdrawal effects

These are psychological disturbances experienced when a drug is removed. These cannot be so easily observed or measured in the way that many physical withdrawal effects can, but they must not be underestimated. Psychological withdrawal includes intense craving, intense emotional experiences such as unmasking of grief, inability to cope, altered mood and depression, which may be prolonged and severe. It tends to be of long duration and contributes markedly to relapse back to drug use.

The harms relating to psychoactive drug use and dependence

The risks and harms that drug use and dependence can present to the individual and society vary with the drug taken, the individual and the circumstances in which the drugs are taken. It is not possible to list all possible consequences from drug use/misuse in this chapter. The risks are categorized below.

Health problems

These affect the individual drug user and include physical and psychological health problems, which can be large and complex. As well as being caused by the individual substances concerned, health problems may relate to the method of administration. For example, injecting drug use is associated with damage to the circulatory system. Blood-borne virus infection (e.g. with HIV, hepatitis B and hepatitis C) is associated with the sharing of injecting equipment. Pharmacists are largely involved in preventing or reducing the harm from drug dependence. Hence the role of the pharmacist in drug dependence contributes towards individual and public health and safety.

Social problems

The social problems should not be underestimated and often drive people to seek treatment. Social problems may include poverty (e.g. social deprivation, exclusion or failure in education, inability to obtain or sustain employment, spending of income on drugs), damage to family relationships, difficulties forming relationships, exclusion from society and homelessness.

Drug-related crime

Drug-related crime includes not only the criminal activities committed against the Misuse of Drugs Act (see below) for which the individual is punished, but also crime that impacts on communities and society at large. The latter may relate to the acquisition of drugs or the effects of drugs, e.g. burglary to obtain money to buy drugs, robbery, violence associated with drunkenness, drunk/drug driving. Drug-related crime is of concern to

society and is one of the reasons why treatment of drug problems and drug dependence is a key public health issue (see Ch. 13). Additionally, there is evidence that treatment of drug dependence contributes towards a very marked reduction in drug-related crime. Hence, treatment benefits not only the individual in terms of improved health but also society by making communities safer.

Drug users are often at greater risk than non-drug users of being victims of crime, e.g. violence associated with debt to drug dealers, prostitution, robbery and mugging if homeless or intoxicated.

Legislation

Misuse of Drugs Act

The Misuse of Drugs Act 1971 classifies drugs into Class A, Class B and Class C. The purpose of this legislation is to define the penalties imposed for the illegal undertaking of various activities, e.g. possession, supply, import, and export. These are summarized in Table 50.2. This classification system is different from the Misuse of Drugs Regulations that largely govern dispensing and other activities of the pharmacist.

Road Traffic Act

This 1988 Act makes it illegal to be in charge of a motor vehicle if 'unfit to drive through drink or drugs'. This includes both illicit substances and prescribed medicines. Drivers are required by law to notify the Driving and Vehicle Licensing Agency (DVLA) if there is any reason that the safety of their driving may be impaired, e.g. the misuse of drugs, the need for medicines that impair reactions or cause sedation. The responsibility for notification lies with the patient, not healthcare professionals.

The management of drug use and dependence

Pharmacists are primarily involved with the treatment of dependence rather than interventions aimed at recreational and non-problematic drug use. The prevalence of drug dependence on a population basis is relatively small compared with national statistics that estimate numbers of people who have

Table 50.2 Classification of some commonly misused substances according to the Misuse of Drugs Act 1971

Class	Drugs	Maximum penalties
A	Cocaine including crack cocaine, diamorphine (heroin), dipipanone, ecstasy, LSD, methadone, morphine, opium, pethidine	7 years imprisonment and/or unlimited fine for possession. Life imprisonment and/or fine for supply[a]
B[b]	Most amphetamines[c], cannabis[d], codeine, dihydrocodeine, methylphenidate	5 years imprisonment and/or fine for possession. 14 years imprisonment and a fine for supply
C	Benzodiazepines, anabolic steroids and growth hormones	2 years imprisonment and/or fine for possession. 14 years imprisonment and/or fine for supply

[a]The term 'supply' includes drug trafficking and unauthorized production.
[b]If Class B drugs are prepared for injection they become Class A.
[c]Unless prepared for injection when amphetamines become Class A.
[d]Pure cannabinoids are Class A drugs.

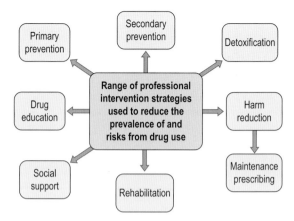

Figure 50.1 • The range of professional intervention strategies used to reduce or manage drug use and dependence.

ever tried drugs. However, the extent of harm from drug dependence can be large; hence the need for effective strategies to support people in changing their drug use. Since the 1990s, treatment, criminal justice and prevention initiatives in the UK have been guided by government drugs strategies.

Figure 50.1 illustrates the range of methods used in preventing, reducing and controlling drug use and dependence and managing the adverse consequences.

Primary prevention

Primary prevention is concerned with preventing people from starting to use drugs. Target groups include vulnerable groups such as school children, children in care and young people who have left education. Health promotion and education campaigns are used to warn about the harm that can result from drug use and dependence using. Primary prevention also includes legislation, as the illegal nature of many drugs may prevent some people from using

them. It is difficult to evaluate the impact of primary prevention activities. Reliable research in this area can also be difficult to undertake. This does not mean that primary prevention activities should not be used. They are very important for informing children and young people about drugs and their effects, in a factually correct and not 'scaremongering' way.

Secondary prevention

Secondary prevention is aimed at people who use drugs by discouraging further use. Examples of secondary prevention are giving advice to prevent problems such as overheating and dehydration to ecstasy users, discouraging heroin smokers from progressing to injecting, and warning of the risks and guiding on the use of CNS depressant drugs (such as heroin and methadone) by stimulant users (such as ecstasy and amphetamine) when depressant drugs are used to assist with the 'come down' following CNS stimulation.

Drug education

Drug education is a tool used in primary and secondary prevention campaigns and formats include leaflets, booklets, films, online information and posters. People who are dependent on drugs may also benefit from drug education as they may not be fully informed on the drugs they use or may consider using, e.g. long-term risks and overdose prevention. Drug education is also a key part of harm reduction, giving people information to assist them in minimizing risks from drug taking, e.g. safer injecting information. Drug education may be provided by a range of people, e.g. teachers, youth workers, health promotion workers, medical and nursing staff and police officers and should always be appropriate for the target group. For example, advice given to dependent heroin smokers would differ from that aiming to prevent heroin use in school children. Pharmacists may be asked to provide talks and should only deliver such talks if they feel competent to do so and capable of answering questions. Advice and information from a credible source such as publications by drug charities and health promotion units and the support of the local drugs service should be sought.

Social support

Social support refers loosely to non-medical/pharmacological interventions that can be made. These may include practical advice and assistance (e.g. seeking housing, benefits advice, and provision of hostel accommodation) and use of psychological tools such as motivational interviewing. Motivational interviewing aims to assist people in examining their drug use and the impact it has on their lives and those of others to move people towards a psychological state, where they are motivated to change their behaviour and attempt to change their drug use. Pharmacists should be aware of the need for a holistic approach to care, to improve outcomes. Some pharmacists with a special interest (PwSI) who have specialized in drug misuse have developed skills in motivational interviewing and other psychological support tools.

Detoxification

Detoxification aims for the person to become abstinent from the drug on which they are dependent by the gradual removal of the drug or substitute therapy. Examples include the use of diazepam at gradually reducing doses in benzodiazepine dependence and the use of nicotine replacement therapy.

Rehabilitation

Rehabilitation may include a detoxification process followed by a period of social support and intensive psychotherapy to facilitate sustained change. Alternatively, it may comprise the social support and intensive psychotherapy phase only, with successful detoxification being a requirement for entry on the programme. Rehabilitation is usually provided within a 'therapeutic community' – participants live in the environment where treatment is given, often for several months. The outcomes from various drug rehabilitation programmes show improvements in drug use, physical health, psychological health and involvement in crime.

Harm reduction

Harm reduction is a generic term to describe the range of interventions used to reduce the adverse consequences of drug dependence experienced by both individual drug users and society. Strategies prioritize goals in treatment, recognizing that, whereas abstinence from drug use may be the end goal, in some cases and for some drugs, it is not always immediately achievable. Instead, the risks and harm to the individual and others are reduced, by a process of prioritization, which the individual is involved in defining. Harm reduction engages drug users with service providers, enabling for example, motivational interventions. Harm reduction is, for most, an important route to abstinence.

Examples of harm reduction interventions include the provision of sterile injecting equipment and information to drug injectors to prevent the sharing of injecting equipment (to prevent the transmission of HIV, hepatitis B and C). Minimizing the prevalence of such diseases also protects the non-injecting community.

Harm reduction also includes the provision of substitute therapies with the aim of reducing illicit drug use and reducing drug-related crime. Substitute therapy is provided, either at an adequate maintenance dose or as a detoxification agent. Pharmacists are frequently involved in the provision of harm reduction services.

Service providers

Drug and alcohol services in the UK can be broadly grouped according to their different sources of funding.

Statutory sector

The statutory sector comprises NHS and local authority services and includes prevention initiatives and services that provide harm reduction and abstinence-directed care. A large amount of NHS drug treatment is provided in GP surgeries, either by GPs alone or in partnership with GP liaison workers from specialist drugs services. This is often termed 'shared care'. Community drug teams (CDTs) are attached to NHS trusts. CDTs may provide primary care drug treatment, either through GP liaison work or with their own clinicians running special clinics, similar to outpatient clinics. CDT services are typically provided by doctors and psychiatric nurses but some employ pharmacists to advise on or undertake prescribing and manage on-site dispensing. Statutory sector needle exchanges also exist.

NHS services also include secondary care, where treatment such as inpatient detoxification from alcohol and other drugs is provided, typically over a short time period such as 2 weeks.

Voluntary sector

Voluntary sector ('third sector') services are particularly prevalent in the substance misuse field. Voluntary sector services receive funding from a range of sources (e.g. NHS, criminal justice money, local authorities, grants and donations) and are usually registered charities, with paid workers and/or volunteers operating under a management committee structure. Workers may come from a range of backgrounds, e.g. nursing, social work and community work. Some projects employ current or ex-drug users. Services may include:

- Support and/or counselling
- Information and advice including harm reduction information
- Needle exchange
- Preparation for rehabilitation or inpatient detoxification and aftercare
- Client advocacy
- Complementary therapies
- Support to and liaison with GPs
- Specialist services such as women-only sessions
- Outreach and detached street-based work
- Prescribing services
- Input into multidisciplinary groups funded by the statutory service such as pregnancy clinics for drug-using women.

Other voluntary sector services offer spiritual and practical support, e.g. hostel accommodation and self-help groups. The voluntary sector also may represent drug users' views in advocacy, policy and service planning.

Private sector

The private sector includes ultra-rapid detoxification units, inpatient detoxification clinics, private primary care doctors and residential rehabilitation providers, private psychotherapists and alternative therapy providers. Funding for some of these treatments may come through the statutory sector but they are most often paid for by the patients or their families. Some pharmacists work in private sector treatment facilities advising on prescribing and dispensing. Private services offer a wide range of choice to patients but access is obviously limited by ability to pay. Ultra-rapid detoxification is not recommended for safety reasons.

Pharmaceutical care

This section focuses on pharmaceutical care of drug users, specifically looking at aspects of good pharmacy practice.

The role of the pharmacist in drug dependence

Community pharmacists

Community pharmacists are ideally placed to contribute to the care of drug users. In addition to the health gains for the patient, there are several advantages for drug users, the community and pharmacists from providing care:

- Extended opening hours: most pharmacies are open at least part of the weekend and some evenings, when specialist drugs services may be closed
- Accessibility
- Expert advice
- Discretion: pharmacies provide a confidential service exchange
- Network of service
- Job satisfaction: the pharmacist may be the only healthcare professional with whom some drug users have regular contact. Over time, improvements in health can often be seen in

people receiving substitute therapies, bringing job satisfaction.

The two most common services provided by community pharmacists to prevent and reduce harm are needle exchange and dispensing services.

Hospital pharmacists

Hospitals should have guidelines for the admission and discharge of drug users to ensure that any ongoing prescribing is continued. There should also be policies and specialist support available to ensure treatment can be initiated if a need is identified.

Hospital pharmacists may contribute to the formulation of such guidelines. Issues to include are:

- Admissions: how to ensure the safe and prompt continuation of substitute prescribing with attention paid to acute and out of hours admissions
- Discharge: how to ensure safe continuation of substitute prescribing on discharge without a break in care or doubling up of prescribing. Liaison with the patient's nominated community pharmacist is important
- Initiation of substitute therapy. For example, if a heroin-dependent person is admitted to a ward unplanned via accident and emergency, it will be necessary to control withdrawal symptoms that onset quickly (typically within 4–6 h)
- Appropriate referral to service providers: Guidance on identifying patients at particular risk and rapid referral from hospital to primary care services is recommended.

Hospital pharmacists play a key role in advising on co-prescribing for people on substitute therapies such as methadone. Many drug interactions can occur. Treatments for epilepsy and HIV/AIDS in particular must be carefully considered.

Specialist pharmacists (PwSI)

There are pharmacists who specialize in drug dependency, many of whom come under the umbrella term of 'pharmacist with a special interest' (PwSI). Some provide services from community pharmacies, whereas others may be based in GP surgeries or specialist drugs services. They may be prescribers, or provide support to clinical colleagues, e.g. by advising on prescribing or providing drug information. They may also oversee dispensing and liaise with (other) community pharmacists. Others undertake strategic roles such as coordinating local pharmacy needle exchange services or overseeing the pharmacy contribution to shared care.

Needle and syringe exchange

Background

Needle and syringe exchange programmes (NSPs) began in the UK in the mid-1980s in response to the threat from HIV. NSPs were started in many countries in order to enable safe injecting of drugs. Research projects found that NSPs were effective in reducing the transmission of HIV without causing an increase in injecting drug use.

In the early 1990s, hepatitis C (HCV) was identified. This blood-borne virus is highly transmissible among injectors. It has been shown to be spread through the sharing of injecting paraphernalia, including needles and syringes, but also probably other items used in the preparation of illicit injections play a role, for example mixing water, shared makeshift filters used to remove insoluble materials and contaminated swabs. It is important that NSPs are widely available in order to limit the spread of blood-borne viruses.

Practical issues in NSP provision

Training

Before setting up an NSP service, NSP pharmacists and their staff should undertake training on issues relating to needle exchange. Specialist agencies may be able to offer training for pharmacists and their staff.

Hepatitis B vaccination

Although here are no vaccines for hepatitis C or HIV, it is a wise health and safety precaution for all staff involved in NSP to be vaccinated against hepatitis B (HBV).

Needle exchange procedure

Needle exchange involves supplying clean, sterile injecting equipment in exchange for used equipment, which is returned in a sealed sharps container. Practitioners should provide advice and check injecting sites, with referral to medical services when problems such as abscesses are identified.

NSP are usually coordinated within the health locality, so local policies and procedures should exist and in order to minimize risk support and guidance should be available to pharmacists. Adequate storage facilities are essential. Used equipment returned to the pharmacy in a sharps bin should be placed in a larger bin by the client, stored in a separate area from clean equipment and away from medicines. These bins are sealed when full and collected for incineration by clinical waste disposal companies.

To maximize the public health benefits, injecting drug users need to be able to use a clean set of equipment for each injection and every set of equipment supplied should be returned for incineration. In order to try to meet this aim, adequate amounts of injecting equipment should be supplied, bearing in mind that some crack cocaine injectors may be injecting very frequently (e.g. 15 times per day or more). Capping of numbers of sets of equipment allowed is not advocated and dilutes harm reduction effectiveness. A sharps bin should be supplied with every exchange. The return of equipment should be strongly encouraged. Written advice on safe disposal accompanied by verbal emphasis is important. However, if a person requests needle exchange but has no used equipment to return, it is advocated that supply is provided, as the health risks of not supplying are great. Pharmacy staff should not open disposal bins to count the number of sets returned.

Record-keeping and audit

Records need to be kept in order to audit the pharmacy NSP. In order to encourage use, needle exchange should be provided on an anonymous basis (no names recorded). Attractions of pharmacy-based NSPs are their anonymity and low threshold access. Too many obstacles will discourage use. One of the benefits of pharmacy NSPs is their ability to attract hard-to-reach clients. In some schemes, pharmacies issue cards which give the service user an identification number or code. This can be used to record service usage but it also allows discreet service provision, as the person only needs to show the card to indicate that they require needle exchange. This can be helpful in a crowded pharmacy. The advantage of having a record for each service user is that it can quickly

be seen if someone returns used equipment or not. Those who do not can be targeted with information and firm requests to return equipment. The disadvantage is that in a busy pharmacy, this system can be too time-consuming. Additionally, some people do not want to carry a card, fearing that it identifies them as an injector. As a basic requirement, the daily number of sets of injecting equipment supplied and the approximate number returned should be recorded and data compiled for weekly or monthly audit purposes. Data should be returned to the scheme coordinator where one exists. Pharmacies with poor return rates should seek the advice of specialist drugs agencies and the scheme coordinator on strategies to increase return rates and be proactive in encouraging returns.

Risk management

A written procedure for needle exchange should be in place and followed. Body fluid spillage kits should be kept in all pharmacies as a matter of routine, irrespective of whether the pharmacy is part of an NSP, and staff should be trained in their use. In the event of an incident (e.g. a patient bleeds or vomits on the floor), the kit should be used.

Chain mail gloves should be kept in needle exchange pharmacies for use in the event of loose used injecting equipment within the pharmacy requiring disposal. If any event occurs they should be documented as part of the pharmacy's critical incident scheme. Procedures should then be reviewed to see if anything could be done to avoid such an incident in the future (see Ch. 11).

Links with specialist services

Pharmacy NSP providers should have links with local drugs agencies and know what services are provided. Knowledge of other local services means that the pharmacist can advise when a need is identified or an opportunity arises. Often younger, newer injectors and women use pharmacy NSP because of the low threshold and discretion. The pharmacist may be the only healthcare professional these service users have contact with and should consider themselves a gateway to specialist services. Some specialist agencies may be able to supply pharmacists with targeted written information for drug injectors, such as safer injecting leaflets, and with free condoms to reduce sexually transmitted diseases. Safer injecting leaflets should not be available for self-selection but should be targeted at injectors.

Use of pharmacotherapies in drug dependence

The term pharmacotherapy in this context refers to any drug treatment used to assist in the management of drug dependence or symptoms of withdrawal. Substitute therapy refers to drug treatment that replaces an illegal drug with a legal one of the same or similar pharmacological class. For example methadone is a substitute for opiates such as heroin. Non-substitute drugs may also be used to control withdrawal symptoms (e.g. lofexidine to manage opiate withdrawal) and to manage symptoms secondary to withdrawal (e.g. loperamide to manage diarrhoea associated with opiate withdrawal).

Role of pharmacotherapy

Pharmacotherapy can be mistaken both by patients and by professionals as an all-encompassing solution. Alone it cannot stop someone using drugs but it can facilitate change in motivated people by providing what many describe as 'breathing space'. For example substitute therapy can prevent withdrawal symptoms thus giving the person a chance to sever links with illicit drug suppliers. Substitute therapy also removes the need to commit crime to obtain money for drugs. Pharmacotherapy therefore has benefits for both the individual and society.

Evidence shows maintenance doses of substitute drug treatment alone improve patient physical health and mental health outcomes, reduce drug-related deaths and improve social functioning. However, outcomes can be enhanced with appropriate 'wrap around' services providing support and counselling, where the person freely is willing to take part.

The psychoactive and non-psychoactive effects of substitute therapies are not usually the same as the illicit drugs they replace and an awareness of this in the patient at the start of treatment is important. For example, orally taken methadone does not produce euphoria and it can cause lethargy and a feeling of 'heaviness' not associated with heroin use.

All who receive pharmacotherapy, especially in the early stages of treatment, may not achieve complete abstinence from illicit drug use. Ideally, maintenance therapy at an adequate dose may be necessary, prior to planned detoxification and aftercare. This maintenance stage may last for many years.

Methadone

Methadone is used as a substitute drug in opiate dependence. Its long half-life (24–48 h) makes it suitable for once-daily dosing in the majority of cases, although a few patients prefer to divide the dose. Providing it is given in adequate doses and for a satisfactory length of time, there is substantial evidence to suggest that methadone treatment has several benefits:

- Improved physical health
- Improved psychological health
- Reduced illicit drug consumption
- Reduced incidence and frequency of injecting episodes
- Reduced drug-related crime.

The benefits extend beyond the individual patient into the community. Less injecting reduces the risks of blood-borne virus transmission.

Failure to reduce or prevent illicit drug consumption is associated with maintenance doses of methadone less than 60 mg/day and premature pressure to abstain from methadone (Ward et al. 1999). Withdrawal of treatment should begin only when the patient is willing to attempt this, as motivation is the key to success. In detoxification, the speed of dose reduction largely depends on how well the patient is coping. Reductions should be calculated as a percentage of the dose; hence towards the smaller end of the scale, dosing will be reduced by smaller quantities. For some people, the small doses can be the hardest to reduce.

It is important to discuss with patients potential overdose risks from combining CNS depressants, including alcohol. Healthcare teams need to understand that some illicit drug use may continue, especially at the early stages of treatment. Several information leaflets are available, which explain this to patients, e.g. the 'Methadone Briefing' from Exchange Supplies (see: http://www.drug-library.eu/library/books/methadone/intro.html) or the Department of Health-supported Exchange Supplies *Going Over* DVD.

Pharmacists should have a good understanding of the clinical aspects relating to methadone treatment before they begin providing methadone dispensing services. This should be gained as part of a CPD plan if needed.

Safe storage in the home

If take-home doses are dispensed, pharmacists should discuss safe storage of methadone and other drugs in the home with patients, especially those with children.

Other treatments

Buprenorphine is a partial agonist, used as an opiate substitution therapy instead of methadone. Its use has become more widespread. The patient needs clear advice on initiation and counselling on the risks of attempting to overcome the antagonist properties, for example by using large amounts of opiate. This may present an overdose risk. Buprenorphine is used in sublingual tablet form and has a long half-life, which facilitates daily or even every second day administration. The patient must not take the first dose of buprenorphine until they are experiencing opiate withdrawal symptoms to avoid precipitated withdrawal. More information will be given in the manufacturer's data sheet.

Lofexidine and naltrexone are also used in the management of opiate withdrawal. The former reduces some of the physical withdrawal effects from opiates by acting on the noradrenergic system, while the latter is an opiate antagonist used in relapse prevention. There are also recognized regimens to assist withdrawal for those with stimulant, benzodiazepine and alcohol dependence. When a person is dependent on more than one drug, withdrawal should be done one drug at a time.

Urine screening and responding to symptoms

People receiving treatment for drug dependence may have their urine screened. This is done to check for evidence of compliance with prescribed regimens or to confirm the consumption of illicit drugs. Pharmacists should undertake training in this area of toxicology, as some over the counter and prescribed medicines can interfere with urine screens, giving false results.

Pharmaceutical dispensing services

Shared care

Shared care with regard to substance misuse is a partnership between the GP, pharmacist, key worker and patient, to manage dependence within a formalized, structured scheme. Pharmacists participating in such schemes receive additional remuneration. Examples of schemes in the UK include those in Glasgow and Berkshire. Daily dispensing of controlled drugs is often advocated by prescribers. This means that the pharmacist is likely to be the healthcare professional with the most frequent contact with the patient. Pharmacists can play an important role in monitoring the patient's health.

One of the benefits of shared care is that the workload of providing care is distributed locally. This prevents one or two pharmacies becoming overburdened and allows patients access to care within their communities. Participation of all or the majority of community pharmacies in the area is therefore vital for the scheme to succeed.

Before joining a shared-care scheme, pharmacists should consider any changes within the pharmacy that may be necessary. For example is there enough space in the controlled drug cabinet to store dispensed controlled drugs waiting for collection? Consider the layout of the premises. What can be done to ensure an appropriate area is available to allow a respectful service to be provided? Is there a private area for supervised consumption?

Supervised consumption

Many shared-care schemes require daily dispensing and supervision of consumption of all or most doses of substitute therapy, at least for the first 3–6 months of treatment. Supervised consumption was introduced because of leakage of methadone and other drugs to the illicit market contributing to overdoses in people who had not been prescribed the drugs.

Supervised consumption is a contentious area (see Ch. 48). Some patients view it as a useful part of treatment, whereas others dislike it. Supervised consumption can cause the patient much embarrassment.

To assist with organization, it is suggested that pharmacists prepare all daily dispensed prescriptions the day before or at the start of the week.

Doses should be packaged appropriately in individually labelled containers and stored in the controlled drug cupboard, or as legislation dictates, with the prescription attached. When the patient presents for supervised consumption, the pharmacist should recheck the dispensed item. The patient should then be given the substance to be consumed together with a drink of water. The water helps take the taste of the medicine away, rinses the mouth (methadone is acidic, which could damage tooth enamel) and helps ensure the dose has been swallowed. Disposable cups should be used. The pharmacist should take the opportunity for discussion with the patient to assess their well-being and offer any advice as the opportunity arises. Over time, a good rapport and therapeutic relationship can develop with patients.

Confidentiality

Communication between healthcare professionals is key in shared care. However, patient confidentiality must be borne in mind. Information should only be shared on a need-to-know basis and with consent. Such consent is usually obtained at the start of treatment as part of a shared care agreement. The patient should be involved in negotiations about care and treatment changes. Patient's wishes should only be breached when a severe risk to health or well-being is considered to exist if confidentiality is not broken. All matters relating to the upholding or breaching of confidentiality should be documented.

Contracts

Some shared-care schemes advocate the use of contracts, which clearly state what is expected of the patient and what the patient can expect from the service. Often they dictate standards of behaviour and include clauses requiring the patient to fulfill certain criteria, including restricting the times when patients can collect prescriptions. It is debated whether contracts should be used specifically for patients with drug problems. They imply that it is expected that the person will not behave appropriately and as such stereotypes patients. Contracts are not routinely used within pharmacy health care for other patients and it can be argued that using one for drug users is unfair and discriminatory. Pharmacies should have practice leaflets as a matter of routine which are available to all pharmacy users. These may include a statement that all pharmacy customers have a right to privacy and respect and all pharmacy staff have a right to be treated with courtesy. If individuals present any problems, the pharmacist should deal with these individually. This applies to any customers who cause difficulty within the pharmacy. Pharmacies should have a complaints procedure which can be useful for reviewing response to such incidents.

Restricted collection hours for drug users should also be considered with caution. Pharmacists are required to dispense prescriptions with 'reasonable promptness'. Refusing to dispense a prescription during opening hours because a person has not arrived within a designated collection time may be considered discriminatory and is certainly unfair.

Locums

All standard operating procedures for pharmacy services should be documented and available for locums (see Ch. 11). This includes needle exchange and supervised consumption.

KEY POINTS

- Pharmacists can make an important contribution to the care and support of people with drug misuse problems
- Treatment of substance misuse benefits not only the patient but the community as well by reducing blood-borne virus transmission and drug-related crime
- Pharmacists should seek adequate continuous professional development to increase their competence in providing services to drug users. This should include clinical and therapeutic knowledge of treatment in this area as well as service provision skills
- Pharmacists should seek to be informed on local specialist services for drug users and have good professional links with such treatment providers
- Pharmacists should treat all pharmacy users with respect. This includes not discriminating on the basis of a person's disease state or drug dependence
- Local pharmacy scheme coordinators can be of great benefit in supporting pharmacists who provide services to drug users

Monitoring the patient

51

Alison Littlewood

STUDY POINTS

- The Yellow Card reporting scheme
- The pharmacist's role in adverse drug reaction reporting
- The medicines use review/prescription intervention service

Introduction

Monitoring the patient may conjure up visions of healthcare professionals, including pharmacists, taking samples of blood from the patient, recording measurements or merely observing them in order to manage a medical condition. While these are important examples of how monitoring may be achieved, there are other schemes that are used specifically in relation to monitoring patients and their medication.

Pharmacovigilance is the science and activities relating to the detection, assessment, understanding and prevention of adverse effects or any other drug-related problem. This has become increasingly important in evaluating medicines and providing checks, controls and warnings to healthcare professionals and patients.

The yellow card scheme

The Medicines and Healthcare products Regulatory Agency (MHRA) is the government agency which is responsible for assessing the safety, quality and efficacy of a wide range of materials from medicines and medical devices to blood and therapeutic products that are derived from tissue engineering. The MHRA authorizes and regulates their sale or supply for human use in the UK (see Ch. 4).

Medicines are controlled as soon as they are first discovered and undergo clinical trials, but it is recognized that only the most common or predictable adverse drug reactions (ADRs) will be detected by the time the drug is marketed and some adverse reactions may not be seen until a very large number of people have received the medicine.

As part of its activities, the MHRA operates post-marketing surveillance and other systems for reporting, investigating and monitoring adverse reactions to medicines and adverse incidents involving medical devices. Included in this remit, the MHRA and the Commission on Human Medicines (CHM) run the UK's national reporting system for ADRs – called the Yellow Card Scheme (YCS).

The YCS was introduced in 1964 initially to provide doctors or dentists with a route to report a suspicion that a medicine could have harmed a patient. The YCS gets its name from the colour of the original document used for reporting the ADR. These 'cards' have become increasingly more accessible and can be sourced by a variety of methods (Box 51.1). There is also a Yellow card freephone line. The fundamental principles of the scheme have not changed. Proof of a causal link between a medicine or a combination of medicines does not need to be established, so the reports are suspected ADRs. In the UK, the MHRA collates data on ADRs via the YCS from a wide range of healthcare professionals working in the NHS or from private healthcare providers. These now include doctors, dentists, pharmacists (from 1997), nurses, midwives and health

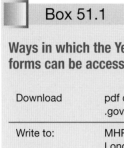

Box 51.1

Ways in which the Yellow Card reporting forms can be accessed

Download	pdf copy (http://www.mhra.gov.uk/)
Write to:	MHRA, CHM Freepost, London, SW8 5BR or CHM's Yellow Card centres
Copies included in:	The British National Formulary (BNF), BNF for children (cBNF), the ABPI Medicines Compendium the MIMS Companion
Available from:	Pharmacies, GP surgeries

visitors (from 2002) and also HM Coroners. Reports are received directly from them and via pharmaceutical companies. The scheme is voluntary for healthcare professionals (HCPs) but pharmaceutical companies holding marketing authorizations have a statutory obligation to report ADRs to the MHRA.

Following pilot schemes in 2005–2006, direct reports from patients, parents and carers are now accepted. The Yellow Card report forms for patients are different from those for healthcare professionals. Standard report forms are shown in Figures 51.1 and 51.2.

There have been over 600 000 reports received since the YCS was set up. Yellow Card reports are collected on all types of medicines irrespective of legal status. These include:

- Prescription medicines
- Medicines you can buy without a prescription over-the-counter (OTC)
- Herbal and other complementary remedies.

However, additional criteria have also been applied when products have been selected for intensive monitoring, and include:

- A new vaccine
- A biosimilar product
- Addition of paediatric use
- A different formulation for an existing route
- A new combination of active substances
- Administration by a new route which is significantly different from existing routes
- A novel drug delivery system

- A change or addition of a therapeutic indication that
  - may alter the established risk/benefit profile of that drug
  - is likely to result in a significantly different population being exposed to the drug.

HCPs are asked to report all suspected ADRs for these products as opposed to focussing only on serious reactions for established products.

It has been suggested that the capacity of the scheme to identify ADRs should be strengthened by including other categories such as:

- Off label use of licensed products
- Delayed drug effects
- Products whose legal status has changed.

The Commission and the MHRA monitored intensively products carrying a black triangle symbol (▼) in the BNF. This symbol identified newly licensed medicines where the drug was a new active substance.

A product retained black triangle status until the safety of the drug or product was well established, which was usually following 2 years of post-marketing experience. There were generally 250–300 drugs under intensive surveillance (Black Triangle List). In July 2012, new pharmacovigilance legislation came into effect across the EU and a European Additional Monitoring list was published in April 2013. A medicine can be included on the list when it is approved for the first time or at any time during its lifecycle and will remain under additional monitoring usually for five years. The list will be reviewed every month.

The Black Triangle will now be used by all EU Member States and from the autumn of 2013 medicines under additional monitoring will have an inverted Black Triangle displayed in their patient information leaflet and in the information for healthcare professionals, called the summary of product characteristics, together with a short sentence:

▼ This medicinal product is subject to additional monitoring.

There are a number of problems associated with the YCS but the major one has been, and continues to be, under-reporting. An internet electronic Yellow Card is available (http://www.mhra.gov.uk) to enable all reporters to submit ADR reports via the MHRA website in a paperless way.

The online reporting forms have been designed to improve clarity and usability by incorporating 'drop-down' menus and dictionaries for technical terms. They allow a reporter to save a partially

In Confidence

YellowCard
It's easy to report online: www.mhra.gov.uk/yellowcard

COMMISSION ON HUMAN MEDICINES (CHM)

MHRA

SUSPECTED ADVERSE DRUG REACTIONS

If you suspect an adverse reaction may be related to one or more drugs/vaccines/complementary remedies, please complete this Yellow Card. See 'Adverse reactions to drugs' section in BNF or **www.mhra.gov.uk/yellowcard** for guidance. Do not be put off reporting because some details are not known.

PATIENT DETAILS Patient Initials:_____ Sex: M / F   Ethnicity:_____   Weight if known (kg):_____

Age (at time of reaction):_____   Identification number (e.g. Your Practice or Hospital Ref):_____

SUSPECTED DRUG(S)/VACCINE(S)

Drug/Vaccine (Brand if known)	Batch	Route	Dosage	Date started	Date stopped	Prescribed for

SUSPECTED REACTION(S)   Please describe the reaction(s) and any treatment given:

Outcome
Recovered ☐
Recovering ☐
Continuing ☐
Other ☐

Date reaction(s) started:_____   Date reaction(s) stopped: _____

Do you consider the reactions to be serious? Yes / No

If yes, please indicate why the reaction is considered to be serious (please tick all that apply):
Patient died due to reaction ☐   Involved or prolonged inpatient hospitalisation ☐
Life threatening ☐   Involved persistent or significant disability or incapacity ☐
Congenital abnormality ☐   Medically significant; please give details: _____

OTHER DRUG(S) (including self-medication and complementary remedies)

Did the patient take any other medicines/vaccines/complementary remedies in the last 3 months prior to the reaction? Yes / No
If yes, please give the following information if known:

Drug/Vaccine (Brand if known)	Batch	Route	Dosage	Date started	Date stopped	Prescribed for

Additional relevant information e.g. medical history, test results, known allergies, rechallenge (if performed), suspect drug interactions. For congenital abnormalities please state all other drugs taken during pregnancy and the last menstrual period.

Please list any medicines obtained from the internet:

REPORTER DETAILS
Name and Professional Address:_____

Postcode:_____ Tel No:_____
Email:_____
Speciality:_____
Signature:_____ Date:_____

CLINICIAN (if not the reporter)
Name and Professional Address:_____

Postcode:_____ Tel No:_____
Email:_____
Speciality:_____
Date:_____

Information on adverse drug reactions received by the MHRA can be downloaded at **www.mhra.gov.uk/daps**
Stay up-to-date on the latest advice for the safe use of medicines with our monthly bulletin *Drug Safety Update* at
www.mhra.gov.uk/drugsafetyupdate

Please attach additional pages if necessary. Send to: FREEPOST YELLOW CARD (no other address details required)

Figure 51.1 • Standard Yellow Card report form for reporting suspected adverse drug reactions by healthcare professionals. (Crown Copyright 2012).

FREEPOST YELLOW CARD

SECOND FOLD HERE

GUIDELINES FOR YELLOW CARD REPORTING

Please use the Yellow Card Scheme to tell us about:
- **All** suspected adverse drug reactions **for new medicines** - identified by the black triangle ▼ symbol.
- **All** suspected adverse drug reactions occurring **in children**, even if a medicine has been used off-label.
- **All serious*** suspected adverse drug reactions for established vaccines and medicines, including unlicensed medicines, herbal remedies, and medicines used off-label.

*Reactions which are fatal, life-threatening, disabling or incapacitating, result in or prolong hospitalisation, or medically significant are considered serious.

If you are unsure, please report anyway

For more information contact:
- The Yellow Card Information Service on Freephone 0800 731 6789
- Visit the Yellow Card website - www.mhra.gov.uk/yellowcard

FIRST FOLD HERE

Figure 51.1 • Continued

Tear along the dotted line

YellowCard* report

Confidential

Use blue or black ink. Complete all the lines marked with ✳ and give as much other information as you can

1 About the suspected side effect

✳ **What were the symptoms of the suspected side effect, and how did it happen?** If there isn't enough space here, attach an extra sheet of paper.

How bad was the suspected side effect?   Tick the box that best describes how bad the symptoms were

✳ ☐ Mild ☐ Unpleasant, but did not affect everyday activities ☐ Bad enough to affect everyday activities ☐ Bad enough to see a doctor
☐ Bad enough to be admitted to hospital   ☐ Caused very serious illness   ☐ Caused death ☐ Other

When did the side effect start?

How is the person feeling now? Tick the box that best describes whether the person still has symptoms of the suspected side effect.

✳ ☐ Better (no more symptoms) ☐ Getting better ☐ Still has symptoms ☐ More seriously ill ☐ Died ☐ Other

Can you give any more details?   For example, did the person take or receive any other treatment for the symptoms?
Did they stop taking the medicine as a result of the side effect?

2 About the person who had the suspected side effect

Who had the suspected side effect?

✳ ☐ You ☐ Your child ☐ Someone else

Information about the person Supply as much information as you can, even if you prefer not to give a name.

First name or initials   Family name   ☐ Male ☐ Female

✳ Age   Weight   ☐ kg ☐ stones/pounds   Height   ☐ metres ☐ feet/inches

Any other relevant information? For example, does the person have any medical conditions or allergies?

Make sure you have completed all the lines marked ✳   **Please turn over →**

Figure 51.2 • Standard Yellow Card report form for reporting suspected adverse drug reactions by patients, parents and carers. (Crown Copyright 2010).

3 About the medicine(s) which might have caused the side effect

Give details of the medicine you suspect of causing the side effect.

✱ **Name of the medicine** ☐ prescription ☐ bought in pharmacy ☐ bought elsewhere

Dosage (for example, one 250 mg tablet, twice a day) ☐ bought on the internet

What was it taken for?

Start date: End date: Did you stop because of side effects? ☐ Yes ☐ No

If you (or the person you're reporting for) were taking any other medicine at the same time (which might have caused an interaction), give details of it. If you need to give details of more than one other medicine, attach an extra sheet of paper.

Name of other medicine ☐ prescription ☐ bought in pharmacy ☐ bought elsewhere

Dosage (for example, one 250 mg tablet, twice a day) ☐ bought on the internet

What was it taken for?

Do you think this medicine might also have caused the side effect? ☐ Yes ☐ No ☐ Possibly

Start date: End date: Did you stop because of side effects? ☐ Yes ☐ No

Have you taken any other medicines or herbal remedies (as well as the above) within the last 3 months? ☐ Yes ☐ No

4 About your doctor *(optional)*

Would you like a copy of this report to be sent to your doctor?

☐ Yes ☐ No **If Yes, give the doctor's name and address.**

If you want us to send a copy of this report to any other healthcare professional, attach a separate sheet with their contact details.

If we need more medical information (such as test results), do we have your permission to contact your doctor directly for it?

☐ Yes ☐ No

Doctor's name

Address

Postcode

5 About you – the person making the report

We need contact details – please supply a full postal address, even if you prefer not to give a phone number or email address.

✱ Title First name or initials Family name

✱ Address

✱ Postcode

Telephone number Email address

Please sign and date this form I agree that the Medicines and Healthcare products Regulatory Agency (MHRA) can contact me to discuss the suspected side effect, and to ask for more information that might help understanding of the case.

✱ Signed Date

Return addressed to: FREEPOST YELLOW CARD. (No other address details are required) © Crown Copyright 2010

Figure 51.2 • Continued

completed report at any point so that it can be finished and submitted at a convenient time or later when more information had been received concerning the ADR. This method is being strongly promoted to encourage spontaneous reporting. The MHRA and CHM also have five Yellow Card centres whose role focusses on increasing awareness of ADRs and the YCS and follow-up of reports in their areas as this has been shown to improve the number and quality of reports. In the period 1 November 2001 to 31 December 2006, reporting of ADRs initially increased by approximately 5% each year compared with the same period in the previous year, but numbers have remained static, at approximately 25 000 reports per year since then.

In a 2-year study period between 1 October 2005 and 30 September 2007, the YCS received 26 129 reports from all patients and HCPs. Table 51.1 provides details on the specialty of the reporters for reports received during this period. Patient reporting has been supported by the distribution of improved Yellow Cards to all GP surgeries, community pharmacies and other NHS outlets across the UK and the freephone line. The patient electronic Yellow Card has been updated and can also be accessed through the website. The study showed that patients had adopted paper, internet and telephone methods of reporting, whereas HCPs appeared to prefer to submit paper reports. However, this may have changed in the interim.

Since the scheme was opened to them, there has been a steady increase in the number of ADR reports received from patients. The patient report form uses a different format and less technical terms than those used by HCPs. In 2011, an evaluation of the pharmacovigilance impact of patient reporting of ADRs to the UK YCS noted that patient reports add value to the scheme because they report different types of drugs and reactions to reports from HCPs. They tend to provide more detail on the impact of the ADR on daily life and activities and the reports are of an equivalent level of seriousness to those of HCPs in generating new potential signals. Information collected through the YCS is an important means of monitoring drug safety in clinical practice and many important early warnings of new ADRs have been identified in addition to increasing the knowledge of known ADRs.

All data are closely scrutinized by the MHRA/CHM to determine whether a potential health threat is emerging and further investigation is required or more immediate action needs to be taken. In some cases, marketing authorization for the drug is withdrawn by the regulatory authority when the risks are considered to outweigh the benefits or the company may voluntarily suspend or withdraw the product. In several instances, a drug has continued to be available following amendments to the summary of product characteristics (SPC) and patient information leaflet (PIL) indicating restrictions in use, reduction in dosages and special warnings and precautions. Some examples can be seen in Table 51.2. Complete listings of the suspected ADRs reported to the MHRA through the YCS by HCPs and patients are provided in drug

Table 51.1 Analysis of YCS reports between October 2005 and 30 September 2007

Type of reporter	No. during period	Percentage of all reports
All healthcare professionals	20 949	80.2
Patients	5180	19.8
Total	26 129	

Breakdown of HCP reporters	Subgroup	(%)
Doctors (65)	GP	51
	Hospital	8
	Physician	6
Pharmacists (13)	Community	6
	Hospital	5
	Not specified	2
Other health professionals (22)	Nurses	11
	Other HCP	10
	Dentist	1

analysis prints (DAPs). Drug analysis prints can be accessed from the MHRA website.

It is recognized that there are a number of problems with spontaneous reporting systems such as this. Under-reporting arises because HCPs or patients do not recognize an ADR if it is unknown or difficult to spot. Conversely, there may be a bias to report ADRs that are well publicized. The true incidence of a particular ADR cannot be determined, since there is a lack of information on the total number of patients exposed to the drug. The quality of the data reported is variable and some important details may be omitted and the report only indicates that an ADR is suspected, which does not imply causality, and false positives are mixed with true effects. The YCS is also poor at detecting long delayed reactions.

In addition, reporting systems in different countries differ and it was difficult to compare reports of ADRs across international boundaries. However, the WHO set up its Collaborating Centre for International Drug Monitoring after the thalidomide disaster. Since 1978, the programme has been carried out by the Uppsala Monitoring Centre

Table 51.2 Safety issues which Yellow Card reports have helped to identify

Year	Medicine	Safety issue	Resulting action or advice
1995	Quinolone antibiotics	Tendonitis, tendon rupture	Improved warnings
1996	Alendronate (Fosamax)	Severe oesophageal reactions	Warnings and revised dosing instructions
1998	Sertindole (Serdolect)	Sudden cardiac death	Drug withdrawn[a]
1999 and 2007	*Aristolochia* in Chinese herbal remedies	Renal failure. Transitional cell carcinoma	*Aristolochia* banned. Reminder issued
2000	Cisapride (Prepulsid, Alimix)	Serious cardiovascular reactions	Use of cisapride suspended in the UK[b]
2003	Aspirin	Reye's Syndrome in children under 16 years	Statutory label warning
2003	Kava-kava	Hepatotoxicity	Supply of Kava-kava prohibited in the UK
2004	Rosuvastatin (Crestor)	Rhabdomyolysis	Revised dosing instructions and improved warnings
2006	Linezolid (Zyvox)	Optic neuropathy	Improved warnings and monitoring recommendations
2008	Varenicline (Champix)	Depression, suicidal thoughts and behaviour	Warnings issued and monitoring of patients with history of psychiatric illness advised
2011	Citalopram and escitalopram	QT interval elongation	New maximum daily dose restrictions (including in elderly patients), contraindications and warnings
2012	Sitaxentan (Thelin)	Worldwide withdrawal from the market	Worldwide withdrawal from the market
2012	Dabigatran (Pradaxa)	Serious haemorrhage	Contraindications clarified and reminder to monitor renal function
2012	Simvastatin	Drug interactions	Updated warnings and contraindications with maximum dose recommendations

[a]Sertindole was reinstated in 2002 with increased warnings.
[b]Cisapride licences have been cancelled.

(UMC) in Sweden, which is able to apply techniques to identify signals of ADRs that require further investigations using reports from over 100 member nations.

Patient or consumer reporting schemes are known to be operating in 46 countries.

The role of the pharmacist

Pharmacists have an important contribution to make in the prevention, identification, documentation and reporting of ADRs and in strengthening Yellow Card reporting. Currently, the proportion of Yellow Cards received from pharmacists remains around 13%, whereas the proportion of patient reports submitted over a similar time period is almost 20%.

The new medicine service (NMS) was launched in October 2011 and commissioned until December 2013. In the first 9 months, the NMS had a marked effect on reporting by community pharmacists with a significant increase of 120% compared with the same period in the previous year.

It is important that pharmacists are not reluctant to report suspected ADRs because they are often the HCP most able to identify ADRs and to play an active role in their prevention.

On a daily basis, the pharmacist becomes aware of factors that could indicate an ADR is occurring such as:

- Excessive therapeutic effects of medicines
- Abnormal laboratory values
- Medications prescribed or purchased to treat 'side-effects'
- Drugs being discontinued but alternatives with the same indication being prescribed or purchased.

Their role as prescribers means they are more closely involved with the patient and the choice of medication. The expanding range of over-the-counter (OTC) medicines and the increasing number of medicines whose legal status has changed means that the responsibility of providing guidance to patients on the safe use of medicines frequently falls to the pharmacist (see Ch. 21). This also means that they should be advising patients to contribute to the YCS by completing forms themselves or encouraging patients to do so.

The future

For the future, it is hoped that the information collected by the YCS can be used by researchers to help studies that will advance knowledge in the safe use of medicines. Examples of research applications that have been accepted, include acute renal toxicity reported to the YCS and pharmacogenetics of antimicrobial drug-induced liver injury.

International collaboration is also important to improve patient safety and public health. In conjunction with the launch of the new EU pharmacovigilance legislation, the European Medicines Agency (EMA) is responsible for a centralized system for reporting suspected adverse drug reaction

cases to common medicines and active substances used in nationally-authorized medicines in the EU. The system will publish regular reports and in doing so, provide better prevention, detection and assessment of ADRs throughout the EU. Similarly, pharmacovigilance methods are being applied to public health programmes to supplement existing knowledge on adverse effects of newly introduced medicines for conditions such as malaria, tuberculosis and HIV.

The medicines use review (MUR)/prescription intervention service

Background

The community pharmacy contractual framework (CPCF) for England and Wales was introduced in April 2005. The CPCF comprises 'Essential', 'Advanced' and 'Enhanced' service tiers. The medicines use review (MUR)/prescription intervention service is included under 'Advanced' services.

Although there are two service titles, in reality there is only one service, and the same premises and pharmacist accreditation requirement apply to both but the trigger which initiates provision is different. The MUR is a national service in which accredited pharmacists are remunerated to discuss the patient's medication both prescribed and non-prescribed and support them in getting the most from their medicines.

The pharmacist reviews the patient's use, experience and taking of medicines together with identifying side-effects and interactions. The regular MUR is a routine consultation not triggered by a problem with the patient's adherence to their regimen. Prescription interventions involve the same review, but are triggered by a significant issue, such as an adherence problem, that comes to light during the dispensing of a prescription. The pharmacist aims to resolve any issues around poor or ineffective drug use by the patient and in this way, uses a different approach to patient monitoring and patient safety. Following the first year of implementation, the national evaluation of the CPCF in 2007 indicated that 60% of pharmacies were providing the MUR service. The MUR was seen as the first opportunity for the pharmacist to demonstrate the added value that their input could make to patient care. Since then, the directions applying to MURs have been amended to incorporate a revised reporting form and GP (or equivalent) notification requirements. Uptake of the service has steadily increased and statistics now show that around 9000 pharmacies claim MUR payments, with an average of 20–25 MURs carried out per claiming pharmacy, each month.

Accreditation

A pharmacy can only provide advanced services if it is satisfactorily providing all the essential services in the CPCF. In order to provide MUR services, certain criteria must be met by both the pharmacy from which the service is taking place and the pharmacist who is providing the service.

Pharmacy criteria

As well as providing essential services, a pharmacy must have a consultation area:

- Where the patient and pharmacist can sit down together
- Where the patient and pharmacist can talk together without being overheard by other visitors to the pharmacy or staff undertaking normal duties
- Which is clearly designated for confidential consultations, distinct from the general public areas of the pharmacy.

If there is no space for a consultation room, pharmacists may conduct an MUR when the pharmacy is closed, making the whole pharmacy the consultation room. A request form has to be submitted to the Commissioning body in order to do this.

Pharmacists' criteria

Pharmacists must successfully undertake a competency assessment to gain accreditation before providing MURs and send a copy of the certificate to the PCO before they can begin to offer the service.

Any higher education institution (HEI) can provide training and competency assessments for the MUR service. A national competency framework is used as the basis for these assessments. The framework is not designed to be an exhaustive list of competencies that might be required to undertake MUR, but consists of those key elements that can be assessed in a robust and reliable manner.

There are a number of providers who run courses and/or competency assessments. Additionally, some academic institutions that provide postgraduate clinical programmes, such as diplomas, have ensured their courses develop and test the skills of students in order to meet the requirements of the MUR competencies. A list of providers across the UK is available from the Pharmaceutical Services Negotiating Committee (PSNC) website (www.psnc.org.uk).

A pharmacist registered with a primary care organization in England has to register separately in Wales – and a pharmacist registered with a local health board in Wales has to register separately in England.

A pharmacist must also apply to the PCO for permission to conduct MURs in special circumstances, e.g. at a patient's own home, at a residential home, at an external clinic or on the phone. A separate request has to be made for each category of patient on each occasion.

Carrying out an MUR

Although it could be considered to be a simple task to carry out an MUR once the criteria for the premises and pharmacist have been satisfied, it still requires a considerable amount of planning and preparation to achieve a satisfactory result.

Patient selection – there are specified criteria that determine which patients are suitable for selection:

- An MUR can be conducted with patients on multiple medicines and those with long-term conditions
- Regular MURs, initiated by the pharmacist, must only be provided for patients who have been using the pharmacy for the dispensing of prescriptions for at least the previous 3 months
- The next regular MUR can be conducted 12 months after the last MUR.

In addition, national target groups were introduced in October 2011 and at least 50% of all MURs undertaken by each pharmacy in each year should be on patients in these groups. The national target groups and other patient groups suitable for MURs can be seen in Box 51.2.

It is important to note that the MUR covers all the patient's medicines not just those that are specified for the target group. Patients on only one

Box 51.2

National target groups and other patient groups suitable for MURs

- Patients taking high risk medicines, e.g. NSAIDs, anticoagulants (including low molecular weight heparin), antiplatelets, diuretics
- Patients with respiratory disease (specifically those who are taking a medicine that is on the asthma and COPD list for the NMS)
- Patients recently discharged from hospital who had changes made to their medicines while they were in hospital (within 4 weeks and up to 2 months of discharge at time of review).

Other groups

- Patients over 75 on four or more medications
- Any patient taking five or more medicines
- Patients with known toxicities
- Patients with known compliance issues
- Patients with repeat prescriptions, which contain several items for different durations.

medicine may have an MUR if that medicine is one of those specified in the high risk group.

Patients who have been recruited to the new medicine scheme (NMS) because they have been prescribed a new medicine for the management of a long-term condition on discharge from hospital should not have an MUR.

Local criteria

Most PCOs, working with their community pharmacies, may identify priority groups who would be appropriate for MURs, based on the needs of the local health economy. Many pharmacists have or are looking to have areas of specialized interest and MURs provide them with an excellent opportunity to use this expertise in certain patient groups.

Pharmacists do not only select suitable patients themselves, they may accept referrals for MUR from the local surgery, other HCPs, e.g. district and practice nurses, key workers and social services. In this way, one of the perceived positive aspects for the CPCF, to allow the extended role of the community pharmacist to align with local health needs, may be achieved. The pharmacist can accept requests directly from patients for an MUR as long as the national criteria are met.

Prescription intervention

It should be noted that the patient selection criteria do not apply in the case of a 'prescription intervention', where the requirement for a MUR to be undertaken is initiated by the pharmacist identifying a significant problem during the dispensing of regular prescriptions. In particular, the requirement to have provided pharmaceutical services for a minimum of 3 months is removed. In these cases, the initiating issue which led to the need for a prescription intervention is discussed with the patient as part of the MUR.

Engaging the patient

Since the service was introduced, engaging with patients to invite them to attend for the MUR has proved to be a problem. Patients must give written consent to an MUR using nationally approved wording to permit their information to be shared with the GP, PCO and the NHS Business Services Authority (NHSBSA).

Initially uptake was poor because few patients had heard of the service and awareness of its purpose was low. Surveys had indicated that patients supported the concept of pharmacists helping them to understand what their medicines were for but patients were less inclined to attend an appointment to discuss their medicines. Many did not perceive that an annual MUR was required.

Similarly, GPs and other relevant professionals had received little information about the service, availability was not, and is still not guaranteed from all pharmacies, and there were a number of other problems with the paperwork resulting in reluctance to signpost the service to patients.

Since that time, steps have been taken locally and nationally to develop and provide support for those offering the MUR service. These resources can be accessed from the PSNC website. In July 2012, the new NHS MUR requirements were started, with specific changes made to the structure of the MUR process. Pharmacists have realized that they have to proactively engage patients to emphasize the benefits of the service and arrange appointments. To incorporate MURs into the daily work of the pharmacy without additional pharmacist cover is difficult. Experience has now shown that the most successful MUR schemes use skill mix with pharmacy staff assisting with planning and preparatory work for the MUR. Pharmacy staff require an understanding of what MURs are all about, but once this has been established, they can work together to:

- Identify appropriate patients
- Alert the pharmacist when a potential MUR candidate has presented a prescription or is about to receive the dispensed items
- Organize the appointment system when the MUR pharmacist is available
- Keep interruptions to a minimum during the interview.

Bringing in an extra pharmacist on 1 or 2 days per week is another option.

The patient interview

Despite pharmacists having extensive experience in communicating with patients, many have found the MUR interview difficult. Eliciting the information required to capture all that is required for the national dataset can be time-consuming and is important, as this must be kept for every MUR completed for 2 years.

With experience, pharmacists have realized that the key areas they need to address are to:

- look through the patient medication record (PMR) beforehand
- note any listed medical conditions
- prepare a structured format for the session including suitable questions
- have specific PILs available if necessary.

This is in addition to all the general issues of putting the patient at ease, revising the purpose of the interview, active listening and appropriate responses to any comments or questions from the patient.

Completing the MUR

Since July 2012, there is no longer a requirement to use the previous MUR form. A PSNC MUR worksheet is available (see Fig. 51.3) but the pharmacist can adopt any method for creating a record as long as it includes the nationally agreed MUR dataset and ensures that ongoing care is provided.

The patient no longer needs to be provided with a copy of the full MUR form, but pharmacists may provide them with a summary of the key points discussed during the MUR. If there are no items to consider, the pharmacist needs only to store the data and include it in a quarterly activity report to the PCO.

These changes have made the system more efficient and acceptable to all those involved.

Interactions with GPs

The MUR was the first community pharmacy service where a formal communication between the pharmacist and the GP was required to notify a GP practice that an MUR had been carried out on a patient. However, it has been agreed that this information was not useful and consequently an approved MUR Feedback Form (accessed from the PSNC website) is now provided to the patient's GP practice, only where there is an issue for them to consider. The pharmacist may also feel it is necessary to discuss urgent issues with the GP directly.

The future

The potential outcomes from MURs and the NMS include improved attainment of health goals and quality of life through better use of medicines, reduced wastage and more effective use of resources. It is possible that patients will make fewer visits to the surgery and have reduced unplanned hospital admissions. To some extent, these outcomes have been accepted, although a major flaw has been the lack of measurements and monitoring of the quality of the service. The introduction of targeted MURs has provided evidence that they can provide better control and improve symptom management of respiratory conditions.

MURs are one of the biggest innovations in community pharmacy in the last few years. They require community pharmacists to undertake functions complementing the work of GPs and other healthcare workers and align them to local health priorities. Pharmacy has to continue to demonstrate that services such as the MUR and NMS are valuable in delivering medicines' optimization. Improvement in patient knowledge ensures better medicines safety, a more rational approach to the use of medication and better monitoring.

MUR statistics collated for England are available to view on the PSNC website (www.psnc.org.uk).

NHS Medicines Use Review service worksheet

PHARMACY
the Heart of our Community

Confidential

PSNC

Patient name:		DOB:		The mandatory MUR dataset also requires you to record the patient's address, gender, NHS number (where available), ethnicity and registered GP practice. This data can be recorded in the patient's PMR.
Pharmacist name:		Date:		

Suggested questions	Medicines not listed on the patient's PMR	Dosage	Notes
1. How are you getting on with your medicines?			
2. How do you take or use each of these medicines?			
3. Are you having any problems with your medicines, or concerns about taking or using them?	**Consultation notes**		
Group Q4 & Q5 by therapeutic areas			
4. Do you think they are working? *Prompt: is this different from what you were expecting?*			
5. Do you think you are getting any side effects or unexpected effects?			
6. People often miss taking doses of their medicines, for a wide range of reasons. Have you missed any doses of your medicine, or changed when you take it? *Prompt: when did you last miss a dose?*			
7. Do you have anything else you would like to know about your medicines or is there anything you would like me to go over again? *Prompt: Are you happy with the information you have on your medicines?*			

Target group:	☐ Respiratory	☐ High risk medicine	☐ Post-discharge	☐ Not in a target group

Total number of medicines being used by patient:	Prescribed		OTC & complementary therapies	

Matters identified during the MUR: or   ☐ No matters identified during the MUR

☐ Patient not using a medicine as prescribed (non-adherence)   ☐ Problem with pharmaceutical form of a medicine or use of a device

☐ Patient reports need for more information about a medicine or condition   ☐ Patient reports side effects or other concern about a medicine

☐ Other matter and / or notes on above

Action taken / to be taken by pharmacist:

☐ Information /advice provided   ☐ Yellow card report submitted to MHRA   ☐ Patient referred to GP or other healthcare professional

☐ Other action and / or notes on above

Post-MUR the pharmacist believes there will be an improvement in the patient's adherence as a result of the following: (Where appropriate more than one may apply)

☐ Better understanding/reinforcement of why they are using the medicine/what it is for   ☐ Better understanding/reinforcement of side effects and how to manage them

☐ Better understanding/reinforcement of when/how to take the medicines   ☐ Better understanding/reinforcement of the condition being treated

Healthy living advice provided: (More than one may apply)   or   ☐ Healthy living advice not applicable

☐ Diet & nutrition   ☐ Smoking   ☐ Physical activity   ☐ Alcohol   ☐ Sexual health   ☐ Weight management

☐ Other:

Other notes:

Figure 51.3 • NHS medicines use review (MUR) service worksheet.

KEY POINTS

- The MHRA is responsible for assessing safety, quality and efficacy of medicines and medical devices in the UK
- Post-marketing surveillance aims to detect ADRs which did not show during pre-marketing testing
- The YCS was introduced for doctors and dentists in 1964 to report suspected ADRs
- The YCS has been extended to other HCPs, including pharmacists and patients
- New pharmacovigilance legislation was introduced across the EU and a European Additional Monitoring list to identify drugs for intensive monitoring replacing the Black Triangle list
- When an ADR is identified, the drug may be voluntarily or compulsorily withdrawn or it may continue in use with amended SPC or PIL
- Under-reporting appears to be a problem with ADRs
- MUR is an advanced service in the pharmacy contract in England and Wales, but was slow to become established
- For accreditation to carry out MUR, the pharmacy and pharmacist must meet set criteria, the pharmacist applying to the PCO for permission
- There are national target groups for selection of patients for MUR
- Apart from comprehensive preparation, the pharmacist needs to employ effective communication skills
- The MUR feedback form is to be sent to the GP practice only when there is an issue to consider

Appendices

Appendix 1: Abbreviations and terms used in this book

Introduction

As different countries both inside and outside the UK have different health services and different pharmacy structures, we wanted to use some general terms which you can then use to identify the relevant organization in your country.

We have also used some common abbreviations throughout this book.

General terms

The regulator or regulating body

This is the organization in your country or state, which recognizes your training qualifications and authorizes you to practice, e.g. the General Pharmaceutical Council in the UK.

The commissioner or commissioning body

This is the organization which pays money to a pharmacy or pharmacist to deliver a service, e.g. dispensing prescriptions, needle exchange. Examples of commissioners include in the UK: NHS, Local Health Boards and local authorities.

The professional body

This is the organization in your country, which provides professional guidance and a voice for the pharmacy profession, e.g. the RPS in the UK. In some countries, the regulator and the professional body may be the same organization.

Abbreviations

Abbreviation	What it stands for
ADR	Adverse drug reaction
BNF	British National Formulary
CD	Controlled drug
CPD	Continuing professional development
DH	Department of Health
FtP	Fitness to practice
GP	General Practitioner
GPhC	General Pharmaceutical Council
GSL	General Sales List
MUR	Medicines Use Review
NHS	National Health Service
NICE	National Institute for Health and Care Excellence
NSF	National Service Framework
OTC	Over-the-Counter
PM	Pharmacy Medicine
PGD	Patient Group Direction
PMR	Patient Medication Record
POM	Prescription only Medicine
RPS	Royal Pharmaceutical Society of Great Britain
SOP	Standard Operating Procedure
WHO	World Health Organization

Appendix 2: Medical abbreviations

Megan R. Thomas

Introduction

Abbreviations are widely used throughout all areas of life. While some abbreviations are so well known as to be accepted as part of everyday conversation, other abbreviations are very specific to a particular profession or even a specialty within a profession. This can easily lead to confusion, as the meaning of the abbreviation may not be immediately clear. As many abbreviations have a number of different interpretations, it is important to consider them within context. For instance, 'aka' is widely understood to mean 'also known as', but can also stand for 'above knee amputation'. It would be easy to recommend that abbreviations were never used, but with the sheer volume of information that requires recording and the often linguistically challenging terminology, their use is inevitable. Listed below are some of the more widely used medical abbreviations, including a section concerning physical examination findings. A useful web-based resource offers over 200 000 medical, pharmaceutical, biomedical and healthcare acronyms and abbreviations and can be found at http://www.medilexicon.com/. However, it is best, as with all things in life, *never to assume*.

Common medical abbreviations

AAA	Abdominal aortic aneurysm
Ab	Antibody, abortion
Abd	Abdomen
ABG	Arterial blood gas
ABO	Blood group classification
ABX	Antibiotic
ACTH	Adrenocorticotrophic hormone
AD(H)D	Attention deficit (hyperactivity) disorder
ADH	Antidiuretic hormone
ADL	Activities of daily living
ADR	Adverse drug reaction
A&E	Accident and emergency
AED	Antiepileptic drug
AF	Anterior fontanelle, atrial fibrillation
AFB	Acid fast bacilli
AFL	Atrial flutter
AFO	Ankle-foot orthosis
AFP	Alpha-fetoprotein
A/G	Albumin/globulin ratio
Ag	Antigen
AIDS	Acquired immunodeficiency syndrome
aka	Also known as
AKA	Above knee amputation
ALL	Acute lymphocytic leukaemia
ALT	Alanine aminotransferase
ALTEs	Acute life-threatening episodes
AMA	Against medical advice
AML	Acute myeloid leukaemia
amnio	Amniocentesis
ANA	Antinuclear antibody
ANF	Antinuclear factor
AOB	Alcohol on breath
AP	Anteroposterior
A&P	Anterior and posterior
A(P)LS	Advanced (paediatric) life support
appt	Appointment

AR	Aortic regurgitation		c	Cum (with)
A-R	Apical-radial pulse		C_1	First cervical vertebra, etc.
ARDS	Adult respiratory distress syndrome		Ca	Calcium
ARF	Acute renal failure		CA, Ca, ca	Cancer, carcinoma
AS	Aortic stenosis		CAB(G)	Coronary artery bypass (graft)
ASAP	As soon as possible		CAD	Coronary artery disease
ASCVD	Arteriosclerotic cardiovascular disease		CAPD	Continuous ambulatory peritoneal dialysis
ASD	Atrial septal defect		C(A)T	Computed (axial) tomography
ASHD	Atherosclerotic heart disease		cath	Catheter
ASO(T)	Antistreptolysin O (titre)		CBC	Complete blood count
AV	Arteriovenous, atrioventricular		CBG	Capillary blood gas
A&W	Alive and well		CC	Chief complaint
AXR	Abdominal X-ray		CCF	Congestive cardiac failure
Ba	Barium		CCU	Coronary care unit, clean catch urine
Bact	Bacteriology		CDs	Controlled drugs
BaE	Barium enema		CDH	Congenital diaphragmatic hernia, congenital dislocated hips
BBA	Born before arrival		CF	Cystic fibrosis
BBB	Bundle branch block, blood–brain barrier		CHD	Congenital heart disease
BCC	Basal cell carcinoma		CHF	Congestive heart failure
BCG	Bacillus Calmette–Guérin vaccine (against tuberculosis)		CIBD	Chronic inflammatory bowel disease
			CLL	Chronic lymphocytic leukaemia
BEAM	Brain electrical activity mapping		CMV	Cytomegalovirus
Beta-HCG	Human chorionic gonadotrophin		CN	Cranial nerves
BID	Brought in dead		CNS	Central nervous system
b.i.d.	Twice a day		CO	Carbon monoxide, cardiac output
bil	Bilateral		c/o	Complains of
bili	Bilirubin		COAD	Chronic obstructive airway disease
BKA	Below knee amputation		co-arct	Coarctation of the aorta
B(P)LS	Basic (paediatric) life support		COLD	Chronic obstructive lung disease
BM	Bowel movement, bone marrow, blood sugar, breast milk		COPD	Chronic obstructive pulmonary disease
BMR	Basal metabolic rate		CP	Chest pain, cerebral palsy
BNO	Bowels not open		CPAP	Continuous positive airways pressure
BOM	Bilateral otitis media		C(P)K	Creatinine (phospho)kinase
BOR	Bowels open regularly		CPR	Cardiopulmonary resuscitation
BP	Blood pressure		CRF	Chronic renal failure
BPD	Bipolar disorder, borderline personality disorder, bronchopulmonary dysplasia		CRP	C-reactive protein
			C&S	Culture and sensitivity
			CSF	Cerebrospinal fluid
BPH	Benign prostatic hypertrophy		C section	Caesarean section
bpm	Beats per minute		CTS	Carpal tunnel syndrome
BS	Bowel sounds, breath sounds, blood sugar		CVA	Cerebrovascular accident, costovertebral angle
BSA	Body surface area		CVP	Central venous pressure
BSER	Brain stem-evoked response		CVS	Cardiovascular system, chorionic villus sampling
BTL	Bilateral tubal ligation			
BUN	Blood urea nitrogen		Cx	Cervix, cervical
BW	Birth weight, body weight		CXR	Chest X-ray
Bx	Biopsy		D(x)	Diagnosis

D&C	Dilatation and curettage	FFA	Free fatty acids
DH	Drug history	FFP	Fresh frozen plasma
DIC	Disseminated intravascular coagulation	FH	Family history
		FISH	Fluorescent in situ hybridization
diff	Differential blood count	FOB	Faecal occult blood, foot of the bed
DIP	Distal interphalangeal joint	FROM	Full range of movement
DKA	Diabetic ketoacidosis	FSH	Follicle stimulating hormone
DM	Diabetes mellitus	FTNVD	Full-term normal vaginal delivery
DNA	Did not attend (outpatient)	FTT	Failure to thrive
DNR	Do not resuscitate	FU	Follow-up
DOA	Dead on arrival	FUO	Fever of unknown origin
DOB	Date of birth	FVC	Forced vital capacity
DOE	Dyspnoea on exertion	Fx	Fracture
DPL	Diagnostic peritoneal lavage	GA	General anaesthetic
DPT	Diphtheria, pertussis, tetanus vaccine	GCS	Glasgow coma scale
DSA	Digital subtraction angiography	GFR	Glomerular filtration rate
DTR	Deep tendon reflexes	GI(T)	Gastrointestinal (tract)
DTs	Delirium tremens	GN	Glomerulonephritis
DU	Duodenal ulcer	G6PD	Glucose-6-phosphate dehydrogenase
D&V	Diarrhoea and vomiting	G&S	Group and save
DVT	Deep vein thrombosis	GSW	Gun shot wound
D/W	Discussed with	GTN	Glyceryl trinitrate
DXT	Deep X-ray treatment	GTT	Glucose tolerance test
ECF	Extracellular fluid	GU	Genitourinary, gastric ulcer
ECG	Electrocardiogram	GYN, gynae	Gynaecology
ECMO	Extracorporeal membrane oxygenation	Hb, Hgb	Haemoglobin
		HC	Head circumference
ECT	Electroconvulsive therapy	Hct	Haematocrit
EDD	Expected date of delivery (baby)	HCVD	Hypertensive cardiovascular disease
EEG	Electroencephalogram	HDL	High density lipoprotein
ELBW	Extremely low birth weight	HDN	Haemolytic disease of the newborn
EMG	Electromyogram	HDU	High-dependency unit
EMU	Early morning urine	Hep	Hepatitis
ENT	Ear, nose and throat	HFO	High-frequency oscillation
EOM	Extraocular muscles	HH	Hiatus hernia
Ep	Epilepsy	HI	Haemagglutination inhibition, head injury
ERCP	Endoscopic retrograde cholangiopancreatography	HIE	Hypoxic ischaemic encephalopathy
ERG	Electroretinogram	HIV	Human immunodeficiency virus
ESM	Ejection systolic murmur	HL	Hodgkin's lymphoma
ESR	Erythrocyte sedimentation rate	HLA	Human leukocyte antigen
ET	Endotracheal	HMD	Hyaline membrane disease
ETA	Expected time of arrival	HO	History of
EUA	Examination under anaesthetic	HOCM	Hypertrophic obstructive cardiomyopathy
exc	Excision		
FB	Finger breadths, foreign body	H&P	History and physical
FBC	Full blood count	HPI	History of presenting illness
FBS	Fasting blood sugar	HR	Heart rate
FDPs	Fibrin degradation products	HRT	Hormone replacement therapy
FEV$_1$	Forced expiratory volume (in 1 second)	HSM	Hepatosplenomegaly

HSP	Henoch–Schönlein purpura, hereditary spastic paraparesis	jt	Joint
HT	Hypertension	JVP	Jugular venous pulse
ht	Height	KO	Keep open
HUS	Haemolytic uraemic syndrome	KO'd	Knocked out
HVS	High vaginal swab	KUB	Kidneys, ureters, bladder
Hx	History	L$_1$	First lumbar vertebra, etc.
IA	Intra-arterial	LA	Local anaesthetic, left atrium
IABP	Intra-aortic balloon pump, intra-arterial blood pressure	Lab	Laboratory
		labs	Results of tests
IBS	Irritable bowel syndrome	lac	Laceration
ICF	Intracellular fluid	LAD	Left anterior descending (coronary artery), left axis deviation
ICM	Infracostal margin		
ICP	Intracranial pressure	lat	Lateral
ICS	Intercostal space	LBBB	Left bundle branch block
ICU	Intensive care unit	LBW	Low birth weight
ID	Intradermal, initial dose	LD	Lethal dose
I&D	Incision and drainage	LDH	Lactate dehydrogenase
IDD	Insulin-dependent diabetic	LDL	Low density lipoprotein
IDM	Infant of a diabetic mother	LFTs	Liver function tests
Ig	Immunoglobulin	LH	Luteinizing hormone
IHD	Ischaemic heart disease	LIH	Left inguinal hernia
IM	Intramuscular	LMN	Lower motor neurone
imp	Impression	LMP	Last menstrual period
IMV	Intermittent mandatory ventilation	LN	Lymph node
inf	Inferior	LOC	Loss of consciousness
inj	Injury, injection	LP	Light perception, lumbar puncture
INR	International normalized ratio (prothrombin time)	LSCS	Lower segment caesarean section
		LSE	Left sternal edge
I&O	Intake and output	Lt	Left
IO	Intraosseous	LUQ	Left upper quadrant
IOP	Intraocular pressure	LV	Left ventricle
IP	Intraperitoneal, inpatient	LVF	Left ventricular failure
IPPV	Intermittent positive pressure ventilation	LVH	Left ventricular hypertrophy
		LVOT	Left ventricular outflow tract
IRDS	Idiopathic respiratory distress syndrome	LWBS	Left without being seen
		MAOIs	Monoamine oxidase inhibitors
IVC	Inferior vena cava	MAP	Mean arterial pressure
ISQ	No change (in status quo)	MCH	Mean corpuscular haemoglobin
ITP	Idiopathic thrombocytopenic purpura	MCHC	Mean corpuscular haemoglobin concentration
ITU	Intensive therapy unit		
IUD	Intrauterine device, intrauterine death	MCT	Medium chain triglyceride
		MCU	Micturating cystourethrogram
IUGR	Intrauterine growth retardation	MCV	Mean corpuscular volume
IV, iv	Intravenous	mets	Metastasis
IVH	Intraventricular haemorrhage	MI	Mitral incompetence or insufficiency, myocardial infarction
IVP	Intravenous pyelogram		
IVU	Intravenous urography	MMR	Mumps, measles, rubella vaccine
Ix	Investigations	MR	Mitral regurgitation
J	Jaundice	MRI	Magnetic resonance imaging
JRA	Juvenile rheumatoid arthritis	MRSA	Meticillin-resistant *Staphylococcus aureus*

MS	Mitral stenosis, morphine sulphate, multiple sclerosis
MSU	Midstream urine
MVA	Motor vehicle accident
N	Normal
NAD	Nothing abnormal detected, no active disease, no acute distress
NAI	Non-accidental injury
NBI	No bony injury
NBM	Nil by mouth
NCPAP	Nasal continuous positive airways pressure
Neb	Nebulizer
NEC	Narcotizing enterocolitis
Neuro	Neurology
NF	Neurofibromatosis
NFR	Not for resuscitation
NG	New growth
NG(T)	Nasogastric (tube)
NHL	Non-Hodgkin's lymphoma
NICU	Neonatal intensive care unit
NIDDM	Non-insulin-dependent diabetes mellitus
NKA	No known allergies
NMR	Nuclear magnetic resonance
NPA	Nasopharyngeal aspirate
NPN	Non-protein nitrogen
NPO	Nothing orally
NSR	Normal sinus rhythm, no sign of recurrence
NTD	Neural tube defect
N&V	Nausea and vomiting
NWB	Non-weight-bearing
O	Oedema
O/A	On admission
OA	Osteoarthritis
Obs-Gyn/gynae	Obstetrics and gynaecology
OD	Overdose, right eye
OGD	Oesophagogastroduodenoscopy
OOB	Out of bed
op	Operation
OP	Outpatient
OPA	Outpatient appointment
OPD	Outpatient department
open + shut	Inoperable case
OPV	Oral polio vaccine
OR	Operating room
ortho	Orthopaedics
OS	Left eye
O_2sat	Oxygen concentration
OT	Occupational therapy

OTC	Over the counter (medicine)
OU	Both eyes
P	Pulse
PA	Posteroanterior, pulmonary artery
$PaCo_2$	Partial pressure of carbon dioxide in arterial blood
Paeds	Paediatrics
PaO_2	Partial pressure of oxygen in arterial blood
Pap	Papanicolaou smear
path	Pathology
PBI	Protein bound iodine
PC	Presenting complaint
PCA	Patient-controlled analgesia
PCO_2	Partial pressure of carbon dioxide
PCR	Polymerase chain reaction
PCV	Packed cell volume
PD	Peritoneal dialysis
PDA	Persistent ductus arteriosus
PE	Physical examination, pulmonary embolus
PEEP	Positive end expiratory pressure
PEFR	Peak expiratory flow rate
PERRLA	Pupils equal, round, react to light and accommodation
PET	Positron emission tomography
PF(R)	Peak flow (rate)
PFO	Persistent foramen ovale
PFT	Pulmonary function tests
PG	Prostaglandin
PH	Past history
PHT	Pulmonary hypertension
PID	Pelvic inflammatory disease, prolapsed intervertebral disc
PIP	Proximal interphalangeal joint
PKU	Phenylketonuria
Plt	Platelets
PM	Post mortem
PMD	Post micturition dribbling
PMH	Past medical history
PMS	Premenstrual syndrome
PND	Paroxysmal nocturnal dyspnoea
PO	Per oral
PO_2	Partial pressure of oxygen
POD	Postoperative day
post op	After operation
PP	Private patient
PPD	Purified protein derivative (of tuberculin)
PPHN	Persistent pulmonary hypertension of the newborn

PR	Per rectum, pulmonary regurgitation	RR	Respiratory rate
		RS	Respiratory system
pre op	Before operation	RSV	Respiratory syncytial virus
prep	Prepare for surgery	rt	Right
prn	As required	RT	Radiotherapy
PROM	Premature rupture of membranes, prolonged rupture of membranes, passive range of movement, patient reported outcome measure	RTA	Road traffic accident
		RUQ	Right upper quadrant
		RV	Residual volume, right ventricle
		RVH	Right ventricular hypertrophy
		RVT	Renal vein thrombosis
PS	Pulmonary stenosis	Rx	Prescription
PSM	Pansystolic murmur	s	Without
Psych	Psychiatry	SA	Sino-atrial
Pt	Patient	Sab	Spontaneous abortion
PT	Physiotherapy, prothrombin time	SAH	Subarachnoid haemorrhage
PTA	Prior to admission	SB	Stillbirth, short of breath
PTC	Percutaneous transhepatic cholangiogram	S/B	Seen by
		SBE	Subacute bacterial endocarditis
PTCA	Percutaneous transluminal coronary angioplasty	SBFT	Small bowel follow through
		SBO	Small bowel obstruction
PTH	Parathyroid hormone	SBS	Short bowel syndrome
PTT	Partial thromboplastin time	SC	Subcutaneous
PUO	Pyrexia of unknown origin	SCC	Sickle cell crisis, squamous cell carcinoma
PV	Per vagina		
PVC	Premature ventricular contraction	SCBU	Special care baby unit
PVD	Peripheral vascular disease	SCID	Severe combined immunodeficiency
PVL	Periventricular leukomalacia	SGA	Small for gestational age
PVR	Pulmonary vascular resistance	SH	Social history, serum hepatitis
RA	Rheumatoid arthritis, right atrium	SIADH	Syndrome of inappropriate antidiuretic hormone
RAIU	Radioactive iodine uptake		
RBBB	Right bundle branch block	SIDS	Sudden infant death syndrome
RBC	Red blood cell, red blood count	SL	Sublingual
RBS	Random blood sugar	SLE	Systemic lupus erythematosus
RCA	Right coronary artery	S(A)LT	Speech (and) language therapist
RCC	Red cell count	SOA	Swelling of the ankles
RDS	Respiratory distress syndrome	SOB(OE)	Short of breath (on exertion)
rehab	Rehabilitation	SOL	Space occupying lesion
REM	Rapid eye movement	spec	Specimen
RF	Renal failure, rheumatic fever, rheumatoid factor	SPECT	Single photon emission computed tomography
		SR	Sinus rhythm
RHD	Rheumatic heart disease	S&S	Signs and symptoms
Rh neg. (Rh−)	Rhesus factor negative	SSS	Sick sinus syndrome
Rh pos. (Rh+)	Rhesus factor positive	stat	Immediately
RLF	Retrolental fibroplasia	STD	Sexually transmitted disease
RLQ	Right lower quadrant	SVC	Superior vena cava
RN	Registered nurse	SVD	Spontaneous vaginal delivery
R/O	Rule out	SVT	Supraventricular tachycardia
ROM	Range of movement, ruptured membranes	SW	Social worker
		Sx	Symptoms
ROP	Retinopathy of prematurity	SXR	Skull X-ray
ROS	Review of systems		

T	Temperature		UAC	Umbilical artery catheter
T_1	First thoracic vertebra, etc.		UC	Ulcerative colitis, umbilical cord
T_3	Triiodothyronine		U&Es	Urea and electrolytes
T_4	Levothyroxine (thyroxine)		UMN	Upper motor neurone
T&A	Tonsillectomy and adenoidectomy		UR(T)I	Upper respiratory (tract) infection
Tabs	Tablets		U/S	Ultrasound
TB	Tuberculosis		UTA	Unable to attend (outpatient appointment)
TBA	To be arranged, to be administered		UTI	Urinary tract infection
TBI	Total body involvement		VA	Visual acuity
T&C	Type and crossmatch		VD	Venereal disease
TCI	To come in		VDRL	Venereal disease research laboratory
TED stocking	Thromboembolic deterrent stocking		VE	Vaginal examination
temp	Temperature		vent	Ventilator
TFTs	Thyroid function tests		VEP	Visual evoked potential
TGA	Transposition of great arteries		VF(ib)	Ventricular fibrillation
THR	Total hip replacement		VF	Visual fields
TIA	Transient ischaemic attack		VLBW	Very low birth weight
tib and fib	Tibula and fibula		VMA	Vanilmandelic acid
TIBC	Total iron binding capacity		VMI	Very much improved
TKVO	To keep vein open		VP	Venous pressure, ventriculoperitoneal
TL	Tubal ligation		VPB	Ventricular premature beats
TLC	Tender loving care, total lung capacity		VQ scan	Ventilation perfusion scan
			VS	Vital signs
TLE	Temporal lobe epilepsy		VSD	Ventricular septal defect
TMJ	Temporomandibular joint		VT	Ventricular tachycardia
TOF	Tetralogy of Fallot, tracheo-oesophageal fistula		VZIG	Varicella zoster immune globulin
			WBC	White blood count
TOP	Termination of pregnancy		WBS	Whole body scan
TORCH screen	Toxoplasma, rubella, cytomegalovirus, herpes simplex infection screen		WC	Wheelchair
			WNL	Within normal limits
			WPW	Wolff–Parkinson–White
			WR	Ward round, Wasserman reaction
TPN	Total parenteral nutrition		wt	Weight
TPR	Temperature, pulse, respirations		X-match	Crossmatch
TR	Tricuspid regurgitation		XR	X-ray
Trachy	Tracheostomy		y.o.	Year-old
TS	Tricuspid stenosis			
TSH	Thyroid stimulating hormone			
TTAs	To take away (discharge medicines)			

Common abbreviations used to document physical examination findings

TTN	Transient tachypnoea of the newborn		AAL	Anterior axillary line
			AB	Apex beat
TTOs	To take out (discharge medicines)		HO	Hernial orifices
			HS	Heart sounds
TURP	Transurethral resection of prostate		ICS	Intercostal space
			MAL	Mid-axillary line
TVH	Total vaginal hysterectomy		MCL	Mid-clavicular line
Tx	Treatment		N/P	Not palpable
UA	Uric acid, urinalysis			

°	Absent	Δ	Diagnosis
° JAClCyL	No jaundice, anaemia, clubbing, cyanosis or lymphadenopathy	†	Died
		ΔΔ	Differential diagnosis
° LKKS	No liver, kidney, kidney, spleen palpable	#	Fracture
		−ve	Negative
O/E	On examination	+ve	Positive
PAL	Posterior axillary line	↔	No change
S_1	First heart sound	1°	Primary
S_2	Second heart sound	2°	Secondary
TGR	Tenderness, guarding and rebound	Σ	Sigmoidoscopy
VF	Vocal fremitus	∴	Therefore
VR	Vocal resonance	1/7	One day
∵	Because	2/52	2 weeks
↑BP	High blood pressure	3/12	3 months

Appendix 3:
Latin terms and abbreviations

Introduction

Prescriptions written in the UK should be written in English and the use of Latin is strongly discouraged. However, the use of some Latin terms persists and abbreviations are often used, especially to indicate the frequency of dosing. Abbreviations may have different meanings in different countries. Great care is required to avoid errors arising through misunderstanding.

The following lists include terms which may be encountered in current practice. For more comprehensive lists, see previous editions of this book, Carter (1975) and the *Pharmaceutical Handbook* (Wade 1980).

Dosage forms

Latin name	Abbreviation	English name
Auristillae	aurist.	ear drops
Capsula	caps.	capsule
Cataplasma	cataplasm.	poultice
Collunarium	collun.	nosewash
Collutorium	collut.	mouthwash
Collyrium	collyr.	eye lotion
Cremor	crem.	cream
Guttae	gtt.	drops
Haustus	ht.	draught

Latin name	Abbreviation	English name
Liquor	liq.	solution
Lotio	lot.	lotion
Mistura	mist.	mixture
Naristillae	narist.	nose drops
Nebula	neb.	spray solution
Oculentum	oculent.	eye ointment
Pasta	past.	paste
Pigmentum	pig.	paint
Pulvis	pulv.	powder
Pulvis conspersus	pulv. consp.	dusting powder
Trochiscus	troch.	lozenge
Unguentum	ung.	ointment
Vapor	vap.	inhalation
Vitrella	vitrell.	glass capsule (crushable)

Terms used in prescriptions

Latin	Abbreviation	English name
ante cibum	a.c.	before food
ante meridiem	a.m.	before noon
Ana	aa.	of each
Ad	ad	to

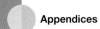

Latin	Abbreviation	English name
ad libitum	ad lib.	as much as desired
Alternus	alt.	alternate
Ante	ante	before
applicandus	applic.	apply
aqua	aq.	water
bis	b.	twice
bis die	b.d.	twice daily
bis in die	b.i.d.	twice daily
calidus	calid.	warm
cibus	cib.	food
compositus	co.	compound
concentratus	conc.	concentrated
cum	c.	with
dies	d.	a day
destillatus	dest.	distilled
dilutus	dil.	diluted
duplex	dup.	double
ex aqua	ex aq.	in water
fiat	ft.	let it be made
fortis	fort.	strong
hora	h.	at the hour of
hora somni	h.s.	at bedtime
inter cibos	i.c.	between meals
inter	int.	between
mane	m.	in the morning
more dicto	m.d.	as directed
more dicto utendus	m.d.u.	to be used as directed
mitte	mitt.	send
nocte	n.	at night
nocte et mane	n. et m.	night and morning
nocte maneque	n.m.	night and morning
nomen proprium	n.p.	the proper name
nocte	noct.	at night

Latin	Abbreviation	English name
omnibus alternis horis	o.alt.hor	every other hour
omni die	o.d.	every day
omni mane	o.m.	every morning
omni nocte	o.n.	every night
parti affectae	p.a.	to the affected part
parti affectae applicandus	part. affect.	apply to the affected part
partes aequales	p.aeq.	equal parts
post cibum	p.c.	after food
post meridiem	p.m.	afternoon
partes	pp.	parts
pro re nata	p.r.n.	when required
parti dolente	part. dolent.	to the painful part
quarter die	q.d.	four times daily
quarter die sumendus	q.d.s.	take four times daily
quarter in die	q.i.d.	four times daily
quaque	qq.	every
quaque hora	qq.h.	every hour
quarta quaque hora	q.qq.h.	every fourth hour
	q.q.h.	every fourth hour
quantum sufficiat	q.s.	sufficient
recipe	R_x	take
secundum artem	sec. art.	with pharmaceutical skill
semisse	ss.	half
si opus sit	s.o.s.	if necessary
signa	sig.	label
statim	stat.	immediately
sumendus ter	sum. t.	take thrice
ter de die	t.d.d.	three times daily
ter die sumendus	t.d.s.	take three times daily

Latin	Abbreviation	English name
ter in die	t.i.d.	three times daily
Tussis	tuss.	a cough
tussi urgente	tuss. urg.	when the cough troubles
ut antea	u.a.	as before
ut dictum	ut. dict.	as directed
ut directum	ut. direct.	as directed
Utendus	utend.	to be used

Table A3.1 Roman numerals: Roman symbol and corresponding Latin names for the cardinal and ordinal numbers and their adverbs

Arabic number	Roman symbol	Cardinals	Ordinals	Adverbs
1	I	*unus*	*primus, -a, -um*	*semel* (once)
2	II	*duo*	*secundus or alter*	*bis* (twice)
3	III	*tres, tria(n.)*	*tertius*	*ter* (three times)
4	IV	*quattuor*	*quartus*	*quater* (four times)
5	V	*quinque*	*quintus*	*quinquies*
6	VI	*sex*	*sextus*	*sexies*
7	VII	*septem*	*septimus*	*septies*
8	VIII	*octo*	*octavus*	*octies*
9	IX	*novem*	*nonus*	*novies*
10	X	*decem*	*decimus*	*decies*
11	XI	*undecim*	*undecimus*	*undecies*
12	XII	*duodecim*	*duodecimus*	*duodecies*
14	XIV	*quattuordecim*	*quartis decimus*	*quattuordecies*
15	XV	*quindecim*	*quintus decimus*	*quindecies*
20	XX	*viginti*	*vicesimus*	*vicies*
50	L	*quinquaginta*	*quinquagesimus*	*quinquagies*
100	C	*centum*	*centesimus*	*centies*

Appendix 4:
Key references and further reading

Introduction

This section includes guides to further reading and the references used in some chapters. Several books are referred to many times, especially pharmacopoeias and similar 'official' books. Others are important textbooks, including the two companion volumes to this book. These have been grouped together in the first section. This is followed by a chapter by chapter listing of other suggested reading to expand on the individual chapters and the references cited within the chapters, where appropriate.

Frequently used references

Allen, L.V., Popovich, N.G., Ansel, H.C., 2004. Ansel's pharmaceutical dosage forms and drug delivery systems, 8th edn. Lippincott Williams & Wilkins, Philadelphia.

Aulton, M.E., 2007. Aulton's pharmaceutics: the design and manufacture of medicines, 3rd edn. Churchill Livingstone, Edinburgh.

Aulton, M.E., Taylor, K., 2013. Aulton's pharmaceutics: the design and manufacture of medicines, 4th edn. Churchill Livingstone, Edinburgh.

British National Formulary, current edition. British Medical Association and Royal Pharmaceutical Society, London.

British National Formulary for children, current edition. London: British Medical Association, Royal Pharmaceutical Society and Royal College of Paediatrics and Child Health.

British Pharmaceutical Codex 1973 Pharmaceutical Press, London.

British Pharmacopoeia, current edition. Stationery Office, London.

Committee of Inquiry Into Pharmacy: a report to the Nuffield Foundation 1986 Nuffield Foundation, London.

Department of Health. Online. Available: <www.dh.gov.uk>.

Department of Health, DH, 2000. An organisation with a memory: a report from an expert working group on learning from adverse events in the NHS. Department of Health, London.

European Pharmacopoeia, current edition and supplements. Maisonneuve, Saint Ruffine.

Farwell J. 1995 Aseptic dispensing for NHS patients (the Farwell Report). Stationery Office, London.

General Pharmaceutical Council. Online. Available: <www.pharmacyregulation.org>.

General Pharmaceutical Council. GPhC Standards of conduct, ethics and performance. Online. Available: <www.pharmacyregulation.org>.

Handbook of pharmaceutical excipients, current edition. Pharmaceutical Press, London.

Marriott, J.F., Wilson, K.A., Langley, C.A., et al. 2006. Pharmaceutical compounding and dispensing. Pharmaceutical Press, London.

Martindale: The Complete Drug Reference. Pharmaceutical Press, London.

Martindale: The Extra Pharmacopoeia. Pharmaceutical Press, London.

Medicines compendium, current edition. Datapharm Publications, London.

Medicines Control Agency, 2002. Rules and guidance for pharmaceutical manufacture. Stationery Office, London.

Medicines and Healthcare Regulatory Authority, MHRA. Online. Available: <www.MHRA.gov.uk>.

National Institute for Health and Care Excellence, NICE. Online. Available: <www.nice.gov.uk>.

National Prescribing Centre. Online. Available: <www.npc.co.uk>.

Pharmaceutical codex, 11th edn. 1979 Pharmaceutical Press, London.

Pharmaceutical codex, 12th edn. 1994 Pharmaceutical Press, London.

Pharmaceutical Services Negotiating Committee. Online. Available: <www.psnc.org.uk>.

Stephens, M., 2002. Hospital pharmacy. Pharmaceutical Press, London.

Stone, P., Curtis, S.J., 2002. Pharmacy practice, 3rd edn. Pharmaceutical Press, London.

United States pharmacopoeia, current edition. Mack, Easton.

Wade, E. (Ed.), 1980. Pharmaceutical handbook, 19th edn. Pharmaceutical Press, London.

Walker, R., Whittlesea, C., 2012. Clinical pharmacy and therapeutics, 5th edn. Churchill Livingstone, Edinburgh.

Waterfield, J., 2008. Community pharmacy handbook. Pharmaceutical Press, London.

Section One: An introduction to pharmacy and its place in society

Chapter 1: The role of pharmacy in health care

Bond, C., 2000. Evidence-based pharmacy. Pharmaceutical Press, London.

Clinical Resources Audit Group, l996. Clinical pharmacy in the hospital pharmaceutical service: a framework for practice. Stationery Office, Edinburgh.

Department of Health, DoH, 1996. Choice and opportunity. Primary care: the future. Stationery Office, London.

Department of Health, DH, 2001. Response to the report of the public inquiry into children's heart surgery at the Bristol Royal Infirmary, 1984–1995. Stationery Office, London.

Department of Health, DH, 2002. Pharmacy in the future: implementing the NHS plan – a programme for pharmacy in the National Health Service. Stationery Office, London.

Royal Pharmaceutical Society of Great Britain, l996. Pharmacy in a new age: the new horizon. Royal Pharmaceutical Society of Great Britain, London.

Scottish Executive, 2002. The right medicine: a strategy for pharmaceutical care in Scotland. Stationery Office, London.

Weller P.J. (ed.) Pharmacists' directory and yearbook, current edition. Royal Pharmaceutical Society of Great Britain, London.

Chapters 2 and 3: Socio-behavioural aspects of health, illness and treatment with medicines

Abraham, C., Conner, M., Jones, F., et al. 2008. Health psychology: topics in applied psychology. Hodder Education, London.

Allardt E. 1973. About dimensions of welfare – Research Group for Comparative Sociology. Research Report No. 1. University of Helsinki, Helsinki.

Bernstein, L., Bernstein, R.S., 1985. Emotions in illness and treatment Interviewing: a guide for health professionals, 4th edn. Appleton-Century Crofts, New York.

Bissell, P., Traulsen, J.M., 2005. Sociology and pharmacy practice. Pharmaceutical Press, London.

Bond, C. (Ed.), 2004. Concordance. Pharmaceutical Press, London.

Britten, N., Stevenson, F.A., Barry, C.A., et al. 2000. Misunderstandings in prescribing decisions in general practice: qualitative study. British Medical Journal 320, 484–488.

Charles, C., Gafni, A., Whelan, T., 1997. Shared decision-making in the medical encounter: what does it mean? (or it takes at least two to tango). Social Science and Medicine 44, 681–692.

Charles, C., Gafni, A., Whelan, T., 1999. Decision making in the physician-patient encounter: revisiting the shared decision making model. Social Science and Medicine 49, 651–661.

Cleary, P.D., McNeil, B.J., 1988. Patient satisfaction as an indicator of quality care. Inquiry 25, 25–26.

Donabedian A. 2005 [1966]. Evaluating the quality of medical care. Reprinted in The Milbank Quarterly 83(4): 691–729.

FIP (International Pharmaceutical Federation). Standards for quality of pharmacy services. Online. Available: <www.fip.org>.

Florence, A.T., Taylor, K.M.G., Harding, G., 2001. Pharmacy practice. Taylor and Francis, London.

Friedman, M., Rosenman, R.H., 1974. Type A behaviour and your heart. Random House, New York.

Gard, P., 2000. A behavioural approach to pharmacy practice. Wiley Blackwell, Oxford.

Hope, T., 1996. Evidence based patient choice. King's Fund, London.

Kasl, S.V., Cobb, S., 1966. Health behaviour, illness behaviour and sick role behaviour. Archives of Environmental Research 12, 246–247.

Kosma, C.M., Reeder, C.E., Schultz, R.E., 1993. Economic, clinical and humanistic outcomes: a planning model for pharmacoeconomic research. Clinical Therapeutics 15 (6), 1121–1132.

Lewis, R., Maude, A., 1952. Professional people. Phoenix House, London.

Lilja J., Larsson S., Hamilton D., 1996. Drug communication. How cognitive science can help the health professionals. In: Pharmaceutical Sciences No. 24. Kuopio University Publications, Kuopio.

Maj-Britt Hedvall, Mikael Paltschik, 1991. Intrinsic service quality determinants for pharmacy customers. International Journal of Service Industry Management 2 (2), 38–48.

Marmot, M., Wilkinson, R.G., 2005. Social determinants of health, 2nd edn. Oxford University Press, Oxford.

Maslow, A.H., 1943. A theory of human motivation. Psychological Review 50, 370–396.

Maslow, A.H., 1954. Motivation and personality. Harper and Row, New York.

Miller, D.F., Price, J.H., 1998. Dimensions of community health, 5th edn. McGraw-Hill, Boston.

Montagne, M., 1996. The Pharmakon Phenomenon: Cultural perceptions of drugs and drug use. In: Davis, P. (Ed.), Contested ground – Public purpose and private interest in the regulation of prescription drugs. Oxford University Press, Oxford.

Panton, R., Chapman, S., 1998. Medicines management. Pharmaceutical Press, London.

Parasuraman, A., Zeithmal, V.A., Beery, L.L., 1988. SERVQUAL: A multiple-item scale for measuring consumer perceptions of service quality. Journal of Retailing 64 (1) Spring.

Parsons, T., 1979. Definitions of health and illness in the light of American values and social structure. In: Jaco, E., Gartley, E. (Eds.), Patients, physicians and illness: a source book in behavioural science and health, 3rd edn. Collier-Macmillan, London.

Quick, J.D., 1997. Management sciences for health: managing drug supply, 2nd edn. Kumarian Press, Hartford.

Rogers, E.M., 1995. Diffusion of Innovations, 5th edn. Free Press, New York.

Rose, G., 1985. Sick individuals and sick populations. International Journal of Epidemiology 14, 32–38.

Rosenstock, I., 1974. [1966] Historical origins of the health belief model. Health Education Monographs 2 (4), 328–335.

Royal Pharmaceutical Society of Great Britain, 1997. From compliance to concordance: achieving shared goals in medicine taking. RPSGB, London.

Sarafino, E.P., 2005. Health psychology: biopsychosocial interactions, 5th edn. John Wiley, New York.

Smith, F.J., 2002. Research methods in pharmacy practice. Pharmaceutical Press, London.

Smith, M.C., Knapp, D.A., 1992. Pharmacy, drugs and medical care, 5th edn. Williams and Wilkins, Baltimore.

Smith, M.C., Wertheimer, A.I., 2002. Social and behavioural aspects of pharmaceutical care. Pharmaceutical Products Press, New York.

Taylor, K., Nettleton, S., Harding, G., 2003. Sociology for pharmacists, 2nd edn. Taylor and Francis, London.

Taylor, K.M.G., Nettleton, S., Harding, G., 2003. Sociology for pharmacists, 2nd edn. Taylor and Francis, Andover.

World Health Organization, WHO 1948 Definition of health. Online. Available: <www.who.int/about/definition/en/print.html>.

World Health Organization, WHO 1978 Declaration of Alma-Ata. International Conference on Primary Health Care, Alma-Ata, USSR, 6–12 September. Online. Available: <www.searo.who.int/LinkFiles/Health_Systems_declaration_almaata.pdf>.

World Health Organization, WHO 2003 International conference on Primary healthcare, Alma Ata: 25th anniversary. Report by the Secretariat. WHO Press, Geneva.

Section Two: Protecting the public

Chapter 4: Control of medicines

Department of Health, DoH, 1998. A review of the prescribing, supply and administration of drugs – a report of the supply and administrations of medicines under group protocols. HMSO, London.

Department of Health, DoH, 1999. Review of prescribing, supply and administration of medicines – final report. HMSO, London.

Department of Health, DH, 2005. Supplementary prescribing by nurses and pharmacists within the NHS in England: a guide for implementation. HMSO, London.

Department of Health, DH, 2006. Improving patients' access to medicines: a guide to implementing nurse and pharmacist independent prescribing within the NHS in England. HMSO, London.

Royal Pharmaceutical Society, 2006. Better management of minor ailments: using the pharmacist. Pharmaceutical Press, London.

Chapter 5: Control of health professionals and their staff

General Dental Council. Online. Available: <www.gdc-uk.org>.

General Medical Council. Online. Available: <www.gmc-uk.org>.

Health and Care Professions Council. Online. Available: <www.hcp-uk.org>.

Nursing and Midwifery Council. Online. Available: <www.nmc-uk.org>.

Chapter 6: Continuing professional development and revalidation

Department of Health, DoH, 1998. The new NHS: a first class service. Stationery Office, London.

Department of Health, DH, 2007. Trust, assurance and safety – the regulation of health professionals in the 21st century. HMSO, London.

Pharmacists and Pharmacy Technicians Order, 2007. HMSO, London.

Royal Pharmaceutical Society CPD recording site. Online. Available: <www.uptodate.org.uk>.

Wilkie, V., 2012. Leadership and management for all doctors. British Journal of General Practice 62, 230–231.

Chapters 7 and 8: Ethics – the theory and ethics in practice and ethical dilemmas

Aggarwal, R., Bates, I., Davies, J.G., et al. 2002. A study of academic dishonesty among students at two schools of pharmacy. Pharmaceutical Journal 269, 529–533.

Beauchamp, T.L., Childress, J.F., 2001. Principles of biomedical ethics, 5th edn. Oxford University Press, New York.

Belmont Report 1979 Ethical principles and guidelines for the protection of human subjects of research. National Commission for the Protection of Human Subjects of Biomedical and Behavioral Research, 18 April. Online. Available: <www.hhs.gov/ohrp/humansubjects/guidance/belmont_html>.

Benson, A., 2006. Pharmacy values and ethics: a qualitative mapping of the perceptions and experiences of UK pharmacy practitioners. Centre for Public Policy, Department of Education and Professional Studies. King's College London, London.

Benson, A., Cribb, A., Barber, N., 2007. Respect for medicines and respect for people: mapping pharmacist practitioners' perceptions and experiences of ethics and values. Royal Pharmaceutical Society of Great Britain, London.

Berwick, D., Davidoff, F., Hiatt, H., et al. 2001. Refining and implementing the Tavistock principles for everybody in health care. Commentary: Justice in health care a response to Tavistock. British Medical Journal 323, 616–620.

British Medical Association, BMA, 1995. Core values of the medical profession in the 21st century – survey report. British Medical Association, London.

Department of Health, DH, 2008. White Paper: Pharmacy in England. Building on strengths – delivering the future. HM Government, London.

EthicsWeb.ca. Online. Available: <www.ethicsweb.ca/> (accessed 14 October 2008).

Ethox Centre, Department of Public Health and Primary Health Care, University of Oxford. Online. Available: <www.ethox.org.uk/> (accessed 14 October 2008).

Gillon, R., 1985. Medical oaths, declarations, and codes. British Medical Journal 290, 1194–1195.

Gillon, R., 1999. Philosophical medical ethics. John Wiley, Chichester.

Hawksworth, G., 2003. From the president: a personal professional pledge. Pharmaceutical Journal 271, 849–850.

Hawksworth, G., 2004. The president promotes a personal professional pledge for pharmacists. Pharmaceutical Journal 272, 684–685.

Hawley, G., 2007. Ethics in clinical practice: an interprofessional approach. Pearson Education, Harlow.

Hill, T.E., Zweig, A., 2002. Kant: groundwork for the metaphysics of morals. Oxford University Press, Oxford.

Hope, T., Savulescu, J., Hendrick, J., 2008. Medical ethics and law, the core curriculum, 2nd edn. Churchill Livingstone, Edinburgh.

Hurwitz, B., Richardson, R., 1997. Swearing to care: the resurgence in medical oaths. British Medical Journal 315, 1671–1674.

Internet Encyclopaedia of Philosophy. Online. Available: <www.iep.utm.edu/> (accessed 14 October 2008).

Kennedy Institute of Ethics Georgetown University. Online. Available: <http://bioethics.georgetown.edu/> (accessed 14 October 2008).

Leathard, A., McLaren, S., 2007. Ethics: contemporary challenges in health and social care. Policy Press, Bristol.

Rennie, S.C., Crosby, J.R., 2001. Are tomorrow's doctors honest? A questionnaire study exploring the attitudes and reported behaviour of medical students to fraud and plagiarism. British Medical Journal 322, 274–275.

Rogers, R., John, D., 2006. Paternalism to professional judgement – the history of the code of ethics. Pharmaceutical Journal 276, 721–723.

Schwartz, L., Preece, P.E., Hendry, R.A., 2002. Medical ethics: a case-based approach. Saunders, Edinburgh.

Smith, R., Hiatt, H., Berwick, D., 1999a. Shared ethical principles for everybody in health care: a working draft from the Tavistock group. British Medical Journal 318 (7178), 248–251.

Smith, R., Hiatt, H., Berwick, D., [Tavistock group], 1999b. A shared statement of ethical principles for those who shape and give health care: a working draft from the Tavistock group. Annals of Internal Medicine 130 (2), 143–147.

Sritharan, K., Russell, G., Fritz, Z., et al. 2001. Medical oaths and declarations. British Medical Journal 323, 1440–1441.

Stanford Encyclopaedia of Philosophy. Online. Available: <http://plato.Stanford.edu/contents.html> (accessed 14 October 2008).

Thimbleby, C.E.H., 2003. Drug tariff. Do we have to dispense a prescription item at a loss? Pharmaceutical Journal 271, 47.

Thompson, M., 2003. An introduction to philosophy and ethics. Hodder Murray, Manchester.

Tonks, A., 2002. What's a good doctor and how do you make one? British Medical Journal 325, 711.

Vardy, P., Grosch, P., 1999. The puzzle of ethics. Fount, London.

Wingfield, J., 2007a. New emphasis in the code of ethics. Pharmaceutical Journal 279, 237–240.

Wingfield, J., 2007b. Consent: the heart of patient respect. Pharmaceutical Journal 279, 411–414.

Wingfield, J., 2007c. When confidences should be kept and what constitutes an exception. Pharmaceutical Journal 279, 533–536.

Wingfield, J., Badcott, D., 2007. Pharmacy ethics and decision making. Pharmaceutical Press, London.

Chapter 9: Clinical governance

Dean, B., 2000. What is clinical governance? Pharmacy in Practice 10, 182–184.

Department of Health, DH, 1998. A first class service: Quality in the new NHS. Stationery Office, London.

Department of Health, DH, 2000. An organisation with a memory. Stationery Office, London.

Department of Health, DH, 2001. Clinical governance in community pharmacy. Stationery Office, London.

Department of Health, DH, 2004. Building a safer NHS for patients: Improving medication safety. DoH, London.

NHS, 1999. Clinical Governance in the new NHS. Stationery Office, London.

NHS Executive and National Prescribing Centre, 2000. Competencies for pharmacists working in primary care. Online. Available: <www.npc.co.uk/publications/CompPharm/competencies.htm>.

Royal Pharmaceutical Society of Great Britain, 2000. Pharmacy audit support pack. Online. Available: <www.rpsgb.org/registrationandsupport/audit>.

Royal Pharmaceutical Society of Great Britain, 2005. Scottish Executive 2005 Audit to excellence. CD-ROM. Online. Available: <www.rpsgb.org/registrationandsupport/audit>.

Chapter 10: Risk management

Department of Health, DH, 2000. An organisation with a memory: a report from an expert working group on learning from adverse events in the NHS. DoH, London.

Department of Health, DH, 2004. Building a safer NHS for patients: improving medication safety (a report by the Chief Pharmaceutical Officer). DoH, London.

National Patient Safety Agency, 2007a. Design for patient safety: a guide to the design of the dispensing environment. National Patient Safety Agency, London.

National Patient Safety Agency, 2007b. Healthcare risk assessment made easy. National Patient Safety Agency, London.

National Patient Safety Agency, 2008. Exploring incidents – improving safety: a guide to root cause analysis from the NPSA. E-learning programme. Online. Available: <www.msnpsa.nhs.uk/rcatoolkit/course/iindex.htm>.

Reason, J., 2000. Human error: models and management. British Medical Journal 320, 768–770.

Chapter 11: Standard operating procedures

General Pharmaceutical Council, GPhC, 2010. Guidance for Responsible Pharmacists. Online. Available: <http://www.pharmacyregulation.org/sites/default/files/GPhC%20Responsible%20pharmacist%20guidance.pdf>.

General Pharmaceutical Council, GPhC, 2010. Standards for owners and superintendent pharmacists of retail pharmacy businesses. Online. Available: <http://pharmacyregulation.org/sites/default/files/Standards%20for%20owners%20and%20superintendent%20pharmacist%20of%20retail%20pharmacy%20businesses%20s.pdf>.

National Pharmacy Association, NPA, 2003. The NPA guide to standard operating procedures a step-by-step approach for community pharmacy. NPA, St Albans.

Pharmaceutical Services Negotiating Committee. Tips on Standard Operating Procedures (SOPs). Online. Available: <www.psnc.org.uk>.

Pharmaceutical Society of Northern Ireland. Standards on sale and supply of medicines. Online. Available: <www.psni.org.uk/responsiblepharmacist>.

Chapter 12: Audit

Healthcare Commission National Clinical Audit, 2008. Online. Available: <www.healthcarecommission.org.uk>.

National Institute for Health and Clinical Excellence, 2002. Principles for best practice in clinical audit. Radcliffe Medical Press, Oxford.

NHS Clinical Governance Support Team, 2005. A practical handbook for clinical audit. Online. Available: <www.cgsupport.nhs.uk/downloads/Practical_Clinical_Audit_Handbook_vl_l.pdf>.

Royal Pharmaceutical Society of Great Britain Clinical Audit Unit. Online. Available: <www.rpsgb.org/registrationandsupport/audit/> (accessed 14 October).

Chapter 13: Public health

Acheson D. 1998. Independent inquiry into inequalities in health: report. Stationery Office, London.

Dahlgren, G., Whitehead, M., 1991. Policies and strategies to promote social equity in health. Institute of Future Studies, Stockholm.

Department of Health, 2004. Choosing health: making healthy choices easier. Stationery Office, London. Online. Available: <www.dh.gov.uk/en/Publicationsandstatistics/Publications/PublicationsPolicyAndGuidance/DH> 4094550.

Department of Health, 2005. Choosing health through pharmacy: a programme for pharmaceutical public health 2005–2015. Stationery Office, London. Online. Available: <www.dh.gov.uk/en/Publicationsandstatistics/Publications/PublicationsPolicyAndGuidance/DH_4107494>.

Marmot, M.G., Shipley, M.J., Rose, G., 1984. Inequalities in death: specific explanations of a general pattern. Lancet I, 1003–1006.

Marmot, M.G., Davey Smith, G., et al. 1991. Health inequalities among British civil servants: the Whitehall II study. Lancet 337, 1387–1393.

NHS Health Scotland, 2004. Online. Available: <www.healthscotland.com>.

Walker, R., 2000. Pharmaceutical public health: the end of pharmaceutical care? Pharmaceutical Journal 264, 340–341.

Section Three: Delivering professional pharmacy practice

Chapter 14: Structure and organization of pharmacy

British National Formulary, BNF. Online. Available: <www.bnf.org/>.

British Pharmacopeia Commission. British Pharmacopeia. Online. Available: <www.pharmacopoeia.co.uk/>.

NHS Careers, Working as a hospital pharmacist. Online. Available: <www.nhscareers.nhs.uk/explore-by-career/pharmacy-careers/pharmacist/hospital-pharmacist/>.

NHS The NHS in England. The NHS structure explained. Online. Available: <www.nhs.uk/NHSEngland/thenhs/about/Pages/nhsstructure.aspx>.

Pharmaceutical Services Negotiating Committee. Online. Available: <www.psnc.org.uk/pages/about_community_pharmacy.html>.

Royal Pharmaceutical Society. Online. Available: <www.rpharms.com>.

Chapter 16: Information retrieval in pharmacy practice

Allwood, M., Stanley, A.P., Wright, P. (Eds.), 2002. The cytotoxics handbook, 4th edn. Radcliffe Medical Press, Oxford.

Anon, 1995. An introduction to assessing medical literature. MeReC Briefing 9, 1–8.

Applebe, G.E., Wingfield, J., 2009. Dale and Applebe's pharmacy law and ethics. Pharmaceutical Press, London.

Aronson, J.K., Dukes, M.N.G., 2006. Meyler's side-effects of drugs: the international encyclopedia of adverse drug reactions and interactions, 15th edn. Elsevier, Amsterdam.

Ashley, C., Currie, A., 2009. The renal drug handbook. Radcliffe Medical Press, Oxford.

Baxter, K., 2007. Stockley's drug interactions, 8th edn. Pharmaceutical Press, London.

Brazier, H., McCabe, G., 1998. Making the most of Medline. Hospital Medicine 59 (10), 756–761.

Covell, D.G., Uman, G.C., Manning, P.R., 1985. Information needs in office practice: are they being met? Annals of Internal Medicine 103, 596–599.

Ely, J.W., Osheroff, J.A., Bell, M.H., et al. 1999. Analysis of questions asked by family doctors regarding patient care. British Medical Journal 319, 358–361.

Ely, J.W., Osheroff, J.A., Ebell, M.H., et al. 2002. Obstacles to answering doctors' questions about patient care with evidence: qualitative study. British Medical Journal 324, 710–713.

Gardner, M., 1997. Information retrieval for patient care. British Medical Journal 314, 950–954.

Gray, A., Wright, J., Goodey, V., et al. 2011. Injectable drugs guide. Pharmaceutical Press, London.

Greenhalgh, T., 1997. Assessing the methodological quality of published papers. British Medical Journal 315, 305–308.

Guillebaud J. Contraception: your questions answered. Churchill Livingstone, Edinburgh.

Hands, D., Judd, A., Golightly, P., et al. 1999. Drug information and advisory services – past, present and future. Pharmaceutical Journal 262, 160–162.

Impicciatore, P., Pandolfini, C., Casella, N., et al. 1997. Reliability of health information for the public on the world wide web: systematic survey of advice on managing fever in children at home. British Medical Journal 314, 1875–1881.

Kumar, P.J., Clark, M.L., 2012. Clinical medicine. Elsevier, Oxford.

McRibbon, K.A., Wilczynski, N.L., Walker-Dilks, C.J., 1996. How to search for and find evidence about therapy. Evidence-Based Medicine 1 (3), 70–72.

Malone, P., 1998. Drug information technology and Internet resources. Journal of Pharmacy Practice 11, 196–218.

Mason, P., 2011. Dietary Supplements. Pharmaceutical Press, London.

Morgan D. 2010. Formulary of Wound Management Products. Euromed Communications, Surrey.

North-Lewis, P., 2008. Drugs and the liver: a guide to drug handling in liver dysfunction. Pharmaceutical Press, London.

Porter, R.S., 2008. Merck manual of diagnosis and therapy. Merck and Co, West Point.

Regnard, C.F.B., Dean, M., 2010. A guide to symptom relief in palliative care. Radcliffe Medical Press, Oxford.

Rubin, P., Ramsay, M., 2007. Prescribing in pregnancy. Blackwell, Oxford.

Schaefer, C., Peters, P.W.J., Miller, R.K., 2007. Drugs during pregnancy and lactation. Elsevier, Edinburgh.

Shaughnessy, A.F., Slawson, D.C., Bennett, J.H., 1994. Becoming an information master: a guidebook to the medical information jungle. Journal of Family Practice 39, 489–499.

Slawson, D.C., Shaughnessy, A.F., 1997. Obtaining useful information from expert based sources. British Medical Journal 314, 947–949.

Slawson, D.C., Shaughnessy, A.F., Bennett, J.H., 1994. Becoming a medical information master: feeling good about not knowing everything. Journal of Family Practice 39, 505–513.

Smith, R., 1996. What clinical information do doctors need? British Medical Journal 313, 1062–1068.

Straus, S.E., Glasziou, P., Richardson, W.S., et al. 2011. Evidence-based medicine: how to practice and teach it. Churchill Livingstone, Edinburgh.

Sweetman, S.C., 2011. Martindale: the complete drug reference. Pharmaceutical Press, London.

Taylor, D., Paton, C., Kapur, R., 2012. Maudsley prescribing guidelines in psychiatry. Blackwell, Oxford.

Walker, R., Whittlesea, C., 2007. Clinical pharmacy and therapeutics, 5th edn. Churchill Livingstone, Edinburgh.

Williamson, E.M., Driver, S., Baxter, K., 2013. Stockley's herbal medicines interactions: a guide to the interactions of herbal medicines. Pharmaceutical Press, London.

Winter, M.E., 2009. Basic clinical pharmacokinetics. Lippincott Williams & Wilkins, London.

Wright, S.G., LeCroy, R.L., Kendrach, M.G., 1998. A review of the three types of biomedical literature and the systematic approach to answer a drug information request. Journal of Pharmacy Practice 11, 148–162.

Chapter 17: Communication skills for pharmacists and their team

Argyle, M., 1983. The psychology of interpersonal behaviour, 4th edn. Penguin, Harmondsworth.

Beardsley, R.S., Kimberlin, C.L., Tindall, W.N., 2007. Communication skills in pharmacy practice, 5th edn. Lippincott Williams & Wilkins, Baltimore.

Burnard, P., 1997. Effective communication skills for health professionals, 2nd edn. Chapman and Hall, London.

Dickson, D., Hargie, O., Morrow, N., 1997. Communication skills training for health professionals, 2nd edn. Chapman and Hall, London.

Kurtz, S.M., Silverman, J.D., 1996. The Calgary-Cambridge referenced observation guides: an aid to defining the curriculum and organizing the teaching in communication training programmes. Medical Education 30 (2), 83–89.

Ley, P., 1988. Communicating with patients. Croom Helm, London.

Pease, B., Pease, A., 2006. The definitive book of body language. Bantam Books, Atlanta.

U.S. Pharmacopeia Medication counseling behaviour guidelines. Online. Available: <www.usp.org>.

Chapter 18: Concordance

Berry, D., 2004. Risk, Communication and Health Psychology. Open University Press, Maidenhead.

Bond, C. (Ed.), 2004. Concordance – a partnership in medicine taking. Pharmaceutical Press, London

Britten, N., Stevenson, F.A., Barry, C.A., et al. 2000. Misunderstandings in prescribing decisions in general practice: qualitative study. British Medical Journal 320, 484–488.

Chewning, B., Bylund, C.L., Shah, B., et al. 2012. Patient preferences for shared decisions: a systematic review. Patient Education and Counseling 86, 9–18.

Clyne W., Granby T., Picton C. 2007 A competency framework for shared decision-making with patients – achieving concordance for taking medicines. Keele: NPC Plus; January. Online. Available: <www.npc.nhs.uk/non_medical/resources/competency_framework_2007.pdf>.

Coulter, A., 1997. Partnerships with patients: the pros and cons of shared clinical decision-making. Journal of Health Services Research and Policy 2, 112–121.

Coulter, A., Ellins, J., Swain, D., et al. 2006. Assessing the quality of information to support people in making decisions about their health and healthcare. The Picker Institute, Oxford.

General Pharmaceutical Council, 2010. Standards of conduct, ethics and performance. GPhC, London.

Gigerenzer, G., Edwards, A., 2003. Simple tools for understanding risks: from innumeracy to insight. British Medical Journal 327, 741–744.

Haynes R.B., Montague P. Oliver T. et al. 2001 Interventions for helping patients to follow prescriptions for medications (Cochrane Review). In: The Cochrane Library, Issue 2. Oxford Update Software, Oxford.

Joosten, E.A.G., De-Fuentes-Merillas, L., de Weert, G.H., et al. 2008. Systematic review of the effects of shared decision-making on patient satisfaction, treatment adherence and health status. Psychotherapy and Psychosomatics 77, 219–226.

Kurtz, S., Silverman, J.D., Bendon, J., et al. 2003. Marrying Content and Process in Clinical Method Teaching: Enhancing the Calgary-Cambridge Guides. Academic Medicine 78, 802–809.

Lewin, S.A., Skea, Z.C., Entwistle, V., et al. 2001. Interventions for providers to promote a patient-centred approach in clinical consultations. Cochrane Database of Systematic Reviews (4): CD003267.

Marinker M., Blenkinsopp A., Bond C. et al. 1997. From Compliance to Concordance – achieving shared goals in medicine taking. A joint report by the Royal Pharmaceutical Society of Great Britain and Merck, Sharpe & Dohme. Royal Pharmaceutical Society, London.

National Institute for Health and Clinical Excellence, 2009. Medicines adherence: involving patients in decisions about prescribed medicines and supporting adherence (CG76). NICE, London.

O'Connor, A.M., Stacey, D., Entwistle, V., et al. 2003. Decisions aids for people facing health treatment or screening decisions. Cochrane Database Systematic Review (1): CD001431.

Ottawa Health Research Institute 2007 Patient Decision Aids. Online. Available: <http://decisionaid.ohri.ca/index.html> 12 August.

Raynor, D.K., Blenkinsopp, A., Knapp, P., et al. 2007. A systematic review of quantitative and qualitative research on the role and effectiveness of written information available to patients about individual medicines. Health Technology Assessment 11, 5.

Simpson, S.H., Eurich, D.T., Majumdar, S.R., et al. 2006. A meta-analysis of the association between adherence to drug therapy and mortality. British Medical Journal 333, 15.

Stevenson, F.A., Cox, K., Britten, N., et al. 2004. A systematic review of the research on communication between patients and health care professionals about medicines: the consequences for concordance. Health Expectations 7, 235–245.

Stewart, M.A., 1995. Effective physician-patient communication and health outcomes: a review. Canadian Medical Association Journal 152, 1423–1433.

Weiss, M.C., 2007. The informed patient: friend or foe? Pharmaceutical Journal 278, 143–146.

Weiss, M.C., Britten, N., 2003. What is concordance? Pharmaceutical Journal 271, 493.

Chapter 19: Pharmaceutical calculations

Ansel, H.C., 2009. Pharmaceutical calculations, 13th edn. Lippincott Williams & Wilkins, Baltimore.

Rees, J.A., Smith, I., Smith, B., 2010. Introduction to pharmaceutical calculations, 3rd edn. Pharmaceutical Press, London.

Smith, I., Rees, J.A., 2005. Pharmaceutical calculations workbook. Pharmaceutical Press, London.

Winfield, A.J., Edafiogho, I.E., 2005. Calculations for pharmaceutical practice. Churchill Livingstone, Edinburgh.

Section Four: Access to medicines and their selection

Chapter 20: The prescribing process and evidence-based medicine

Barber, N., 1995. What constitutes good prescribing? British Medical Journal 310, 923–925.

Department of Health, 2006. Improving patients' access to medicines: A guide to implementing nurse and pharmacist independent prescribing within the NHS in England. HMSO, London.

Eccles, M., Freemantle, N., Mason, J., 1998. North of England evidence-based guideline development project. British Medical Journal 317, 526–530.

MeReC, 1995. Evidence based medicine. MeReC Bulletin 6 (12), 45–48.

National Prescribing Centre, 2012. A single competency framework for all prescribers. NPC, London.

Chapter 21: Prescribing for minor ailments

Briggs, G.G., Freeman, R.K., Yaffe, S.J., 2008. Drugs in pregnancy and lactation: a reference guide to fetal and neonatal risk, 8th edn. Lippincott Williams & Wilkins, Philadelphia.

Chapter 22: Drug evaluation and pharmacoeconomics

Briggs, A.H., O'Brien, B.J., 2001. The death of cost-minimization analysis? Health Economics 10, 179–184.

Drummond, M.F., Sculpher, M.J., Torrance, G.W., et al. 2005. Methods for the economic evaluation of health care programmes, 3rd edn. Oxford University Press, Oxford.

Elliot, R., Payne, K., 2004. Essentials of economic evaluation in healthcare. Pharmaceutical Press, London.

Heart Protection Study Collaborative Group, 2005. Cost-effectiveness of simvastatin in people at different levels of vascular disease risk: economic analysis of a randomized trial in 20,536 individuals. Lancet 365, 1779–1785.

Hughes, D.A., 2004. Modelling in health economics. In: Walley, T., Haycox, A., Boland, A. (Eds.), Pharmacoeconomics. Churchill Livingstone, Edinburgh.

Hughes, D.A., Vilar, F.J., Ward, C.C., et al. 2004. Cost-effectiveness analysis of HLA B*5701 genotyping in preventing abacavir hypersensitivity. Pharmacogenetics 14 (6), 335–342.

Lowson, K.V., Drummond, M.F., Bishop, J.M., 1981. Costing new services: long-term domiciliary oxygen therapy. Lancet 1 (8230), 1146–1149.

National Institute for Health and Clinical Excellence 2004 Guide to the methods of technology appraisal. Prescribing Support Unit. Online. Available: <www.ic.nhs.uk/services/prescribing-support-unit-psu>.

Scottish Intercollegiate Guidelines Network 2008 SIGN Guideline 50. A guideline developer's handbook, revised edn. Online. Available: <www.sign.ac.uk/guidelines/fulltext/50/index.html> (accessed 14 October 2008).

Scottish Medicines Consortium. Online. Available: <www.scottishmedicines.org.uk/smc>.

Walley, T., Haycox, A., Boland, A., 2003. Pharmacoeconomics. Churchill Livingstone, Edinburgh.

Chapter 23: Formularies in pharmacy practice

Cambridgeshire Primary Care Trust Formulary, latest update. Online. Available: <www.cambsphn.nhs.uk/default.asp?id=149> (accessed 14 October 2008).

Central Services Agency Northern Ireland COMPASS therapeutic notes. Online. Available: <www.centralservicesagency.com/display/compass> (accessed 14 October 2008).

Furniss L. 2000 Formularies in primary care. Primary Care Pharmacy 1(2): 37–39. Online. Available: <www.pharmj.com/PrimaryCarePharmacy/200003/medicines/formularies.html> (accessed 14 October 2008).

Health Solutions Wales. Online. Available: <www.hsw.wales.nhs.uk/page.cfm?orgid=166&pid=3997> (accessed 14 October 2008).

Information Services Division (Scotland). Online. Available: <www.isdscotland.org/isd/1038.html> (accessed 14 October 2008).

Lothian Joint Formulary. Online. Available: <www.ljf.scot.nhs.uk/> (accessed 14 October 2008).

National Prescribing Centre 2007 Managing medicines across a health community: making area prescribing committees fit for purpose. NHS Tayside Area Prescribing Guide (TAPG). Online. Available: <www.nhstaysideadtc.scot.nhs.uk/approved/formular/formular.htm>.

National Institute for Health and Clinical Excellence December, 2012. Developing and updating local formularies Available at: <www.nice.org.uk/mpc/goodpracticeguidance/GPG1.jsp> (accessed February 2013).

Pegler S. 2007 Whatever the appeal of drug lunches, take STEPS to avoid indigestion! Pharmaceutical Journal 278: 612–614 Online. Available: <www.pharmj.com/pdf/articles/pj_20070526_steps.pdf>.

Prescribing Support Unit Items. Measures of prescribing: Online. Available: <www.ic.nhs.uk/services/prescribing-support-unit-psu/measures>.

Prescribing Indicators. Online. Available: <www.ic.nhs.uk/our-services/prescribing-support-unit/indicators>.

Prescription Pricing Division (England). Online. Available: <www.ppa.org.uk/index.htm>. (accessed 14 October 2008).

Twycross, R., Wilcock, A., Charlesworth, S., et al. 2002. Palliative care formulary, 2nd edn. Radcliffe Publishing, Oxford.

Chapter 24: Complementary and alternative medicine

Ang-Lee, M.K., Moss, J., Yuan, C.-S., 2001. Herbal medicines and perioperative care. Journal of the American Medical Association 286, 208–216.

Barnes, J., Anderson, L.A., Phillipson, J.D., 2007. Herbal medicines. A guide for healthcare professionals, 3rd edn. Pharmaceutical Press, London.

Commission of the European Communities, 2002/0008. Proposal for amending the directive 2001/83/EC as regards traditional herbal medicinal products. The European Commission, Brussels.

Department of Health, 2001. Government response to the House of Lords Select Committee on Science and Technology's report on complementary and alternative medicine. Stationery Office, London.

Directive 2004/24/EC of the European Parliament and of the Council of 31 March 2004 amending, as regards traditional herbal medicinal products, Directive 2001/83/EC on the Community code relating to medicinal products for human use. Online. Available: <http://europa.eu.int/eur-lex/lex/LexUriServ/LexUriServ.do?uri=CELEX:32004L0024:HTML>, EN.

Eisenberg, D.M., Davis, R.B., Ettner, S.L., et al. 1998. Trends in alternative medicine use in the United States,

1990–1997. Results of a national follow-up survey. Journal of the American Medical Association 280, 1569–1575.

Ernst, E., White, A., 2000. The BBC survey of complementary medicine use in the UK. Complementary Therapies in Medicine 8, 32–36.

Gunther, S., Patterson, R.E., Kristal, A.R. et al. 2004. Demographic and health-related correlates of herbal and specialty supplement use. Journal of the American Dietetic Association 104 (1), 27–34.

House of Lords Select Committee on Science and Technology, 2000. Session 1999–2000, 6th report. Complementary and alternative medicine. Stationery Office, London.

Kayne, S., 2002. Complementary therapies for pharmacists. Pharmaceutical Press, London.

MCA (Now MHRA), 2002. Safety of herbal medicinal products, July. Online. Available: <http://64.233.183.104/search?q=cache>: DYdaAUqZ2P4J: <www.mhra.gov.uk/home/idcplg%3FIdcService%3DGET_FILE%26dID%3D665%26noSaveAs%3D0%26Rendition%3DWEB+safety+of+herbal+medicinal+products&hl=en&ct=clnk&cd=2&gl=u> (accessed 14 February 2007).

Mills S., Peacock W. 1997 Professional organisation of complementary and alternative medicines in the United Kingdom 1997. A report to the Department of Health. University of Exeter, Exeter.

Mintel Oxygen 2009 Complementary Medicines Market, UK.

Thomas, K.J., Nicholl, J.P., Coleman, P., 2001. Use and expenditure on complementary medicine in England: a population based survey. Complementary Therapies in Medicine 9, 2–11.

Traditional ethnic medicines, 2001. Public health and compliance with medicines law. London: Medicines Control Agency. Online. Available: <www.mca.gov.uk>.

UK Government. The Medicines for Human Use (Marketing Authorisations, etc.) Regulations (S1 1994/3144) 1994. Stationery Office, London.

UK Government. The Medicines for Human Use (Marketing Authorisations, etc.) Amendment Regulations (S1 2000/292) 2000. Stationery Office, London.

UK Government. The Medicines for Human Use (Marketing Authorisations, etc.) Amendment Regulations (S1 2005/768) 2005. Stationery Office, London.

UK Government. The Medicines (Aristolochia and Mu Tong etc.) (Prohibition) Order (S1 2001/1841) 2001. Stationery Office, London.

Zollman, C., Vickers, A., 1999. What is complementary medicine? British Medical Journal 319, 693–696.

Chapter 25: Communication skills: advice and information on the selection of medicines

Beardsley, R.S., Kimberlin, C.L., Tindall, W.N., 2007. Communication skills in pharmacy practice, 5th edn. Lippincott Williams & Wilkins, Baltimore.

Dickson, D., Hargie, O., Morrow, N., 1997. Communication skills training for health professionals, 2nd edn. Chapman and Hall, London.

Egan, G., 1990. The Skilled Helper, 4th edn. Brooks/Cole, Pacific Grove.

Ley, P., 1988. Communicating with patients. Croom Helm, London.

Tindall, W.N., Beardsley, R.S., Kimberlin, C.L., 2002. Communication skills in pharmacy practice, 4th edn. Lippincott Williams & Wilkins, Baltimore.

U.S. Pharmacopeia Medication Counseling Behaviour Guidelines. Online. Available: <www.usp.org> (accessed 15 October 2008).

Chapter 26: Patient charges for medicines and their impact on access

Austvoll-Dahlgren, A., Aaserud, M., Vist, G., et al. 2008. Pharmaceutical policies: Effects of cap and co-payment on rational drug use. Cochrane Database of Systematic Reviews (1): CD007017.

Cox, E.R., Henderson, R.R., 2002. Prescription use behaviour among Medicare beneficiaries with capped prescription benefits. Journal of Managed Care Pharmacy 8, 360–364.

Cox, E.R., Jernigan, C., Joel Coons, S.J., et al. 2001. Medicare beneficiaries' management of capped prescription benefits. Medical Care 39, 296–301.

Lexchin, J., Grootendorst, P., 2004. Effects of prescription drug user fees on drug and health services use and on health status in vulnerable populations: a systematic review of the evidence. International Journal of Health Services 34, 101–122.

Rice, T., Matsuoka, K.Y., 2004. The impact of cost-sharing on appropriate utilization and health status: a review of the literature on seniors. Medical Care Research and Review 61, 415–452.

Safran, D.G., Neuman, P., Schoen, C., et al. 2005. Prescription drug coverage and seniors: Findings from a 2003 national survey. Health Affairs Web Exclusive W5 (April), 152–166.

Schafheutle, E.I., 2009. The impact of prescription charges on asthma patients is uneven and unpredictable: evidence from qualitative interviews. Primary Care Respiratory Journal 18, 266–272.

Schafheutle, E.I., Hassell, K., Noyce, P.R., 2004. Coping with prescription charges in the UK. International Journal of Pharmacy Practice 12, 239–246.

Schafheutle, E.I., Hassell, K., Noyce, P.R., et al. 2002. Access to medicines: cost as an influence on the views and behaviour of patients. Health and Social Care in the Community 10, 187–195.

Soumerai, S.B., McLaughlin, T.J., Ross-Degnan, D., et al. 1994. Effect of limiting Medicaid drug-reimbursement benefits on the use of psychotropic agents and acute mental health services by patients with schizophrenia. New England Journal of Medicine 331, 650–655.

Tamblyn, R., Laprise, R., Hanley, J.A., et al. 2001. Adverse events associated with prescription drug cost-sharing among poor and elderly persons. Journal of the American Medical Association 285, 421–429.

Weiss, M.C., Hassell, K., Schafheutle, E.I., et al. 2001. Strategies used by General Practitioners to minimise the impact of the prescription charge. European Journal of General Practice 7, 23–26.

Chapter 27: The prescription

Department of Health, 1998. Review of prescribing supply and administration of medicines. Initial report (Crown review). Department of Health, London.

Department of Health, 1999. Review of prescribing supply and administration of medicines. Final report (Crown review). Department of Health, London.

Drug tariff, current edition. Stationery Office. Online. Available: <www.ppa.org.uk/ppa/edt_intro.htm> (accessed 16 October 2008).

Editorial, 2001. Consultation on SOPs for dispensing. Pharmaceutical Journal 266, 616–619.

National Prescribing Centre, 1999. Signposts for prescribing nurses. Prescribing Nurse Bulletin 1 (1), 1–4.

Chapter 28: Veterinary pharmacy

British Small Animal Veterinary Association. Online. Available: <www.bsava.com>.

British Veterinary Association. Online. Available: <www.bva.co.uk>.

Food Standards Agency. Online. Available: <www.food.gov.uk/business-industry/farmingfood/vetmeds/>.

Health and Safety Executive. Online. Available: <www.hse.gov.uk>.

Kahn, C.M., Line, S., 2005. The Merck veterinary manual, 9th edn. Merck, London.

National Office of Animal Health. Online. Available: <www.noah.co.uk>.

Pharmaceutical Society of Northern Ireland. The Veterinary Medicines Regulations Medicines for Veterinary Use.

Royal Pharmaceutical Society, including the Veterinary Pharmacists' Group. Online. Available: <www.rps.org.uk>.

Veterinary Medicines Directorate. Online. Available: <www.vmd.defra.gov.uk>.

Section Five: Medicines and their preparation

Chapter 31: Labelling of dispensed medicines

Information leaflet pictograms. Online. Available: <www.fip.org/pictograms>.

Chapter 32: Packaging

Royal Pharmaceutical Society, 1990. Working Party Report. Labelling of dispensed medicines. Pharmaceutical Journal 245, 128–129.

Chapter 33: Solutions

Diluent directories (internal and external), current edition. National Pharmaceutical Association, NPA, St Albans.

Chapter 36: External preparations

Benson, H.A.E., Watkinson, A.C., 2012. Topical and transdermal drug delivery: principles and practice. Wiley-Blackwell, Hoboken.

Walters, K.A., Roberts, M.S., 2007. Dermatologic, cosmeceutic, and cosmetic development: therapeutic and novel approaches: absorption efficacy and toxicity. Informa Healthcare, New York.

Williams, A.C., 2003. Transdermal and topical drug delivery. Pharmaceutical Press, London.

Chapter 37: Suppositories and pessaries

Allen, L.V., 2007. Suppositories. Pharmaceutical Press, London.

Pharmaceutical Society of Great Britain, 1980. Pharmaceutical handbook, 19th edn. Pharmaceutical Press, London.

Chapter 39: Oral unit dosage forms

Podczeck, F., Jones, B., 2004. Pharmaceutical capsules, 2nd edn. Pharmaceutical Press, London.

Section Six: Specialized pharmacy products and services

Chapter 40: Production of sterile products

Beaney, A.M., 2005. Quality assurance of aseptic preparation service, 4th edn. Pharmaceutical Press, London.

European Commission, 2005. The rules governing medicinal products in the European Union EU guidelines to good manufacturing practice for medicinal products for human and veterinary use, Vol IV. European Commission, Brussels.

MHRA, 2007. Rules and guidance for pharmaceutical manufacturers and distributors 2007 – the 'Orange guide'. Pharmaceutical Press, London.

Midcalf, B., Phillips, M., Neiger, J.S., et al. 2004. Pharmaceutical isolators. Pharmaceutical Press, London.

Chapter 41: Parenteral products

Akers, M.J., Larrimore, D.S., Guazzo, D.M., 2002. Parenteral quality control: sterility, pyrogens, particulate and package integrity testing, 3rd edn. Marcel Dekker, New York.

Avis, K.E., Lieberman, H.A., Lachman, L. (Eds.),, 1992. Pharmaceutical dosage forms: parenteral medications, Vol. 1, 2nd edn. Marcel Dekker, New York.

British Standards Institute 1989 British Standard 2463, Part 2. British Standards Institute, London.

British Standards Institute 2004 BS EN ISO 1135–1134: 2004. British Standards Institute, London.

Collentro, W.V., 2008. Pharmaceutical water: systems design, operation and validation, 2nd edn. Interpharm Press, Buffalo Grove.

DeLuca, P.P., Boylan, J.C., 1992. Formulation of small volume parenterals, 2nd edn. In: Avis, K.E., Lieberman, H.A., Lachman, L. (Eds.), Pharmaceutical dosage forms: parenteral medications. Marcel Dekker, New York.

Demorest, L.J., Hamilton, J.G., 1992. Formulation of large volume parenterals, 2nd edn. In: Avis, K.E., Lieberman, H.A., Lachman, L. (Eds.), Pharmaceutical dosage forms: parenteral medications. Marcel Dekker, New York.

Levchuk, J.W., 1992. Parenteral products in hospital and home care pharmacy practice, 2nd edn. In: Avis, K.E., Lieberman, H.A., Lachman, L. (Eds.), Pharmaceutical dosage forms: parenteral medications. Marcel Dekker, New York.

Pharmaceutical codex, 1994. Solution properties, 12th edn. Pharmaceutical Press, London. pp. 49–67.

Turco, S., 1994. Sterile dosage forms: their preparation and clinical application, 4th edn. Lippincott Williams & Williams, Baltimore.

Williams, K.L., 2001. Endotoxins, pyrogens, LAL testing and depyrogenation, 2nd edn. Marcel Dekker, New York.

Chapter 42: Ophthalmic products

Royal Pharmaceutical Society, 2001. Guidance for use of ophthalmic preparations in hospital and care homes. Pharmaceutical Journal 267, 307.

Chapter 43: Inhaled route

ABPI compendium of patient information leaflets current edition. Datapharm, London.

BTS/SIGN Asthma Guideline 2011 (January 2012 revision). Online. Available: <www.brit-thoracic.org.uk/guidelines/asthma-guidelines.aspx>.

EMC Medicines. Electronic medicines compendium. Online. Available: <http://emc.medicines.org.uk>.

Murphy, A., 2006. Asthma in focus. Pharmaceutical Press, London.

National Institute for Health and Clinical Excellence. Chronic obstructive pulmonary disease. Online. Available: <http://guidance.nice.org.uk>.

National Prescribing Centre, 1998. Chlorofluorocarbon (CFC) free inhalers. MeReC Bulletin 9 (5), 17–20.

NICE CG101. Chronic Obstructive Pulmonary Disease. Online. Available: <http://guidance.nice.org.uk/CG101/NICEGuidance/pdf/English>.

Purewal, T.S., Grant, D.J.W., 2002. Metered dose inhaler technology. Interpharm Press, Buffalo Grove, IL.

SIGN Guideline British guideline on the management of asthma. Online. Available: <www.sign.ac.uk/guidelines>.

Chapter 44: Parenteral nutrition and dialysis

Ashley, C., Currie, A., Renal, U.K., Pharmacy Group, UKRPG, 2009. The renal drug handbook, 3rd edn. Radcliffe Medical Press, Oxford.

Ashley, C., Morlidge, C., Renal, U.K., Pharmacy Group, UKRPG, 2008. Introduction to renal therapeutics. Pharmaceutical Press, London.

Austin, P., Stroud, M., 2007. Prescribing adult intravenous nutrition. Pharmaceutical Press, London.

Walker, R., Edwards, C., 2003. Clinical pharmacy and therapeutics, 3rd edn. Churchill Livingstone, Edinburgh.

Wood, S., 1995. Home parenteral nutrition: quality criteria for clinical services and the supply of nutrient fluids and equipment. British Association for Parenteral and Enteral Nutrition, Maidenhead.

Chapter 45: Radiopharmacy

Sampson, C.B. (Ed.), 1999. Textbook of radiopharmacy: theory and practice, 3rd edn. Gordon and Breach Science, Amsterdam.

Chapter 46: Specialized services

Allwood, M., Stanley, A.P., Wright, P. (Eds.), 2002. The cytotoxics handbook, 4th edn. Radcliffe Medical Press, Oxford.

Beaney, A.M., (formerly from NHS Quality Control Committee), 2006. The quality assurance of aseptic services, 4th edn. Pharmaceutical Press, London.

British Oncology Pharmacy Association, 2004. Position statement on care of patients receiving oral anticancer drugs. Pharmaceutical Journal 272, 423–424.

Department of Health and Social Security 1976 Breckenridge working party: report of the working party on addition of drugs to intravenous infusion fluids. HC (76)9. HMSO, London.

International Society of Oncology Pharmacy Practitioners (ISOPP) Guidelines on safe handling and other information. Online. Available: <www.isopp.org>.

Management and Awareness of Risks of Cytotoxic Handling (MARCH) guidelines. Online. Available: <www.marchguidelines.com>.

Needle, R.A., 1995. Survey of hospital centralized intravenous additive services. Pharmaceutical Journal 225, 326–327.

Needle, R.A., 2007. CIVAS handbook. Pharmaceutical Press, London.

Pharmaceutical Society, 1983. Working party report: guidelines for the handling of cytotoxic drugs. Pharmaceutical Journal 230, 230–231.

Society of Hospital Pharmacists of Australia, 2007. Standards of practice for the provision of oral chemotherapy for the treatment of cancer. Journal of Pharmacy Practice and Research 37, 147–150.

Trissel, L.A., 2006. Handbook on injectable drugs, 14th edn. American Society of Health-System Pharmacists, Bethesda.

Section Seven: Pharmacy services

Chapter 48: Public health and pharmacy interventions

Fraser Guidelines. Online. Available: <www.gpnotebook.co.uk>.

National Pharmacy Association. Online. Available: <www.npa.co.uk>.

Pharmaceutical Services Negotiating Committee. Online. Available: <www.psnc.org.uk>.

Royal Pharmaceutical Society. Online. Available: <www.rpharms.com>.

Chapter 49: Pharmacy services for vulnerable patients

Department of Health, 2000. No Secrets: Guidance on developing and implementing multi-agency policies and procedures to protect vulnerable adults from abuse. DH, London.

Department of Health, 2001. National Service Framework for older people. DH, London.

Department of Health, 2001. The Bristol Royal Infirmary Inquiry Report. London: The Stationery Office Limited.

Department of Health, 2004. National Service Framework for children young people and maternity services. DH, London.

Department for Education, 2010. First and Second Serious Case Review Reports relating to Peter Connelly ('Baby P'). London: Haringey Local Safeguarding Children Board. Online. Available: <www.education.gov.uk>.

Department of Health (updated 2010). Working together to safeguard children: A guide to inter-agency working to safeguard and promote the welfare of children. DH, London.

Department of Health, 2011. Safeguarding adults: The role of health service practitioners. DH, London.

Department of Health (regular updates). The green book. DH, London.

House of Commons Health Committee, 2003. The Victoria Climbié Inquiry Report. London: The Stationery Office Limited. Online. Available: <www.publications.parliament.uk>.

Royal Pharmaceutical Society, 2011. Protecting vulnerable adults a professional practice quick reference guide.

Royal Pharmaceutical Society, 2011. Protecting children and young people a professional practice quick reference guide.

UK Government, 1997. 'Who decides?', Consultation paper. Lord Chancellor's Department, London.

Chapter 50: Substance use and misuse

Berridge, V., Edwards, G., 1998. Opium and the people, 2nd edn. Free Association Books, London.

Department of Health (England) and the devolved administrations (2007). Drug Misuse and Dependence: UK Guidelines on Clinical Management. London: Department of Health (England), the Scottish Government, Welsh Assembly Government and Northern Ireland Executive. Online. Available: <www.nta.nhs.uk/uploads/clinical_guidelines_2007.pdf>.

Driver and Vehicle Licensing Agency, 2008. At a glance guide to medical aspects of fitness to drive. DVLA, Swansea. Online. Available: <www.dvla.gov.uk./medical/ataglance>. aspx (accessed 15 October 2008).

DrugScope U.K. charity. Supporting professionals. Online. Available: <www.drugscope.org.uk/>

Gelder, M., Mayou, R., Harrison, P., 2006. Misuse of alcohol and drugs. The shorter Oxford textbook of psychiatry, 5th edn. Oxford University Press, Oxford.

Gossop, M., 2007. Living with drugs, 6th edn. Ashgate, Aldershot.

Gossop M., Marsden J., Stewart D. 2001. NTORS (National Treatment Outcome Research Study) after five years: changes in substance use, health and criminal behaviour during the five years after intake.

Home Office 2010 Current strategy. Online. Available: <www.homeoffice.gov.uk/drugs/drug-strategy-2010>.

Ksobiech, K., 2003. A meta-analysis of needle sharing, lending, and borrowing behaviors of needle exchange program attenders. AIDS Education and Prevention 15 (3), 257–268.

MacDonald, M., Law, M., Kaldor, J., et al. 2003. Effectiveness of needle and syringe programmes for preventing HIV transmission. International Journal of Drug Policy 14, 353–357.

Mathei, C., Shkedy, Z., Denis, B., et al. 2006. Evidence for a substantial role of sharing of injecting paraphernalia other than syringes/needles to the spread of hepatitis C among injecting drug users. Journal of Viral Hepatitis 13 (8), 560–570.

National Addiction Centre (Crown copyright), London. Online. Available: <www.erpho.org.uk/Download/Public/5367/1/ntors5yr.pdf> (accessed 15 October 2008).

National Treatment Agency publication Best Practice Guidance for Commissioners and Providers of Pharmaceutical Services for Drug Users (February 2006). Online. Available: <www.nta.nhs.uk/uploads/nta_best_practice_pharma_services_for_drug_users_pharmguide06.pdf>.

Neale, J., 1999. Drug users' views of substitute prescribing conditions. International Journal of Drug Policy 10, 247–258.

Release: Drugs the Law and Human Rights. Online. Available: <www.release.org.uk/>.

Roberts, K., Bryson, S.M., 1999. The contribution of Glasgow pharmacists to the management of drug misuse. Hospital Pharmacist 6, 244–248.

Sheridan, J., Strang, J., 2002. Drug misuse and community pharmacy. Taylor and Francis, Andover.

Stimson, G.V., Des Jaríais, D.C., Ball, A., 1998. Drug injecting and HIV infection. Taylor and Francis, London.

The Alliance. Online. Available: <www.m-alliance.org.uk>

Walker, M., 2001. Shared care of opiate misusers in Berkshire. Pharmaceutical Journal 266, 547–552.

Ward, J., Hall, W., Mattick, R., 1999. Role of maintenance treatment in opioid dependence. Lancet 353, 221–226.

Wills, S., 2005. Drugs of abuse, 2nd edn. Pharmaceutical Press, London.

World Health Organization, 2007. Expert Committee on Drug Dependence 34th Report. WHO, Geneva.

World Health Organization 2010 Online. Available: <http://apps.who.int/classifications/icd10/browse/2010/en#>.

Chapter 51: Monitoring the patient

MHRA Black Triangle list. Online. Available: <www.mhra.gov.uk>.

MHRA Yellow Card Scheme. Online. Available: <http://yellowcard.mhra.gov.uk>.

Pharmaceutical Services Negotiating Committee (PSNC) Online. Available: <www.psnc.org.uk>.

Randall, M., Neil, K.E., 2004. Disease management. Pharmaceutical Press, London.

Sexton, J., Nickless, G., Green, C., 2006. Pharmaceutical care made easy. Pharmaceutical Press, London.

World Health Organization. WHO regional monitoring center. Online. Available: <www.who-umc.org>.

Appendix 3: Latin terms and abbreviations

Carter, S., 1975. Dispensing for pharmaceutical students, 13th edn. Pitman Medical, London.

Wade, E. (Ed.), 1980. Pharmaceutical handbook, 19th edn. Pharmaceutical Press, London

Index

Note: Page numbers followed by "*f*" "*t*" and "*b*" refers to figures, tables and boxes respectively.

Pharmaceutical Practice

Content Strategist: *Pauline Graham*
Content Development Specialist: *Fiona Conn*
Project Manager: *Julie Taylor*
Designer/Design Direction: *Christian Bilbow*
Illustration Manager: *Jennifer Rose*
Illustrator: *Robert Britton*